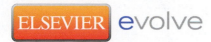

YOU'VE JUST PURCHASED
MORE THAN
A TEXTBOOK!*

Evolve Student Resources for *Gardenhire: Rau's Respiratory Care Pharmacology, 9th Edition*, include the following:

- Interactive Drug Cards
- WorkBook Answer Key

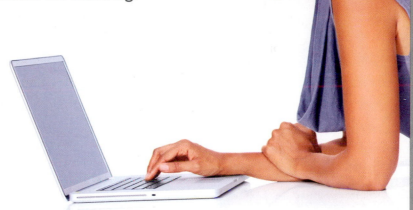

Activate the complete learning experience that comes with each *NEW* textbook purchase by registering with your scratch-off access code at

http://evolve.elsevier.com/Gardenhire/

If you purchased a used book and the scratch-off code at right has already been revealed, the code may have been used and cannot be re-used for registration. To purchase a new code to access these valuable study resources, simply follow the link above.

REGISTER TODAY!

You can now purchase Elsevier products on Evolve!
Go to evolve.elsevier.com/html/shop-promo.html to search and browse for products.

* Evolve Student Resources are provided free with each *NEW* book purchase only.

NINTH EDITION

RAU'S Respiratory Care Pharmacology

DOUGLAS S. GARDENHIRE, EdD, RRT-NPS, FAARC
Chair and Clinical Associate Professor
Department of Respiratory Therapy
Lewis School of Nursing and Health Professions
Georgia State University
Atlanta, Georgia

ELSEVIER

ELSEVIER

3251 Riverport Lane
St. Louis, Missouri 63043

RAU'S RESPIRATORY CARE PHARMACOLOGY, NINTH EDITION   ISBN: 978-0-323-29968-8

Previous editions copyrighted 2012, 2008, 2002, 1998, 1994, 1989, 1984, 1978

Library of Congress Cataloging-in-Publication Data

Gardenhire, Douglas S., author.
   Rau's respiratory care pharmacology / Douglas S. Gardenhire.—Ninth edition.
      p. ; cm.
   Respiratory care pharmacology
   Includes bibliographical references and index.
   ISBN 978-0-323-29968-8 (pbk. : alk. paper)
   I. Title. II. Title: Respiratory care pharmacology.
   [DNLM: 1. Respiratory Therapy. 2. Respiratory System Agents—pharmacology. 3. Respiratory Tract Diseases—drug therapy.   WF 145]
   RM388
   615.8'36—dc23
                                                             2015031220

Executive Content Strategist: Sonya Seigafuse
Content Strategist: Billie Sharp
Content Development Specialist: Charlene Ketchum
Publishing Services Manager: Julie Eddy
Senior Project Manager: Mary G. Stueck
Design Direction: Xiaopei Chen

Printed in the United States of America

Last digit is the print number: 9 8 7 6 5 4 3

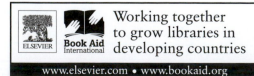

To Erlene and the late Paul D. Cares,
your love of education should be dispensed as a medication to all!

CONTRIBUTORS

Ahmed S. BaHammam, MD, FACP
Professor of Medicine
University Sleep Disorders Center
College of Medicine and National
  Plan for Science and Technology
King Saud University
Riyadh, Saudi Arabia
Chapter 23: Sleep and Sleep Pharmacology

Henry Cohen, MS, PharmD, FCCM, BCPP, CGP
Professor of Pharmacy Practice
Arnold & Marie Schwartz College of
  Pharmacy and Health Sciences
Long Island University;
Chief Pharmacotherapy Officer
Director of Pharmacy Residency
  Programs (PGY-1 and PGY-2)
Kingsbrook Jewish Medical Center
Department of Pharmacy Services
Brooklyn, New York
Chapter 21: Vasopressors, Inotropes, and Antiarrhythmic Agents
Chapter 22: Drugs Affecting Circulation: Antihypertensives, Antianginals, Antithrombotics

Michelle Friedman, B.S., Pharm.D.
Department of Pharmacy
Kingsbrook Jewish Medical Center
Brooklyn, New York
Chapter 22: Drugs Affecting Circulation Antihypertensives, Antianginals, Antithrombotics

Lynda T. Goodfellow, EdD, RRT, AE-C, FAARC
Professor, Department of Respiratory
  Therapy
Georgia State University
Atlanta, Georgia
Chapter 16: Selected Agents of Pulmonary Value

Markus Henke, MD, Privatdozent
Assistant Professor, Department of
  Pulmonary Medicine
Asklepios Fachkliniken München-
  Gauting
Comprehensive Pneumology Center
  (CPC)
Member of the German Center for
  Lung Research (DZL)
Robert-Koch-Allee 2
Gauting, Germany
Chapter 9: Mucus-Controlling Drug Therapy

David N. Neubauer, MD
Associate Professor, Department of
  Psychiatry
Johns Hopkins University School of
  Medicine
Baltimore, Maryland
Chapter 23: Sleep and Sleep Pharmacology

Seithikurippu R. Pandi-Perumal, MSc
President and Chief Executive Officer
Somnogen Canada, Inc.
Toronto, Canada
Chapter 23: Sleep and Sleep Pharmacology

Susan L. Pendland, MS, PharmD
Adjunct Associate Professor,
  Department of Pharmacy Practice
University of Illinois at Chicago
Chicago, Illinois;
Clinical Staff Pharmacist
Saint Joseph Berea Hospital
Berea, Kentucky
Chapter 14: Antimicrobial Agents

Ruben D. Restrepo, MD, RRT
Professor of Respiratory Care
University of Texas Health Science
  Center
San Antonio, Texas
Chapter 17: Neonatal and Pediatric Aerosolized Drug Therapy
Chapter 19: Diuretic Agents

Bruce K. Rubin, MEngr, MD, MBA, FRCPC, FAARC
Jessie Ball duPont Distinguished
  Professor and Chair, Department
  of Pediatrics
Professor of Biomedical Engineering
Virginia Commonwealth University
  School of Medicine;
Physician in Chief, Children's
  Hospital of Richmond
Virginia Commonwealth University
Richmond, Virginia
Chapter 9: Mucus-Controlling Drug Therapy

Christopher A. Schriever, MS, PharmD, AAHIVE
Clinical Assistant Professor
University of Illinois at Chicago
  College of Pharmacy
Rockford, Illinois
Chapter 14: Antimicrobial Agents

Diana Marcela Serrato, BSRC, CRT, MSCE
Clinical Instructor
Universidad Santiago de Cali
Cali, Colombia
Chapter 17: Neonatal and Pediatric Aerosolized Drug Therapy

Samantha Smalley, Pharm.D., BCPS
NYU Langone Medical Center
Department of Pharmacy
New York, New York
Chapter 21: Vasopressors, Inotropes, and Antiarrhythmic Agents

Darko Todorov, Pharm.D., BCPS
Department of Pharmacy
Kingsbrook Jewish Medical Center
Brooklyn, New York
Chapter 22: Drugs Affecting Circulation Antihypertensives, Antianginals, Antithrombotics

Chanie Wassner, Pharm.D.
Department of Pharmacy
Kingsbrook Jewish Medical Center
Brooklyn, New York
Chapter 22: Drugs Affecting Circulation Antihypertensives, Antianginals, Antithrombotics

ANCILLARY CONTRIBUTOR

Sandra T. Hinski, MS, RRT-NPS
Faculty, Respiratory Care Division
Gateway Community College
Phoenix, Arizona

REVIEWERS

Allen W. Barbaro, MS, RRT
Department Chair, Respiratory Care
  Education
St. Luke's College
Sioux City, Iowa

Lisa Conry, MA, RRT
Instructor, Respiratory Care
Spartanburg Community College
Spartanburg, South Carolina

Cindy Duncan, BS, RRT
Instructor/Clinical Coordinator—
  Respiratory Care Program
St. Luke's College–UnityPoint Health
Sioux City, Iowa

Jennifer L. Keely, MEd, RRT-ACCS
Assistant Clinical Professor
Respiratory Therapy Program
Department of Clinical and
  Diagnostic Sciences
School of Health Professions
University of Missouri
Columbia, Missouri

**Sara Wing Parker, MPH, RRT-NPS,
  AE-C**
Clinical Instructor
Respiratory Therapy Program
University of Missouri
Columbia, Missouri

PREFACE

Rau's Respiratory Care Pharmacology, ninth edition, provides the most exhaustive and up-to-date information pertaining to the field of respiratory care pharmacology. The importance of this text stems from the ever-changing nature of the field. The improvement of existing drugs and the creation of new drugs that use the direct access the lungs provide to the human body have expanded the types of drugs respiratory therapists are using today and will use in the future. This book provides the respiratory therapy student with a strong foundation of the drugs presently used in respiratory care. It also serves as a valuable resource for the respiratory care practitioner.

ORGANIZATION

The text is organized into three specific, fully referenced, and comprehensive sections to allow the reader easy access to a particular section of interest. Unit One covers the basics of respiratory care pharmacology, including the principles of drug action, the basic methods of drug administration, the standard drug calculations, and the effects of drugs on body systems. Unit Two covers the drugs most frequently delivered to patients by respiratory therapists, and Unit Three covers the drugs used to treat critical care and cardiovascular patients, featuring an entirely new chapter on the role of the respiratory therapist in the emerging area of sleep and sleep pharmacology.

DISTINCTIVE FEATURES

- For more than 30 years, *Rau's Respiratory Care Pharmacology* has been the preeminent respiratory care pharmacology text. In their passion for excellent patient care in the field of respiratory care, Dr. Gardenhire and his team of notable contributors are committed to engaging the reader.
- The up-to-date material reflects changes in the field and prepares students for careers as respiratory therapists in today's health care environment.
- Comprehensive coverage provides the most thorough explanations of any respiratory care pharmacology text on the market.
- Pharmacokinetic principles are discussed as they relate to respiratory agents, drug administration, and a range of specific drugs used in respiratory care and their effects on body systems.
- Consistent organization throughout and helpful learning tools give students the optimum opportunity for knowledge and growth.
- A thoroughly revised Student Workbook provides extra opportunities for review and self-assessment.

NEW TO THIS EDITION

- Improved readability provides greater comprehension of this difficult material.
- Respiratory Care Assessment boxes list before, during, short-term, and long-term instructions and contraindications for the various drug groups. The Respiratory Care Assessment box is the "one-stop shop" for clinical assessment tips and techniques.
- Expansion of Evolve Learning Resources for respiratory therapy students includes lecture notes, animations of respiratory-related processes, electronic flashcards to assist study efforts, and an expansive audio glossary of pharmacologic terms and trade and generic drug names.
- Expansion of Evolve Teaching Resources for instructors allows them to customize their course further by providing ideas for classroom activities and discussion and giving basic structure to their class with objective-driven lesson plans.
- Two appendices include a conversion chart for units and systems of measurement from customary U.S. imperial measures to the metric system as well as a list of the most commonly prescribed respiratory medications and acceptable mixtures.
- New drug cards have been created to provide detailed information on agents in a simple accessible form.

PEDAGOGIC FEATURES

- A consistent approach within each chapter begins with Chapter Outlines, measurable Objectives, and Key Terms with definitions identifying key information. Key pharmacologic agents are covered, noting the dosage and administration, mode of action, pharmacokinetics, and hazards and side effects. Each chapter ends with a series of Self-Assessment Questions and a Clinical Scenario to help readers assess their comprehension of the material. Answers are provided in Appendix A at the back of the book.
- Learning Objectives that parallel the levels tested by the NBRC examinations help identify important information that goes beyond memorization and recall.
- Key Terms with definitions provide easy access to the pharmacologic vocabulary the respiratory therapy student should embrace.
- Full-color illustrations throughout highlight special features and draw out relevant details.
- Key Points boxes, located throughout each chapter, highlight concepts with which the reader should become familiar while working through the material.

ANCILLARIES

For the Instructor

For the ninth edition, the Evolve Resources for *Rau's Respiratory Care Pharmacology* provide an interactive learning environment designed to work in coordination with the textbook. It features an all new Instructor Resource Manual with content topics, competencies, teaching focus, lists of resources and materials, key terms with page references, a critical thinking question, and lesson plans that align each chapter's learning objectives with class activities and discussions and reference other resources such as the Test Bank, PowerPoints, and Animations.

The Test Bank includes more than 600 questions. There are more than 500 PowerPoint slides that include embedded animations and Automated Response System questions. Evolve may be used to publish the class syllabus, outlines, and lecture notes; set up "virtual office hours" and e-mail communication; share important dates and information through the online class calendar; and encourage student participation through chat rooms and discussion boards. Evolve allows instructors to post examinations and manage their grade books online. For more information, visit http://evolve.elsevier.com/Gardenhire/Rau/respiratory/ or contact an Elsevier sales representative.

For the Student

The *Workbook for Rau's Respiratory Care Pharmacology* has been completely rewritten to provide a variety of exercises for each of the 23 chapters in the book. The ninth edition was reviewed and extensively revised to correspond with the learning objectives. All answers are referenced back to the text for ease in further review. Examples include NBRC-type questions, critical thinking exercises, case studies, definitions, and appropriate content review to help break down the difficult concepts in the textbook. The workbook creates a more complete learning package for students and allows the student more exposure to different questions in addition to what is available in the text. The answers for the exercises are located on the Evolve Teaching Resources. Ask your instructor for details.

The Evolve Student Resources include lecture notes, animations of respiratory-related processes, electronic flashcards to assist study efforts, and an expansive audio glossary of pharmacology terms and trade and brand drug names.

The continuing developments in respiratory drugs and in related critical care drug groups challenge practitioners, students, and authors alike with increasing complexity and scope of material. Every effort has been made to ensure the accuracy of information on drugs in this text. However, practitioners are urged to review the manufacturer's detailed literature when administering a drug and to keep informed of new information on drug therapy.

ACKNOWLEDGMENTS

The ninth edition of *Rau's Respiratory Care Pharmacology* is a dedication to all who have a thirst for knowledge and wish to share it with those who want the same. As with previous editions, this edition benefits from the substantial contributions of individuals who are each experts in various areas of pharmacology and aerosol medicine. Their names and affiliations, too numerous to list here, are found in the list of Contributors. They have graciously provided invaluable material for this new revision of the text. I thank all of them for their wisdom and kindness in preparing their chapter.

Many thanks will continue to be in order for Joseph L. Rau, PhD, RRT, FAARC, a great mentor and colleague who only occurs once in a lifetime. The title of this text is only a small way that I repay you for all that you have provided me in my years at Georgia State University

Thank you to my former student Sandra T. Hinski, MS, RRT, an instructor at Gateway Community College in Phoenix, Arizona, for her writing and dedication to the workbook and ancillary material. You have grown so much since your graduation, and I am happy to call you a colleague and a better yet—a friend!

I am grateful to the reviewers who provided me direction and clarification from their experiences in the classroom and the hospital. I also appreciate the efforts of all those who work so tirelessly behind the scene to make sure this book makes it to market. A big hug goes out to Charlene Ketchum for her ability to keep me on task and move this project forward, no matter the time or the place she is in!

Thank you to my wife, Robin, and my two beautiful daughters, Ali and Ella, for always being there for me. It is the three of you who push me to be better each day.

Finally, I must recognize all students and therapists who have and will continue to learn from this textbook. Thank you for allowing me to be a small part of your career!

Douglas S. Gardenhire, EdD, RRT-NPS, FAARC

"There are many problems, but I think there is a solution to all these problems; it's just one, and it's education."

Malala Yousafzai
Human Rights and Education Advocate
Youngest-ever Nobel Prize Laureate

CONTENTS

UNIT ONE

Basic Concepts and Principles in Pharmacology

CHAPTER 1

Introduction to Respiratory Care Pharmacology

Douglas S. Gardenhire

CHAPTER OUTLINE

OBJECTIVES

After reading this chapter, the reader will be able to:

1. Define *pharmacology*
2. Define *drugs*
3. Describe how drugs are named
4. List the various sources of drug information
5. List the various sources used to manufacture drugs
6. Describe the process for drug approval in the United States
7. Define *orphan drugs*
8. Differentiate between prescription drugs and over-the-counter (OTC) drugs
9. Apply the various abbreviations and symbols used in prescribing drugs
10. Describe the therapeutic purpose of each of the major aerosolized drug groups
11. Identify related drug groups in respiratory care

KEY TERMS AND DEFINITIONS

Acute respiratory distress syndrome (ARDS) Respiratory disorder characterized by respiratory insufficiency that may occur as a result of trauma, pneumonia, oxygen toxicity, gram-negative sepsis, and systemic inflammatory response.

Aerosolized agents Group of aerosol drugs for pulmonary applications that includes adrenergic, anticholinergic, mucoactive, corticosteroid, antiasthmatic, and antiinfective agents and surfactants instilled directly into the trachea.

Airway resistance (R_{aw}) Measure of the impedance to ventilation caused by the movement of gas through the airway.

Brand name See Trade name.

Chemical name Name indicating the chemical structure of a drug.

Chronic obstructive pulmonary disease (COPD) Disease process characterized by airflow limitation that is not fully reversible, is usually progressive, and is associated with an abnormal inflammatory response of the lung to noxious particles or gases. Diseases that cause airflow limitation include chronic bronchitis, emphysema, asthma, and bronchiectasis.

Code name Name assigned by a manufacturer to an experimental chemical that shows potential as a drug. An example is aerosol SCH 1000, which was the code name for ipratropium bromide, a parasympatholytic bronchodilator (see Chapter 7).

Cystic fibrosis (CF) Inherited disease of the exocrine glands, affecting the pancreas, respiratory system, and apocrine glands. Symptoms usually begin in infancy and are characterized by

KEY TERMS AND DEFINITIONS—cont'd

increased electrolytes in the sweat, chronic respiratory infection, and pancreatic insufficiency.

Drug administration Method by which a drug is made available to the body.

Generic name Name assigned to a chemical by the United States Adopted Name (USAN) Council when the chemical appears to have therapeutic use and the manufacturer wishes to market the drug.

Nonproprietary name Name of a drug other than its trademarked name.

Official name In the event that an experimental drug becomes fully approved for general use and is admitted to the *United States Pharmacopeia–National Formulary (USP-NF)*, the generic name becomes the official name.

Orphan drug Drug or biologic product for the diagnosis or treatment of a rare disease (affecting fewer than 200,000 persons in the United States).

Pharmacodynamics Mechanisms of drug action by which a drug molecule causes its effect in the body.

Pharmacogenetics Study of the interrelationship of genetic differences and drug effects.

Pharmacognosy Identification of sources of drugs, from plants and animals.

Pharmacokinetics Time course and disposition of a drug in the body, based on its absorption, distribution, metabolism, and elimination.

Pharmacology Study of drugs (chemicals), including their origins, properties, and interactions with living organisms.

Pharmacy Preparation and dispensing of drugs.

Pneumocystis jiroveci (formerly *carinii*) Organism causing Pneumocystis pneumonia in humans, seen in immunosuppressed individuals, such as those infected with human immunodeficiency virus (HIV).

Prescription Written order for a drug, along with any specific instructions for compounding, dispensing, and taking the drug. This order may be written by a physician, osteopath, dentist, veterinarian, and others but not by chiropractors or opticians.

Pseudomonas aeruginosa Gram-negative organism, primarily a nosocomial pathogen. It causes urinary tract infections, respiratory system infections, dermatitis, soft tissue infections, bacteremia, bone and joint infections, gastrointestinal infections, and various systemic infections, particularly in patients with severe burns and in patients who are immunosuppressed (e.g., patients with cancer or acquired immunodeficiency syndrome [AIDS]).

Respiratory care pharmacology Application of pharmacology to the treatment of pulmonary disorders and, more broadly, critical care. Chapter 1 introduces and defines basic concepts and selected background information useful in the pharmacologic treatment of respiratory disease and critical care patients.

Respiratory syncytial virus (RSV) Virus that causes the formation of syncytial masses in cells. This leads to inflammation of the bronchioles, which may cause respiratory distress in young infants.

Therapeutics Art of treating disease with drugs.

Toxicology Study of toxic substances and their pharmacologic actions, including antidotes and poison control.

Trade name Brand name, or proprietary name, given to a drug by a particular manufacturer.

PHARMACOLOGY AND THE STUDY OF DRUGS

KEY POINT

Key terms in the study of pharmacology are introduced, including *drug* and *pharmacology*. The study of **respiratory care pharmacology** is broadly defined as the application of pharmacology to cardiopulmonary disease and critical care.

The many complex functions of the human organism are regulated by chemical agents. Chemicals interact with an organism to alter its function, providing methods of diagnosis, treatment, or prevention of disease. Such chemicals are termed *drugs*. A drug is any chemical that alters the organism's functions or processes. Examples include oxygen, alcohol, lysergic acid diethylamide (LSD), heparin, epinephrine, and vitamins. The study of drugs (chemicals), including their origins, properties, and interactions with living organisms, is the subject of **pharmacology**.

Pharmacology can be subdivided into the following more specialized topics:

Pharmacy: The preparation and dispensing of drugs
Pharmacognosy: The identification of sources of drugs, from plants and animals

Pharmacogenetics: The study of the interrelationship of genetic differences and drug effects
Therapeutics: The art of treating disease with drugs
Toxicology: The study of toxic substances and their pharmacologic actions, including antidotes and poison control

The principles of drug action from dose administration to effect and clearance from the body are the subject of processes known as **drug administration, pharmacokinetics,** and **pharmacodynamics.** These processes are defined and presented in detail in Chapter 2. Table 1-1 summarizes key developments in the regulation of drugs in the United States.

NAMING DRUGS

KEY POINT

Each drug has five different names: chemical, code, official, generic, and trade (or brand). Sources of drug information include references, such as the *Physicians' Desk Reference (PDR)* and the *United States Pharmacopeia–National Formulary (USP-NF),* textbooks, such as Goodman & Gilman's *The Pharmacological Basis of Therapeutics,* and subscription services, such as *Drug Facts and Comparisons* and *Clinical Pharmacology* by Gold Standard.

TABLE 1-1	Legislation Affecting Drugs
1906	First *Food and Drugs Act* is passed by Congress; the *USP* and the *NF* were given official status.
1914	*Harrison Narcotic Act* is passed to control the importation, sale, and distribution of opium and its derivatives as well as other narcotic analgesics.
1938	*Food, Drug, and Cosmetic Act* becomes law. This is the current federal *Food, Drug, and Cosmetic Act* to protect the public health and to protect physicians from irresponsible drug manufacturers. This act is enforced by the FDA.
1952	*Durham-Humphrey Amendment* defines the drugs that may be sold by the pharmacist only on prescription.
1962	*Kefauver-Harris Amendment* is passed as an amendment to the *Food, Drug, and Cosmetic Act* of 1938. This law requires proof of the safety and efficacy of all drugs introduced since 1938. Drugs in use before that time have not been reviewed but are under study.
1970	*Controlled Substances Act* becomes effective; this act lists requirements for the control, sale, and dispensation of narcotics and dangerous drugs. Five schedules of controlled substances have been defined. Schedule I to Schedule V generally define drugs of decreasing potential for abuse, increasing medical use, and decreasing physical dependence. Examples of each schedule are as follows:
Schedule I	All nonresearch use is illegal; examples—heroin, marijuana, LSD, peyote, and mescaline.
Schedule II	No telephone prescriptions, no refills; examples—opium, morphine, certain barbiturates, amphetamines.
Schedule III	Prescription must be rewritten after 6 months or five refills; examples—certain opioid doses, anabolic steroids, and some barbiturates.
Schedule IV	Prescription must be rewritten after 6 months or five refills; penalties for illegal possession differ from those for Schedule III drugs; examples—phenobarbital, barbital, chloral hydrate, meprobamate (Equanil, Miltown), and zolpidem (Ambien).
Schedule V	As for any nonopioid prescription drug; examples—narcotics containing nonnarcotics in mixture form, such as cough preparations or Lomotil (diphenoxylate [narcotic; 2.5 mg] and atropine sulfate [nonnarcotic]).
1972	*Drug Listing Act* requires drug establishments that are engaged in the manufacturing, preparation, propagation, processing, or compounding of a drug to register their establishments and list all of their commercially marketed drug products with the FDA. This requirement includes establishments that repackage or change the container, labeling, or wrapper of any drug package in the distribution of the drug from the original place of manufacture to the person who makes final delivery or sale to the customer.
1983	*Orphan Drug amendments* provided incentives for the development of drugs that treat diseases that affect fewer than 200,000 patients in the United States.
1984	*Drug Price Competition and Patent Restoration Act* provided abbreviated new drug application for generic medication. Allowed the patent to be extended for up to 5 years owing to loss of marketing because of FDA reviews.
1992	*Prescription Drug User Fee Act* was reauthorized in 2007. User fees are paid for certain new drug applications by manufacturers.
1994	*Dietary Supplement Health and Education Act* established standards of dietary supplements. Specific ingredient and nutrition labels must be included on each package.
2002	*Bioterrorism Act* provided more stringent control on biologic agents and toxins.
2007	*FDA Amendments Act* gave the FDA greater authority over drug labeling, marketing, and advertising. Made clinical trial information more visible to the public.
2012	*FDA Safety and Innovation Act (FDASIA)* provided the FDA with power to collect fees (reauthorization from 2007), expedite agents of clinical significance, learn from patients first hand, and protect the global drug supply chain. All are efforts to make medications safer for U.S. citizens.

For more information, access the FDA website at www.fda.gov.
FDA, Food and Drug Administration; *LSD,* lysergic acid diethylamide; *NF, National Formulary; USP, United States Pharmacopeia.*

A manufacturer of a drug or pharmacologic agent must complete numerous steps set forth by the U.S. Food and Drug Administration (FDA). Along the way, each agent picks up various labels rather than a single name. An agent that becomes officially approved for general clinical use in the United States will have accumulated at least five different names, as follows:

Chemical name: The name indicating the drug's chemical structure.
Code name: A name assigned by a manufacturer to an experimental chemical that shows potential as a drug. An example is aerosol SCH 1000, which was the code name for ipratropium bromide, a parasympatholytic bronchodilator (see Chapter 7).

Generic name: The name assigned to a chemical by the United States Adopted Name (USAN) Council when the chemical appears to have therapeutic use and the manufacturer wishes to market the drug. Instead of a numeric or alphanumeric code, as in the code name, this name often is loosely based on the drug's chemical structure. For example, isoproterenol has an isopropyl group attached to the terminal nitrogen on the amino side chain, whereas metaproterenol is the same chemical structure as isoproterenol except that a dihydroxy attachment on the catechol nucleus is now in the so-called meta position (carbon-3,5 instead of carbon-3,4). The generic name is also known as the **nonproprietary name**, in contrast to the brand name.

Official name: In the event that an experimental drug becomes fully approved for general use and is admitted to the *United States Pharmacopeia–National Formulary (USP-NF)*, the generic name becomes the official name. Because an officially approved drug may be marketed by many manufacturers under different names, it is recommended that clinicians use the official name, which is nonproprietary, and not brand names.

Trade name: This is the **brand name**, or proprietary name, given by a particular manufacturer. For example, the generic drug named albuterol is currently marketed by Schering-Plough as Proventil-HFA, by GlaxoSmithKline as Ventolin-HFA, and by Teva as Proair HFA.

Following is an example of the various names for the drug zafirlukast, an agent intended to control asthma:

Chemical name: 4-(5-cyclopentyloxy-carbonylamino-1-methyl-indol-3-ylmethyl)-3-methoxy-*N*-o-tolylsulfonylbenzamide
Code name: ICI 204,219
Generic name: Zafirlukast
Official name: Zafirlukast
Trade (or brand) name: Accolate (AstraZeneca)

SOURCES OF DRUG INFORMATION

The USP-NF is a book of standards containing information about medications, dietary supplements, and medical devices. The FDA considers this book the official standard for drugs marketed in the United States.

Another source of drug information is the *Physicians' Desk Reference (PDR)*. Although prepared by manufacturers of drugs and potentially lacking the objectivity of the USP-NF, this annual volume provides useful information, including descriptive color charts for drug identification, names of manufacturers, and general drug actions.

The Drug Listing Act of 1972 requires registered drug establishments to provide the FDA with a current list of all drugs manufactured, propagated, prepared, processed, or compounded for commercial distribution. Drug products are identified and reported using a unique, three-segment number, called the National Drug Code (NDC), which serves as a product identifier for drugs. If searching for specific product information on drugs used in the United States you may search the NDC database at http://www.accessdata.fda.gov/scripts/cder/ndc/.

A comprehensive and in-depth discussion of general pharmacologic principles and drug classes can be found in several texts. Two examples are the following (see References for a complete listing):

- *Goodman & Gilman's The Pharmacological Basis of Therapeutics*, ed. 11[1]
- *Basic and Clinical Pharmacology*, ed. 11[2]

An excellent way to obtain information on drug products and new releases is the monthly subscription service provided as *Drug Facts and Comparisons*, published by Facts & Comparisons.[3]

SOURCES OF DRUGS

Although the source of drugs is not a crucial area of expertise for the respiratory care clinician, it can be extremely interesting. Recognition of naturally occurring drugs dates back to Egyptian papyrus records, to the ancient Chinese, and to the early Central American civilizations, and is still seen in remote regions of modern America, such as Appalachia.

For example, the prototype of cromolyn sodium was khellin, found in the eastern Mediterranean plant *Ammi visnaga*; this plant was used in ancient times as a muscle relaxant. Today, its synthetic derivative is used as an antiasthmatic agent. Another example is curare, derived from *Chondrodendron tomentosum* (a large vine) and used by South American Indians to coat their arrow tips for lethal effect. Its derivative is now used as a neuromuscular blocking agent. Digitalis is obtained from the foxglove plant (*Digitalis purpurea*) and was reputedly used by the Mayans for relief of angina. This cardiac glycoside is now used to treat heart conditions. The notorious poppy seed (*Papaver somniferum*) is the source of the opium alkaloids, immortalized in *Confessions of an English Opium-Eater*.[4]

Today, the most common source of drug preparation is chemical synthesis. Plants, minerals, and animals have often contributed to the synthesis of drug preparation. Examples of these sources include the following:

- *Animal:* Thyroid hormone, insulin, pancreatic dornase
- *Plant:* Khellin (*Ammi visnaga*); atropine (belladonna alkaloid); digitalis (foxglove); reserpine (*Rauwolfia serpentina*); volatile oils of eucalyptus, pine, anise
- *Mineral:* Copper sulfate, magnesium sulfate (Epsom salts), mineral oil (liquid hydrocarbons)

PROCESS FOR DRUG APPROVAL IN THE UNITED STATES

 KEY POINT

The process of drug approval in the United States is lengthy and expensive and involves multiple phases.

The process by which a chemical moves from the status of a promising potential drug to one fully approved by the FDA for general clinical use is, on the average, long, costly, and complex. Cost estimates vary, but in the 1980s it took an average of 13 to 15 years from chemical synthesis to marketing approval by the FDA, with a cost of $350 million in the United States.[5] In a study done in 2003 by DiMasi and associates,[6] it was calculated that companies spend over $800 million on research and development and on preclinical and postclinical trials of a new drug in the current market. In a recent study by Adams and Brantner[7] that

| BOX 1-1 | Major Steps in the Process of Marketing a Drug in the United States |

BOX 1-1   Major Steps in the Process of Marketing a Drug in the United States

Isolation and Identification of the Chemical
Animal studies
General effects
- Special effects on organ systems
- Toxicology studies

Investigational New Drug (IND) Approval
Phase 1 studies: Small number, healthy subjects
Phase 2 studies: Small number, subjects with disease
Phase 3 studies: Large, multicenter studies

New Drug Application (NDA)
Reporting system for first 6 months

BOX 1-2   Alphanumeric Coding System of the FDA

Chemical/Pharmaceutical Standing
1 = New chemical entity
2 = New salt form
3 = New dosage form
4 = New combination
5 = Generic drug
6 = New indication

Therapeutic Potential
A = Important (significant) therapeutic gain over other drugs
AA = Important therapeutic gain, indicated for a patient with AIDS; fast-track
B = Modest therapeutic gain
C = Important options; little or no therapeutic gain

replicated DiMasi's calculations, they estimated companies now spend over $1 billion to bring a new drug to market.

The major steps in the drug approval process have been reviewed by Flieger[8] and by Hassall and Fredd.[9] Box 1-1 outlines the major steps of the process.

Chemical Isolation and Identification

Because a drug is a chemical, the first step in drug development is to identify a chemical with the potential for useful physiologic effects. This step is exemplified by the plant product paclitaxel, which is derived from the needles and bark of the western yew tree *(Taxus brevifolia)*. Paclitaxel showed antitumor activity, making it attractive for investigation as an anticancer drug. As the first step in the process of drug approval, the exact structure and physical and chemical characteristics of paclitaxel were established. Paclitaxel was subsequently developed and marketed as Taxol by Bristol-Myers Squibb.

Animal Studies

Once an active chemical is isolated and identified, a series of animal studies examines its general effect on the animal and effects on specific organs, such as the liver or kidneys. Toxicology studies to examine mutagenicity, teratogenicity, effect on reproductive fertility, and carcinogenicity are also performed.

Investigational New Drug Approval

At this point, an Investigational New Drug (IND) application is filed with the FDA for the chemical being examined. The IND application includes all of the information previously gathered and plans for human studies. These studies proceed in three phases and usually require about 3 years to complete.

Phase 1

The drug is investigated in a small group of healthy volunteers to establish its activity. This investigation is the basis

for the pharmacokinetic description of the drug (rates of absorption, distribution, metabolism, and elimination).

Phase 2

The drug is next investigated as a treatment in a small number of individuals with the disease the drug is intended to treat.

Phase 3

The drug is investigated in large, multicenter studies to establish safety and efficacy.

New Drug Application

After a successful IND process, a New Drug Application (NDA) is filed with the FDA, and, on approval, the drug is released for general clinical use. A detailed reporting system is in place for the first 6 months to track any problems that arise with the drug's use. The drug is no longer experimental (investigational) and can be prescribed for treatment of the general population by physicians.

Because of the involved, lengthy, and expensive process of obtaining approval through the FDA to market a new drug in the United States, the process is often criticized.

FDA New Drug Classification System

Because some drugs are simply released in new forms or are similar to previously approved agents, the FDA has a classification system to help identify the significance of new products.[10] An alphanumeric code is given to provide this information (Box 1-2).

Orphan Drugs

 KEY POINT

Certain drugs used for rare diseases, which may not return the cost of their development, are termed *orphan drugs*.

TABLE 1-2 Examples of Orphan Drugs of Interest to Respiratory Care Clinicians

DRUG	PROPOSED USE
Acetylcysteine	Intravenous administration for moderate to severe acetaminophen overdose
α_1-Proteinase inhibitor (Prolastin)*	Replacement therapy for congenital α_1-proteinase (α_1-antitrypsin) deficiency
Beractant (Survanta)*	Prevention or treatment of RDS in newborns
CF transmembrane conductance regulator	Treatment of CF
Dornase alfa (Pulmozyme)*	Treatment of CF: reduction of mucus viscosity and increase in airway secretion clearance
Nitric oxide gas (INOmax)*	Treatment of persistent pulmonary hypertension of newborns or of ARDS in adults
Tobramycin solution for inhalation (TOBI)*	Treatment of *Pseudomonas aeruginosa* in CF or bronchiectasis
Pentamidine isethionate	Prevent *Pneumocystis jiroveci* (formerly *carinii*) pneumonia in high-risk patients

ARDS, Acute respiratory distress syndrome; *CF*, cystic fibrosis; *RDS*, respiratory distress syndrome.
*Use has been approved by the FDA.

An **orphan drug** is a drug or biologic product for the diagnosis or treatment of a rare disease. *Rare* is defined as a disease that affects fewer than 200,000 persons in the United States. Alternatively, a drug may be designated as an orphan if it is used for a disease that affects more than 200,000 persons but there is no reasonable expectation of recovering the cost of drug development. Table 1-2 lists several orphan drugs of interest to respiratory care clinicians.

THE PRESCRIPTION

KEY POINT

The selling of many drugs requires a health care prescriber's order, known as the *prescription*, and may involve Latin terms and abbreviations.

The **prescription** is the written order for a drug, along with any specific instructions for compounding, dispensing, and taking the drug. This order may be written by a physician, osteopath, dentist, veterinarian, and other health care practitioners, such as a physician assistant and nurse practitioner, but not by chiropractors or opticians. Today, although many prescriptions are written and distributed by electronic means, it is important to note that written prescriptions are

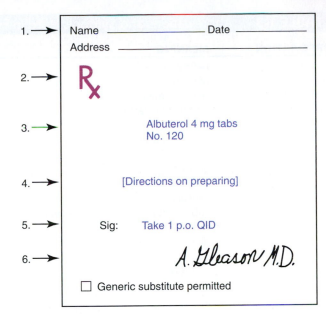

Figure 1-1 Parts of a prescription.
1. Patient's name and address and the date the prescription was written.
2. ℞ (meaning "recipe" or "take thou") directs the pharmacist to take the drug listed and prepare the medication. This is referred to as the *superscription*.
3. The inscription lists the name and quantity of the drug being prescribed.
4. When applicable, the healthcare prescriber includes a subscription, which is directions to the pharmacist on how to prepare the medication. For example, a direction to make an ointment, which might be appropriate for certain medications, would be "ft ung." In many cases, with precompounded drugs, counting out the correct number is the only requirement.
5. *Sig (signa)* means "write." The transcription or signature is the information the pharmacist writes on the label of the medication as instructions to the patient.
6. Name of the prescriber: Although the healthcare prescriber signs the prescription, the word "signature," as described in Part 5, denotes the directions to the patient, not the prescriber's name.

still used. The detailed parts of a prescription are shown in Figure 1-1. It should be noted that Latin and English, as well as metric and apothecary measures, are used for drug orders.

The directions (*4* in Figure 1-1) to the pharmacist for mixing or compounding drugs have become less necessary with the advent of the large pharmaceutical firms and their prepared drug products. The importance of these directions is in no way diminished, however, because misinterpretation is potentially lethal when dealing with drugs.

Since passage of the Controlled Substances Act of 1971, healthcare practitioners must include their registration number provided by the Drug Enforcement Administration (DEA) (usually termed a *DEA registration number*) when prescribing narcotics or controlled substances. Any licensed physician may apply for a DEA registration number.

Table 1-3 lists the most common abbreviations seen in prescriptions.

TABLE 1-3	Abbreviations and Symbols Used in Prescriptions*		
ABBREVIATION	**MEANING**	**ABBREVIATION**	**MEANING**
ā	before	ol	oil
āā	of each	OS	left eye
ac	before a meal	OU	both eyes
ad lib	as much as desired	P̄	after
alt hor	every other hour	part aeq	equal parts
aq dest	distilled water	pc	after meals
bid	twice daily	pil	pill
C, cong	gallon	placebo	I please (inert substitute)
c̄	with	po	per os (by mouth)
cap	capsule	prn	as needed
cc	cubic centimeter (another term for mL)	pr	rectally
dil	dilute	pulv	powder
dtd	give such doses	q	every
elix	elixir	qh	every hour
emuls	emulsion	qid	four times daily
et	and	qod	every other day
ex aq	in water	qd	every day
ext	extract	q2h	every 2 hours
fld	fluid	q3h	every 3 hours
ft	make	q4h	every 4 hours
gel	a gel, jelly	qs	as much as required (quantity sufficient)
g	gram	qt	quart
gr	grain	Rx, ℞	take
gtt	a drop	s̄	without
hs	at bedtime	sig	write
IM	intramuscular	sol	solution
IV	intravenous	solv	dissolve
L	liter	sos	if needed (for one time)
lin	liniment	spt	spirit
liq	liquid, solution	sp frumenti	whiskey
lot	lotion	s̄s̄	half
M	mix	stat	immediately
mist, mixt	mixture	syr	syrup
mL	milliliter	tab	tablet or tablets
nebul	a spray	tid	three times daily
non rep	not to be repeated	tr, tinct	tincture
npo	nothing by mouth	ung	ointment
O, ō	pint	ut dict	as directed
OD	right eye	vin	wine

*Not all of these abbreviations are considered safe practice; however, they may still be seen occasionally.

Over-the-Counter Drugs

 KEY POINT

An over-the-counter (OTC) drug does not require a prescription for purchase.

Many drugs are available to the general population without a prescription; these are referred to as *over-the-counter (OTC)* products. Although the strength and amount per dose may be less than that of a prescription formulation, OTC drugs can be hazardous in normal amounts if their effects are not understood. In addition, when taken in large quantities, OTC products may increase the risk of hazard to the consumer. For example:

Consider OTC preparations containing epinephrine. For patients with mild asthma, racemic epinephrine is available OTC as an inhalation solution known as Asthmanefrin. Racemic epinephrine can provoke cardiac arrhythmia or hypertension, and, in particular, can exacerbate these conditions if they preexist in a patient. Dependence on OTC preparations may encourage "self-treatment" that could mask or complicate a serious medical condition.

Generic Substitution in Prescriptions

A healthcare prescriber can indicate to the pharmacist that generic substitution is permitted in the filling of a prescription. In such a case, the pharmacist may provide any manufacturer's version of the prescribed drug and not a specific brand. This practice is intended to save money because the manufacturer of the generic substitute has not invested considerable time and money in developing the original drug product, and presumably the generic substitute is less expensive to the consumer than the original proprietary brand.

RESPIRATORY CARE PHARMACOLOGY: AN OVERVIEW

KEY POINT

Aerosolized agents are central to respiratory care in pulmonary diseases. This group of drugs includes adrenergic, anticholinergic, mucoactive, corticosteroid, antiasthmatic, and antiinfective agents and surfactants instilled directly into the trachea. Other drug groups important in respiratory care include cardiovascular, antiinfective, neuromuscular blocking, and diuretic agents.

Helping people with pulmonary diseases, such as **cystic fibrosis (CF)**, or pulmonary derangements, such as **acute respiratory distress syndrome (ARDS)**, defines a spectrum of pharmacologic care from maintenance support of a person with stable disease through intervention for a critically ill patient. The respiratory system cannot be dissociated from the cardiac and vascular systems, given the interlinked function of these systems. As a result, respiratory care pharmacology involves a relatively broad area of drug classes.

Aerosolized Agents Given by Inhalation

Drugs delivered by oral inhalation or nasal inhalation are intended to provide a local topical treatment of the respiratory tract. The following are advantages of this method and route of delivery:

- Aerosol doses are smaller than doses used for the same purpose and given systemically.
- Side effects are usually fewer and less severe with aerosol delivery than with oral or parenteral delivery.
- The onset of action is rapid.
- Drug delivery is targeted to the respiratory system, with lower systemic bioavailability.
- The inhalation of aerosol drugs is painless, relatively safe, and may be convenient depending on the specific delivery device used.

The classes of aerosolized agents (including surfactants, which are directly instilled into the trachea), their uses, and individual agents are summarized in Table 1-4.

TABLE 1-4	Common Agents Used in Respiratory Therapy	
DRUG GROUP	**THERAPEUTIC PURPOSE**	**AGENTS**
Adrenergic agents	*β-Adrenergic:* Relaxation of bronchial smooth muscle and bronchodilation, to reduce **airway resistance (R_{aw})** and to improve ventilatory flow rates in airway obstruction resulting from **chronic obstructive pulmonary disease (COPD)**, asthma, CF, acute bronchitis	Albuterol Arformoterol Formoterol Indacaterol Levalbuterol Metaproterenol Olodaterol Salmeterol Vilanterol
	α-Adrenergic: Topical vasoconstriction and decongestion Used to treat upper airway swelling	Racemic epinephrine
Anticholinergic agents	Relaxation of cholinergically induced bronchoconstriction to improve ventilatory flow rates in COPD and asthma	Aclidinium bromide Ipratropium bromide Tiotropium bromide Umeclidinium bromide
Mucoactive agents	Modification of properties of respiratory tract mucus; current agents reduce viscosity and promote clearance of secretions	Acetylcysteine Dornase alfa
Corticosteroids	Reduction and control of airway inflammatory response usually associated with asthma (lower respiratory tract) or with seasonal or chronic rhinitis (upper respiratory tract)	Beclomethasone dipropionate Budesonide Ciclesonide Flunisolide Fluticasone furoate Fluticasone propionate Mometasone furoate
Antiasthmatic agents	Prevention of onset and development of the asthmatic response through inhibition of chemical mediators of inflammation	Cromolyn sodium Montelukast Omalizumab Zafirlukast Zileuton

Continued

TABLE 1-4	Common Agents Used in Respiratory Therapy—cont'd	
DRUG GROUP	**THERAPEUTIC PURPOSE**	**AGENTS**
Antiinfective agents	Inhibition or eradication of specific infective agents, such as *Pneumocystis jiroveci* (**formerly** *carinii*) (pentamidine), **respiratory syncytial virus (RSV)** (ribavirin), ***Pseudomonas aeruginosa*** in CF or influenza A and B	Aztreonam Pentamidine Ribavirin Tobramycin Zanamivir
Exogenous surfactants	Approved clinical use is by direct intratracheal instillation for the purpose of restoring more normal lung compliance in RDS of newborns	Beractant Calfactant Lucinactant Poractant alfa
Prostacyclin analogs	Clinically indicated to treat pulmonary hypertension for the purpose of decreasing shortness of breath and increasing walking distance	Iloprost Treprostinil

CF, Cystic fibrosis; *RDS,* respiratory distress syndrome.

Related Drug Groups in Respiratory Care

Additional groups of drugs important in critical care are the following:

- *Antiinfective agents,* such as antibiotics or antituberculous drugs
- *Neuromuscular blocking agents,* such as curariform agents and others
- *Central nervous system agents,* such as analgesics and sedatives/hypnotics
- *Antiarrhythmic agents,* such as cardiac glycosides and lidocaine
- *Antihypertensive and antianginal agents,* such as β-blocking agents or nitroglycerin
- *Anticoagulant and thrombolytic agents,* such as heparin or streptokinase
- *Diuretics,* such as the thiazides or furosemide

? SELF-ASSESSMENT QUESTIONS

Answers can be found in Appendix A.
1. What is the definition of the term *drug?*
2. What is the difference between the generic name and trade name of a drug?
3. What part of a prescription contains the name and amount of the drug being prescribed?
4. A physician's order reads as follows: "gtt iv of racemic epinephrine, c̄3 cc of normal saline, q4h, while awake." What has been ordered?
5. The drug salmeterol was released for general clinical use in the United States in 1994. Where would you look to find information about this drug such as the available dosage forms, doses, properties, side effects, and action?

📖 CLINICAL SCENARIO

Answers can be found in Appendix A.

A 24-year-old man played golf on a newly mown course. He had exhibited allergies in the past few years and was diagnosed as having asthma. He did not have a regular physician or medical treatment site, and he was not taking any medications to control his asthma and allergies. He began to experience difficulty breathing later in the day, with wheezing and some shortness of breath on mild exertion. He visited his local drugstore and purchased Primatene Mist. On use, he obtained immediate relief for his breathing, but his heart rate increased from 66 beats/min to 84 beats/min, and he felt shaky. By midnight, his wheezing had returned. He continued using the Primatene Mist through the next morning. The relief he experienced with the drug diminished during the afternoon, and a friend found him later that evening with audible wheezing, gasping for air, and in severe respiratory distress. He was rushed to a local emergency department, where he went into respiratory arrest approximately 5 minutes after arrival.

Using the SOAP method, assess this clinical scenario.

REFERENCES

1. Brunton LL, Chabner B, Knollman B, editors: *Goodman & Gilman's the pharmacological basis of therapeutics,* ed 12, New York, 2011, McGraw-Hill Medical Publishing.
2. Katzung BG, Masters SB, Trevor AJ, editors: *Basic and clinical pharmacology,* ed 12, New York, 2012, Lange Medical Books/McGraw-Hill.
3. *Drug facts and comparisons,* St. Louis, 2014, *Facts & Comparisons,* Wolters Kluwer Health.
4. De Quincey T: *Confessions of an English opium-eater* (Dover Thrift Editions), Mineola, N.Y., 1995, Dover Publications.
5. Gale EA, Clark A: A drug on the market? *Lancet* 355:61, 2000.
6. DiMasi JA, Hansen RW, Grabowski HG: The price of innovation: new estimates of drug development costs. *J Health Econ* 22:151, 2003.
7. Adams CP, Brantner VV: Spending on new drug development. *Health Econ* 19:130, 2010.
8. Flieger K: How experimental drugs are tested in humans. *Pediatr Infect Dis J* 8:160, 1989.
9. Hassall TH, Fredd SB: A physician's guide to information available from the FDA about new drug approvals. *Am J Gastroenterol* 84:1222, 1989.
10. Covington TR: The ABCs of new drugs. *Facts and Comparisons Newsletter* 10:73, 1991.

CHAPTER 2

Principles of Drug Action

Douglas S. Gardenhire

CHAPTER OUTLINE

OBJECTIVES

After reading this chapter, the reader will be able to:

1. Define key terms that pertain to principles of drug action
2. Define the *drug administration phase*
3. Describe the various routes of administration available
4. Define the *pharmacokinetic phase*
5. Discuss the key factors in the pharmacokinetic phase (e.g., absorption, distribution, metabolism, and elimination)
6. Describe the first-pass effect
7. Differentiate between systemic and inhaled drugs in relation to the pharmacokinetic phase
8. Explain the lung availability/total systemic availability (L/T) ratio
9. Define the *pharmacodynamic phase*
10. Discuss the importance of structure-activity relationships
11. Discuss the role of drug receptors
12. Discuss the importance of dose-response relationships
13. Describe the importance of pharmacogenetics

KEY TERMS AND DEFINITIONS

Agonist Chemical or drug that binds to a receptor and creates an effect on the body.

Antagonist Chemical or drug that binds to a receptor but does not create an effect on the body; it blocks the receptor site from accepting an agonist.

Bioavailability Amount of drug that reaches the systemic circulation.

Drug administration Method by which a drug is made available to the body.

Enteral Use of the intestine.

First-pass effect Initial metabolism in the liver of a drug taken orally before the drug reaches the systemic circulation.

Hypersensitivity Allergic or immune-mediated reaction to a drug, which can be serious, requiring airway maintenance or ventilatory assistance.

Idiosyncratic effect Abnormal or unexpected reaction to a drug, other than an allergic reaction, compared with the predicted effect.

Inhalation Taking a substance, typically in the form of gases, fumes, vapors, mists, aerosols, or dusts, into the body by breathing in.

Local effect Limited to the area of treatment (e.g., inhaled drug to treat constricted airways).

Lung availability/total systemic availability ratio (L/T ratio) Amount of drug that is made available to the lung out of the total available to the body.

Parenteral Administration of a substance in any way other than the intestine, most commonly an injection (e.g., intravenous, intramuscular, subcutaneous, intrathecal, or intraosseous).

Pharmacodynamics Mechanisms of drug action by which a drug molecule causes its effect in the body.

Continued

Pharmacogenetics Study of genetic factors and their influence on drug response.

Pharmacokinetics Time course and disposition of a drug in the body, based on its absorption, distribution, metabolism, and elimination.

Receptor Cell component that combines with a drug to change or enhance the function of the cell.

Structure-activity relationship (SAR) Relationship between a drug's chemical structure and the outcome it has on the body.

Synergism Drug interaction that occurs from two or more drug effects that are greater than if the drugs were given alone.

Systemic effect Pertains to the whole body, whereas the target for the drug is not local, possibly causing side effects (e.g., capsule of acetaminophen for a headache).

Tachyphylaxis Rapid decrease in response to a drug.

Therapeutic index (TI) Difference between the minimal therapeutic and toxic concentrations of a drug; the smaller the difference, the greater chance the drug will be toxic.

Tolerance Decreasing intensity of response to a drug over time.

Topical Use of the skin or mucous membrane (e.g., lotion).

Transdermal Use of the skin (e.g., patch).

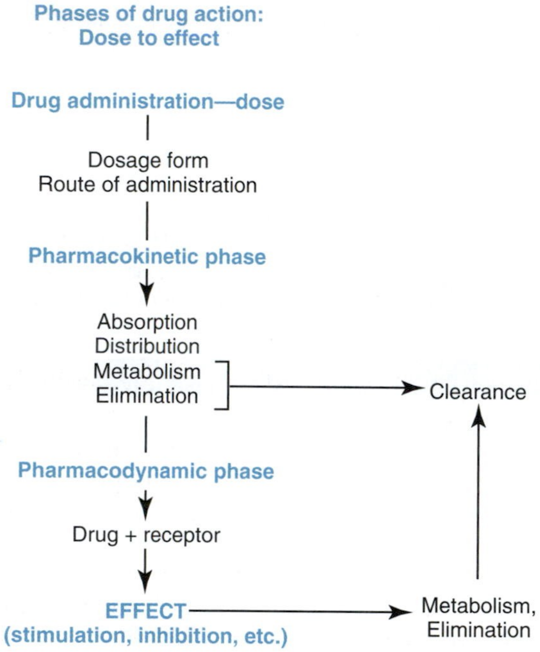

Phases of drug action:
Dose to effect

Drug administration—dose
|
Dosage form
Route of administration

Pharmacokinetic phase
↓
Absorption
Distribution
Metabolism ——→ Clearance
Elimination
|
Pharmacodynamic phase
↓
Drug + receptor
↓
EFFECT ——→ Metabolism,
(stimulation, inhibition, etc.)   Elimination

Figure 2-1 Conceptual scheme illustrating the major phases of drug action in sequence, from dose administration to effect in the body. (From Katzung BG, Masters SB, Trevor AJ, editors: *Basic and clinical pharmacology*, ed. 12, New York, 2012, McGraw Hill Medical.)

The entire course of action of a drug, from dose to effect, can be understood in three phases: the drug administration, pharmacokinetic, and pharmacodynamic phases. This useful conceptual framework, based on the principles offered by Ariëns and Simonis,[1] organizes the steps of a drug's action from **drug administration** (method by which a drug dose is made available to the body) through effect and ultimate elimination from the body. This framework is illustrated in Figure 2-1, which provides an overview of the interrelationship of the three phases of drug action, each of which is discussed in this chapter.

    KEY POINT

Principles of drug action encompass three major topic areas: drug administration, pharmacokinetics, and pharmacodynamics.

DRUG ADMINISTRATION PHASE

!   **KEY POINT**

The *drug administration* phase identifies drug dosage forms and routes of administration. The *pharmacokinetic phase* describes the factors determining drug absorption, distribution in the body, metabolism, breakdown of the active drug to its metabolites, and elimination of the active drug and inactive metabolites from the body.

Drug Dosage Forms

The drug administration phase entails the interrelated concepts of drug formulation (e.g., compounding a tablet for particular dissolution properties) and drug delivery (e.g., designing an inhaler to deliver a unit dose). Two key topics of this phase are the drug dosage form and the route of administration. The *drug dosage form* is the physical state of the drug in association with nondrug components. Tablets, capsules, and injectable solutions are common drug dosage forms. The *route of administration* is the portal of entry for the drug into the body, such as oral (enteral), injection, or inhalation. The form in which a drug is available must be compatible with the route of administration desired. The injectable route (e.g., intravenous route) requires a liquid solution of a drug, whereas the oral route can accommodate capsules, tablets, or liquid solutions. Some common drug formulations for each of the common routes of drug administration are listed in Table 2-1.

Drug Formulations and Additives

A drug is the active ingredient in a dosage formulation, but it is usually not the only ingredient in the total formulation. For example, in a capsule of an antibiotic, the capsule itself is a gelatinous material that allows the drug to be swallowed. The capsule material disintegrates in the stomach, and the active drug ingredient is released for absorption. The rate at which the active drug is liberated from a capsule or tablet can be controlled during the formulation process by altering drug particle size or by using a specialized coating or formulation matrix. Aerosolized agents for inhalation and treatment of the respiratory tract also contain ingredients other than the active drug, such as preservatives,

TABLE 2-1	Common Drug Formulations for Various Routes of Administration			
ENTERAL	**PARENTERAL**	**INHALATION**	**TRANSDERMAL**	**TOPICAL**
Tablet	Solution	Gas	Patch	Powder
Capsule	Suspension	Aerosol	Paste	Lotion
Suppository	Depot	—	—	Ointment
Elixir	—	—	—	Solution
Suspension	—	—	—	—

TABLE 2-2	Three Different Dosage Forms for the Bronchodilator Drug Albuterol, Indicating Ingredients Other Than Active Drug		
DOSAGE FORM	**ACTIVE DRUG**	**INGREDIENTS**	
Nebulizer solution	Albuterol sulfate	Benzalkonium chloride, sulfuric acid	
Respimat	Albuterol-ipratropium	Benzalkonium chloride, edetate disodium hydrochloric acid	
Tablets	Albuterol sulfate	Lactose, butylparaben, sugar	
MDI HFA	Albuterol	1,1,1,2-Tetrafluoroethane, ethanol, oleic acid	

HFA, Hydrofluoroalkane; *MDI,* metered dose inhaler.

propellants for metered dose inhaler (MDI) formulations, dispersants (surfactants), and carrier agents for dry powder inhalers (DPIs). Table 2-2 presents the various formulations with different ingredients for the beta (β)-adrenergic bronchodilator albuterol. In the nebulizer solution, benzalkonium chloride is a preservative, and sulfuric acid adjusts the pH of the solution. In the hydrofluoroalkane (HFA)-MDI, a hydrofluoroalkane is used as a propellant.

Routes of Administration

Advances in drug formulation and delivery systems have yielded a wide range of routes by which a drug can be administered. In the following discussion, routes of administration have been divided into five broad categories: enteral, parenteral, transdermal, inhalation, and topical.

Enteral

The term **enteral** refers literally to the small intestine, but the enteral route of administration is more broadly applicable to administration of drugs intended for absorption anywhere along the gastrointestinal tract. The most common enteral route is by mouth (oral) because it is convenient, is painless, and offers flexibility in possible dosage forms of the drug, as seen in Table 2-1. The oral route requires the patient to be able to swallow; therefore, airway-protective reflexes should be intact. If the drug is not destroyed or inactivated in the stomach and can be absorbed into the bloodstream, distribution throughout the body and a **systemic effect** can be achieved. Other enteral routes of administration include suppositories inserted in the rectum, tablets placed under the tongue (sublingual), and drug solutions introduced though an indwelling gastric tube.

Parenteral (Injectable)

Technically, the term **parenteral** means "besides the intestine," which implies any route of administration other than

enteral. However, the parenteral route commonly refers to injection of a drug. Various options are available for injection of a drug, the most common of which are the following:

- *Intravenous (IV):* Injected directly into the vein, allowing nearly instantaneous access to systemic circulation. Drugs can be given as a bolus, in which case the entire dose is given rapidly, leading to a sharp increase in the drug's plasma concentration, or a steady infusion can be used to avoid this precipitous increase.
- *Intramuscular (IM):* Injected deep into a skeletal muscle. Because the drug must be absorbed from the muscle into the systemic circulation, the drug effects occur more gradually than with intravenous injection, although typically more rapidly than by the oral route.
- *Subcutaneous (SC):* Injected into the subcutaneous tissue beneath the epidermis and the dermis.
- *Intrathecal (IT):* Injected into the arachnoid membrane of the spinal cord to diffuse throughout the spinal fluid.
- *Intraosseous (IO):* Injected into the marrow of the bone.

Transdermal

An increasing number of drugs are being formulated for application to the skin (i.e., **transdermal** administration) to produce a systemic effect. The advantage of this route is that it can supply long-term continuous delivery to the systemic circulation. The drug is absorbed percutaneously, obviating the need for a hypodermic needle and decreasing the fluctuations in plasma drug levels that can occur with repeated oral administration.

Inhalation

Drugs can be given by **inhalation** for either a systemic effect or a local effect in the lung. Two of the most common drug formulations given by this route are gases, which usually are given by inhalation for anesthesia (a systemic effect), and aerosolized agents intended to target the lung or respiratory tract in the treatment of respiratory disease (**local effect**). The technology and science of aerosol drug delivery to the respiratory tract continue to develop and are described in detail in Chapter 3. Box 2-1 provides a summary of devices commonly used for inhaled aerosol drug delivery. The general rationale for aerosolized drug delivery to the airways for treating respiratory disease is the local delivery of the drug to the target organ, with reduced or minimal body exposure to the drug and, it is hoped, reduced prevalence or severity of possible side effects.

Topical

Drugs can be applied directly to the skin or mucous membranes to produce a local effect. Such drugs are often formulated to minimize systemic absorption. Examples of **topical** administration include the application of corticosteroid cream to an area of contact dermatitis (e.g., poison ivy rash), administration of an eye drop containing a β-adrenergic antagonist to control glaucoma, and instillation of nasal drops containing an α-adrenergic agonist to relieve congestion.

PHARMACOKINETIC PHASE

The *pharmacokinetic phase* refers to the time course and disposition of a drug in the body, based on its absorption, distribution, metabolism, and elimination. Once presented to the body as described in the drug administration phase, a drug crosses local anatomic barriers to varying extents depending on its chemical properties and the physiologic environment of the body compartment it occupies. For a systemic effect, it is desirable for the drug to get into the bloodstream for distribution to the body; for a local effect, this is not desirable and can lead to unwanted side effects throughout the body. Absorption, distribution, metabolism, and elimination are the factors influencing and determining the course of a drug after it is introduced to the body. In essence, **pharmacokinetics** describes what the body does to a drug, and **pharmacodynamics** describes what the drug does to the body.

Absorption

When given orally for a systemic effect, a pill must first dissolve to liberate the active ingredient. The free drug

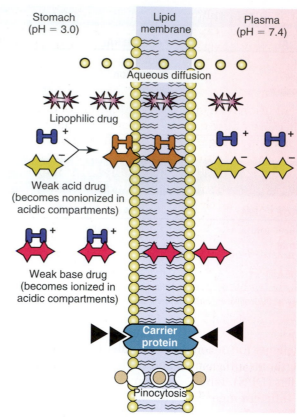

Figure 2-2 Pathways by which drugs can traverse lipid membranes and enter the circulation. A membrane separating an acidic compartment (stomach) and a neutral compartment (plasma) is shown to illustrate that only the nonionized forms of weak acids or weak bases cross these lipophilic barriers more readily than ionized forms.

must then reach the epithelial lining of the stomach or intestine and traverse the lipid membrane barriers of the gastric and vascular cells before reaching the bloodstream for distribution throughout the body. The lining of the lower respiratory tract also presents barriers to drug absorption. This mucosal barrier consists of five identifiable elements:

1. Airway surface liquid
2. Epithelial cells
3. Basement membrane
4. Interstitium
5. Capillary vascular network

After traversing these layers, a drug can reach the smooth muscle or glands of the airway. The mechanisms by which drugs move across membrane barriers include aqueous diffusion, lipid diffusion, active or facilitated diffusion, and pinocytosis. Generally, a drug must be sufficiently water-soluble to reach a lipid (cell) membrane and sufficiently lipid-soluble to diffuse across the cell barrier. Figure 2-2 illustrates these basic mechanisms.

Aqueous Diffusion

Aqueous diffusion occurs in the aqueous compartments of the body, such as the interstitial spaces or within a cell.

Transport across epithelial linings is restricted because of small pore size; capillaries have larger pores, allowing passage of most drug molecules. Diffusion occurs by a concentration gradient.

Lipid Diffusion

Lipid diffusion is an important mechanism for drug absorption because of the many epithelial membranes that must be crossed if a drug is to distribute in the body and reach its target organ. Epithelial cells have lipid membranes, and a drug must be lipid-soluble (nonionized, nonpolar) to diffuse across such a membrane. Lipid-insoluble drugs tend to be ionized, or have positive and negative charges separated on the molecule (polar), and are water-soluble.

Many drugs are weak acids or weak bases, and the degree of ionization of these molecules is dependent on the pK_p (the pH at which the drug is 50% ionized and 50% nonionized), the ambient pH, and whether the drug is a weak acid or base. The direction of increasing ionization is opposite for weak acids and weak bases while the ambient pH changes.

Weak acid: Because an acid contributes protons (H^+ ions), the protonated form is neutral, or nonionized.

Drug neutral $\leftrightarrow$ Drug$^-$ anion + H^+ Proton (protonated)

Drug$^+$ cation $\leftrightarrow$ Drug neutral + H^+ Proton (protonated)

Weak base: Because a base accepts protons (H^+ ions), the unprotonated form is neutral, or nonionized.

- The protonated weak acid is neutralized by the addition of H^+ ions in an acidic environment, is nonionized, and is lipid-soluble.
- The protonated weak base gains a charge by adding H^+ ions in an acidic environment, is ionized, and is not lipid-soluble.

Figure 2-2 conceptually illustrates the principle of lipid diffusion and absorption for weak acids and bases.

Some drugs, such as ethanol, are neutral molecules and are always nonionized. They are well absorbed into the bloodstream and across the blood-brain barrier. Other drugs, such as ipratropium bromide and *d*-(+)-tubocurarine, are quaternary amines, have no unshared electrons for reversible binding of H^+ ions, and are permanently positively charged. Ipratropium is not lipid-soluble and does not absorb and distribute well from the mouth or the lung with oral inhalation. A secondary or tertiary amine, such as atropine, can give up its H^+ ion and become nonionized, increasing its absorption, distribution, and consequent side effects in the body.

Carrier-Mediated Transport

Special carrier molecules embedded in the lipid membrane can transport some substances, such as amino acids, sugars, or naturally occurring peptides, and the drugs that resemble these substances. In some instances, a drug can compete with the endogenous substance normally transported by the carrier.

Pinocytosis

Pinocytosis refers to the incorporation of a substance into a cell by a process of membrane engulfment and transport of the substance within vesicles, allowing translocation across a membrane barrier.

Factors Affecting Absorption

The route of administration determines which barriers to absorption must be crossed by a drug. These barriers can affect the drug's time to onset and time to peak effect. Intravenous administration bypasses the need for absorption from the gastrointestinal tract seen with oral administration, generally gives a very rapid onset and peak effect, and provides 100% availability of the drug in the bloodstream. The term **bioavailability** indicates the proportion of a drug that reaches the systemic circulation. For example, the bioavailability of oral morphine is 0.24 because only about a quarter of the morphine ingested actually arrives in the systemic circulation. Bioavailability is influenced not only by absorption but also by inactivation caused by stomach acids and by metabolic degradation, which can occur before the drug reaches the main systemic compartment. Another important variable governing absorption and bioavailability is blood flow to the site of absorption.

Distribution

To be effective at its desired site of action, a drug must have a certain concentration. An antibiotic is investigated for its *minimal inhibitory concentration (MIC)*—the lowest concentration of a drug at which a microbial population is inhibited. *Drug distribution* is the process by which a drug is transported to its sites of action, is eliminated, or is stored. When given intravenously, most drugs distribute initially to organs that receive the most blood flow. After this brief initial distribution phase, subsequent phases of distribution occur on the basis of the principles of diffusion and transport outlined earlier and the drug's physical and chemical nature and ability to bind to plasma proteins. The initial distribution phase is clinically important for lipophilic anesthetics (e.g., propofol and thiopental) because they produce rapid onset of anesthesia as a function of the high blood flow to the brain, and their effects are quickly terminated during redistribution to other tissues. The binding of drugs to plasma proteins can also be clinically relevant in rare instances, such as when a large portion of a drug is inactive because it is bound to plasma proteins but subsequently becomes displaced (and thus active) by a second drug that binds to the same proteins.

The plasma concentration of a drug is partially determined by the rate and extent of absorption versus the rate of elimination for a given dose amount. The volume of the compartment in which the drug is distributed also determines the concentration achieved in plasma. Compartments and their approximate volumes in a 70-kg adult are given in Table 2-3.

Volume of Distribution

Suppose a certain drug that distributes exclusively in the plasma compartment is administered intravenously. If a 10-mg bolus of the drug is given, and the volume of the patient's plasma compartment is 5 L, the concentration in the plasma (barring degradation or elimination) would be 2 mg/L. In this simple example, the *volume of distribution* (V_D) is the same as the volume of the plasma compartment. In practice, drug distribution is usually more complex, and the actual tissue compartments occupied by the drug are unknown. Nonetheless, V_D describes a useful mathematical equation relating the total amount of drug in the body to the plasma concentration:

$$\text{Volume of distribution } (V_D) = \frac{\text{Drug amount}}{\text{Plasma concentration}}$$

EXAMPLE

> If 350 mg of theophylline results in a concentration in the plasma of 10 mg/L (equivalent to 10 mcg/mL), the volume of distribution (V_D) is calculated as:
>
> $$V_D = \frac{350 \text{ mg}}{10 \text{ mg/L}}$$
>
> $$V_D = 35 \text{ L}$$

The drug can be absorbed and distributed into sites other than the vascular compartment, which is only approximately 5 L, and the calculated volume of distribution can be much larger than the blood volume, as in the case of theophylline, which has a V_D of 35 L in a 70-kg adult. For this reason, V_D is referred to as the *apparent volume of distribution* to emphasize that V_D does not refer to an actual physiologic space. Drugs such as fluoxetine (an antidepressant) and inhaled anesthetics are sequestered in peripheral tissues and can have apparent volumes of distribution many times greater than the entire volume of the body.

In a clinical setting, V_D is rarely measured but is nonetheless important for estimating the dose needed for a given therapeutic level of drug. By rearranging the equation for V_D, the drug amount should equal the V_D multiplied by the concentration.

TABLE 2-3	Volumes (Approximate) of Major Body Compartments
COMPARTMENT	**VOLUME (L)**
Vascular (blood)	5
Interstitial fluid	10
Intracellular fluid	20
Fat (adipose tissue)	14-25

EXAMPLE

> To achieve a concentration of theophylline of 15 mg/L with a V_D of 35 L, we calculate a dose of:
>
> $$\text{Drug amount (drug dose)} = \text{Plasma concentration} \times V_D$$
>
> $$\text{Dose} = 15 \text{ mg/L} \times 35 \text{ L}$$
>
> $$\text{Dose} = 525 \text{ mg}$$

The following points should be noted:

- The preceding calculation assumes that the dose is completely available to the body. This may be true if a dose is given intravenously, but there may be less than 100% bioavailability if a dose is given orally.
- This is a *loading dose,* and subsequent doses to maintain a level of concentration depend on the rate of absorption versus the rates of metabolism and excretion (discussed in the next sections).
- V_D may change as a function of age or disease state.
- The concept of V_D is not directly helpful in topical drug administration and delivery of aerosolized drugs intended to act directly on the airway surface. V_D for topical deposition in the airway is not measured, and the drug is deposited locally in the respiratory tract, with some drugs absorbed from the airway into the blood.

Metabolism

 KEY POINT

The liver is a primary site of drug metabolism and biotransformation, and the kidneys are the primary site of drug excretion, although both drugs and metabolites can also be excreted in the feces.

The processes by which drug molecules are metabolized, or biotransformed, constitute a complex area of biochemistry that is beyond the scope of this text. Common pathways for the biotransformation of drugs are listed in Box 2-2. Generally, phase 1 biochemical reactions convert the active drug to a more polar (water-soluble) form, which can be excreted by the kidney. Drugs that are transformed in a phase 1 reaction may be transformed further in a phase 2 reaction, which combines (conjugates) a substance (e.g., glucuronic acid) with the metabolite to form a highly polar conjugate. For some drugs, biotransformation is

BOX 2-2	Common Pathways for Drug Metabolism

Phase 1
- Oxidative hydroxylation
- Oxidative dealkylation
- Oxidative deamination
- N-oxidation
- Reductive reactions
- Hydrolytic reactions (e.g., esterase enzymes)

Phase 2
- Conjugation reactions (e.g., glucuronide or sulfate)

accomplished by just phase 1 or phase 2 metabolism without prior transformation by the other phase. Metabolites are often less biologically active than the parent drug. Nevertheless, some drugs are inactive until metabolized (e.g., enalapril) or produce metabolites that are more toxic than their progenitors (e.g., breakdown products of acetaminophen).

Site of Drug Biotransformation

The liver is the principal organ for drug metabolism, although other tissues, including the lung, intestinal wall, and endothelial vascular wall, can transform or metabolize drugs. For example, epinephrine, a weak base, is absorbed into the intestinal wall, where sulfatase enzymes inactivate it as the drug diffuses into the circulation. The liver contains intracellular enzymes that usually convert lipophilic (lipid-soluble) drug molecules into water-soluble metabolites that are more easily excreted. The major enzyme system in the liver is the cytochrome P450 oxidase system (CYP). There are many forms of cytochrome P450, which are hemoproteins with considerable substrate versatility and the ability to metabolize new drugs or industrial compounds. The various forms of cytochrome P450 have been divided into about a dozen subcategories, termed *isoenzyme families*. The four most important isoenzyme families for drug metabolism have been designated *CYP1*, *CYP2*, *CYP3*, and *CYP4*. A given drug may be metabolized predominantly by only one member of an isoenzyme family, whereas another drug may be metabolized by multiple enzymes in the same family or by several distinct enzymes across families. Knowing which particular CYP enzyme metabolizes a drug can be important for predicting drug interactions, as further described subsequently.

Enzyme Induction and Inhibition

Chronic administration or abuse of drugs that are metabolized by the enzyme systems in the liver can induce (increase) or inhibit the levels of the enzymes (enzyme induction and inhibition). Examples of drugs or agents that can induce or inhibit CYP enzymes are listed in Table 2-4.

Enzyme induction can affect the therapeutic doses of drugs required. Rifampin can induce CYP enzymes and increase the metabolism of several drugs, including

warfarin and oral contraceptives. Likewise, cigarette smoking can increase the breakdown of theophylline in patients with chronic lung disease, shortening the half-life of the drug from approximately 7.0 to 4.3 hours. Dosages would need to be adjusted accordingly to maintain a suitable plasma level of theophylline. Conversely, a substantial portion of drug interactions involves inhibition of CYP enzymes. A given drug is not likely to inhibit all the CYP isoenzymes equally. For example, the antibiotic ciprofloxacin is a potent inhibitor of an enzyme in the CYP family that also metabolizes theophylline. Coadministration of ciprofloxacin with theophylline can increase theophylline levels: the opposite effect of cigarette smoking.

First-Pass Effect

Another clinically important effect of the liver on drug metabolism is referred to as the **first-pass effect** of elimination. When a drug is taken orally and absorbed into the blood from the stomach or intestine, the portal vein drains this blood directly into the liver (Figure 2-3). The blood from the liver is drained by the right and left hepatic veins directly into the inferior vena cava and on into the general circulation.

If a drug is highly metabolized by the liver enzymes and is administered orally, most of the drug's activity is terminated in its passage through the liver before it ever reaches the general circulation and the rest of the body. This is the first-pass effect. Examples of drugs with a high first-pass effect are propranolol; nitroglycerin (sublingual administration is preferred to oral); and fluticasone propionate, an aerosolized corticosteroid. The first-pass effect causes difficulties with oral administration that must be overcome by increasing the oral dose (compared with the parenteral dose) or by using a delivery system that circumvents first-pass metabolism. The following routes avoid first-pass circulation through the liver: injection, buccal or sublingual (e.g., tablets), transdermal (e.g., patch), rectal (e.g., suppositories), and inhalation. These routes of administration bypass the portal venous circulation, allowing drugs to be generally distributed in the body before being circulated through the liver and ultimately metabolized. They also bypass metabolic degradation occurring in the gut as a result of specific metabolic enzymes (e.g., CYP3) or bacterial flora.

Elimination

The primary site of drug excretion in the body is the kidney, just as the liver is the site of much drug metabolism. The kidney is important for removing drug metabolites produced by the liver. Some drugs are not metabolized and are eliminated from the circulation entirely by the kidney. The route of elimination becomes important when choosing between alternative therapies because liver or kidney disease can alter the clearance of a drug by these organs. Generally, *clearance* is a measure of the ability of the body to rid itself of a drug. Most often, clearance is expressed as *total systemic* or *plasma clearance* to emphasize that all of the various

TABLE 2-4	Drugs Causing Induction or Inhibition of Cytochrome P450 Enzymes	
CYTOCHROME P450 ISOENZYME	**INDUCERS**	**INHIBITORS**
CYP1A2	Phenytoin	Ciprofloxacin
	Rifampin	Diltiazem
CYP2D6		Ranitidine
		Fluoxetine
CYP3A4	Carbamazepine	Diltiazem
	Corticosteroids	Fluoxetine
	Rifampin	Erythromycin

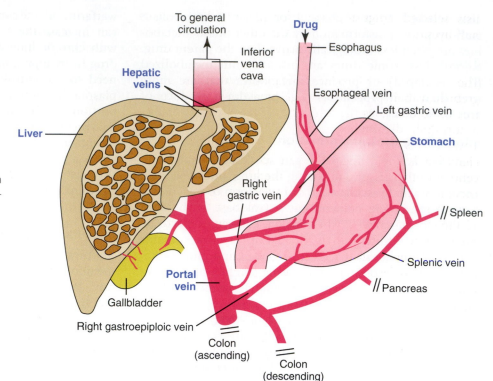

Figure 2-3 Anatomy of venous drainage from the stomach that forms the basis for the first-pass effect of orally administered drugs.

mechanisms by which a given drug is cleared (e.g., metabolism, excretion) are taken into account.

Plasma Clearance

Just as the term V_D is an abstraction that does not usually correspond to any real physiologic volume, so the term *plasma clearance (Cl_p)* refers to a hypothetical volume of plasma that is completely cleared of a drug over a given period. Consequently, Cl_p is usually expressed as liters per hour (L/hr) or, if body weight is taken into account, liters per hour per kilogram. Because Cl_p gives an indication of the quantity of drug removed from the body over a given time, it can be used to estimate the rate at which a drug must be replaced to maintain a steady plasma level.

Maintenance Dose

To achieve a steady level of drug in the body, dosing must equal the rate of elimination:

Dosing rate (mg/hr) =
   $(Cl_P)(L/hr) \times$ Plasma concentration (mg/L)

EXAMPLE

The clearance of theophylline is given as 2.88 L/hr/70 kg. For an average 70-kg adult, to maintain a plasma drug level of 15 mg/L (equivalent to 15 mcg/mL), calculate the dosing rate as follows:

   Dosing rate = 2.88 L/hr × 15 mg/L = 43.2 mg/hr

TABLE 2-5	Plasma Half-Lives of Common Drugs
DRUG	**HALF-LIFE (hr)**
Acetaminophen	2.0
Amoxicillin	1.7
Azithromycin	40.0
Digoxin	39.0
Gabapentin	6.5
Morphine	1.9
Paroxetine	17.0
Terbutaline	14.0

The preceding simplified calculation assumes total bioavailability of the drug, which may not be true for some routes of administration, and is intended for conceptual illustration only. Actual patient treatment must take other factors into account. The drug could be given by constant infusion or divided into dosing intervals (e.g., where half the daily dose is given every 12 hours). When deciding on a dosing interval, it is desirable to know the *plasma half-life.*

Plasma Half-Life

The *plasma half-life* $(T_{1/2})$ (the time required for the plasma concentration of a drug to decrease by one half) is a measure of how quickly a drug is eliminated from the body. More pertinent to dosing schedules, however, $T_{1/2}$ indicates how quickly a drug can accumulate and reach steady-state plasma levels. Drugs with a short $T_{1/2}$ (e.g., amoxicillin) reach steady-state levels quickly and must be given more frequently to maintain plasma levels, whereas the opposite is true of drugs with a long $T_{1/2}$, such as digoxin. Table 2-5 lists selected drugs in common use with their plasma half-lives.

Time-Plasma Curves

The concentration of a drug in the plasma over time can be graphed as a time-plasma curve (Figure 2-4). The shape of this curve describes the interplay of the kinetic factors of absorption, distribution, metabolism, and elimination. These curves can indicate whether the dose given is sufficient to reach and maintain the critical threshold of concentration needed for the desired therapeutic effect. Such a curve can also be plotted for concentrations of an aerosol drug in respiratory tract secretions. However, the duration of the *clinical effect*, rather than the concentration of the drug, is often represented in studies of aerosol drugs, particularly bronchodilators. The clinical effect is more helpful than a blood level in describing the pharmacokinetics of inhaled aerosols, which rely on topical delivery with a local effect in the airway.

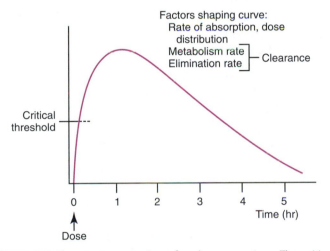

Figure 2-4 Plasma concentration of a drug over time. The critical threshold is the minimal level of drug concentration needed for a therapeutic effect.

Figure 2-5 illustrates hypothetical curves for the peak effect and duration of effect of three bronchodilator drugs on expiratory flow rates. The short-acting curve could represent a drug such as racemic epinephrine, an ultra-short-acting catecholamine bronchodilator. On the basis of its time curve, this agent is too short-acting for maintenance therapy and is not beta-receptor specific. The intermediate curve could represent an agent such as albuterol, with a peak effect of 30 to 60 minutes by inhalation and a duration of action of approximately 4 to 6 hours. These kinetics are useful for as-required bronchodilation or for maintenance therapy if a subject needs the drug four times daily. The kinetics indicate that bronchodilation with albuterol, an intermediate-acting drug, would not be maintained during an entire night. Finally, a long-acting agent such as the bronchodilator salmeterol could provide a 12-hour duration of effect, although time to peak effect is slower (less than 2 hours). These kinetics are useful for convenient twice-daily dosage and around-the-clock bronchodilation. This example illustrates how pharmacokinetics of an inhaled aerosol can help determine the choice of a particular drug for a given clinical application and the dosage schedule needed for the therapeutic effect. Other factors in the choice of a drug, whether inhaled aerosol, oral, or injectable, include the side effect profile, the individual's reaction to the drug, allergies, and compliance factors (patient adherence to dosage instructions) such as delivery formulations and dose timing.

Pharmacokinetics of Inhaled Aerosol Drugs

The inhalation route used for inhaled therapeutic aerosols, together with the physical and chemical nature of the drug, determine the absorption, distribution, metabolism, and elimination of the aerosol drug.

Local versus Systemic Effect

Inhaled aerosols are deposited on the surface of the upper or lower airway and are a form of topically administered

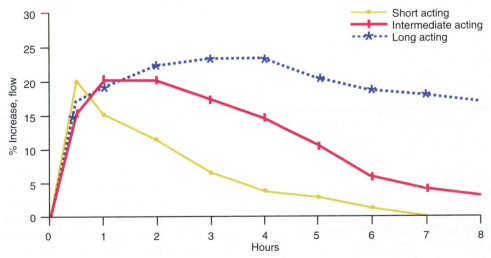

Figure 2-5 Hypothetical time-effect curves for three different bronchodilating agents, illustrating onset, peak effect, and duration.

drug. As topically deposited agents, inhaled aerosols can be intended either for a local effect in the upper or lower airway or for a systemic effect because the drug is absorbed and distributed in the blood. A *local effect* is exemplified by a nasally inhaled vasoconstricting agent (decongestant), such as oxymetazoline (Afrin), or by an inhaled bronchodilator aerosol, such as albuterol (Proventil-HFA, Ventolin-HFA, Proair HFA). A systemic effect might be exemplified by the administration of inhaled zanamivir (Relenza) to treat influenza, inhaled morphine for pain control, or inhaled insulin aerosol for systemic control of diabetes.[2]

Inhaled Aerosols in Pulmonary Disease

Inhaled aerosols used in the treatment of respiratory diseases such as asthma, chronic obstructive pulmonary disease (COPD), or cystic fibrosis (CF) are intended for a local, targeted effect in the lung and airway. The rationale for the inhalation route in therapy of the lung is to maximize lung deposition while minimizing body (systemic) exposure and unwanted side effects. If the ratio of drug in the lung is high relative to the amount of drug in the overall body (systemic drug level), the inhalation route offers an advantage over direct systemic administration (oral, intravenous) in treating the lung.

Distribution of Inhaled Aerosols

KEY POINT

The inhaled route of administration can involve both gastrointestinal and lung distribution. The systemic level of an inhaled drug and possible extrapulmonary side effects depend on both gastrointestinal and lung absorption of the active drug.

Because a portion of an inhaled aerosol is swallowed, the inhalation route leads to gastrointestinal absorption as well as lung absorption of the drug (Figure 2-6). After inhalation of an aerosol by a spontaneously breathing patient with no artificial airway, a proportion of the aerosol impacts in the oropharynx and is swallowed, and a proportion is inhaled into the airway. The traditional percentages given for stomach and airway proportions, based on Newman's classic measures[3] in 1981 with an MDI, are approximately 90% (stomach) and 10% (airway). Similar percentages have been found with other aerosol delivery devices; however, newer devices are able to deliver more to the airway, assuming use of good technique.

Approximately 50% to 60% of the drug impacts in the mouth or oropharynx and contributes to the 90% reaching the stomach. These amounts are used in discussing the pathways of metabolism for an inhaled drug. Although the remaining 10% is traditionally accepted as the proportion of inhaled drug that reaches the lower respiratory tract when delivered with current devices, the exact percentage can vary from 10% to 30% with different delivery devices or techniques of patient use. Lung deposition with an inhaled corticosteroid, budesonide (Pulmicort), has been reported as 15% with a pressurized MDI (pMDI) and 32%

with a DPI[4] (Pulmicort Turbuhaler; AstraZeneca, Wilmington, Delaware). Use of reservoir devices with MDIs or delivery through endotracheal tubes can significantly change oropharyngeal impaction or airway delivery (see Chapter 3).

Oral portion (stomach). The swallowed aerosol drug is subject to gastrointestinal absorption, distribution, and metabolism just like an orally administered drug. The aerosol drug can be absorbed from the stomach and metabolized in the liver (see Figure 2-6), producing a first-pass effect. The drug may also be inactivated in the intestinal wall as it is absorbed into the portal circulation. The site of absorption in the gastrointestinal tract is determined by the principles governing diffusion of drugs through lipid membranes. Generally, if the first-pass metabolism is high, systemic levels are only caused by lung absorption; if the first-pass metabolism is low and the drug is swallowed, there is a higher systemic level from gastrointestinal tract absorption, which may increase side effects in the body. The first-pass metabolism of three common inhaled aerosol drugs is as follows:

- Albuterol: 50%
- Budesonide: 90%
- Terbutaline: 90%

Inhaled portion. It is thought that aerosol drugs interact with the site of action in the airway: secretions in the lumen, nerve endings, cells (e.g., mast cells), or bronchial smooth muscle in the airway wall. The drug may be subsequently absorbed into the bronchial circulation, which drains into the right and left atria of the heart and then into the systemic circulation. The exact mechanism by which an aerosol drug, such as a bronchodilator, reaches the appropriate receptors to exert an effect is not well known. If the inhaled drug is not removed by mucociliary action or locally inactivated, the drug may be absorbed, and this increases the systemic availability of the drug.

Lung Availability/Total Systemic Availability Ratio

KEY POINT

The sources of the total systemic level of a drug are quantified in the lung availability/total systemic availability ratio (L/T ratio)—the higher the ratio, the more the systemic drug level is from the lung, as a result of efficient lung delivery, high first-pass metabolism, or both.

The **lung availability/total systemic availability ratio (L/T ratio)** quantifies the efficiency of aerosol drug delivery to the lung and is based on the distribution to the airway and gastrointestinal tract just described. For an aerosol drug (e.g., a bronchodilator or corticosteroid) that targets the respiratory tract, the L/T ratio can be defined as the proportion of drug available from the lung, out of the total systemically available drug.

The *clinical* or *therapeutic effect* of a bronchoactive aerosol comes from the inhaled drug deposited in the airways. The

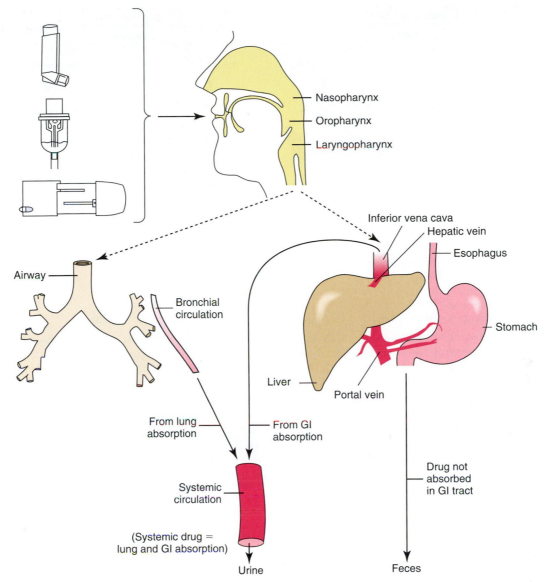

Figure 2-6 Orally inhaled aerosol drugs distribute to the respiratory tract and to the stomach through swallowing of oropharyngeally deposited drug. *Top left:* Inhalation devices include metered dose inhaler *(top)*, nebulizer *(middle)*, and dry powder inhaler *(bottom)*. *GI,* Gastrointestinal.

systemic or *extrapulmonary side effects* come from the total amount of drug absorbed into the system. The total systemic drug level is caused by airway absorption plus the amount absorbed from the gastrointestinal tract. The L/T ratio can quantify and compare the efficiency of drug delivery systems targeting the respiratory tract. Any action that reduces the swallowed portion of the inhaled drug, such as a reservoir device (spacer, holding chamber), or high first-pass metabolism, can increase the L/T ratio. Factors that can increase the L/T ratio are summarized in Box 2-3. A perfectly efficient inhalation device would deliver all of the drug to the lung and none to the oropharynx or gastrointestinal tract, giving a ratio of 1 (lung availability = total systemic availability; all systemic drug comes only from lung absorption).

This concept was proposed in 1991 by Borgström[5] and elaborated on by Thorsson.[6] An example, based on the data of Thorsson for albuterol inhalation using two different

BOX 2-3	Factors Increasing Lung Availability/Total Systemic Availability Ratio With Inhaled Drugs

- Efficient delivery devices (high airway and low gastrointestinal delivery)
- Inhaled drugs with high first-pass metabolism
- Mouthwashing, including rinsing and spitting
- Use of a reservoir device (spacer, holding chamber) to decrease oropharyngeal deposition and swallowed drug amount

delivery devices, is given in Figure 2-7. Using an MDI, approximately 30% of the inhaled drug reaches the lung, with 70% going to the stomach. With complete absorption from the stomach, half of this 70% is broken down in the liver, so that 35% reaches the systemic circulation. The total amount of the original 100% dose reaching the circulation

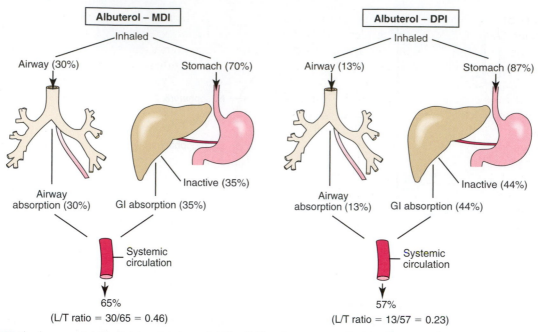

Figure 2-7 The lung availability/total systemic availability *(L/T)* ratio can quantify the efficiency of aerosol drug delivery to the respiratory tract by partitioning relative amounts from the gastrointestinal tract and from the respiratory tract (see text for explanation). *DPI,* Dry powder inhaler; *GI,* gastrointestinal; *MDI,* metered dose inhaler. (Data from Thorsson L: Influence of inhaler systems on systemic availability, with focus on inhaled corticosteroids, *J Aerosol Med* 8[suppl 3]:S29, 1995.)

TABLE 2-6	Lung Availability/Total Systemic Availability Ratios for Several Inhaled Drugs With Various Aerosol Delivery Devices*			
DRUG	**DEVICE**	**LUNG DEPOSITION (%)**	**L/T RATIO**	**SUBJECTS**
Albuterol	pMDI	18.6	0.36	Patients—good coordinators
		7.2	0.17	Patients—poor coordinators
	BAI (pMDI)	20.8	0.41	Patients—poor coordinators
	Turbuhaler	23.2	0.45	Healthy volunteers
Budesonide	pMDI (CFC)	15	0.66	Healthy subjects
	Turbuhaler	32	0.87	Healthy subjects
	MDI (HFA)†	59	0.92	Patients

Data from Borgström L: Local versus total systemic bioavailability as a means to compare different inhaled formulations of the same substance, *J Aerosol Med* 11:55, 1998.

BAI, Breath-actuated inhaler; *CFC,* chlorofluorocarbon; *HFA,* hydrofluoroalkane; *L/T ratio,* lung availability/total systemic availability; *pMDI,* pressurized metered dose inhaler.

*All drug amounts are expressed as percentages of metered or nominal dose.

†Data from Harrison LI: Local versus total systemic bioavailability of beclomethasone dipropionate CFC and HFA metered dose inhaler formulations, *J Aerosol Med* 15:401, 2002 [erratum in *J Aerosal Med* 2003; 16:97].

is 65% (lung, 30%; stomach and liver, 35%). Because 30% of the 65% comes from the lung, this gives an L/T ratio of 30/65 = 0.46.

The data for the DPI, using a Rotahaler (GlaxoSmith-Kline, Research Triangle Park, North Carolina), which is no longer available, gives an L/T ratio of 0.23 (lung, 13%; stomach and liver, 44%). On the basis of these ratios, inhalation of albuterol via an MDI gives more efficient lung delivery with less systemic availability compared with inhalation via a DPI such as the Rotahaler. With the MDI, 46% of the systemic exposure is from the lung, whereas with the DPI, 23% is from the lung. A high L/T ratio is desired;

Table 2-6 gives examples of various L/T ratios, along with lung deposition for several drugs and delivery devices.

The L/T ratio is determined by the rate of first-pass metabolism and the efficiency of the inhalation device in placing the drug in the airway. A high L/T ratio can be achieved even with poor lung delivery and efficient stomach absorption if there is a high first-pass effect on the swallowed drug. Comparisons of L/T ratios must be between the *same* drugs with different delivery devices. Two drugs with different first-pass metabolism rates can have different L/T ratios even if the airway deposition or delivery device is the same. A good example is provided in Table 2-6 by comparing albuterol and budesonide, both administered with a Turbuhaler DPI. Albuterol and budesonide have first-pass metabolism rates of 50% and 90%, respectively. With approximately the same lung delivery of 22% to 23% for both drug-device systems, the L/T ratio is 0.45 for albuterol but 0.87 for budesonide. The improved L/T ratio of budesonide compared with albuterol is not caused by a difference in device efficiency but by the higher rate of metabolism of budesonide that reduces systemic blood levels from gastrointestinal absorption. The L/T ratio also suggests that aerosol delivery devices should be evaluated together with the drug to be used. "Each combination of active drug and device is a unique pharmaceutical formulation, as both the drug itself and the device can influence the overall properties of the formulation."[5] The L/T ratio does not determine whether systemic toxicity or side effects will occur. First, systemic effects depend on the amount of active drug absorbed into the system, whether from the lung or gastrointestinal tract. An inhaled corticosteroid, such as flunisolide, is rapidly metabolized in a first-pass effect. As a result, the swallowed portion gives minimal systemic levels. Good absorption of the aerosol drug from the lungs in sufficiently high doses could cause systemic effects, however. Second, delivery to the oropharynx and gastrointestinal tract by a less efficient aerosol delivery device or method may be irrelevant if the drug is largely inactivated when taken orally and causes no local oropharyngeal effects. Catecholamine bronchodilators would be examples of such a drug. The L/T ratio indicates clearly how close an aerosol drug delivery system comes to the ideal of having all of the systemic drug exposure come from only the lung dose.

PHARMACODYNAMIC PHASE

KEY POINT

Pharmacodynamics describes the mechanism of activity by which drugs cause their effects in the body. The principal concept is the drug target protein (e.g., drug receptor).

The mechanism of drug action by which a drug molecule causes its effect in the body is the pharmacodynamic phase. Most drugs exert their effects by binding to protein targets and subsequently modulating the normal function of these proteins, usually inducing physiologic changes that affect multiple tissues and organ systems. The relevant protein targets include receptors, enzymes, ion channels, and carrier molecules. A **receptor** is any cell component that combines with a drug to change or enhance the function of the cell. In addition, some drugs exert their main therapeutic effect by interacting with DNA rather than by binding directly to proteins. The chemotherapeutic agent cisplatin inhibits cell division by binding to and disrupting cancer cell DNA, and the antiviral drug ganciclovir inhibits herpes virus replication by insinuating itself in the viral DNA and stopping further transcription.

Structure-Activity Relationships

The matching of a drug molecule with a receptor or enzyme in the body is based on a structural similarity between the drug and its binding site. The relationship between the chemical structure of a drug and its clinical effect or activity is termed the **structure-activity relationship (SAR)**. Isoproterenol and albuterol are examples of two aerosol bronchodilators whose differing structures cause different pharmacokinetic activity and tissue responses.

The structures of isoproterenol and albuterol are illustrated in Figure 2-8, with a summary of two critical differences in their pharmacokinetic profile and one critical difference in their side effects (heart rate increase). Although the two structures are very similar, and both are in the same family of β-adrenergic bronchodilators (see Chapter 6 for a discussion of this class of drugs), they are different. Isoproterenol is a catecholamine, which is metabolized rapidly because it is absorbed in the airway by the enzyme catechol O-methyltransferase (COMT), giving it a short duration of action. Albuterol, a saligenin, is not a substrate for the enzyme COMT but is instead metabolized through sulfate conjugation, a slower process. This difference is caused by the substitution of $HOCH_2$ for the OH group at the carbon-3 position. In addition, the structures of the two side chains

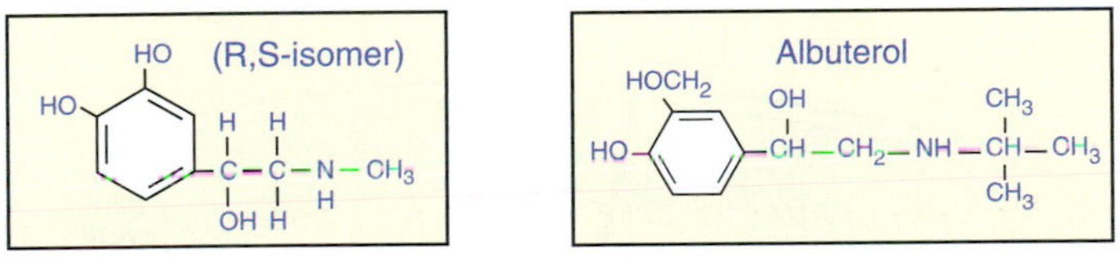

Structure:	Catecholamine	Saligenin (Catecholamine analogue)
Pharmacokinetics:	Peak effect: 20 min Duration: 1.5-2 hr	Peak effect: 30-60 min Duration: 4-6 hr
Side effect:	Increased heart rate	Little/no change in heart rate
Class of drug:	Adrenergic bronchodilator	Adrenergic bronchodilator
Therapeutic effect:	Relax airway, smooth muscle	Relax airway, smooth muscle

Figure 2-8 Structure-activity relationships (SARs) for two drugs representing the same class of bronchodilator. Racemic epinephrine and albuterol are both β-adrenergic agents, with minor structural differences leading to significantly different clinical effects.

are sufficiently different to change their receptor selectivity. Isoproterenol matches to receptors found in the airway (β_2 receptors) and the heart (β_1 receptors), whereas albuterol is more selective for receptors in the airway only. In recommended doses, albuterol has little or no effect on heart rate; however, isoproterenol usually causes an increase in heart rate.

Nature and Type of Drug Receptors

 KEY POINT

Two mechanisms of drug-receptor action form the basis for the effects of two drug classes in respiratory care: intracellular receptor binding and modified gene transcription by lipid-soluble drugs (glucocorticoids) and receptors linked to their effector systems by G proteins (β-adrenergic bronchodilators).

At present, drugs having the greatest relevance to respiratory therapy act through receptor proteins, although enzymes are important targets for some antibiotics, antiviral drugs, and antihypertensive drugs. Receptors for many drugs have been biochemically purified and directly characterized, whereas in the past such receptors were only indirectly inferred from drug action and differences of action between similar drugs.

Drug Receptors

Most drug receptors are proteins, or polypeptides, whose shape and electric charge provide a match to a drug's corresponding chemical shape or charge. Drug-receptor proteins include receptors on cell surfaces and within the cell.

The process by which attachment of a drug to its receptor results in a clinical response involves complex molecular mechanisms. This process sends a signal from the drug chemical into an intracellular sequence that controls cell function. Usually the drug attaches to a receptor protein that spans the cell membrane, and so the process is one of "transmembrane signaling."

Four mechanisms for transmembrane signaling are well understood. Each mechanism can transduce signals for a group of different drug receptors and for different drugs. The four mechanisms are as follows:

1. Lipid-soluble drugs cross the cell membrane and act on intracellular receptors to initiate the drug response. *Examples:* Corticosteroids, vitamin D, thyroid hormone.
2. The drug attaches to the extracellular portion of a protein receptor, which projects into the cell cytoplasm (a "transmembrane protein") and activates an enzyme system, such as tyrosine kinase, in the intracellular portion to initiate an effect. *Examples:* Insulin, platelet-derived growth factor (PDGF).
3. The drug attaches to a surface receptor that regulates the opening of an ion channel. *Examples:* Acetylcholine receptors on skeletal muscle, γ-aminobutyric acid (GABA).

4. The drug attaches to a transmembrane receptor that is coupled to an intracellular enzyme by a G protein (guanine nucleotide–regulating protein). *Examples:* β-adrenergic agents, acetylcholine at parasympathetic nerve endings.

The first, third, and fourth mechanisms are reviewed in more detail in the next paragraphs because these are the basis for the activity of drugs commonly used in respiratory care.

Lipid-Soluble Drugs and Intracellular Receptor Activation

Intracellular receptor activation by lipid-soluble drugs is the basis on which corticosteroids, an important class of drugs in respiratory care, cause a cell response. Examples of corticosteroid drugs are inhaled beclomethasone and flunisolide and oral prednisone. In this drug-receptor mechanism, the drug is sufficiently lipid-soluble to cross the lipid bilayer of the cell membrane, diffuse into the cytoplasm, and attach to an intracellular polypeptide receptor. The drug-receptor complex translocates to the cell nucleus and binds to specific DNA sequences termed *hormone response elements,* which can either stimulate or repress the transcription of genes in the nucleus. An example of such drug-receptor signaling is illustrated in Figure 2-9 for glucocorticoid drugs, such as inhaled flunisolide or oral prednisone. The glucocorticoid diffuses across the cell membrane and attaches to a receptor in the cytoplasm. Attachment of the

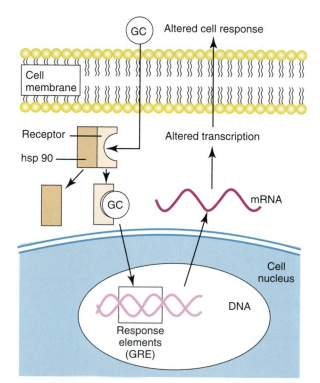

Figure 2-9 Diagram of the mechanism of action for lipid-soluble drugs, such as glucocorticoids, which bind to intracellular receptors and then modify cell nuclear transcription. *GC,* Glucocorticoid; *GRE,* glucocorticoid response element; *hsp 90,* heat shock protein 90.

drug to the receptor causes displacement of certain proteins, termed *heat shock proteins,* and a change in the receptor configuration to an active state. The newly coupled drug-receptor complex moves or *translocates* to the nucleus of the cell, where it pairs with other drug-receptor complexes, which then bind to a glucocorticoid response element (GRE) of the cell's DNA. This binding initiates or represses cell response and transcription of target genes (see Chapter 11 for a discussion of the mechanism and effects of glucocorticoids).

Drugs that act by diffusing into the cell and regulating gene responses have longer periods for observed responses, ranging from 30 minutes to several hours. Typically, there is also a persistence of effect for hours or days, even after the drug has been eliminated from the body.

Drug-Regulated Ion Channels

Another process of drug signal transduction regulates the flow of ions, such as sodium or potassium, through cell membrane channels. This can be seen in Figure 2-10. The drug binds to a receptor on the cell membrane surface. The receptor has a portion above or on the surface of the cell membrane and extends through the membrane into the cytoplasm of the cell. When activated by the drug (or by an endogenous ligand), the receptor opens an ion channel to allow increased transmembrane conductance of an ion.

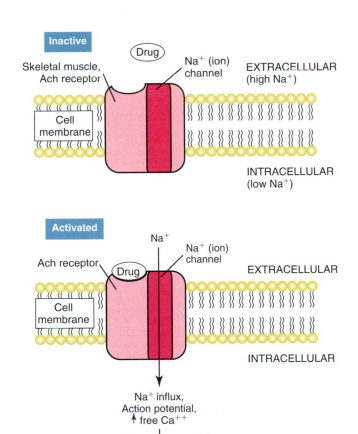

Figure 2-10 Illustration of the drug signal mechanism that regulates ion channel flow to cause a drug response, such as that of acetylcholine (*Ach*) or nicotine in stimulating skeletal muscle fibers to contract.

An example of such a receptor is that for acetylcholine, a neurotransmitter, on skeletal muscle. This acetylcholine receptor is termed a *nicotinic receptor* because it responds to the substance nicotine as well as acetylcholine. Attachment of acetylcholine or nicotine opens an ion channel and allows the high sodium (Na^+) concentration in extracellular fluid to flow into the lower concentration of the cell. This produces a reversal of voltage, or *depolarization,* and a corresponding muscle twitch. Acetylcholine is the neurotransmitter for voluntary muscle contraction and movement, and stimulation by nicotine can increase skeletal muscle tremor.

Receptors Linked to G Proteins

G protein–linked receptors mediate bronchodilation and bronchoconstriction in the airways in response to endogenous stimulation by the neurotransmitters epinephrine and acetylcholine. These same airway responses can be elicited by adrenergic bronchodilator drugs (discussed in Chapter 6) or blocked by acetylcholine-blocking (anticholinergic) agents, such as ipratropium bromide (discussed in Chapter 7). G proteins and G protein–linked receptors also mediate the effects of other chemicals, including the effects of histamine and glucagon, and the phototransduction of light in retinal rods and cones. Drug-receptor signaling with G protein–linked receptors involves three main components: the *drug receptor, G protein,* and *effector system.* When a drug attaches to a G protein–linked receptor, these three components interact to cause a cellular response to the drug. The effector system triggers the cell response by activating or inhibiting a *second messenger* within the cell. Figure 2-11 shows the main elements of a G protein–linked receptor. Each of the major elements in this signaling mechanism complex is described briefly, along with the dynamics of their interaction.

Receptors that couple with G proteins have been well characterized and show a similar structure in which a polypeptide chain crosses the cell membrane seven times, giving a serpentine appearance to the receptor. The polypeptide chain has an amino (NH_2, or N) terminal site outside the cell membrane and a carboxyl (COOH, or C) terminus inside the cell. Although the seven transmembrane segments of the receptor are illustrated in Figure 2-12 as side by side, the receptor appears to form a cylindrical structure if viewed perpendicular to the surface of the cell membrane, with the transmembrane loops forming the sides of the cylinder. The drug usually couples to the receptor at a site surrounded by the transmembrane regions of the receptor protein; that is, within the interior of the cylinder. The receptor activates a G protein on the cytoplasmic (inner) surface of the cell membrane. The site of the interaction of the G protein with the receptor polypeptide is thought to be at the third cytoplasmic loop of the receptor chain.

G proteins are so termed because they are a family of guanine nucleotide–binding proteins with a three-part, or *heterotrimeric,* structure. The three subunits of the G protein are designated by the Greek letters alpha (α), beta (β), and gamma (γ). The α subunit differentiates members of the G

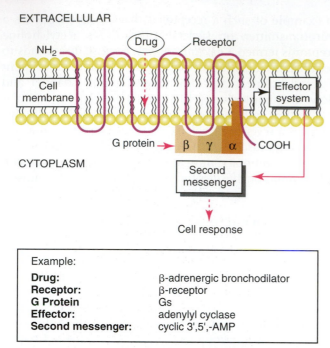

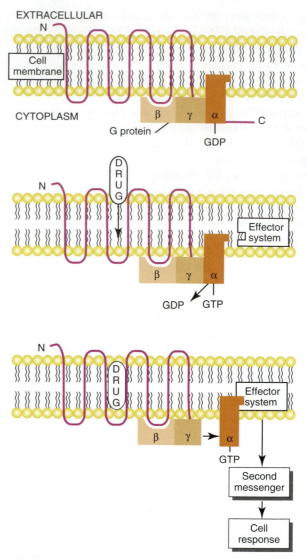

Figure 2-11 Simplified diagram of the components by which a G protein–linked receptor causes a cell response: drug, receptor, G protein, effector system, and second messenger. Each of these components is identified in this example of a β-adrenergic bronchodilator drug and the β receptor, which is a G protein–linked receptor. *Gs,* Stimulatory G protein.

Figure 2-12 Sequential diagram of G protein–linked receptor activation and G protein function in linking a drug signal to a cell response.

protein family. On the basis of the α subunit, the G protein is classified into subgroups, such as Gs, which *stimulates* an effector system, and Gi, which *inhibits* the effector system. Other types of G proteins have been identified as well; they are not reviewed in this chapter.

The activated G protein changes the activity of an *effector system,* which may be either an enzyme, which catalyzes the formation of a *second messenger,* or an ion channel, which allows the outflow of K^+ ions from the cell. One of the second messengers is the well-known cyclic adenosine 3′,5′-monophosphate (cAMP). The effector enzyme for increasing cAMP is adenylyl cyclase (previously termed adenyl cyclase), which converts adenosine triphosphate (ATP) to cAMP. The G protein that stimulates adenylyl cyclase is the Gs (for *stimulatory*) protein. β receptors, which couple with β-adrenergic bronchodilators, activate Gs proteins. Another G protein, Gi (for *inhibitory*), inhibits the activation of adenylyl cyclase; Gi proteins are activated by cholinergic (muscarinic) agonists such as acetylcholine or the drug methacholine.

The dynamics of cell signaling by G protein–linked receptors are illustrated schematically in Figure 2-12. When there is no drug attached to the receptor site, the α subunit of the G protein is bound to guanosine diphosphate (GDP), and the G protein is in an inactive state. When a drug attaches to the receptor, there is a change in the receptor conformation that causes the release of GDP and the binding of guanosine triphosphate (GTP) to the α subunit. This is the active state for the G protein. The GTP-bound α subunit dissociates, or *unlinks,* from the β-γ portion and

couples with the effector system to stimulate or inhibit a second messenger within the cell. The GTP bound to the α subunit is hydrolyzed by a GTPase enzyme, dissociates from the effector, and reassociates with the β-γ dimer. The G protein–linked receptor is then ready for reactivation.

Details on specific G proteins, their effector systems, and their second messengers are presented for neurotransmitters such as epinephrine and acetylcholine in the nervous system (see Chapter 5) and for the classes of drugs that link to such receptors, such as adrenergic bronchodilators (see Chapter 6) and anticholinergic bronchodilators (see Chapter 7).

Dose-Response Relationships

 KEY POINT

Various terms describe the dose-response relationship of drugs, while they combine with their corresponding receptors, and drug interactions: potency; maximal effect; therapeutic index (TI); agonists and antagonists; synergism; additivity; potentiation; and reaction types such as idiosyncratic, hypersensitivity, tolerance, and tachyphylaxis.

The response to a drug is proportional to the drug concentration. As drug concentration increases, the number of receptors occupied increases, and the drug effect also increases up to a maximal point; this is graphed as a dose-response, or concentration-effect, curve (Figure 2-13). Increasing amounts of a drug increase the response in a fairly direct fashion; however, the rate of response usually diminishes as the dose increases, until a plateau of maximal effect is reached. Such a convex, or *hyperbolic*, curve is normally transformed mathematically by using the logarithm of the dose so that a sigmoid curve is obtained. The linear midportion of a sigmoid curve allows easier comparison of the dose-response curve for different drugs. In particular, the dose at which 50% of the response to the drug occurs is indicated in Figure 2-13 and is referred to as the ED_{50},

the dose of drug that produces 50% of the maximal effect. This value may also be denoted as the EC_{50}, for effective concentration giving 50% of maximal response.

Potency versus Maximal Effect

Dose-response curves are the basis for defining and illustrating several concepts used to characterize and compare drugs. Two concepts that allow comparison of drugs are potency and maximal effect, both illustrated in Figure 2-14.

1. *Potency:* Refers to the concentration (EC_{50}) or dose (ED_{50}) of a drug producing 50% of the *maximal response* of the drug. The potency of two drugs, A and B, can be compared on the basis of the ED_{50} values of the two drugs: relative potency, A and B = ED_{50} (B)/ED_{50} (A).
2. *Maximal effect:* The greatest response that can be produced by a drug, a dose above which no further response can be elicited.

The lower the ED_{50} for a given drug, the more potent the drug is, as seen in Figure 2-14. Curves for drugs A and B show different potencies. If the ED_{50} for drug B is 5 mg and

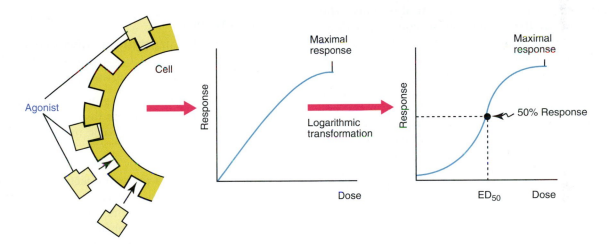

Figure 2-13 Illustration of the dose-response curve *(left)*, showing an increasing effect that ultimately plateaus, and its logarithmic transformation to produce a sigmoid curve *(right)*. ED_{50}, Drug dose that produces 50% of the maximal effect.

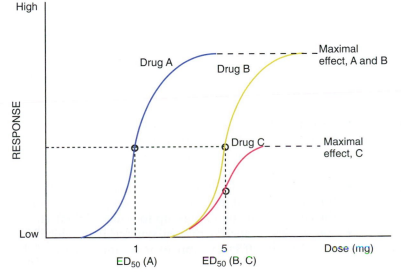

Figure 2-14 The potency of a drug is defined as the dose producing 50% of the drug's maximal effect. Drug *A* is more potent than drug *B*; however, drugs *B* and *C* are equally potent, although drug *C* has less maximal effect than drug *B*.

for drug *A* is 1 mg, then drug *A* is five times more potent than drug *B*:

$$ED_{50}(B)/ED_{50}(A) = 5 \text{ mg}/1 \text{ mg} = 5$$

Drug *B* requires five times the amount of drug *A* to produce 50% of its maximal effect. Potency is not the same as maximal effect, also illustrated in Figure 2-14. Potency is relatively defined using the ED_{50} values of two drugs, whereas maximal effect is absolutely defined as a physiologic or clinical response. The curves indicate that drugs *B* and *C* have the same potency; that is, the same dose produces 50% of the maximal response. However, drug *B* has a greater maximal effect than drug *C*. Because the ED_{50} is the dose causing a response that is half the maximal response of the *same* drug, two drugs can have different maximal responses but the same ED_{50} (and the same potency), as seen in Figure 2-14.

Therapeutic Index

The **therapeutic index (TI)** can be defined as the ratio of the lethal dose for 50% of the test population (LD_{50}) to the ED_{50} for a given drug, with ED_{50} and LD_{50} indicating half of the test subjects rather than a 50% clinical response. The TI is also based on the dose-response curve of a drug. However, instead of a graded clinical or physiologic response, such as an increase in heart rate, we substitute an all-or-nothing response of improvement for each subject, or toxicity or death for each subject. In this case the ED_{50} represents the dose of the drug at which half of the test subjects improve. Similarly, the LD_{50} is the lethal dose for 50% of the test population. Doses are established for a test population of animals (as illustrated in Figure 2-15).

The ratio of the dose that is toxic to 50% of test subjects to the dose that provides relief to 50% of the subjects is the clinical TI. This index represents the safety margin of the

drug. The smaller the TI, the greater is the possibility of crossing from a therapeutic effect to a toxic effect. Theophylline is a drug used in respiratory care that has a narrow therapeutic margin. As a result, toxic side effects can be seen at close to therapeutic dose levels in some individuals.

Agonists and Antagonists

An **agonist** is a drug or chemical that binds to a corresponding receptor (has affinity) and *initiates* a cellular effect or response (has efficacy). An **antagonist** is a drug or chemical that is able to bind to a receptor (has affinity) but causes no response (zero efficacy). Because the antagonist drug is occupying the receptor site, it can prevent other drugs or an endogenous chemical from reaching and activating the receptor site. By doing so, an antagonist *inhibits* or *blocks* the agonist at the receptor. Agonists are divided further into *full* and *partial agonists*. A full agonist is a drug that gives a higher maximal response than a partial agonist. The dose-response curves for a partial agonist and a full agonist are represented in Figure 2-16. Both have receptor affinity, but a partial agonist has less efficacy than a full agonist.

Drug Interactions

The concept of drug antagonism just discussed is an example of a drug interaction in which one drug can block the effect of another. Mechanisms of drug antagonism are as follows:

- *Chemical antagonism:* Direct chemical interaction between a drug and biologic mediator that inactivates the drug. An example is chelation of toxic metals by a chelating agent.
- *Functional antagonism:* Can occur when two drugs each produce an effect and the two effects cancel each other. For example, methacholine can stimulate parasympathetic (muscarinic) receptors in the airways, causing bronchoconstriction; epinephrine can stimulate β_2 receptors in the airways, causing bronchodilation.
- *Competitive antagonism:* Occurs when a drug has affinity for a receptor but no efficacy and at the same time blocks the active agonist from binding to and stimulating the receptor. For example, fexofenadine is a competitive antagonist to histamine on specific receptors (H_1) on bronchial smooth muscle and the nasopharynx and is used to treat allergies to pollens.

The following terms are used to describe positive interactions between two drugs:

- *Synergism:* Occurs when two drugs act on a target organ by different mechanisms of action, and the effect of the drug pair is greater than the sum of the separate effects of the drugs.
- *Additivity:* Occurs when two drugs act on the same receptors, and the combined effect is the simple linear sum of the effects of the two drugs, up to a maximal effect.
- *Potentiation:* A special case of synergism in which one drug has no effect but can increase the activity of the other drug.

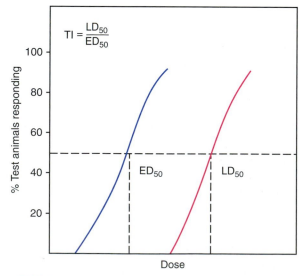

Figure 2-15 Therapeutic index *(TI)*, defined as the ratio of the dose that is lethal for 50% of test animals *(LD$_{50}$)* to the dose causing improvement in 50% of test animals *(ED$_{50}$)*.

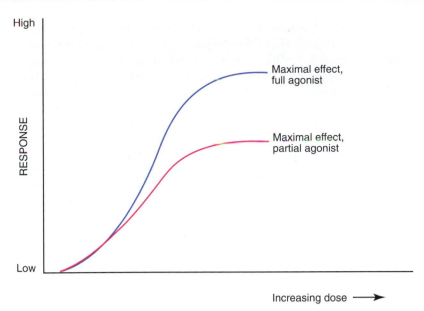

Figure 2-16 Dose-response curves for full and partial agonists, illustrating the greater maximal effect of the full agonist.

Terms for Drug Responsiveness

Individuals exhibit variation in their responses to drugs; the dose-response curves previously illustrated represent an average of an entire group. The following terms are encountered in pharmacology to describe individual reactions to drugs:

- *Idiosyncratic effect*: Effect that is the opposite of, or unusual, or an absence of effect, compared with the predicted usual effect in an individual.
- *Hypersensitivity*: Allergic or immune-mediated reaction to a drug, which can be serious, requiring airway maintenance or ventilatory assistance.
- *Tolerance*: Decreasing intensity of response to a drug over time.
- *Tachyphylaxis*: Rapid decrease in responsiveness to a drug.

PHARMACOGENETICS

KEY POINT

Pharmacogenetics refers to hereditary differences in the way the body handles specific drugs.

The well-described variations among patients in responses to drugs are being increasingly traced to hereditary differences. The study of these hereditary or genetic differences is referred to as **pharmacogenetics**. These genetic variations may not be manifested as an "abnormality" until the patient is challenged with a drug, at which time the irregularity in the pharmacokinetic or pharmacodynamic response is revealed. Genetic differences affecting drug metabolism have been most extensively studied, although variation in target proteins may be equally important.

Several examples can be given from drugs commonly seen in respiratory and critical care:

- *Isoniazid*: Antituberculosis drug that varies in its rate of metabolism and inactivation among individuals, with rapid and slow inactivators seen. The proportion of rapid versus slow inactivators is about 50/50 among white and black individuals, but Inuit and some Asian people tend to be rapid inactivators.
- *Succinylcholine*: Neuromuscular paralyzing agent used during surgery. Succinylcholine is normally metabolized by a butyrylcholinesterase enzyme (pseudocholinesterase). Approximately 1 in 3000 individuals has a genetically determined variant of this enzyme. As a result, a patient may take several hours to recover from the drug rather than the several minutes usually seen, and may also begin to breathe spontaneously. Mechanical ventilatory support would be required until spontaneous breathing is adequate.
- *Isoflurane*: Inhalation anesthetic that (similar to several other related anesthetics) can cause malignant hyperthermia in genetically susceptible individuals. Patients with an atypical variant of a calcium release channel can die as a result of this serious complication of general anesthesia, which involves a rapid increase in body temperature and increased oxygen consumption.

SELF-ASSESSMENT QUESTIONS

Answers can be found in Appendix A.
1. If a drug is in liquid solution, what routes of administration are available for its delivery, considering only its dosage form?
2. Although generic drug equivalents all have the same amount of active drug, do formulations of the same drug from different manufacturers all have the same ingredients?
3. If 200 mg of a drug results in a plasma concentration of 10 mg/L, what is the calculated volume of distribution (V_D)?

Continued

4. If the V_D of a drug such as phenobarbital is 38 L/70 kg, and an effective concentration is 10 mg/L, what loading dose would be needed for an average adult (assuming total bioavailability)?

5. If an inhaled aerosol has zero gastrointestinal absorption of an active drug and only lung absorption, what is the L/T ratio?

6. True or False: A patient uses a reservoir device with an inhaled aerosol, and there is no swallowed portion of the drug; therefore, there are no systemic side effects.

7. Which receptor system signal mechanism is responsible for the effects caused by β-receptor activation, such as those seen with adrenergic bronchodilators (e.g., albuterol)?

 ## CLINICAL SCENARIO

Answers can be found in Appendix A.

A resident orders racemic epinephrine, a bronchodilator, to be given qid to a 67-year-old man. The patient has had chronic obstructive pulmonary disease (COPD) for the past 10 years and was admitted to the hospital the previous evening with a respiratory infection. At 8:00 AM, you administer the prescribed usual recommended dose of aerosol treatment by nebulizer. After the treatment, the patient's respiratory rate is reduced from 26 breaths/min to 18 breaths/min, and there is less use of accessory muscles. Wheezing on auscultation is also decreased, although you hear adequate breath sounds bilaterally. He seems less short of breath. At 10:00 AM,

he is exhibiting moderate respiratory distress, using accessory muscles, complaining of dyspnea, and having increased wheezing on auscultation. His next aerosol treatment is due at noon. He admits to no chest pain; wheezes and breath sounds can be auscultated over the entire thorax. You review the pharmacokinetics of racemic epinephrine and find the following:

- Onset: 3 to 5 minutes
- Peak effect: Approximately 15 minutes
- Duration: Approximately 2 hours or less

Using the SOAP method, assess this clinical scenario.

REFERENCES

1. Holford N: Pharmacokinetics and pharmacodynamics: Rational dosing and the time course of drug action. In Katzung BG, Masters SB, Trevor AJ, editors: *Basic and clinical pharmacology*, ed 11, New York, 2009, McGraw Hill Medical.

2. Heinemann L, Pfutzner A, Heise T: Alternative routes of administration as an approach to improve insulin therapy: update on dermal, oral, nasal and pulmonary insulin delivery. *Curr Pharm Des* 7:1327, 2001.

3. Newman SP, Pavia D, Moren F, et al: Deposition of pressurized aerosols in the human respiratory tract. *Thorax* 36:52, 1981.

4. Thorsson L, Edsbäcker S, Conradson TB: Lung deposition of budesonide from Turbuhaler is twice that from a pressurised metered-dose inhaler P-MDI. *Eur Respir J* 7:1839, 1994.

5. Borgström L: A possible new approach of comparing different inhalers and inhaled substances. *J Aerosol Med* 4:A13, 1991. (abstract).

6. Thorsson L: Influence of inhaler systems on systemic availability, with focus on inhaled corticosteroids. *J Aerosol Med* 8(Suppl 3):S29, 1995.

CHAPTER 3

Administration of Aerosolized Agents

Douglas S. Gardenhire

CHAPTER OUTLINE

OBJECTIVES

After reading this chapter, the reader will be able to:

1. Define terms that pertain to administration of aerosol agents
2. Define *aerosol therapy*
3. Select an appropriate aerosol medication nebulizer on the basis of particle size distributions
4. Discuss aerosol particle size and deposition in the lungs
5. Differentiate between the types of aerosol devices
6. Describe the clinical applications of aerosol devices
7. Recommend the use of various aerosol devices

KEY TERMS AND DEFINITIONS

Aerodynamic diameter of a particle Diameter of a unit-density (1 g/cc) spherical particle having the same terminal settling velocity as the measured particle.

Aerosol Suspension of liquid or solid particles 0.001 to 100 micrometers (µm) in diameter in a carrier gas.

Aerosol therapy Delivery of aerosol particles to the lungs.

Cascade impactor Device that uses multiple steps in determining size of aerosol particles.

Chlorofluorocarbon (CFC) Liquefied gas (e.g., Freon) propellant used to administer medication from a metered dose inhaler (MDI).

Dead volume Amount of solution that remains in the reservoir of a small volume nebulizer once sputtering begins, causing a decrease in aerosolization.

Deposition Process of particles depositing out of suspension to remain in the lung.

Heterodisperse In reference to the size of particles in an aerosol, meaning the particles are of different sizes.

Hydrofluoroalkane (HFA) Nontoxic liquefied gas propellant used to administer medication from an MDI.

In vitro Mechanically simulating the clinical setting; testing in a laboratory.

In vivo Testing done on animals or humans; clinical testing.

Monodisperse In reference to the size of particles in an aerosol, meaning all particles are the same size.

Nebulizer Device used for making a fine spray or mist, also known as an aerosol generator.

Penetration Refers to the depth within the lung reached by particles.

Polydisperse In reference to the size of particles in an aerosol, meaning many different particle sizes.

Continued

KEY TERMS AND DEFINITIONS—cont'd

Reservoir device Global term describing or referring to extension, auxiliary, or add-on devices attached to MDIs for administration. This term can include "spacer" and "valved holding chamber" (defined subsequently).

Spacer Simple tube or extension device with no one-way valves to contain the aerosol cloud; its purpose is simply to extend the MDI spray away from the mouth.

Stability Describing the tendency of aerosol particles to remain in suspension.

Valved holding chamber Spacer device with the addition of a one-way valve to contain and hold the aerosol cloud until inspiration occurs.

Aerosol therapy refers to the delivery of aerosol particles to the respiratory tract. At the present time, there are three main uses of aerosol therapy in respiratory care:

1. Humidification of dry inspired gases using bland aerosols
2. Improved mobilization and clearance of respiratory secretions, including sputum induction, using bland aerosols of water and hypertonic or hypotonic saline
3. Delivery of aerosolized drugs to the respiratory tract

Chapter 3 presents information for delivery of aerosolized drugs to the respiratory tract. As outlined in Chapter 2, the first prerequisite for a drug to exert a therapeutic effect at the target organ is an effective dosage form and route of administration for the target organ. Aerosol generation and delivery to the lung is a complex topic. Development of both the technology and the scientific basis of inhaled aerosol administration are ongoing. This chapter reviews physical principles of aerosol delivery to the airways and aerosol-generating devices for inhalation of drugs. Research findings on aerosol delivery devices and methods of administration are summarized. The general advantages supporting the use of aerosolized drug therapy in respiratory care and the disadvantages with this method of drug delivery are summarized in Box 3-1.

PHYSICAL PRINCIPLES OF INHALED AEROSOL DRUGS

 KEY POINT

An *aerosol* is a suspension of solid or liquid particles whose *deposition* in the respiratory tract is determined by *inertial impaction, gravitational settling (sedimentation),* and, perhaps less importantly, *diffusion (brownian motion)*.

The term *aerosol* has been used since the beginning of the twentieth century; however, inhaled agents used for medicinal purposes date back 4000 years ago.[1] The following definitions apply to inhaled therapeutic aerosols:

Aerosol: Suspension of liquid or solid particles between 0.001 and 100 micrometers (μm) in diameter in a carrier gas.[2] For pulmonary diagnostic and therapeutic applications, the particle size range of interest is 1 to 10 μm. Particles in this size range are small enough to exist as a suspension and to enter the lung and large enough to deposit and contain the required amount of an agent.[3,4]

BOX 3-1   Advantages and Disadvantages Seen With Aerosol Delivery of Drugs

Advantages
- Aerosol doses are smaller than doses for systemic treatment
- Onset of drug action is rapid
- Drug delivery is targeted to the respiratory system for local pulmonary effect
- Systemic side effects are fewer and less severe than with oral or parenteral therapy
- Inhaled drug therapy is painless and relatively convenient
- The lung provides a portal to the body for inhaled aerosol agents intended for systemic effect (e.g., pain control, insulin)

Disadvantages
- Numerous variables affect dose of aerosol drug delivered to airways
- Dose estimation and dose reproducibility are inconsistent
- Many patients have difficulty in coordinating hand action and breathing with metered dose inhalers (MDIs)
- Many physicians, nurses, and therapists lack knowledge of device use and administration protocols
- Standardized technical information on aerosol-producing devices is lacking for practitioners and patients
- Numerous device types and variability of use are confusing to patients and practitioners

---

Stability: Describing the tendency of aerosol particles to remain in suspension.

Penetration: Referring to the depth within the lung reached by particles.

Deposition: Describing the process by which particles deposit out of suspension to remain in the lung.

Aerosol-generating devices for orally inhaled drugs have typically had an efficiency of 10% to 15%; that is, only 10% to 15% of a given dose from a device usually reaches the lower respiratory tract, regardless of the device type. Newer aerosol-generating devices are proving to be exceptions to this lack of efficiency, with 30% to 50% or more of the dose reaching the lungs.

Aerosol Particle Size Distributions

 KEY POINT

A major factor in lung penetration by aerosols is particle size, which is best characterized by the *mass median aerodynamic diameter (MMAD)* for inhaled drugs because particle mass is a function of the third power of the particle radius. The particle size of interest for pulmonary applications is in the range of 1 to 10 μm, and the fine particle fraction (FPF) is considered to include particles less than 5 μm in size.

Aerosol particles produced for inhalation into the lungs via inhalant devices such as metered dose inhalers (MDIs), small volume nebulizers (SVNs), and dry powder inhalers (DPIs) include a range of sizes (**polydisperse** or **heterodisperse**) rather than a single size (**monodisperse**).

Count mode: Most frequently occurring particle size in the distribution.

Count median diameter (CMD): Particle size above and below which 50% of the particles are found (i.e., the size that evenly divides the number of particles in the distribution).

Mass median diameter (MMD) or mass median aerodynamic diameter (MMAD): Particle size above and below which 50% of the mass of the particles are found (i.e., the size that evenly divides the mass of the particles in the distribution).

Geometric standard deviation (GSD): Measure of the dispersion of a distribution (i.e., the scattering of values from the average), calculated as the ratio of particle size below which 84% of the particles occur to the particle size below which 50% occur, in a log-normal distribution. This ratio determines how spread out the particles are in relationship to their size.

MMD or MMAD indicates where the mass of drug is centered in a distribution of particle sizes. Aerosol particles are three-dimensional and have volume. Aerosol particles are assumed to be roughly spherical, and the relationship of volume (or mass, if all particles have equal densities) to diameter in a sphere is given by the following formula:

$$V = (\tfrac{4}{3})\pi r^3$$

V = volume; r = radius

The volume increases or decreases as the third power of the radius of the particle, as seen in the preceding formula. As a result, the bulk of drug mass is centered in the larger particle sizes. Because it is the mass of the drug entering the lung on which the therapeutic effect is based, it is necessary to know where the mass is centered in a range of particle sizes to know whether that distribution will be efficient for penetration into the respiratory tract and delivery of an adequate dose.

EXAMPLE

Two hypothetical SVNs, *A* and *B*, have the following specifications from the manufacturer:

A	*B*
CMD = 1.9 μm	*CMD = 1.7 μm*
MMAD = 3.4 μm	*MMAD = 7.9 μm*
GSD = 1.2	*GSD = 1.6*

Although nebulizer *B* has a smaller CMD compared with nebulizer *A*, which appears to indicate that it gives smaller particles, it is evident from the respective MMADs that nebulizer *B* has more particles in a larger size range (≥5 μm) compared with nebulizer *A*. Nebulizer *A* produces particles whose mass centers within a lower size range (1-5 μm) and would be the better nebulizer for treatment of the lower respiratory tract.

Inspect aerosol products for their MMAD because this is the best way to determine whether the nebulizer would be better suited for the upper or lower airway.

Aerosol generators should be characterized using the MMD for the center of distribution and either the standard deviation or GSD to indicate the range of variability of particle size.

Measurement of Particle Size Distributions

Several physical methods are used to measure aerosol particle size distributions, including *cascade impaction* and, less commonly, *laser scattering*. The **cascade impactor** measures what is termed the *aerodynamic diameter of aerosols* because the measurement is based on the aerodynamic behavior (sedimentation velocity and impaction characteristics) of the particles in the cascade impactor. Measuring particle size with the *laser-scattering method*, the instrument determines the relationship between the intensity and the angle of light scattered from a particle, then calculates the particle size based on the Mie-scattering theory. The **aerodynamic diameter of a particle** is the diameter of a unit-density (1 g/cc) spherical particle having the same terminal settling velocity as the measured particle.[4,5]

The principle by which a cascade impactor measures the particle size distribution of an aerosol cloud is illustrated in a simplified diagram in Figure 3-1. The *cascade impactor* consists of a series of stages, each of which has progressively smaller orifices through which the aerosol particles must pass. A constant flow draws the particles through the stages. The largest particles are collected on the first stage, and particles not impacting out at this stage move on to the subsequent stages with smaller orifices in the airstream. By means of successively smaller filtration stages, the particles are separated, or *fractionated*, on the basis of size. Any particles leaving the last stage are collected on a final filter.

The amount of aerosol on each stage is measured by weight or, preferably, by spectrophotometry or high-performance liquid chromatography (HPLC). HPLC is considered the most sensitive technique for quantifying the amount of aerosol on each stage. Because each stage is calibrated for a unit-density sphere of specific diameter, the distribution of aerodynamic diameters can be calculated as the percentage of a drug on each stage. The MMAD can be determined as the particle size dividing the drug in half. Sources of error in aerodynamic measures include particle bounce, interstage impaction, possible fragmentation of particles, and particle evaporation or condensation.[5] In addition, **in vitro** methods (mechanically simulating the

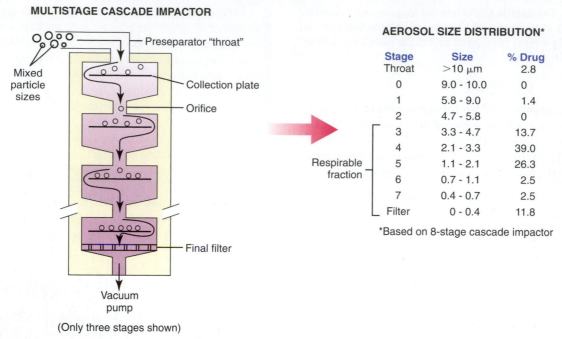

MULTISTAGE CASCADE IMPACTOR

Preseparator "throat"

Mixed particle sizes

Collection plate

Orifice

Final filter

Vacuum pump

(Only three stages shown)

AEROSOL SIZE DISTRIBUTION*

Stage	Size	% Drug
Throat	>10 μm	2.8
0	9.0 - 10.0	0
1	5.8 - 9.0	1.4
2	4.7 - 5.8	0
3	3.3 - 4.7	13.7
4	2.1 - 3.3	39.0
5	1.1 - 2.1	26.3
6	0.7 - 1.1	2.5
7	0.4 - 0.7	2.5
Filter	0 - 0.4	11.8

Respirable fraction (stages 3-7)

*Based on 8-stage cascade impactor

Figure 3-1 The principle of aerodynamic particle size measurement, using multistage cascade impaction. A series of successively smaller orifices and collection plates separate large and smaller particle sizes. Drug amounts *(% Drug)* shown are actual measures of particle sizes for a sample of albuterol (Ventolin) through a Volumatic reservoir. (Data courtesy J.P. Mitchell, Trudell Medical International Aerosol Laboratory, London, Ontario, Canada.)

clinical setting within a laboratory) of aerosol measurement may not reflect conditions in the human lung, such as temperature, humidity, inspiratory flow rates, and exhalation phase. Dolovich[6] reviewed in vitro measures used with MDI and auxiliary devices. Feddah and associates[7] found that MDI formulations did better in vitro than DPI formulations with respect to inhaled doses. The same method of aerosol characterization is not useful or accurate for different methods of aerosol production because of differences in the physical nature of their generation. To determine aerosol particle behavior in animals or humans, **in vivo** methods would be studied.

Particle Size and Lung Deposition

A major factor influencing aerosol deposition in the lung is particle size. The effect of particle size on deposition in the respiratory tract is illustrated in Figure 3-2.

The upper airway (nose and mouth) is efficient in filtering particulate matter, so that generally there is 100% deposition in the nose and mouth of particles larger than 10 μm to 15 μm. Particles sized from 5 to 10 μm tend to deposit out in the upper airways and the early airway generations, whereas particles from 1 to 5 μm in size have a greater probability of reaching the lower respiratory tract (from the trachea to the lung periphery). Larger or coarser aerosol particles (larger than 5 μm in diameter) may be useful for treating the upper airway (nasopharynx and oropharynx). It is impossible to specify exactly where a given size of particle will deposit in the lung. Particle deposition is a function of several mechanisms, including the breathing pattern.

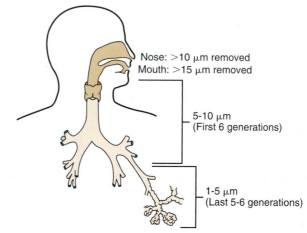

Nose: >10 μm removed
Mouth: >15 μm removed

5-10 μm (First 6 generations)

1-5 μm (Last 5-6 generations)

Figure 3-2 Effect of aerosol particle size on area of preferential deposition within the airway.

For example, tables are often created listing the percentage of droplets of a given size that will deposit in the lung at each bronchial level.[8] Yu and colleagues[9] observed that optimal deposition in the normal human lung is achieved for particles of 3 μm inhaled with low inspiratory flows of less than 1 L/sec (less than 60 L/min) and tidal volumes of 1 L; total lung deposition is divided almost equally throughout the 23 lung generations.

Fine Particle Fraction

The labels *respirable fraction* and *respirable dose* previously were used to refer to the percentage or fraction of aerosol drug mass in a particle size range with a high probability of penetrating into the lower respiratory tract. These generally have been considered to be in the particle size range of less than 5 to 6 µm. There is rarely an absolute correspondence of lower respiratory tract deposition to this particle size range because of age, disease, and breathing patterns, all of which can affect lung deposition. The more descriptive terms *fine particle fraction (FPF)* and *fine particle dose (FPD)* were proposed for use in place of respirable fraction and respirable dose.[10] Agreement was not reached on what size fraction represents the FPF. These terms may be restricted to particles 1 to 3 µm, rather than particles less than 5 to 6 µm.

Particle Size and Therapeutic Effect

Because the respiratory tract apparently functions as a progressive filter of successively smaller particles from the upper airway to the periphery, specific areas of the respiratory tract may be targeted by various aerosol particle sizes. On the basis of the preceding considerations, the respiratory tract might be segmented according to the following particle size ranges.

Particles greater than 10 µm. Particles that are greater than 10 µm are useful to treat the nasopharyngeal and oropharyngeal regions. An example is a nasal spray for perennial rhinitis, such as a corticosteroid.

Particles 5 to 10 µm. Particles 5 to 10 µm may shift deposition to the more central airways, although significant oropharyngeal deposition is expected. An example is a nasal spray, but there is no one standard device that creates this specific particle size. Most aerosol devices use a smaller particle size, which is discussed subsequently.

Particles 2 to 5 µm. As particle size decreases to less than 5 µm, deposition shifts from the oropharynx and large airways to the overall lower respiratory tract (large airways to periphery).[11] This size range is considered useful for the bronchoactive aerosols currently in use. For example, β-adrenergic receptors have been identified throughout the airway, but with greater density in bronchioles. Clay and colleagues[12] showed greater improvement in mid-maximal expiratory flow rates among subjects using a β-adrenergic bronchodilator with an MMAD of 1.8 µm than with an MMAD of 4.6 or 10.3 µm. This finding was confirmed subsequently by Johnson and associates,[13] who found a greater response to the β-adrenergic bronchodilator albuterol (see Chapter 6) with an MMD of 3.3 µm compared with 7.7 µm. Leach[14] found similar results with a **chlorofluorocarbon (CFC)**-MDI of albuterol, where particles averaged 3.5 to 4.0 µm; however, when testing a **hydrofluoroalkane (HFA)**-MDI, particle size decreased to an average of 1.1 µm. In contrast, cholinergic receptors are numerous in proximal bronchial smooth muscle but rare in distal bronchioles.[15]

Particles 0.8 to 3.0 µm. Increased delivery of an aerosol to the lung parenchyma, including the terminal airways and alveolar region, can be achieved with particles less than 3 µm.[11] An MMAD of 1 to 2 µm is suggested for peripheral deposition of the antiinfective drug pentamidine to minimize deposition in and irritation of larger airways and to maximize intraalveolar deposition.[16] However, with the introduction of HFA-MDIs, a finer particle size is seen.[14]

Mechanisms of Deposition

Three physical mechanisms usually are considered for aerosol particle deposition in the human lung:

1. Inertial impaction
2. Gravitational settling (sedimentation)
3. Diffusion (brownian motion).

Inertial impaction. As shown in Figure 3-3, *inertial impaction* is a function of particle size (mass) and velocity and increases with larger size and higher velocities. In the upper airway and early bronchial generations, particle velocity is highest, airflow tends to be turbulent, and total cross-sectional area of the airway is smallest. These factors favor inertial impaction for larger, fast-moving particles on the airway wall, especially at airway bifurcations. Deposition by inertial impaction is expected to occur in the first 10 airway generations.[4]

Gravitational settling. *Gravitational settling*, or *sedimentation*, is a function of particle size and time. Settling is greater for larger particles with slow velocities, which are under the influence of gravity. As particles small enough to escape inertial impaction in earlier airway generations reach the periphery, velocity probably slows, and airflow is less turbulent. There is also a shorter distance to the airway wall in smaller, peripheral airways, favoring impaction resulting from settling (Figure 3-4). The probability of deposition by sedimentation is highest in the last five or six airway generations.[4] Because the process of sedimentation is time-dependent, the end-inspiratory breath hold should maximize deposition in the periphery. The rate of settling is proportional to the square of the particle size. For a 5-µm–diameter particle, the settling rate is reported to be 0.7 mm/sec.[17] The use of a breath hold can increase settling of particles; however, depending on particle size, a particle may not fall out of suspension.

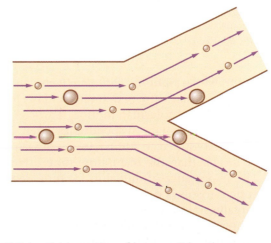

Figure 3-3 Inertial impaction of large particles, the masses of which tend to maintain their motion in straight lines. As airway direction changes, the particles are deposited on nearby walls. Smaller particles are carried around corners by the airstream and fall out less readily. (From Kacmarek RM, Stoller JK, Heuer AJ: *Egan's fundamentals of respiratory care*, ed. 10, St. Louis, 2013, Mosby.)

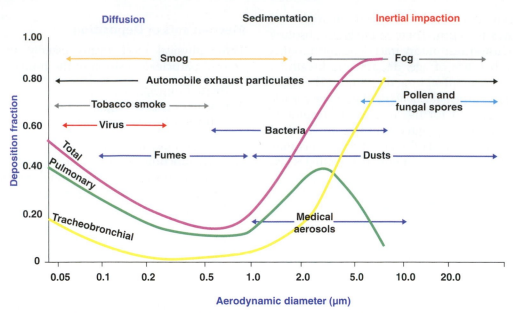

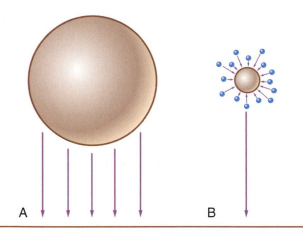

Figure 3-4 Range of particle size for common aerosols in the environment and the influence of inertial impactions, sedimentation, and diffusion. (From Kacmarek RM, Stoller JK, Heuer AJ: *Egan's fundamentals of respiratory care,* ed. 10, St. Louis, 2013, Mosby.)

Figure 3-5 Effect of mass on particle size. Large particles **(A)** are more susceptible to the force of gravity than smaller particles **(B),** which are more affected by the bombardment of molecules deposited by diffusion. (From Kacmarek RM, Stoller JK, Heuer AJ: *Egan's fundamentals of respiratory care,* ed. 10, St. Louis, 2013, Mosby.)

Diffusion (brownian motion).

Diffusion (brownian motion) *Diffusion (brownian motion)* affects particles less than 1 μm in diameter and is a function of time and random molecular motion. Particles 0.1 to 1.0 μm in size may remain suspended or even exhaled because the time required to diffuse to the airway surface tends to be greater than the inspiratory time of a normal breath.[18] The importance of diffusion for lung deposition of therapeutic aerosols is debatable because the size range involved contains so little drug mass and gives such stability. Figure 3-5 shows the relationship between particle size and aerosol deposition in the respiratory tract.

Effect of Temperature and Humidity

Prediction of particle deposition with therapeutic aerosols is complicated further by the fact that the aerosol is generated under relatively dry ambient conditions and then taken into the airway, where temperature and humidity rapidly increase to saturation at 37°C. Inhaled aerosol drugs are not only heterodisperse in size but are also *hygroscopic* (i.e., readily absorbing moisture). Between ambient and BTPS (body temperature, ambient pressure, saturated) conditions, the MMAD of cromolyn sodium powder particles from an MDI increases from 2.31 μm to 3.02 μm.[19,20] Fuller and colleagues[21] measured 50% less aerosol for ventilator delivery through an endotracheal tube (ETT) when using an in vitro model based on a jet nebulizer in warm, humidified air compared with warm, nonhumidified air.

AEROSOL GENERATORS FOR DRUG DELIVERY

KEY POINT

Common devices for the delivery of inhaled aerosol drugs include small volume nebulizers (SVNs), pressurized metered dose inhalers (pMDIs), and dry powder inhalers (DPIs). *Reservoir devices,* such as spacers and holding chambers, can reduce oropharyngeal deposition of a drug and simplify hand-breathing coordination with pMDIs. Proper use of these aerosol-generating devices is necessary to ensure adequate lung delivery, and correct use should be understood by practitioners. Traditional aerosol-generating devices all deliver about 10% to 15% of the dose produced to the lung, although different types of devices vary in their loss patterns.

Lung deposition depends on various factors, such as the aerosol generator, the patient, the drug, and the disease. Depending on the type of SVN used, most of the drug loss with an SVN occurs in the device, whereas the main drug loss with a pressurized metered dose inhaler (pMDI) and

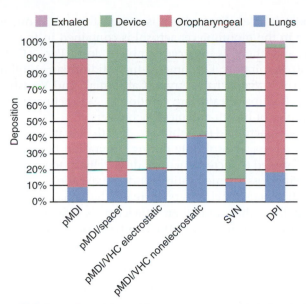

Figure 3-6 Drug deposition with common aerosol inhaler devices. Shown by color are the varying percentages of drug lung deposition and drug loss in the oropharynx, device, and exhaled breath. (From Gardenhire, DS, Ari A, Hess DR, Myers TR: *A guide to aerosol delivery devices for respiratory therapists,* ed. 3, Dallas, 2013, American Association for Respiratory Care.)

DPI is in the oropharyngeal airways. Adding a reservoir device to a pMDI or using a nonelectrostatic valved holding chamber shifts loss from the throat to the reservoir and increases aerosol deposition in the lungs. Lung deposition may range from 1% to 40% with aerosol generators.[22-27] Figure 3-6 indicates the percentages of drug deposition for different aerosol generators, showing that oropharyngeal loss, device loss, and exhalation and ambient loss differ among aerosol device types, as do lung doses.

The overall efficiency in lung deposition of 10% to 15% of the total drug dose is not significantly better than with most pMDIs or DPIs used clinically in the past, as discussed subsequently in the section on clinical application and equivalence of various devices. Nebulizers as well as MDIs and DPIs are undergoing an evolutionary transition toward greater efficiency.

Nebulizers

The term **nebulizer** encompasses various devices that operate on different physical principles to generate an aerosol from a drug solution. The SVN is a type of aerosol generator that converts liquid drug solutions or suspensions into aerosol. SVNs are powered by compressed gas (air or oxygen), a compressor, or an electrically powered device.[27] Because jet nebulizers are often used with infants or with patients in acute respiratory distress, slow breathing and an inspiratory pause may not be feasible or obtainable. One of the main advantages of SVNs is that dose delivery occurs over 60 to 90 breaths, rather than in one or two inhalations. A single ineffective breath does not destroy the efficacy of the treatment. Box 3-2 summarizes the advantages and disadvantages of SVNs.

BOX 3-2 Advantages and Disadvantages of Small Volume Nebulizers

Advantages
- Ability to aerosolize many drug solutions
- Ability to aerosolize drug mixtures (i.e., more than one drug) with suitable testing of drug activity
- Minimal cooperation or coordination required for inhalation
- Useful in very young or very old patients, debilitated patients, and patients in acute distress
- Effective with low inspiratory flows or volumes
- Normal breathing pattern can be used and inspiratory pause (breath hold) not required for efficacy
- Drug concentrations and dose can be modified, if desired

Disadvantages
- Equipment required for use is expensive and cumbersome
- Treatment times are somewhat lengthy, ranging from 5-25 minutes depending on the type of small volume nebulizer used for aerosol drug delivery
- There is variability in performance characteristics among different types, brands, and models
- Contamination is possible with inadequate cleaning
- Assembly and cleaning are required
- Wet, cold spray occurs with mask delivery
- Aerosol drug administration with a face mask may inadvertently deposit in the eyes resulting in eye irritation
- Power source (compressed gas, battery, or electricity) is needed for aerosol drug administration

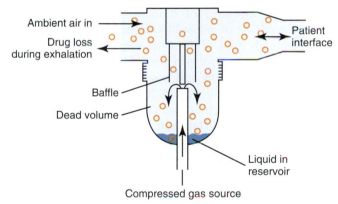

Figure 3-7 Schematic of a small volume jet nebulizer. (Modified from Cairo JM: *Mosby's respiratory care equipment,* ed. 9, St. Louis, 2014, Elsevier.)

Types of Small Volume Nebulizers

SVNs can be classified into three categories:[27]

1. Jet (pneumatic) nebulizers
2. Mesh nebulizers
3. Ultrasonic nebulizers (USNs)

Jet (pneumatic) nebulizers. Jet (pneumatic) nebulizers are small-reservoir, gas-powered (pneumatic) aerosol generators, also referred to as *handheld nebulizers, updraft nebulizers, or unit-dose nebulizers.* The traditional jet nebulizer is commonly used and exhibits a large amount of drug wastage, especially within the device itself; see Figure 3-7 for a generic illustration. Jet nebulizers use a jet-shearing principle for creation of an aerosol from the drug solution. An external source of compressed gas is directed through a narrow orifice inside the reservoir cup. The expanding gas creates a localized negative pressure, drawing the drug solution up feeder tubes. As the liquid enters the gas stream, droplets are formed from gas turbulence and impaction on baffles. Smaller particle sizes are emitted after the baffling process. Larger liquid particles are recirculated back to the reservoir. There is significant evaporation of the aqueous solution with gas-powered nebulization. Nebulizer temperatures can fall from ambient to approximately 10°C within minutes because of the latent heat of vaporization. With evaporation and constant recirculation, drug solute becomes increasingly concentrated, up to 150% to 300% of the original concentration.[28]

Pneumatic jet nebulizers have been conceptualized into four categories:[27-29]

1. Jet nebulizer with reservoir tube
2. Jet nebulizer with collection bag
3. Breath-enhanced jet nebulizer
4. Breath-actuated jet nebulizer

Figure 3-8 illustrates the types of pneumatic jet nebulizers and their aerosol output.

Jet nebulizer with reservoir tube. A jet nebulizer with reservoir tube is the traditional, least expensive, and most widely used nebulizer in which aerosol is produced constantly during inspiration, expiration, and breath hold.[28,30] Although the addition of 6 inches of reservoir tubing reduces the release of aerosol to ambient air during exhalation and breath hold, it does not eliminate ambient contamination. These nebulizers provide a low percentage of the dose to the patient and have been considered to be inefficient because only 10% to 20% of the emitted dose is inhaled. The Misty-neb (Cardinal Health, Dublin, Ohio) and the Neb U mist (Hudson RCI, Durham, N.C.) are examples of this type of jet nebulizer.

Jet nebulizer with collection bag or elastomeric ball. A jet nebulizer with collection bag produces aerosol by continuously filling a collection bag, and no aerosol is lost during expiration because of a one-way inspiratory valve in between the nebulizer and the mouthpiece. Through an inspiratory valve, the patient inhales aerosol from the collection bag and exhales to the atmosphere through the exhalation port placed between the one-way inspiratory valve and the mouthpiece.[27,30] The Circulaire II (Westmed, Inc, Tucson, Arizona) is one model of a jet nebulizer with collection bag. The Circulaire Hybrid (Westmed, Inc, Tucson, Arizona) contains a soft elastomeric ball as the reservoir. The ball is simple to remove and easily washed and dried, which assists in home use.

Breath-enhanced jet nebulizer. Breath-enhanced jet nebulizers allow more aerosol release during inspiration with decreased output during exhalation or breath hold through two one-way valves used to prevent the loss of aerosol to the environment. Although aerosol is produced during inspiration and expiration, the inspiratory valve opens and gas vents through the nebulizer only when the patient inhales. Expired gas is routed through a one-way valve in the mouthpiece; aerosol is contained in the reservoir and there is reduced ambient loss. Pari LC Plus (PARI Respiratory Equipment, Inc, Midlothian, Virginia), NebuTech (Salter Labs, Arvin, California), and Ventstream Pro (Phillips Healthcare, Andover, Massachusetts) are examples of breath-enhanced nebulizers.

Breath-actuated jet nebulizer. Breath-actuated jet nebulizers release aerosol only during inspiration because they are designed to increase aerosol drug delivery to patients by reducing loss of medication during expiration. Although breath-actuated nebulizers increase the inhaled dose by more than threefold, their efficiency is achieved by an increase in dosing time.[30] The two types of breath-actuated nebulizers are:[27]

1. Manual breath-actuated jet nebulizers
2. Mechanical breath-actuated jet nebulizers

Manual breath-actuated jet nebulizer. Manual breath-actuated jet nebulizers represent the first generation of breath-actuated nebulizers, which regulate aerosol production during inspiration and expiration through use of a patient-controlled thumb port. In manual breath-actuated nebulizers, dose delivery occurs only during inspiration; the thumb control is blocked so that there is no nebulization during expiration. Releasing the thumb at the port pauses the nebulization. Even though this type of nebulizers reduce drug loss during expiration, they require good hand-breath coordination and significantly increase the treatment time.[25-27] Figure 3-9 illustrates the relationship of nebulizer generation with a manual breath-actuated jet nebulizer.

Mechanical breath-actuated jet nebulizer. Mechanical breath-actuated jet nebulizers have a breath-actuated valve that is triggered by patients creating an inspiratory force (Figure 3-10). When the breath-actuated valve is triggered, aerosol is produced only during inspiration. This type of nebulizer eliminates the need for a collection bag or reservoir.[27,30] The AeroEclipse II (Trudell Medical International, London, Ontario, Canada) is an example of a mechanical breath-actuated nebulizer. The AeroEclipse II is also available in a reusable nebulizer (R BAN).

Mesh nebulizers. Mesh nebulizers move the liquid formulations through a fine plate or mesh with multiple apertures (small holes) to generate aerosol. These nebulizers have no internal baffling mechanism and create aerosol by using the aperture plate or the ultrasonic horn. The diameter of the apertures determines the size of the particle generated. Mesh nebulizers do not require a gas source because they are powered by electricity, and they leave very little dead volume (0.1 to 0.5 mL) in the nebulizer, so they are very efficient. There are two types of mesh nebulizers on the market:[25-27]

1. Active vibrating mesh nebulizers
2. Passive mesh nebulizers

Active vibrating mesh nebulizer. Active vibrating mesh nebulizers (VMNs) have an aperture plate with 1000 to 4000 funnel-shaped holes on an electroformed sheet that

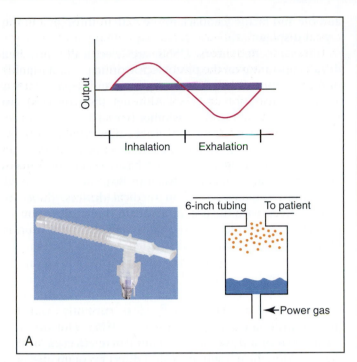

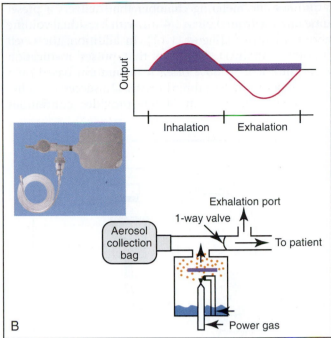

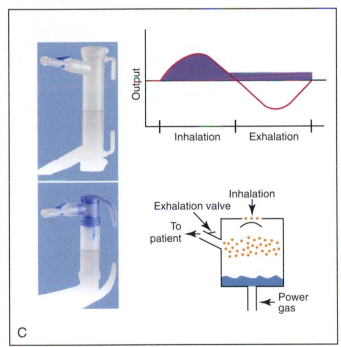

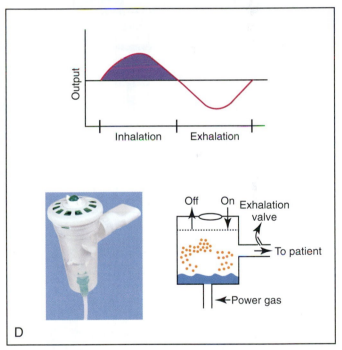

Figure 3-8 Different types of pneumatic jet nebulizer designs and their aerosol output, indicated by *shaded area*. **A,** Pneumatic jet nebulizer with reservoir tube. **B,** Jet nebulizer with collection bag. **C,** Breath-enhanced jet nebulizer. **D,** Breath-actuated jet nebulizer. (Modified from Gardenhire, DS, Ari A, Hess DR, Myers TR: *A guide to aerosol delivery devices for respiratory therapists,* ed. 3, Dallas, 2013, American Association for Respiratory Care.); **A** *inset,* From DeVilbiss Healthcare, Somerset, Pennsylvania; **B** *inset,* From Westmed, Inc., Tucson, Arizona; **C** *inset,* From PARI Respiratory Equipment, Inc., Midlothian, Virginia; **D** *inset,* AeroEclipse II Breath Actuated Nebulizer [BAN], From Trudell Medical International, London, Ontario, Canada.)

is vibrated by a piezo-ceramic element that surrounds the aperture plate.[25-27,31] The Aeroneb Go and Solo (Aerogen, Galway, Ireland), Akita II (Activaero, Dublin, Ohio), and eFlow (PARI Respiratory Equipment, Inc, Midlothian, Virginia) are examples of active VMNs (Figure 3-11).

Passive mesh nebulizer. Passive mesh nebulizers use an ultrasonic horn to push fluid through the mesh. The newest

generation of passive mesh nebulizer is the adaptive aerosol delivery (AAD) system, such as the I-neb (Phillips Healthcare, Andover, Massachusetts). The I-neb is a small, battery-operated, lightweight, and silent aerosol generator designed to deliver a precise and reproducible dose of drug. After aerosol is injected into the breath at the beginning of inhalation, the dosage of the drug is controlled through an AAD disc and specific metering chamber that delivers a preset volume ranging from 0.25 to 1.4 mL with a residual volume of about 0.1 mL[25-27] (Figure 3-12). In addition, the I-neb incorporates an AAD algorithm that pulses medication delivery into 50% to 80% of each inspiration based on a rolling average of the last three breaths. On successful delivery of the medication, the I-neb provides continuous audible and tactile feedback to the patient through a liquid crystal display.[27]

Ultrasonic nebulizers. USNs are electrically powered devices operating on the piezoelectric principle and capable of high output. Particle sizes vary by brand. Figure 3-13 is a generic illustration of a USN. Although these devices have not been used as routinely as other types (described subsequently) for aerosolization of drugs, they have been reintroduced as small, portable units that can operate on direct current (DC) voltage. Such units have several advantages and some disadvantages, as listed in Box 3-3.

At the frequencies used in medical devices, there are several effects with the potential for altering drug activity of the nebulizer solution. Most of the energy produced during ultrasonic nebulization is dissipated as heat. Protein and other heat-sensitive (or *thermolabile*) formulations can be denatured by heat, especially if the melting temperature of the protein is reached. For example, insulin was shown to be inactivated by USN use.[32] Most currently available inhaled drugs are stable with use of a USN.[33] However, the breakdown of a drug can be a cumulative effect of surface denaturation, heat, cavitation, and direct pressure effects in a USN.[33] Drug solutions must be tested by ultrasonic delivery to determine that activity is preserved, particularly when proteins or liposomes are nebulized. The clinician should refer to the manufacturer's directions to help determine which device should be used for each drug.

Nebulizers for ribavirin administration. The small particle aerosol generator (SPAG) device is a large-reservoir nebulizer, capable of holding 300 mL of solution for long periods of nebulization (Figure 3-14). It operates on a jet-shearing principle. The device was used during the clinical trials of the aerosolized antiviral drug ribavirin (Virazole) and is marketed for delivery of that drug by its manufacturer (Valeant Pharmaceuticals International, Aliso Viejo, California). The SPAG unit is described in more detail upon discussion of ribavirin in Chapter 13.

Nebulizers for pentamidine administration. An SVN fitted with inspiratory and expiratory one-way valves and

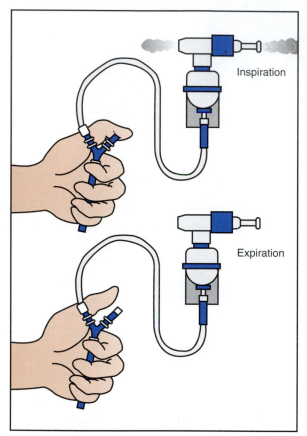

Figure 3-9 Schematic illustration of the function of a manual breath-actuated jet nebulizer. Use of a finger control regulates production during inspiration and expiration. (From Cairo JM: *Mosby's respiratory care equipment*, ed. 9, St. Louis, 2014, Elsevier.)

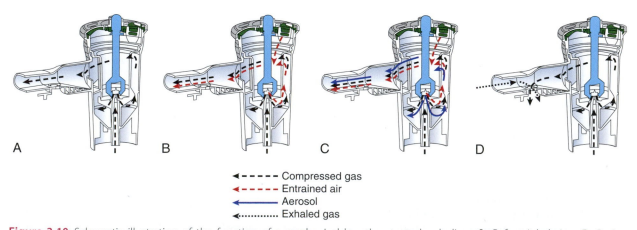

◄------ Compressed gas
◄- - - - Entrained air
◄────── Aerosol
◄·········· Exhaled gas

Figure 3-10 Schematic illustration of the function of a mechanical breath-actuated nebulizer. **A,** Before inhalation. **B,** Patient inhales, and actuator starts to move down. **C,** Negative pressure pulls the diaphragm down (with actuator moved down, sealing around the nozzle cover), producing aerosol. **D,** Patient exhales through valve in mouthpiece. As pressure increases, the diaphragm and actuator move up, stopping aerosol production. (From Trudell Medical International, London, Ontario, Canada.)

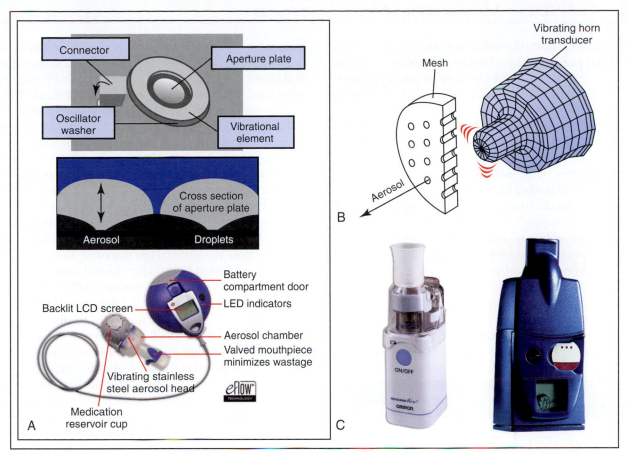

Figure 3-11 Basic configurations of mesh nebulizer. **A,** Active vibrating mesh. **B,** Ultrasonic horn. **C,** Passive mesh. (**A,** Courtesy of PARI Respiratory Equipment, Inc, Midlothian, Virginia. **B** and **C,** Courtesy Omron Healthcare Inc, Bannockburn, Illinois.)

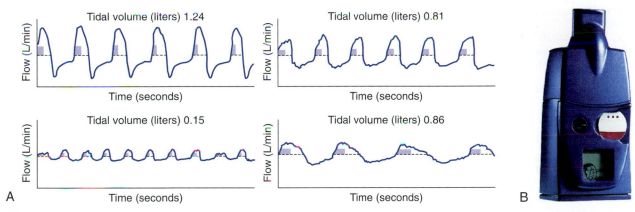

Figure 3-12 **A,** Aerosol is injected into the breath at the beginning of inspiration. Adaptive aerosol drug delivery through a passive mesh nebulizer, such as the I-neb **(B).** (From Cairo JM: *Mosby's respiratory care equipment,* ed. 9, St. Louis, 2014, Elsevier; *photo inset* courtesy Phillips Healthcare, Andover, Massachusetts.)

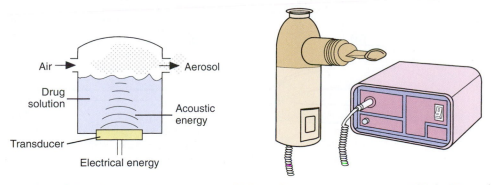

Figure 3-13 Illustration of the principle of ultrasonic nebulization, with an example of a portable device used to aerosolize medications.

with an expiratory filter is used during the administration of aerosolized pentamidine. The one-way valves used with the SVN prevent second-hand exposure of pentamidine by eliminating the contamination of the ambient environment with exhaled aerosol.[27]

Factors affecting jet nebulizer performance. When using a jet nebulizer, it is important to control factors affecting jet nebulizer performance during aerosol drug administration. Various types of jet nebulizers are available on the market, and several studies have indicated that performance varies among manufacturers and among nebulizers from the same manufacturers.[34-36] These factors include residual volume or "dead volume," filling volume, treatment time, flow rate and pressure, output rate, continuous versus inspiratory nebulization, type of power gas, physical nature of the solution to be nebulized, humidity, temperature, and device interface. Some of these factors are reviewed in greater detail subsequently.

Dead volume (residual volume). Jet nebulizers do not aerosolize below a minimal volume, termed the **dead**

volume, which is the amount of drug solution remaining in the reservoir when the device begins to sputter and aerosolization ceases. This volume can vary with the brand of nebulizer, but is on the order of 0.5 to 1.0 mL. This is the primary reason why diluent, which is effectively additional volume, is added to 0.5 mL of a bronchodilator solution, such as albuterol. Adding diluent does not alter the amount of drug (dose) in the nebulizer; it simply "expands" the solution volume. The concentration of the solution is less, not the amount of drug (see Chapter 4 for further discussion). Drug loss with nebulization can also occur into the ambient air. As a result of these factors, the amount of dose available to be inhaled from a nebulizer is considerably less than the dose placed into the reservoir. Kradjan and Lakshminarayan[37] found that under clinical conditions of nebulization until sputter, approximately 35% to 60% of a drug solution was delivered from the nebulizer. Even with vigorous agitation, this amount increased to only 53% to 72%. A study by Shim and Williams[38] found that only 40% to 52% of the total dose was delivered from gas-powered nebulizers. In a positive-pressure circuit, this efficiency may decrease further, to approximately 30% of the total dose.[39] Evaporation of an aqueous solution not only causes cooling of the nebulizer and liquid, but also can increase the concentration of solute in the residual (dead) volume.

Filling volume and treatment time. Based on the work of Hess and associates,[35] Figure 3-15 shows the relationship of volume and flow rate to the time of nebulization, presented as the pooled average performance of 17 nebulizer brands. Increasing the volume increases the time of effective nebulization at any given flow rate. At less than 2 mL, most pneumatic nebulizers do not perform well because the volume is close to the dead volume—that is, the residual amount that does not nebulize. At 6 mL, an excessively long time is required for treatment (more than 10 minutes) with

---

BOX 3-3   Advantages and Disadvantages of Portable Ultrasonic Drug Nebulizers

Advantages
- Small size
- Rapid nebulization with shorter treatment times
- Smaller drug amounts with no diluent for filling volume
- Can be used during car travel or camping

Disadvantages
- Expense
- Fragility, lack of durability
- Requires electrical source (either AC or DC)
- Possible degrading effect on drug must be determined

AC, Alternating current; *DC*, direct current.

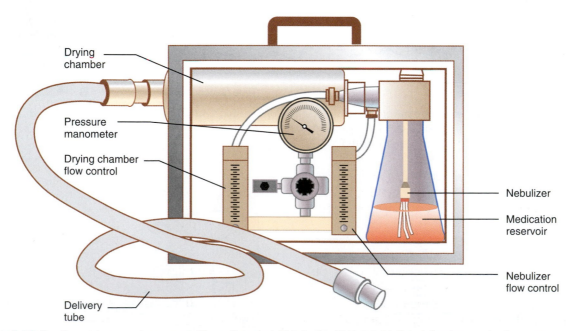

Figure 3-14 Small particle aerosol generator. (From Kacmarek RM, Stoller JK, Heuer AJ: *Egan's fundamentals of respiratory care*, ed. 10, St. Louis, 2013, Mosby.)

Labels on figure: Drying chamber; Pressure manometer; Drying chamber flow control; Delivery tube; Nebulizer; Medication reservoir; Nebulizer flow control

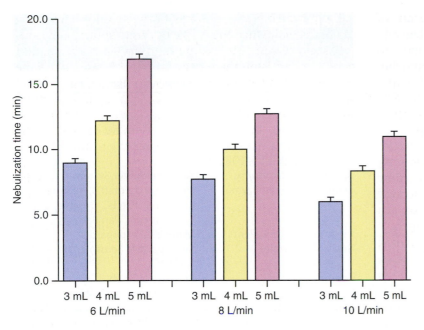

Figure 3-15 Relationship of volume and flow rate to time of nebulization averaged for 17 gas-powered nebulizers. (From Hess D, Fisher D, Williams P, et al: Medication nebulizer performance: effects of diluent volume, nebulizer flow, and nebulizer band, *Chest* 110:498, 1996.)

most brands. Although 5 minutes seems to be a short time, even this can be inconveniently long as a way of taking medication three or four times a day; some patients have difficulty in taking a pill 4 times a day, an approximately 2- to 3-second activity. Patient compliance is directly proportional to convenience. Given the volume requirements of nebulizers for efficient operation and the need for relatively brief treatments, a volume between 3 mL and 5 mL of solution is recommended, unless the nebulizer is specifically designed for a smaller fill volume. Increasing the volume also decreases the concentration of a drug remaining in the dead volume when nebulization ceases.[35] The dose of a drug available to the patient is increased, although treatment times also increase at any given flow rate.

Increasing fill volume increases inhaled efficiency and the dose to the patient. It should be noted that the approved label dose of the drug includes the fill volume that was used in the clinical trials that lead to approval by the U.S. Food and Drug Administration (FDA). Increasing fill volume would increase the dose to the patient and should not be done without consulting with the prescribing physician.

Effect of flow rate and pressure. A second practical question concerns the flow rate at which to power jet nebulizers. The flow rate affects two variables: the length of treatment time and the size of the particles produced. Figure 3-15 illustrates the interaction between volume and flow rate in determining time of nebulization. At a flow rate of 6 L/min, a volume of 3 mL requires less than 10 minutes; at 10 L/min, a volume of 5 mL can be nebulized in approximately 10 minutes. Figure 3-16 shows the effect of flow rates on particle size of the aerosol produced, averaged for the 17 nebulizers studied by Hess and associates.[35] With pneumatically powered nebulizers, increasing the flow rate decreases the particle size and shifts the MMAD lower. On the basis of the results of Hess and colleagues shown in Figures 3-15 and 3-16, average optimal rates are a filling volume of 5 mL and a flow rate of 6 to 8 L/min for many

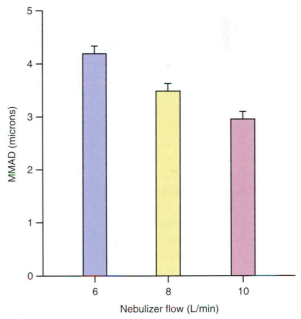

Figure 3-16 Effect of power gas flow rate on the mass median aerodynamic diameter (MMAD) of aerosol particles produced on average by 17 gas-powered nebulizers. (From Hess D, Fisher D, Williams P, et al: Medication nebulizer performance: effects of diluent volume, nebulizer flow, and nebulizer band, *Chest* 110:498, 1996.)

nebulizers. Also, each model of jet nebulizer is designed to work best at a specific flow, ranging from 2 to 8 L/min. It is important to operate a jet nebulizer with a compressor or a gas flow that matches the intended design; at a lower flow or pressure, particle size would increase. If a jet nebulizer designed to operate at 6 to 8 L/min at 50 pounds per square inch (psi) is driven by a compressor producing 13 psi, it will produce a larger particle size, which will influence efficiency.[27]

Type of power gas. Use of gases other than oxygen or air can change the performance characteristics of a nebulizer. Hess and associates[35] showed that the use of heliox (a mixture of helium and oxygen) to nebulize albuterol caused particle size and inhaled drug mass to decrease, along with a more than twofold increase in nebulization time. Increasing the flow of heliox returned output to that seen with air.[40] The flow rate should be increased by 1.5 to 2 times during heliox-driven aerosol drug administration to bring particle size and output back to levels achieved with air or oxygen.[27,41,42] Selection of the appropriate gas to power a nebulizer needs to be done by the practitioner on the basis of patient data or policy and procedure set by the institution. Oxygen has always been used because of its availability; however, using air to control the oxygen a patient receives may be of importance to practitioners.

Device interface. Device interfaces used for aerosol drug administration include mouthpieces and face masks. Ideally, a mouthpiece should be used because studies suggest that the mouthpiece provides greater lung dose than a standard pediatric aerosol mask.[43,44] Also, use of a face mask increases the amount of aerosol deposited on the face, in the eyes, and into the nose, which can be particularly significant for certain drugs such as inhaled corticosteroids. A mouthpiece cannot be used by infants and children, and it is also uncomfortable for longer aerosol therapy. Regardless of the type of device interface used during aerosol therapy, patients should be instructed to inhale through the mouth because the nose tends to filter more aerosol than the mouth.[27]

Type of solution. Droplet size of nebulized solutions is related to surface tension and viscosity of the solution and is partially determined as well by the baffles in the device.[45] Recommended filling volumes and flow rates are suitable for the aqueous bronchodilator solutions usually administered with these devices. However, the volumes and flow rates suggested may require modification for some drug solutions, such as pentamidine or antibiotics, which have different physical characteristics and viscosities. For example, higher viscosity antibiotic solutions of gentamicin or carbenicillin require power gas flow rates of 10 to 12 L/min to produce suitably small aerosol particles for inhalation with some jet nebulizers.[46] Some disposable nebulizers may exhibit greater variability in performance or not achieve adequate output characteristics with new or nonbronchodilator drug solutions. The performance of a jet nebulizer should be tested with various drug solutions, and newly introduced nebulizer drugs should be tested with an intended nebulizer system to ensure adequate performance. It is best to nebulize only drugs that have been manufactured for nebulization; however, it is common to nebulize agents intended for a different route of administration. Nebulizers not tested for performance with a new or unknown drug solution cannot be assumed to produce adequate output and particle sizes. As indicated in Chapter 2 in the review of Lung availability/total systemic availability (L/T) ratios and the pharmacokinetics of inhaled aerosol drugs, efficiency of lung delivery is a function of *both* drug and device. The drug-device combination should be tested before clinical use.

TABLE 3-1	Representative Drug-Device Combinations Tested for Nebulizer Drug Delivery
DRUG	**APPROVED NEBULIZER**
Bronchodilator	Nebulizer type not specified
Acetylcysteine	Nebulizer type not specified
Budesonide (Pulmicort Respules)	Should not be used with ultrasonic nebulizer
Tobramycin (Bethkis, TOBI)	Pari LC
Aztreonam (Cayston)	Altera Nebulizer System
Dornase alfa (Pulmozyme)	Hudson T Up-draft II, Marquest Acorn II, Pari LC, Durable Sidestream, Pari Baby
Pentamidine (NebuPent)	Marquest Respirgard II
Ribavirin (Virazole)	Small particle aerosol generator (SPAG)
Iloprost (Ventavis)	ProDose or I-neb
Treprostinil (Tyvaso)	Tyvaso Nebulizer System

From Gardenhire, DS, Ari A, Hess DR, Myers TR: *A guide to aerosol delivery devices for respiratory therapists,* ed. 3, Dallas, 2013, American Association for Respiratory Care.

Table 3-1 lists some tested and adequate drug-device combinations for nebulizer delivery. Additives to the drug solution can also affect aerosol characteristics and drug delivery.[27] See Box 3-4 for helpful information on the use and cleaning of jet nebulizers.

Pressurized Metered Dose Inhalers

pMDIs have been used since its development by Maison in 1955.[48] These devices are most commonly aerosol generators prescribed for patients with asthma and chronic obstructive pulmonary disease (COPD); they are small, pressurized canisters for oral or nasal inhalation of aerosol drugs and contain multiple doses of accurately metered drug. Advantages and disadvantages of drug delivery by pMDI are listed in Box 3-5.

Technical Description

A pMDI has five major components:

1. Canister
2. Propellant/excipient mixture
3. Drug formulary
4. Metering valve
5. Actuator and dose counter

Figure 3-17 illustrates the major components of a pMDI as well as the function of the metering valve. The characteristics of each pMDI component are described in Table 3-2.

The drug in a pMDI is either a suspension of micronized powder in a liquefied propellant or a solution of the active ingredient in a cosolvent (usually ethanol) mixed with the propellant. Dispersing agents, or *surfactants,* are added to prevent aggregation of drug particles and to lubricate the valve mechanism, thereby maintaining suitable particle sizes in the aerosol plume, aerosol particles discharged

BOX 3-4   Use of Small Volume Nebulizers

Generic Recommendations that Apply to All Nebulizers[27]

1. Read and follow instructions before using nebulizer
2. Ensure that nebulizer is properly assembled in accord with manufacturer's instructions
3. Ensure that nebulizer is cleaned and dried between treatments
4. Ensure that nebulizer is operated in its proper orientation

Critical Steps in Jet Nebulizer Use[27]

1. Assemble all parts of nebulizer before treatment including tubing, nebulizer cup, and mouthpiece or mask
2. Put drug into nebulizer cup
3. Sit in an upright position
4. Connect nebulizer to power source, such as compressed air, oxygen, or a compressor
5. Breathe normally during treatment with occasional deep breaths until sputter occurs or until end of nebulization
6. Keep nebulizer in vertical position during treatment
7. Rinse nebulizer with sterile or distilled water
8. Allow to air dry

Critical Steps in Vibrating Mesh and Ultrasonic Nebulizer Use[27]

1. Correctly assemble nebulizer based on manufacturer's recommendation
2. Follow manufacturer's instructions in performing functionality test before first use of new nebulizer and after each disinfection to verify proper operation
3. Put medicine into medication reservoir. Do not exceed volume recommended by manufacturer
4. Sit in upright position
5. Turn on power
6. Hold nebulizer in position recommended by manufacturer
7. Breathe normally during treatment with occasional deep breaths
8. Turn off unit to avoid waste if treatment must be interrupted
9. Disassemble and clean nebulizer after treatment as recommended by manufacturer
10. When using VMN, do not touch vibrating mesh during cleaning because it will damage unit
11. Disinfect nebulizer according to manufacturer's instructions once or twice a week

Common Errors in Use[27]

- Failure to assemble nebulizer properly
- Wasting dose by tilting some nebulizers
- Failure to keep mouthpiece in mouth during treatment
- Failure to mouth breathe during nebulization

Cleaning Instructions for Small Volume Nebulizers[27]

VMNs and USNs should be cleaned and disinfected based on the manufacturer's recommendations. During the cleaning of vibrating mesh nebulizers, the mesh should not be touched to prevent damage to the unit. For jet nebulizers, the Cystic Fibrosis Foundation guidelines[47] recommend washing the parts of jet nebulizers with soap and hot water after each treatment with care not to damage any parts of the aerosol generator. Also, nebulizers should be cleaned after every treatment given at home. The longer a dirty nebulizer sits and is allowed to dry, the harder it is to clean thoroughly. Rinsing and washing the nebulizer immediately after each treatment reduces infection. Cleaning instructions for the jet nebulizer follow.

Cleaning Instructions for the Jet Nebulizer[27]

Cleaning After Each Use	*Cleaning Once or Twice a Week*
Wash hands before handling equipment	Wash hands before handling equipment
Disassemble parts after every treatment	Disassemble parts after every treatment
Remove tubing from compressor and set aside; tubing should not be washed or rinsed	Remove tubing from compressor and set aside; tubing should not be washed or rinsed
Rinse nebulizer cup and mouthpiece with either sterile water or distilled water	Wash nebulizer parts in warm water with liquid dish soap
Shake off excess water	Disinfect nebulizer based on manufacturer's recommendations; nebulizer parts may be soaked in one of the following solutions:
Air dry on absorbent towel	
Store nebulizer cup in resealable plastic bag	1. 1 part household bleach in 50 parts water for 3 minutes
	2. 70% isopropyl alcohol for 5 minutes
	3. 3% hydrogen peroxide for 30 minutes
	4. 1 part distilled white vinegar in 3 parts hot water for 1 hour (not recommended for patients with cystic fibrosis)
	Rinse parts with sterile or distilled water
	Shake off excess water and place all parts on clean paper towel
	Allow parts to air dry completely on absorbent towel
	Reassemble nebulizer and store in clean dry bag or container

From Gardenhire, DS, Ari A, Hess DR, Myers TR: *A guide to aerosol delivery devices for respiratory therapists*, ed 3, Dallas, Tex., 2013, American Association for Respiratory Care.
USN, Ultrasonic nebulizer; *VMN*, vibrating mesh nebulizer.

BOX 3-5   Advantages and Disadvantages of Pressurized Metered Dose Inhalers

Advantages

- Pressurized metered dose inhalers (pMDIs) are portable, light, and compact
- Drug delivery is efficient
- Treatment time is short
- They are easy to use
- More than 100 doses are available
- Fine particle sizes are available in hydrofluoroalkane (HFA) formulations
- They are difficult to contaminate
- No drug preparation is needed
- It is possible to reproduce emitted doses

Disadvantages

- Complex hand-breathing coordination, proper inhalation pattern, and breath hold are required
- Drug concentrations and doses are fixed
- Canister depletion is difficult to determine accurately
- Reactions to the propellants may occur in small percentage of patients
- High oropharyngeal impaction and loss occur if an extension device is not used
- Foreign body aspiration of coins and debris from mouthpiece can occur*
- Difficult to determine dose remaining in canister without dose counter

*Data from Hannan SE, Pratt DS, Hannan JM, Brienza LT: Foreign body aspiration associated with the use of an aerosol inhaler, *Am J Respir Dis* 129:1205, 1984; Schultz CH, Hargarten SW, Babbitt J: Inhalation of a coin and a capsule from a metered-dose inhaler, *N Engl J Med* 325:432, 1991 (letter).

TABLE 3-2   Basic Components of Pressurized Metered Dose Inhaler

COMPONENT	PARTICULARS
Canister	Inert, able to withstand high internal pressures and use a coating to prevent drug adherence
Propellants	Liquefied compressed gases in which drug is dissolved or suspended
Drug formulary	Particulate suspensions or solutions in presence of surfactant or alcohol that allocates drug dose and specific particle size
Metering valve	Most critical component; crimped onto container and is responsible for metering a reproducible volume or dose; elastomeric valves are responsible for sealing and prevention of drug loss or leakage
Actuator	Frequently referred to as "boot"; partially responsible for particle size based on length and diameter of nozzle of various pMDIs; each boot is unique to a specific pMDI/drug
Dose counter	Provides visual tracking of number of doses remaining in pMDI

From Gardenhire, DS, Ari A, Hess DR, Myers TR: *A guide to aerosol delivery devices for respiratory therapists,* ed. 3, Dallas, 2013, American Association for Respiratory Care.
pMDI, Pressurized metered dose inhaler.

from a pMDI, produced in CFC (e.g., Freon) devices. These surfactants are not soluble in HFA devices.[49] Newman[50] presents a detailed technical description of the complexities involved in producing a pMDI.

Chlorofluorocarbon versus Hydrofluoroalkane Propellants

Historically CFCs and HFAs were the two types of propellants used with pMDIs. In the past, blends of liquefied gas (CFCs) were used with pMDIs to create an aerosol, but because one CFC molecule can destroy 100,000 molecules of stratospheric ozone, the FDA banned the use of CFC–pMDIs. The few remaining CFC aerosol devices were removed from market on December 31, 2013. Hydrofluorocarbons (HFCs), or *HFAs*, were then identified as propellants that were nontoxic to the atmosphere and to the patient and that also had properties suitable for MDI aerosol generation. In particular, HFA 134a has a vapor pressure similar to that of CFC 12. The structure of HFA 134a is illustrated in Figure 3-18 and compared with that of CFC 12. Replacement of CFC propellants has led to overall reengineering of pMDI components (valve, seals, exit orifice, and drug formulation), which has improved pMDI performance. Some of the differences, such as the lower plume force (Figure 3-19) and warmer plume temperature, cause patients who have used CFC-propelled pMDI formulations to think there is reduced or no drug delivery occurring with the HFA formulation of albuterol.[51]

Metered Dose Inhaler

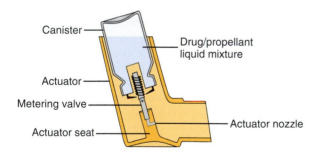

Metering Valve Function

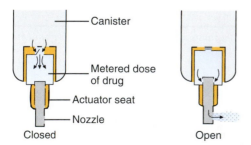

Figure 3-17 Major components of a metered dose inhaler, with an illustration of the function of the metering valve. Oral and nasal adapters are shown.

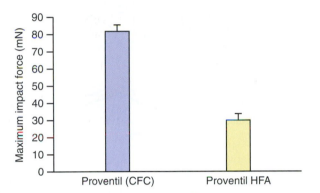

Figure 3-18 Structure and properties of a chlorofluorocarbon (CFC) propellant, CFC 12, and a non-CFC propellant, hydrofluoroalkane (HFA) 134a, used in pressurized metered dose inhaler (pMDI) drug formulations.

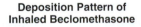

Figure 3-19 Measures of plume force exiting a metered dose inhaler (MDI) for chlorofluorocarbon-propelled and hydrofluoroalkane-propelled albuterol (*Proventil and Proventil HFA*). (Data from Ross DL, Gabrio BJ: Advances in metered dose inhaler technology with the development of a chlorofluorocarbon-free drug delivery system, *J Aerosol Med* 12:151, 1999.)

Equivalence and safety. The efficacy and safety of all reformulated HFA drugs have been studied. It should be noted that the amount of drug may have changed from the CFC form, but many companies have reformulated products to maintain similar strength and dose.

Improved drug delivery with hydrofluoroalkane formulation. Although equivalent drug amounts and effects were found with the drugs, the reengineering of the MDI for HFA propellant has resulted in significant improvements in performance and in particular in lung deposition of the aerosol drug. The traditional amount of 10% for lung deposition has been increased more than fivefold with some HFA formulations.[52] Figure 3-20 illustrates a comparison of lung delivery between HFA-based and CFC-based MDI systems and the increase in lung delivery when the HFA formulation is used.

Types of Pressurized Metered Dose Inhalers

pMDIs can be divided into three categories: (1) conventional pMDIs, (2) breath-actuated pMDIs, and (3) a soft-mist inhaler

Conventional metered dose inhaler. The conventional pMDI has a press-and-breathe design. Figure 3-17 illustrates the components of the conventional pMDI, including canister, medication, propellant/excipient, metering valve, mouthpiece, and actuator. When the canister is depressed into the actuator, the drug-propellant mixture in the metering valve is released under pressure. The liquid propellant rapidly expands and vaporizes, or "flashes," as it ejects from the pressurized valve into ambient pressure. This expansion and vaporization shatter the liquid stream into an aerosol. The initial vaporization of propellant causes cooling of the liquid-gas aerosol suspension, which can be felt if discharged onto the skin; however, HFA versions have a much "warmer" spray temperature. The cold mist from a CFC spray may cause users to stop inhaling as the cold aerosol

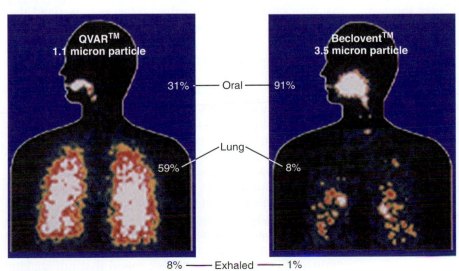

Deposition Pattern of Inhaled Beclomethasone

Figure 3-20 Comparison of lung deposition between chlorofluorocarbon *(right)* and hydrofluoroalkane *(left)* formulations of beclomethasone dipropionate by metered dose inhaler (MDI). (Scintigraph and data courtesy C. Leach, Lovelace Respiratory Research Institute, Albuquerque, New Mexico.)

hits the oropharynx. On release, the metering valve refills with the mixture of drug and propellant from the bulk of the canister and is ready for the next discharge. The metering valve varies from 25 to 100 μL in volume[50] and provides 50 mcg to 5 mg of drug per actuation, depending on the drug formulary.[27]

Breath-actuated metered dose inhaler. A type of device to simplify MDI use is a breath-actuated adapter. In the United States the adrenergic bronchodilator pirbuterol (Maxair, Valent Pharmaceuticals, Montreal, Canada) (see Chapter 6) was marketed as a breath-actuated inhaler. Maxair was removed from the market for containing CFC propellant. It is not known if the device will be returned to the market with an HFA propellant. Breath-actuated inhalers offer an alternative for individuals who find it difficult to coordinate pMDI actuation with inhalation. As described by Newman,[50] Newman and associates,[53] and Baum and Bryant,[54] the pMDI canister is triggered by a spring through a triggering mechanism activated when the patient inhales. Evidence indicates that breath-actuated pMDIs improve the delivery of inhaled medication in patients with poor coordination.[55] However, if the patient has good coordination with the conventional pMDI, the use of a breath-actuated pMDI may not improve drug delivery.[53,55]

Respimat soft mist inhaler. The Respimat (Boehringer Ingelheim Pharmaceuticals, Ridgefield, Conn.) is a propellant-free soft mist inhaler utilizing mechanical energy in the form of a tension spring. Turning the transparent base one-half turn to the right draws a predetermined volume of solution from the medication cartridge through a capillary tube into the micropump. Depressing the dose release button releases energy from the spring, forcing solution to the mouthpiece and producing a soft mist of aerosol lasting 1.5 seconds.[27]

The Respimat will need to be primed before use and when it has not been used for 21 days or more. It is recommended to actuate the inhaler once if it has not been used for three days. Any actuations or repriming after the initial priming will result in loss of medication actuations. The Respimat (Figure 3-21) does not need to be shaken, as it is propellant-free. The device is equipped with a dose indicator and will lock itself after the last dose is used.

Breath-actuated pressurized metered dose inhaler accessory devices. Numerous breath-actuated pMDI devices are available on the market. The MD Turbo (Respirics, Raleigh, North Carolina) and the SmartMist (Aradigm, Hayward, California) are used with most pMDIs because they are able to convert a conventional pMDI to a breath-actuated pMDI through breath-triggering mechanisms.[27]

Factors Affecting Metered Dose Inhaler Performance

The accuracy and consistency of dose from pMDIs may be more sensitive to handling practices than previously thought. Research on the drug content of albuterol sprays by pMDI has shown that various factors affect dose consistency.

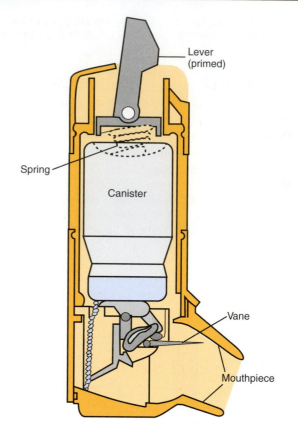

Figure 3-21 Picture of Respimat Soft Mist inhaler. (Boehringer Ingelheim Pharmaceuticals, Ridgefield, Connecticut.)

Loss of dose. *Loss of dose* refers to the loss of drug content in the valve even though propellant may seem to discharge a normal dose. A dose with less than the nominal amount of drug has been noted to occur when first actuating an albuterol MDI that has been stored in the valve-down position, even after only a few hours and with shaking before discharge. The loss of dose ranged from 25% to more than 50% in the studies referenced.[56,57] This loss of dose was not observed with storage in a valve-up position. Other drug formulations may increase or decrease drug concentration in the first discharge after standing unused; this would need to be determined for each product. These findings suggest that the canister be stored valve-up between uses and that a waste dose be discharged if more than 4 hours have elapsed with the valve down when using albuterol by pMDI. The new HFA formulation is not associated with loss of dose.[14]

Shaking the canister. Many of the drugs in MDI formulations are suspensions that can separate from the propellants on standing (*creaming*).[57] This separation should not affect the dose in the valve, which was filled after the previous actuation. However, if the suspended drug is either lighter or heavier than the propellant and separation occurs, a second actuation could deliver more or less concentrated drug if the canister is not shaken to mix the propellant and drug suspension thoroughly. The MDI should be shaken *before* the first actuation after standing, so that the metering valve refills with adequately mixed suspension from the canister. Everard and colleagues[57] found that not shaking an albuterol canister before use and after the canister has been standing upright overnight led to a 26% reduction in total dose and a 36% reduction in particles less than 6.8 μm; this occurred despite wasting two discharges before the measurement. Rubin and Durotoye[58] found similar results with CFC inhalers, but HFA beclomethasone did not seem to be influenced by shaking of the canister.

Timing of actuation intervals. A pause of 1 to 5 minutes has been advocated between each puff of a bronchodilator from an MDI in an attempt to improve distribution of the inhaled drug in the lung.[59] The study by Everard and colleagues[57] found that two actuations of albuterol MDI 1 second apart caused no change in total drug output, although there was a 15.8% decrease in the amount of particles less than 6.8 μm. However, four actuations 1 second apart led to significant reductions in dose output. Concern over cooling of the MDI valve with rapid actuations does not seem to be supported by the results presented by Everard and colleagues.[57] Loss of dose probably occurs as a result of turbulence and coalescence of particles with more than two rapid actuations. Clinically, a pause between puffs from an MDI has not been found to be beneficial in routine maintenance therapy. Pedersen[60] showed no difference in forced expiratory volume in 1 second (FEV_1) with a 3-minute and 10-minute divided dose under nonacute basic maintenance conditions. This was found to be the case for a β agonist (terbutaline) and a corticosteroid (budesonide) when used by preadolescents.[61] However, during asthma exacerbations with acute wheezing, a pause between puffs resulted in significantly improved bronchodilation, with greater effect using a 10-minute pause.[59]

There is no consensus on any of the preceding information covered. It is best to educate the health care practitioner and patient to apply a systematic approach when using an MDI. The better the routine and consistency in using this device, the more likely it is that patients will benefit.

Loss of prime. *Loss of prime* refers to the loss of propellant from the metering valve of the MDI.[62] When this occurs, little or no drug is discharged on actuation; this can be felt and heard by a user. Loss of prime usually takes days or weeks to occur; regular use of the MDI should prevent this. Shaking of the canister and discharge of a waste dose are suggested after long periods of no use to prime the valve with propellant and drug.

Storage temperature. Data indicate that dose delivery from CFC-propelled MDIs of albuterol decreases at lower temperatures. A significant decrease of 65% to 70% of the usual dose has been observed at 10° C. An even greater decrease was observed in a fine particle mass (less than 4.7 μm), with approximately 75% of the usual dose at 10° C and only 25% at −10° C. No medication was delivered at −20° C.[63] In contrast, HFA-propelled albuterol remained constant in total dose over the range of −20° C to 20° C. The fine particle mass of the CFC-free formulation decreased significantly only at −20° C, delivering approximately 60% of the initial FPD. Temperature effects such as these are likely to be relevant only for outdoor use of MDI canisters in extreme weather.

Nozzle size and cleanliness. Aerosol drug delivery with a pMDI is dependent on nozzle size, cleanliness, and lack of moisture.[27] The size of nozzle is specific to the pMDI and influences not only inhaled dose but also particle size. The inverse relationship between the inner diameter and the nozzle extension and the amount of drug delivered to the patient has been documented.[64] According to Niven and colleagues,[64] a nozzle extension with an inner diameter less than 1 mm increases aerosol drug delivery. Because white and crusty residue resulting from crystallization of medication may influence drug delivery the nozzle should be checked and cleaned periodically based on the manufacturer's recommendations.[27]

Breathing technique. The two primary techniques for using a pMDI without a spacer are the *open mouth* technique and the *closed mouth* technique. Actuating the pMDI several centimeters in front of the open mouth theoretically allows for slowing of the particle velocity and evaporation of aerosol droplets, resulting in less oropharyngeal impaction and loss. This maneuver further complicates the use of the pMDI. The manufacturers of pMDIs universally recommend the closed mouth technique for using a pMDI. Although some studies with both children and adults have shown no difference in lung function between an open mouth and a closed mouth technique in use of a bronchodilator,[65,66] others recommend the open mouth technique in an attempt to reduce oropharyngeal deposition and increase lung dose.[67,68] Consequently, the simpler technique should be preferred. If oropharyngeal impaction is undesirable, as in the case of inhaled corticosteroids, or if accurate timing between actuations is a problem, as is sometimes the case for older patients, an extension device (spacer or holding chamber) should be used. More drug—equivalent to the output of a standard SVN—is inhaled from the pMDI with the use of an extension device.[69]

Patient characteristics. Characteristics of the patient using the pMDI lead to a variability of aerosol deposition. For instance, aerosol deposition is lower in infants and children because of differences in their anatomy and physical and cognitive abilities.[27,70]

Correct Use of a Pressurized Metered Dose Inhaler

The effectiveness of treatment with an aerosolized drug delivered by a pMDI depends on correct use of the device. The major problem with pMDI devices is difficulty in patient use.[71] The most common error noted is the failure to coordinate inhalation and actuation of the inhaler (hand-breathing incoordination). Other problems include a too-rapid inspiratory flow rate, inadequate or missing breath hold after inhalation, failure to shake and mix canister contents, cessation of inspiration as the aerosol strikes the throat, actuation of the pMDI at total lung capacity, inhaling through the nose, and exhaling during actuation. Evidence indicates that 50% to 70% of patients do not use pMDIs correctly.[69] In addition, physician, nurse, and respiratory therapist knowledge of correct pMDI use is often inadequate for patient education[69] (Box 3-6).

BOX 3-6   Use of Metered Dose Inhalers[27]

The following instructions for the use of bronchodilator or cortico-steroid aerosols with pMDIs are written in terms that may be helpful for patient education. Package inserts on particular agents should always be checked, and these protocols should be modified as needed, especially for other drug classes.

Generic Recommendations That Apply All pMDIs[27]

1. Remove mouthpiece cover of pMDI from boot
2. Prime pMDI as directed in package insert
3. Clean and dry boot of pMDI based on manufacturer's guidelines
4. Track remaining doses after each use

Critical Steps in Use of the Open Mouth Technique With pMDIs[5]

1. Remove cap, inspect for foreign matter, and push canister into nozzle receptacle of mouthpiece actuator
2. Hold MDI in vertical position, shake inhaler, and, if not used recently, discharge priming dose
3. Exhale to functional residual capacity (easier for subject) or to residual volume
4. Hold MDI about 1 inch in front of open mouth or, alternatively, place in mouth with teeth apart and with tongue flat
5. Begin to breathe in slowly through mouth while actuating inhaler by pressing down on canister. Inspiration should take about 3-4 seconds
6. Continue inhaling to total lung capacity and hold breath for up to 10 seconds (only one puff for inhalation)
7. Exhale normally, shake canister, wait 20-30 seconds to allow valve to refill, and repeat dose if prescribed
8. Keep a diary of number of uses or use a counting device to keep track of number of actuations used

   Note: If you have trouble aiming the MDI at your open mouth, you can place the mouthpiece directly in your mouth and rest it on the lower front teeth without sealing your lips around it. If you find it hard to coordinate breathing and activating the MDI, you may wish to ask your physician to prescribe a reservoir device.

Critical Steps in Use of the Closed Mouth Technique With pMDI[27]

1. Remove mouthpiece cover and check for foreign objects
2. Shake inhaler thoroughly
3. Prime pMDI into air if it is new or has not been used for several days
4. Sit up straight or stand up
5. Exhale all the way out
6. Place pMDI between teeth
7. Ensure that tongue does not block pMDI by keeping it flat under mouthpiece
8. Seal lips
9. Actuate pMDI as you begin to inhale slowly
10. Hold breath for 10 seconds or as long as possible
11. Wait 1 minute before administering another puff of medicine
12. Repeat steps 2 through 10 until dosage prescribed by physician is reached
13. After using a corticosteroid, rinse mouth after last puff of medicine
14. Spit water out and do not swallow any
15. Replace mouthpiece cover on pMDI after each use

Critical Steps in Soft Mist inhaler (Respimat) Use

1. Close mouthpiece cap; press safety catch while pulling off clear base
2. On label of inhaler, write discard date, which is 3 months from date cartridge is inserted into device
3. Remove medication cartridge from box
4. Push narrow end of cartridge into inhaler
5. Return clear base to mouthpiece assembly
6. Hold inhaler upright, with cap closed, to avoid accidental release of dose
7. Turn clear base one-half turn
8. Point inhaler toward ground and press dose release button
9. Continue steps 6 through 8 until mist of medication is seen
10. Once mist is visible, repeat steps 6 through 8 three times
11. Once primed, turn clear base one-half turn and open mouthpiece cap
12. Breathe out, slowly emptying lungs; close lips around mouthpiece without covering air vents
13. Point inhaler to back of throat, keeping inhaler parallel to ground
14. While inhaling slowly and deeply, press dose release button; continue to breathe in slowly for as long as possible
15. Hold breath for 10 seconds or as long as possible
16. Repeat steps 12 through 15 until prescribed dose has been completed
17. When complete, replace mouthpiece cover on inhaler

To Inhale a Corticosteroid

Use the same procedure as described in the use of the open or closed mouth technique with these exceptions:

1. If you use a bronchodilator and a corticosteroid, inhale the bronchodilator first and wait 1-2 minutes before inhaling the corticosteroid
2. Always use an extension or spacer device when inhaling a corticosteroid. If you do not have such a device, try to hyperextend (straighten) your head and neck as much as possible when inhaling (in other words, look at the ceiling)
3. Rinse your mouth and throat with water after finishing

Common Errors in Use

The number of patients using pMDIs incorrectly ranges from 12% to 89%, according to available studies.[6]

- Failure to coordinate actuation with inhalation (27%)
- Too short a period of breath-hold after inhalation (26%)
- Too rapid an inspiratory flow rate (19%)
- Inadequate shaking and mixing of contents before use (13%)
- Abrupt cessation of inspiration as aerosol strikes throat (6%)
- Actuation at total lung capacity (4%)
- Firing actuation into mouth but inhaling through nose (2%)
- Exhaling during actuation
- Placing wrong end of inhaler in mouth, or holding in wrong (nonvertical) position
- Failure to take cap off before use
- Firing of MDI multiple times during a single inhalation
- Covering air vents on specific inhalers (i.e., Respimat)

BOX 3-6   Use of Metered Dose Inhalers—cont'd

Cleaning Instructions for pMDI[27] and Respimat

Cleaning pMDI

Frequency of cleaning: Once a week and as needed

Look at hole where drug sprays out from inhaler

Clean inhaler if you see powder in or around hole

Remove pMDI canister from plastic container so that it does not get wet

Rinse plastic container with warm water and shake out to remove excess water

Dry overnight

Replace canister inside mouthpiece and recap mouthpiece

Cleaning Respimat

Frequency of cleaning: Once a week and as needed

Remove mouthpiece cover

Wipe outside of mouthpiece with damp cloth

Wipe metal piece inside mouthpiece with damp cloth

Clean outside of inhaler with damp cloth when needed

Recap mouthpiece

Store in cool, dry place

Check Canister Fullness

The best approach is to keep a patient log of use, showing date of initial use and subsequent numbers of actuations each day. If a pMDI is used regularly (e.g., two actuations four times daily), the projected date of depletion can be calculated. For occasional use, tallies at the end of the day on a self-stick note kept in a convenient place, such as the bathroom, can be useful. Counting devices can be purchased that count the number of actuations during use. Some manufacturers have a built-in counter on the actuator (e.g., ProAir, Ventolin, and Flovent). Canister flotation in water is no longer recommended; it is imprecise, varies with different drugs, and can clog pMDI nozzles.

MDI, Metered dose inhaler; *pMDI*, pressurized metered dose inhaler.

Accessory Devices for Pressurized Metered Dose Inhalers

Extension, or reservoir, devices were introduced primarily to simplify the complex coordination of aiming, actuating, and breathing with a pMDI. Figure 3-22 illustrates a generic reservoir device. Using accessory devices with pMDIs improves the effectiveness of aerosol drug administration because pMDI accessory devices can modify the aerosol discharged from a pMDI in the following three ways:

1. Such devices allow space and time for more vaporization of the propellants and evaporation of initially large particles to smaller sizes.
2. Reservoirs allow the high initial velocity of particles released from a pMDI to slow before reaching the oropharynx. Particles discharged from the actuator nozzle have velocities exceeding 30 m/sec. By holding the actuator 4 cm in front of the mouth or by using an extension device, this velocity is allowed to slow.[67]
3. As holding chambers for the aerosol cloud release, reservoir devices separate the action of actuation of the canister from inhalation and simplify the coordination required for effective use.

The combined effect of the first two advantages reduces oropharyngeal deposition. This reduces the amount of drug swallowed and absorbed from the gastrointestinal tract and reduces any local oropharyngeal side effects, such as those seen with inhaled corticosteroids. Box 3-7 summarizes the advantages and disadvantages of accessory devices.

Types of pressurized metered dose inhaler accessory devices. Many types of pMDI accessory devices are available on the market. The size ranges from 70 to 80 mL to 750 mL for some European brands; some are available with

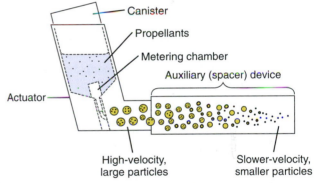

Figure 3-22 The effect of an extension device on aerosol particle size and velocity from a metered dose inhaler (MDI).

a mask. Numerous terms are used to refer to such devices, including *spacer, reservoir, auxiliary device, extension device, holding chamber,* and *add-on device.* Some distinction of terms may be useful to denote significant design differences among these devices. The following terminology is offered, partially based on Dolovich:[72]

Reservoir device: Global term describing or referring to extension, auxiliary, and add-on devices attached to MDIs for administration. This term could include both "spacer" and "holding chamber."

Spacer: Denotes a simple tube or extension device, with no one-way valves to contain the aerosol cloud; its purpose is simply to extend the MDI spray away from the mouth.

Valved holding chamber: Denotes a spacer device with the addition of a one-way valve to contain and hold the aerosol cloud until inspiration occurs.

Design variables. Spacers are simple devices that extend the distance and space between the pMDI and the patient. pMDIs with spacers provide more drug to the patient than pMDIs without spacers. However, valved holding chambers can increase drug delivery, decrease oropharyngeal deposition, and help with coordination. Valves in the holding chamber act as a baffle reducing particle size, which reduces oropharyngeal impaction, and allow the patient to exhale without disrupting the aerosol inside the chamber. Valved holding chambers are superior to spacers.

pMDI accessory devices have several design variables, including volume, shape, direction of pMDI spray, presence of one-way valves, inspiratory flow rate indicators, and presence or absence of an integral (built-in) pMDI actuator. Table 3-3 summarizes these design variables for some reservoir devices available in the United States. Figure 3-23 illustrates differences in the size and design of several units.

Electrostatic charge. An electrostatic charge is inherent on most plastic holding chambers. It has been discovered that by reducing the electrostatic charge, an increase in drug delivery occurs. Simply washing the chamber with water and standard household detergent reduces the electrostatic charge, and the effects can last 30 days. Manufacturers have begun making chambers that are "antistatic." Louca and associates[73] found that the AeroChamber MAX (Monaghan Medical Corp., Plattsburg, New York), a valved holding chamber made from antistatic plastic, performed better

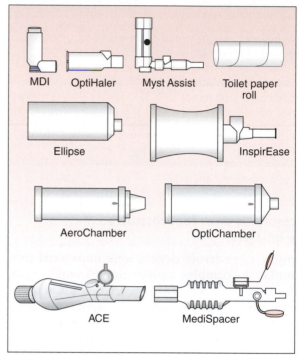

Figure 3-23 Pressurized metered dose inhaler (pMDI) and accessory devices consisting of spacer and holding chambers. All of the accessory devices reduce oropharyngeal deposition. Small volume spacers (OptiHaler and Myst Assist) offer no additional advantage, but large volume spacers (toilet paper roll and Ellipse) improve inhaled aerosol with delay between actuation and inspiration. Only the bag (InspirEase) and valved holding chambers (AeroChamber, OptiChamber, ACE, and MediSpacer) protect the patient from blowing the dose away when the pMDI is actuated during expiration. (From Kacmarek RM, Stoller JK, Heuer AJ: *Egan's fundamentals of respiratory care,* ed 10, St Louis, 2013, Mosby.)

BOX 3-7	Advantages and Disadvantages of Pressurized Metered Dose Inhaler Accessory Devices

Advantages
- Reduced oropharyngeal drug loss
- Separation of pMDI actuation and inhalation steps
- Allows use of MDI during acute airflow obstruction with dyspnea
- Available with mask for children
- No drug preparation required
- Increased inhaled dose by twofold or fourfold compared with pMDI alone

Disadvantages
- Large and cumbersome (some brands)
- Additional expense compared with pMDI alone
- Some assembly required
- Possible source of bacterial contamination with inadequate cleaning
- Patient errors in use of pMDI accessory devices such as firing multiple puffs into chamber before inhaling or a delay between actuation and inhalation

Modified from Gardenhire, DS, Ari A, Hess DR, Myers TR: *A guide to aerosol delivery devices for respiratory therapists,* ed 3, Dallas, 2013, American Association for Respiratory Care.
MDI, Metered dose inhaler; *pMDI,* pressurized metered dose inhaler.

TABLE 3-3	Characteristics of Selected Reservoir Devices Used in the United States, Exemplifying Design Variable Differences

BRAND	VOLUME (APPROXIMATE) (mL)	INSPIRATORY VALVE	SPRAY DIRECTION*	FLOW INDICATOR	INTEGRAL ACTUATOR
AeroChamber Plus	198	One way	Forward	Yes	No[†]
OptiChamber Advantage	218	One way	Forward	No	No[†]
ACE	175	One way	Reverse	Yes	Yes
InspirEase	600	No	Reverse	Yes	Yes
OptiHaler	70	No	Reverse	No	Yes
MediSpacer	160	No	Reverse	Yes	Yes

*Relative to mouth.
[†]Accepts mouthpiece actuator of drug brand.

than other chambers that were washed and rinsed to reduce the electrostatic charge. Reducing electrostatic charge can increase delivery of the aerosolized drug by 70%.[74]

KEY POINT

Reducing electrostatic charge in a reservoir device can significantly increase drug delivery.

Size. The size of a spacer or holding chamber can affect the amount of drug made available to the patient: The larger the spacer, the more drug available. Most spacers in the United States are less than 200 mL. Larger chambers (up to 750 mL) are available outside the United States. There is a tradeoff with inconvenience because the larger and bulkier devices are less likely to be used or taken on travel.

Dose counters. pMDIs look, taste, and feel as if they are working after their label shows that the number of puffs contained were delivered to the patient; this is referred to as "tailing-off effect" with pMDIs, which may last long after the pMDI is empty of its drug.[25,62] It is very important to use dose counters with pMDIs that allow patients and clinicians to determine the number of actuations used and the time when a pMDI should be discarded.[75-77] The FDA also requires new pMDIs to have integrated dose counters and recommends that all pMDIs have dose-counting devices indicating when the pMDI is approaching its last dose. The Ventolin HFA (GlaxoSmithKline) and Flovent HFA (GlaxoSmithKline) have built-in dose counters; mechanical or electronic dose counters are available from third parties that can be attached to a range of pMDIs. Although acceptable performance by and patient satisfaction with pMDIs with dose counters have been confirmed,[78-80] some dose counters may be pMDI specific and may not fit the spacer, which leads to no or partial drug being emitted and a miscount of remaining doses.[81,82] Using a dose counter increases the cost of aerosol therapy and may limit acceptance by patients. In that case, the number of doses remaining in the pMDI should be determined manually. Patients who wish to use a manual method should read the label to determine the total number of doses available in the pMDI and subtract every actuation given from the number of actuations on the label until all have been used. Although manual dose counting is cost-effective, it may be impractical and undependable, especially in use of reliever medications on the go.[27] Note that floating the canister in water to determine the amount of medication remaining in the canister is misleading and can reduce the ability of the pMDI to work properly[77,83,84] and should not be used. For general use instructions, see Box 3-8.

Dry Powder Inhalers

A DPI is similar to a pMDI except that the drug is in powdered form. The main advantage is that the DPI is breath-actuated, meaning that hand-breathing coordination is not needed. The main disadvantage is that the DPI requires a high inspiratory flow rate from the patient to dispense the drug. The flow rate needed is usually 30 to 90 L/min. Children and patients with respiratory disease may be unable to generate the flow needed to use such a device. Box 3-9 lists advantages and disadvantages of DPIs.

Types of Dry Powder Inhalers

DPIs can be divided into three categories based on the design of their dose containers[27,85]: unit-dose DPIs, multiple unit–dose DPIs, and multiple-dose DPIs. All types of DPIs have similar components incorporated with the inhaler, including a drug holder, air inlet, agglomeration compartment, and mouthpiece. Types of DPIs are illustrated in Figure 3-24.

Unit-dose dry powder inhalers. Unit-dose, or single-dose, DPIs have individually wrapped capsules that contain a single dose of medication and deliver powder medication from a punctured capsule. Using a single-dose DPI involves several steps: First, the user places each capsule into the drug holder. Second, the user primes the device by piercing the single-dose capsule and allowing entrance of air into the device for dispersion with inhalation. The Aerolizer (Merck & Co Inc, Whitehouse Station, New Jersey, Neohaler and TOBI Podhaler (Novartis Pharmaceuticals, East Hanover, New Jersey), and HandiHaler (Boehringer Ingleheim Pharmaceuticals Inc, Ridgefield, Connecticut) are examples of single-dose DPIs.[27]

Multiple unit–dose dry powder inhalers. Multiple unit–dose DPIs disperse individual doses that are premetered into blisters; the blister is mechanically punctured when the cover is lifted. The Diskhaler (GlaxoSmithKline, Philadelphia, Pa.) is an example of the multiple unit–dose DPI that requires an inspiratory flow rate greater than 60 L/min to achieve an adequate drug deposition into the lungs.[27] Relenza (zanamivir) is the only Diskhaler currently marketed in the United States.

Multiple-dose dry powder inhalers. Multiple-dose DPIs measure the dose either from a powder reservoir or from blister strips prepared by the manufacturers. The Twisthaler (Merck & Co Inc, Whitehouse Station, New Jersey), the Flexhaler (AstraZeneca, Wilmington, Delaware), and Pressair (Forest Pharmaceuticals, St. Louis, Missouri) have a powder reservoir or storage area, whereas the Advair Diskus (GlaxoSmithKline, Philadelphia, Pennsylvania) contains 60 doses of dry powder medication individually wrapped in blisters. Anoro Ellipta, Breo Ellipta, and Incruse Ellipta (GlaxoSmithKline, Philadelphia, Pennsylvania) contain two double-foil strips with 30 blisters of each medication. The medication's blister wrapping protects the drug from humidity and other environmental factors.[27]

Factors Affecting Dry Powder Inhaler Performance and Drug Delivery

Intrinsic resistance. Intrinsic resistance of the DPI determines how much inspiratory flow must be created in the device to release the correct amount of the drug. Each type of DPI has a different intrinsic resistance to airflow. For instance, the Handihaler has a higher resistance than the

BOX 3-8   Use of Pressurized Metered Dose Inhaler Accessory Devices

The design and use of reservoir devices vary. The following steps are generic and are intended to describe most reservoir devices for handheld use. Specific brand instructions should be reviewed before use or instruction of patients.

Generic Recommendations That Apply to All pMDI Accessory Devices

1. Use nonelectrostatic material or prewash nonconductive material reservoir device
2. To maximize dose, inhale simultaneously or right after actuating MDI
3. Use a single inhalation with each MDI actuation. Multiple MDI actuations followed by a single inhalation reduces the dose available
4. Have small children or infants inhale through device for five or six breaths to maximize emptying of chamber
5. Ensure proper fit of pMDI to spacer or VHC
6. Remove cap from pMDI boot
7. Clean and reassemble pMDI spacers and VHCs based on manufacturer's instructions

Critical Steps in Use of Spacer or Valved Holding Chamber With pMDI[27]

1. Warm pMDI canister to hand or body temperature
2. Take off mouthpiece cover and shake inhaler thoroughly
3. Prime pMDI into air if it is new or has not been used for more than 24 hours
4. Assemble apparatus and check for foreign objects
5. Keep canister in vertical position
6. Sit up straight or stand up
7. Exhale all the way out
8. Follow subsequent instructions based on type of device interface that you use

With Mouthpiece

a. Place mouthpiece of spacer between teeth and seal lips
b. Ensure that tongue does not block pMDI by keeping it flat under mouthpiece
c. Actuate pMDI as soon as you begin to inhale
d. Make sure to breathe in slowly; if device produces a whistle, it means that inspiration is too rapid
e. Move mouthpiece away from mouth and hold breath for 10 seconds or as long as possible

With Mask

a. Hold mask completely over nose and mouth and ensure it fits firmly against child's face
b. Actuate pMDI as the child begins to breathe in
c. Inhale slowly; if the device produces a whistle, it means that inspiration is too rapid
d. Hold mask in place while child takes six normal breaths, including inhalation and exhalation
e. Remove mask from child's face

With Collapsing Bag

a. Open bag to its full size. Press pMDI canister immediately before inhalation
b. Inhale until bag is completely collapsed
c. Breathe in and out of the bag several times to inhale all medication in bag
d. Wait 15-30 seconds if another puff of medicine is needed
e. Repeat steps a through d until dosage prescribed by physician is reached
f. Rinse mouth after treatment if corticosteroid is used
g. Spit water out and do not swallow any
h. Replace mouthpiece cover on pMDI

Common Errors in Use

- Incorrect assembly
- Incorrect (nonvertical) position of pMDI canister on reservoir
- Waiting too long to inhale after actuating pMDI
- Inhaling too rapidly (may reduce dose)
- Firing of multiple puffs into reservoir before inhaling
- Firing of puffs from two different pMDIs before inhaling
- Failure to take mouthpiece cap off before use

Cleaning Instructions for pMDI Chamber and Collapsible Bag Device[27]

Cleaning Chamber Device	*Cleaning Collapsible Bag Device*
Frequency of cleaning: Every 2 weeks and as needed	Frequency of cleaning: Every 2 weeks and as needed
Disassemble device for cleaning	Disassemble device for cleaning
Soak spacer parts in warm water with liquid detergent and gently shake both pieces back and forth	Remove plastic bag assembly from mouthpiece
Shake out to remove excess water. Air dry spacer parts in vertical position overnight	Wash mouthpiece with warm water
Do not towel dry spacer because this would reduce dose delivery owing to static charge	Drip dry overnight
Replace back piece on spacer when it is completely dry	Reassemble device after it is dry
	Plastic bag should not be cleaned but should be replaced every 4 weeks or as needed

MDI, Metered dose inhaler; *pMDI,* pressurized metered dose inhaler; *VHC,* valved holding chamber.

BOX 3-9 Advantages and Disadvantages of Dry Powder Inhaler Devices

Advantages
- Small and portable
- Short preparation and administration times
- Breath actuation; no need for hand-breathing coordination
- No inspiratory hold or head tilt needed
- No CFC propellants (environmentally friendly)
- No cold Freon effect to cause bronchoconstriction or inhibit full inspiration
- Simple determination of remaining drug doses
- Built-in dose counter

Disadvantages
- Only a limited range of drugs is available to date
- Patients are not as aware of the dose inhaled as with an MDI and may distrust delivery
- Moderate to high inspiratory flow rates are needed for powder dispersion
- Relatively high oropharyngeal impaction and deposition can occur
- A device such as the Aerolizer is a single-dose device and must be loaded before each use
- Vulnerable to ambient humidity or exhaled humidity into mouthpiece
- Different DPI needed with different drugs
- Easy for patient to confuse directions for use with other devices

Modified from Gardenhire, DS, Ari A, Hess DR, Myers TR: *A guide to aerosol delivery devices for respiratory therapists*, ed 3, Dallas, Tex., 2013, American Association for Respiratory Care.
CFC, Chlorofluorocarbon; *DPI,* dry powder inhalers; *MDI,* metered dose inhaler.

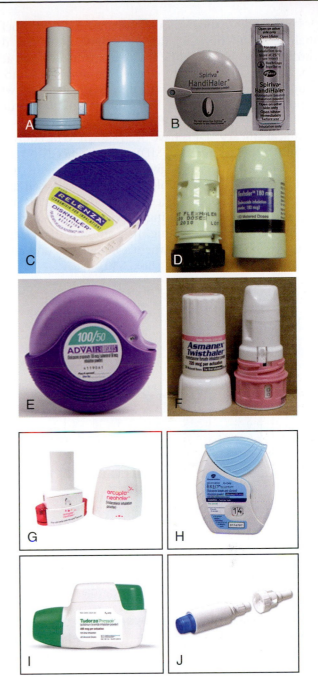

Figure 3-24 Dry powder inhalers (DPIs) available in the U.S. **A,** Unit-dose DPI: Aerolizer (Merck & Co Inc, Whitehouse Station, New Jersey). **B,** Handihaler (Boehringer Ingelheim Pharmaceuticals Inc, Ridgefield, Connecticut). **C,** Multiple unit-dose DPI: Diskhaler (GlaxoSmithKline, used with permission). **D,** Flexhaler (AstraZeneca LP, Wilmington, Delaware). **E,** Multiple-dose DPI: Diskus inhaler (GlaxoSmithKline, used with permission). **F,** Twisthaler (Merck & Co Inc.). (**A,** The FORADIL AEROLIZER photo image is reproduced with permission of Schering Corporation, subsidiary of Merck & Co., Inc. All rights reserved. FORADIL is a registered trademark of Astellas Pharma, Inc. and the trademark of AEROLIZER is a registered trademark of Novartis AG. **F,** The ASMANEX TWISTHALER photo image is reproduced with permission of Schering Corporation, subsidiary of Merck & Co., Inc. All rights reserved. ASMANEX and TWIST-HALER are registered trademarks of Schering Corporation.) **G,** Ellipta. **H,** Arcapta Neohaler. **I,** Tudorza Pressair. **J,** TOBI Podhaler.

Diskus and requires a greater inspiratory effort. The patient's inspiratory effort is important not only in lifting the powder from the drug reservoir, blister, or capsule but also in deaggregating the powder into finer particles.[27]

Inspiratory flow rate. Dispersal of drug powder depends on the energy of the inspiratory flow. A moderate to high inspiratory flow is needed with DPIs to obtain an optimal dose. This requirement affects the use of these devices by young children, especially those less than 5 years old, and by any patient with an acute wheezing episode associated with airflow reduction. Patients should be evaluated for the ability to generate a minimal inspiratory flow before prescription of a DPI. Figure 3-25 illustrates the effect of various inspiratory flows with three DPI devices.

Humidity. Another factor that can affect dose delivery from a DPI is humidity and moisture, which can cause powder clumping and reduce deaggregation and the fine particle mass in the dose. Because a reservoir chamber containing multiple doses for dispensing has less protection from ambient humidity than capsules and drug blisters, DPIs with a reservoir chamber, such as the Twisthaler, Flexhaler, and Pressair, must be kept as dry as possible. In contrast, the Diskus and Ellipta, in which each drug dose is protected inside a blister on a foil strip, showed no change in 8 weeks under such conditions. With any DPI, it is essential that patients not exhale into the device before inhaling; in all devices, including the Diskus, the drug powder is exposed when the device is activated.[74,86] In addition, all DPIs are affected by exhaled air introduced into the mouthpiece, especially after the device is loaded and when the powder is exposed. Therefore patients must be instructed to exhale away from the DPI before inhalation.[27]

Clinical efficacy. DPIs have been shown to be equivalent in efficacy to pressurized pMDIs.[87,88] The need to replace CFC-propelled MDIs has given renewed impetus to the development of DPI technology. In evidence-based guidelines, Dolovich and associates[69] found that a DPI is just as good as a pMDI when selecting a device for inhaled medication in the outpatient setting. It is stressed that selection should be based on the patient's knowledge and understanding of the device's use (Box 3-10).

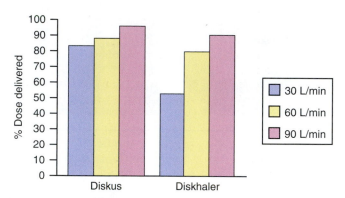

Figure 3-25 Effect of inspiratory flow rate on the percentage of nominal dose delivered by three dry powder inhaler devices. Data were derived in vitro for albuterol. (Modified from Prime D, Grant AC, Slater AL, et al: A critical comparison of the dose delivery characteristics of four alternative inhalation devices delivering salbutamol: pressurized MDI, Diskus inhaler, Diskhaler, and Turbuhaler, *J Aerosol Med* 12:75, 1999.)

SELECTING AN AEROSOL DEVICE

Several important questions arise concerning aerosol devices. How should they be quantitatively described for clinicians? Are there differences in clinical effect with different devices, including spacer and reservoir accessories? What is the correct or optimal use of different types of devices? With all aerosol delivery devices, respiratory care personnel should carefully review instructional materials and package inserts to train patients in their correct use. Knowledge of aerosol delivery devices by medical personnel, together with the ability to teach patients in their correct use, is necessary for effective drug delivery. Respiratory care practitioners have been shown to receive formal education in the use of various aerosol devices more often than nursing staff or physicians. Knowledge and demonstration scores with an MDI, reservoir device, and DPI were higher for respiratory therapists than for registered nurses or physicians in a study by Hanania and associates.[89] Dolovich and colleagues[69] suggest the following eight questions should be asked when selecting an aerosol device:

1. In what devices is the desired drug available?
2. What device is the patient likely to be able to use properly, given age and clinical setting (e.g., home, hospital)?
3. For which device and drug combination is reimbursement available?
4. Which device is least expensive?
5. Can you use the same device for all inhaled drugs that the patient is taking?
6. Which device is the most convenient for the patient or family?
7. How durable is the device?
8. Does the patient or practitioner have a specific device preference?

BOX 3-10   Use of Dry Powder Inhalers

Specific instructions for use of the various DPIs currently available should be reviewed on the package insert before use or patient education.

Generic Recommendations That Apply to All DPIs
1. Read and follow instructions of each DPI for proper assembly
2. Keep DPI in proper orientation during treatment
3. Ensure mouthpiece is clear of all foreign matter
4. Exhale normally *away from the DPI* because humidity reduces inhaled dose
5. Inhale from mouthpiece forcefully to total lung capacity
6. Hold breath up to 10 seconds or as long as possible
7. Remove from mouth and exhale away from device
8. Track doses remaining in the DPI after each use

Manufacturers' recommendations for use are summarized for the unit-dose DPI (Aerolizer, Neohaler, Podhaler, and Handihaler), multiple unit–dose DPI (Diskhaler), and multiple-dose DPI (Diskus, Twisthaler, Flexhaler, Pressair, and Ellipta). As new devices become available in the United States, package inserts will provide instructions for use.

Critical Steps in Use of Unit-Dose DPI
Use of Aerolizer or Neohaler
1. Remove mouthpiece cover
2. Hold base of inhaler and twist mouthpiece counterclockwise
3. Remove capsule of medication from package and place in the base of the inhaler (remove capsule immediately before use; do not store in inhaler)
4. Hold base of inhaler and twist clockwise to close
5. Two buttons are on the sides of the inhaler; press simultaneously to pierce capsule
6. Exhale *away from the inhaler* to functional residual capacity or residual volume
7. Keep head in upright position and hold the device horizontally with lips sealed around mouthpiece
8. Breathe in as deeply as possible, holding breath for about 10 seconds if possible. Breathe out slowly, away from device
9. Open the inhaler to expose the chamber. Examine the capsule, and if powder remains, repeat inhalation. If powder has been completely used, dispose of capsule
10. Close mouthpiece and replace cover

BOX 3-10 Use of Dry Powder Inhalers—cont'd

Use of HandiHaler

1. Before using device, open foil package and remove capsule (remove capsule immediately before use; do not store in inhaler)
2. Pull dust cap upward to open
3. Open mouthpiece and place capsule in chamber
4. Close mouthpiece firmly until you hear it click; leave dust cap open
5. Hold device with mouthpiece up, and press the piercing button once to release the medication
6. Exhale *away from the inhaler* to functional residual capacity or residual volume
7. Place mouthpiece into mouth and close lips tightly around mouthpiece
8. Breathe in slowly at a rate sufficient to hear the capsule vibrate until lungs are at total lung capacity; hold breath for about 10 seconds if possible. Breathe out slowly, away from device
9. To ensure entire dose has been inhaled, repeat steps 6 through 8
10. Open mouthpiece, tip out capsule, and throw it away
11. Close mouthpiece and replace dust cap for storage

Use of Podhaler

1. Hold base of Podhaler and unscrew lid in a counterclockwise direction; set lid aside
2. Stand Podhaler upright in base of case
3. Hold body of Podhaler and unscrew mouthpiece in a counterclockwise direction, setting aside mouthpiece on a clean, dry surface
4. Take blister card and tear precut lines along length and width
5. Peel foil that covers Podhaler capsule on blister card
6. Remove capsule and place in capsule chamber at top of Podhaler
7. Place mouthpiece back on Podhaler and screw mouthpiece in a clockwise direction until tight
8. Hold Podhaler pointing mouthpiece down
9. Place thumb on blue button and press the blue button all the way down once
10. Exhale *away from the inhaler* to functional residual capacity or residual volume
11. Place mouthpiece into your mouth and close lips tightly around mouthpiece
12. Breathe in slowly until lungs are at total lung capacity; hold breath for about 5 seconds if possible; breathe out slowly, away from device
13. To ensure entire dose has been inhaled, repeat steps 10 through 12
14. Unscrew the mouthpiece, remove capsule from chamber, and throw away
15. Repeat steps 4 through 14 three more times until all for doses (four capsules) have been used

Critical Steps in Use of Multiple Unit-Dose DPI[27]
Use of Diskhaler

1. Remove cover of Diskhaler and ensure that device and mouthpiece are clean
2. Extend tray and push ridges to remove tray
3. Load medication disk on rotating wheel
4. Pull cartridge all the way out and then push it all the way in until you see medication disk in dose indicator
5. Keep device flat and lift back of lid until it is lifted all the way up to pierce the medication blister
6. Click back into place
7. Move Diskhaler away from mouth and breathe out as much as possible
8. Place the mouthpiece into mouth
9. Ensure that air hole on mouthpiece is not blocked
10. Inhale as quickly and deeply as possible
11. Move Diskhaler away from mouth and hold breath for 10 seconds or as long as possible
12. Exhale slowly
13. If another dose is needed, pull cartridge out all the way and then push it back in all the way so that next blister can be moved into place; repeat steps 5 through 12
14. Place mouthpiece cover back on after treatment. Keep remaining blisters sealed until inspiration to protect from humidity and loss

Critical Steps in Use of Multiple-Dose DPI
Use of Diskus Inhaler

1. Push thumbgrip away from you to expose mouthpiece
2. Hold Diskus in a level (horizontal) position, slide lever next to mouthpiece away from you until it clicks
3. Hold Diskus level and exhale *away from mouthpiece*
4. Put mouthpiece to lips and inhale steadily and deeply through Diskus
5. Remove Diskus from mouth, hold breath for about 10 seconds if possible, and breathe out slowly *away from device*
6. Close mouthpiece cover by sliding thumbgrip back toward you
7. Rinse mouth with water when using a corticosteroid
8. Do not wash any part of device; keep it dry

Use of Flexhaler[27]

1. Twist cover and lift off
2. Hold mouthpiece of Flexhaler up while loading a dose
3. Do not hold mouthpiece while inhaler is loaded
4. Twist brown grip in one direction as far as it goes, regardless of the way you turn it first
5. Twist grip back in the other direction completely
6. Listen carefully for a click during each of the twisting movements
7. Do not exhale *into* device
8. Place mouthpiece in mouth, seal the mouthpiece with lips, and inhale deeply and forcefully through inhaler
9. Remove inhaler from mouth and hold breath for 10 seconds or as long as possible
10. Exhale but do not blow *into* mouthpiece
11. If more than one dose is required, repeat steps 2 through 10
12. Put the cover back on inhaler and twist shut
13. Rinse mouth with water after each dose to reduce risk of developing thrush; do not swallow rinsing water

Use of Pressair

1. Remove protective cap by squeezing arrows marked on each side of cap and pulling out
2. Hold Pressair outside of mouth, mouthpiece facing you, green button facing straight up
3. Press green button all the way down before inserting into mouth
4. Check control window to make sure color has turned from red to green, meaning dose is ready; if not repeat step 3 until control window turns green

Continued

BOX 3-10   Use of Dry Powder Inhalers—cont'd

5. Exhale completely, not exhaling *into* inhaler
6. Place mouth around mouthpiece and inhale until a click is heard, continuing to inhale all the way even after click is heard
7. Remove inhaler from mouth and hold breath for as long as possible
8. Exhale but do not *into* the mouthpiece
9. Check to make sure control window has turned red, meaning the dose was successful; if not repeat steps 5 through 9
10. When done return cap to mouthpiece

Use of Ellipta
1. Slide cover down until a click is heard and mouthpiece is exposed
2. Holding inhaler away from mouth, exhale completely, not exhaling *into* inhaler
3. Place mouth around mouthpiece and inhale, being careful not to block air vent
4. Remove inhaler from mouth and hold breath for 3 to 4 seconds or as long as possible

5. Exhale but not *into* the mouthpiece
6. When complete slide cover over mouthpiece as far as it will go

Common Errors in Use[27]
- Not inhaling correctly
- Failure to pierce or open drug package
- Using the inhaler in wrong orientation
- Failure to prime
- Exhaling into inhaler at any point in process
- Not exhaling to residual volume before inhalation
- Not inhaling forcefully enough
- Covering inhalation vents
- Inadequate or no breath hold
- Exhaling through mouthpiece after inhalation

Cleaning Instructions: Dry Powder Inhaler
The DPI should not be washed and submerged in water because moisture decreases drug delivery. If necessary, the mouthpiece may be wiped with a dry cloth. Each manufacturing company recommends periodic cleaning and suggests wiping the mouthpiece of the DPI with a clean, dry cloth.[27]

DPI, Dry powder inhaler.

CLINICAL APPLICATION OF AEROSOL DELIVERY DEVICES

Sometimes it seems that with so much information available, it is difficult to decide what is best for patients. Dolovich and colleagues[69] conducted an overview of all pertinent literature to develop recommendations for the clinical use of aerosol devices. The following sections summarize their findings.

Recommendations Based on Clinical Evidence

Aerosol Delivery of Short-Acting β_2 Agonists in the Emergency Department

An MDI with a holding chamber and a nebulizer were equally effective in the treatment of adult and pediatric patients in the emergency department. Both modes of delivery improved symptoms and lung function. There is little information to show that a DPI is as effective as an MDI with a holding chamber or a nebulizer for delivery of short-acting β_2 agonists.

Aerosol Delivery of Short-Acting β_2 Agonists in the Hospital

There was no significant difference in lung function among inpatients treated with either an MDI with a holding chamber or a nebulizer. Reliable studies examining outcomes among inpatients treated with DPIs are lacking. At present, it is better to use an MDI with a holding chamber or a nebulizer to deliver short-acting β_2 agonists.

Intermittent versus Continuous Nebulizer Delivery of β_2 Agonists

There is no difference in effect between intermittent and continuous nebulizer delivery of short-acting bronchodilators. Specifically, there is no change in lung function, asthma scores, or incidence of adverse effects when comparing the two delivery methods. It has been noted that the time required for staff to maintain and administer a continuous aerosol is less than that required with an intermittent nebulizer.

Aerosol Delivery of β_2 Agonists to Patients Receiving Mechanical Ventilation

The quality of evidence concerning the administration of bronchodilators to patients receiving mechanical ventilation is fair. There seems to be no difference in effect regardless of whether a nebulizer or an MDI with a holding chamber is used to deliver bronchodilators to adults or children being mechanically ventilated. Concerning patients receiving noninvasive ventilation, there is little evidence to suggest which formulation is superior. In any case, with invasive and noninvasive ventilation, the technical factors for delivering an aerosolized agent have changed dramatically.

Aerosol Delivery of Short-Acting β_2 Agonists for Asthma in the Outpatient Setting

Among outpatients using either an MDI (with or without a holding chamber) or a DPI, there seems to be no difference in effect on lung function and asthma symptoms. However, the need for a holding chamber is evident; the literature favors the use of this device. Little research has been done on the use of nebulizers in the outpatient setting. Selection of the most appropriate aerosol device for outpatients must be made on a case-by-case basis.

Delivery of Inhaled Corticosteroids for Asthma

Whether an MDI with a holding chamber or a DPI is used, symptom scores and lung function remain the same among adult patients with asthma treated with inhaled cortico-steroids.

Delivery of β₂ Agonists and Anticholinergic Agents for Chronic Obstructive Pulmonary Disease

Evidence gathered in the treatment of patients with COPD shows no difference in effect whether a nebulizer, an MDI with or without a holding chamber, or a DPI is used. Selection of the proper aerosol device depends on numerous factors.

Factors to Consider

There are many factors to consider when selecting the proper aerosol device:

- Patient or clinical preference
- Convenience of device
- Practicality of device
- Durability of device
- Cost and reimbursement
- Drug availability
- Ability of all prescribed drugs to be delivered by same device

After these factors have been addressed and selection has taken place, it is important to educate the patient properly. Education of the patient cannot take place until proper education of the respiratory therapist has been completed.

Lung Deposition and Loss Patterns With Traditional Aerosol Devices

> **KEY POINT**
>
> A traditional aerosol device delivers approximately 10% to 15% of the total dose to the airway. Because total dose amounts differ among the various types of devices for the same drug, these devices do not necessarily deliver equivalent amounts of drug. Newer aerosol devices, as well as some still in development, are more efficient, with resultant lung depositions of 30% to 50% or greater. This improved efficiency in lung delivery will necessitate dose modifications.

Aerosol devices that have traditionally been used in respiratory care deliver approximately 10% to 15% of the total drug dose to the lung. The pattern of loss to the mouth, stomach, and digestive apparatus and through exhalation differs among the device types. Figure 3-6 illustrates the percentage of dose deposited in the lung and the pattern of loss with drug delivery systems that have traditionally been used in respiratory care: an MDI, an MDI with a spacer, an SVN, and a DPI.

Some of the lung deposition data presented in Figure 3-6 are summarized in the following list, along with information from additional studies, including one comparing CFC and HFA formulations. The percentage of lung deposition is much greater with the HFA formulation.

- MDI (CFC, technetium 99m [^{99m}Tc]-labeled Teflon): 8.8%[90]
- MDI (HFA, ^{99m}Tc label): 53%[91]
- MDI and spacer (CFC, ^{99m}Tc-labeled Teflon and Inspir-Ease, Schering Corp., Kennelworth, New Jersey): 14.8%[92]
- SVN (Inspiron Mini-Neb, Bard International of Sunderland, England, ^{99m}Tc label): 12.4%[93]
- DPI (Turbuhaler): 14.8%-27.7%[94]

MDIs and SVNs show the greatest contrast in the loss pattern of aerosol drug. Most of the loss with an MDI occurs in the mouth and stomach (approximately 80%). The loss with an SVN is primarily in the delivery apparatus (66%), with most of that remaining in the nebulizer, whereas an MDI loses approximately 10% in the actuator.

Adding a spacer or holding chamber to an MDI reduces the amount of drug lost in the oropharynx and stomach.[95] The DPI is similar to the MDI in its pattern of aerosol loss.

Equivalent Doses Among Device Types

If traditional MDI, SVN, and DPI devices all deliver approximately the same percentage of total device dose to the lungs, with the exception of HFA formulations, and the nominal dose in the devices differs, then different amounts of drug are placed within the lung. For example, the dose of albuterol, a β-adrenergic bronchodilator, by MDI versus nebulizer is as follows:

- MDI: 2 puffs, or 0.2 mg (200 mg)
- SVN: 0.5 cc, or 2.5 mg (2500 mg)

The ratio of MDI to SVN dose is approximately 1:12. If approximately 10% of the dose reaches the lungs, very different doses are being delivered from these aerosol devices. For example, if we assume that 10% of an albuterol dose reaches the lungs when administered by MDI and SVN, then a lung dose of 20 mcg would be given by MDI versus a lung dose of 250 mcg from an SVN (10% of 200 mcg versus 10% of 2.5 mg). Several studies have examined this question of equipotent doses between delivery devices. An equipotent dose is the dose by each delivery method that produces an equivalent degree of effect (for bronchodilators, this would be bronchodilation).

The standard difference in dose between the MDI and SVN delivery methods for albuterol is in the ratio of 1:12. However, at least two studies suggest MDI/SVN dose ratios of 1:3 and 1:4 to achieve equal bronchodilation or equivalent amounts of drug delivery to the lung.[96,97] An equipotent dose ratio of 1:3 or 1:4 is achieved by increasing the number of puffs from the MDI to 7 or 10 in the two studies.

One of the clearest statements on the question of delivery efficiency among traditional aerosol devices resulted from the study by Zainudin and colleagues.[98] The study examined drug delivery by pMDI (CFC propellants), DPI (Rotahaler), and gas-powered SVN (Acorn). The results are particularly helpful because the investigators used the same dose of 400 mcg of albuterol (salbutamol) in each of the device types[99]; this allowed a direct microgram-for-microgram comparison of the dose from the devices. The percentage of lung deposition is shown in Figure 3-26, with an MDI delivery of 11.2%, a DPI delivery of 9.1%, and an SVN delivery of 9.9%.

The clinical response, measured as the improvement in FEV_1, is also similar, although the change with the MDI (35.6%) is statistically significantly greater than that seen with the DPI (25.2%) or the SVN (25.8%), a result not well explained in the study. These results support the view that the amount of aerosol drug delivered to the lung is similar with any of the three device types, and the clinical response is similar. The amount of bronchodilation obtained is a reflection of the dose of drug given and not the method of delivery.[99,100] As discussed in the following section, the development of aerosol devices that are highly efficient for lung delivery of a drug is likely to lead to changes in recommended doses. For example, the increased efficiency of MDI HFA–propelled beclomethasone, cited in the section on HFA propellants, has resulted in the use of half the dose normally found with MDI CFC–propelled beclomethasone, with equivalent effects. These changes will affect what constitutes equivalent doses between different types of devices.

Lung Deposition With Newer Aerosol Devices

The development of increasingly efficient devices compared with older MDIs, SVNs, and DPIs will cause the traditional figures of 10% to 15% for lung deposition to be revised upward. Unless newer devices completely replace the older, traditional aerosol generators used clinically, there will be a wide variety of lung depositions seen rather than a single range of 10% to 15%. The amount of lung delivery will depend on which device is used. Figure 3-27 graphically compares lung deposition with traditional devices (MDIs, SVNs, and DPIs) with lung deposition with newer devices.

These data are compiled from several studies and for various drugs.[101-103]

One implication of changing and increasing lung deposition amounts is that the total dose from a device must be reduced. With a greater percentage reaching the lung, a lower total dose is needed from the device. Without proportional reduction in total device dose, toxic effects would be possible. Ultimately, the important factor is not the device per se, but rather the amount of drug reaching the lungs when treating pulmonary disease.

Clinical Equivalence of Metered Dose Inhalers and Nebulizers

It is still relatively common in clinical practice to use an SVN instead of an MDI in emergent acute situations requiring aerosol bronchodilator delivery. However, a large and growing body of evidence indicates that an MDI with a spacer or holding chamber is as effective as an SVN in acute airway obstruction. An MDI with a reservoir has been shown to be as effective as an SVN in the treatment of all age groups, from nonventilated preterm infants (with addition of a face mask) to adult patients in emergency departments. Table 3-4 summarizes selected studies supporting the clinical equivalence of either an MDI or an SVN in emergency treatment for various age groups. Amirav and Newhouse[104] published a comprehensive review of studies on this issue. A meta-analysis of studies comparing bronchodilator administration by MDI or "wet nebulizer" (SVN) concluded that either method was equivalent in the treatment of acute airflow obstruction in adults.[105]

Age Guidelines for Use of Aerosol Devices

It cannot be assumed that every patient can correctly use each type of delivery device. The differences, in particular

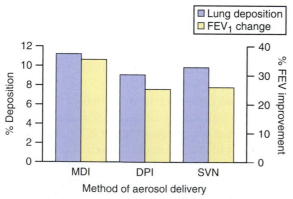

Figure 3-26 Lung deposition and clinical response: Comparison of three bronchodilator delivery methods. Shown are lung deposition (as percentage of total dose) and clinical response (percent improvement in forced expiratory volume in 1 second [FEV_1]) after aerosol delivery of the same dose of albuterol (400 mg) from three types of aerosol devices. (Data from Zainudin BM, Biddiscombe M, Tolfree SE, et al: Comparison of bronchodilator responses and deposition patterns of salbutamol inhaled from a pressurized metered dose inhaler, as a dry powder and as a nebulized solution, *Thorax* 45:469, 1990.)

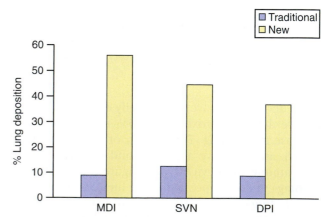

Figure 3-27 Comparison of lung deposition with older traditional aerosol devices (traditional metered dose inhaler [*MDI*], chlorofluorocarbon-MDI; traditional small volume nebulizer [*SVN*], Inspiron MiniNeb; traditional dry powder inhaler [*DPI*], Rotahaler) and with newer devices (new MDI, hydrofluoroalkane-beclomethasone[103]; new SVN, Respimat[102]; new DPI Spiros[101]). See References for further details.

TABLE 3-4	Studies Showing Equivalence of Metered Dose Inhaler With Reservoir or Face Mask to Small Volume Nebulizer for Bronchodilator Administration in Acute Airflow Obstruction for Various Age Groups			
AGE GROUP	**DRUG**	**DOSAGE**	**OUTCOME VARIABLES**	**REFERENCE**
Preterm infants, 47 ± 4.8 days	Albuterol*	MDI/spacer/mask: 2 puffs (200 mcg) q4h	Lung compliance, resistance	Fok et al[116]
		SVN/mask: 0.2 mg × (200 mcg) q4h		
Infants, 16 ± 15 months	Albuterol	MDI/HC/mask: 4 puffs (400 mcg) q20min × 3	Respiratory rate, clinical scores, admissions	Mandelberg et al[117]
		SVN: 2.5 mg q20min × 3		
Children, 5-16 years	Terbutaline	MDI/HC/mask: 3 puffs (0.75 mg) × 1	Lung function, clinical scores	Lin and Hsieh[118]
		SVN/mouthpiece: 0.5 mL (2.5 mg) × 1		
Adults, 64.6 ± 13.3 years	Albuterol	MDI/HC: 2 puffs (200 mcg) q15min × 3	Spirometry, asthma scores	Mandelberg et al[119]
		SVN: 0.5 mL (2.5 mg) q15min × 3		

HC, Holding chamber (valved reservoir); *MDI*, metered dose inhaler; *spacer*, nonvalved reservoir; *SVN*, small volume nebulizer.
*Albuterol is also known as salbutamol outside the United States.

TABLE 3-5	Age Guidelines for Use of Aerosol Delivery Devices
AEROSOL SYSTEM	**AGE**
SVN	≤2 yr
MDI	>5 yr
MDI with reservoir	>4 yr
MDI with reservoir/mask	≤4 yr
MDI with ETT	Neonate and older
Breath-actuated MDI	>5 yr
DPI	≥5 yr

Data from National Asthma Education and Prevention Program, National Heart, Lung, and Blood Institute, National Institutes of Health: National Asthma Education and Prevention Program, Expert Panel Report 3: *Guidelines for the Diagnosis and Management of Asthma*, NIH Publication 08-4051, Bethesda, Md., 2007, National Institutes of Health.
DPI, Dry powder inhaler; *ETT*, endotracheal tube; *MDI*, metered dose inhaler; *SVN*, small volume nebulizer.

the relative advantages and disadvantages of the available devices, can be used as the basis for choosing which type of device best matches a patient's needs. Age is an important factor to consider when selecting an aerosol delivery system. Age guidelines have been provided in the National Asthma Education and Prevention Program Expert Panel Report 3 (NAEPP EPR 3)[106] and are listed in Table 3-5. A consideration that applies to the final decision is discussed by Dolovich and colleagues.[69]

Patient-Device Interface

KEY POINT

The *patient-device interface* is another variable in aerosol delivery to the lung and includes *intermittent positive-pressure breathing (IPPB) administration; face mask administration;* and *delivery to intubated, ventilated patients*, which is complicated by numerous variables.

Most aerosol drug administration is by oral inhalation; that is, the subject inhales the aerosol through the open mouth. However, other types of interface occur in clinical practice and raise questions concerning efficacy and drug delivery. These include positive-pressure aerosol administration with a facemask and administration of aerosolized drugs through ETTs.

Administration by Intermittent Positive-Pressure Breathing

Although administration by intermittent positive-pressure breathing (IPPB) has been a popular form of aerosol therapy, the consensus of research on this method of delivery is that IPPB delivery of aerosolized medication is no more clinically effective than simple spontaneous, unassisted inhalation from SVNs.[107-109] Consequently, if the patient is able to breathe spontaneously without machine support, the use of IPPB for delivery of aerosolized drugs is not supported for general clinical or at-home use.

Face Mask and Blow-by Administration

Use of a facemask with an aerosol generator usually occurs with infants and young children or with debilitated, unresponsive patients. The clinical efficacy of a facemask in a pediatric application has been shown by Restrepo and colleagues[44] and by Lin, Restrepo, and Gardenhire.[110] Lowenthal and Kattan[111] compared facemask and mouthpiece delivery of nebulized albuterol in children and adolescents 6 to 19 years old for emergency department treatment of acute asthma. Their study found that facemask administration did not significantly improve lung function measures, even in subjects with nasal congestion. They speculated that congested nasal passages caused mouth breathing while using the mask. Greater tremor was observed with the facemask group, implying a higher systemic level of drug compared with patients using a mouthpiece.

Lung deposition of drug has also been measured for mouthpiece and facemask administration of aerosol drugs. Most of the available data are for infants and children because this age group is most likely to be treated with a facemask or blow-by for aerosol delivery. Because the use of a mask demonstrates questionable results the use of blow-by provides negligible results. Blow-by is not recommended for any use.[112]

Mechanical Ventilation Administration

Aerosolized drug delivery commonly occurs with intubated neonatal and adult patients during mechanical ventilation. Data quantifying the efficiency of aerosol administration during mechanical ventilation are summarized in a review by Gardenhire.[113] Evaluation of aerosol delivery is complicated by the number of variables introduced if the patient is receiving mechanical ventilation and by the difficulty in quantifying drug delivery accurately. Box 3-11 lists the many variables of administration of an aerosol drug through an ETT to ventilated subjects. The effect of some of these variables, with SVN, VMN, and MDI aerosol administration, has been investigated. The following list summarizes the state of knowledge presented by Gardenhire[113] and Duarte.[114]

- Spontaneous breathing modes provide more aerosol than other controlled ventilator modes.
- In an adult a minimum of 500 mL tidal volume is needed to provide efficacious aerosol delivery.
- The lower the flow the more effective the aerosol delivery.
- Sinusoidal and descending wave forms have better aerosol delivery than square forms.

- A heat and moisture exchanger (HME) should be bypassed when delivering aerosolized agents.
- Heat and humidity decrease aerosol particle delivery to the lungs.
- The literature makes note that a reduction in humidity may increase the number of inhaled particles, but because some nebulizers require a longer time to nebulize, disconnecting a circuit to bypass the humidifier could lead to increased risk of ventilator-associated pneumonia.
- The diameter of the tube plays a role in the impaction of aerosol particles. The narrower the tube (e.g., in pediatrics), the lower the percentage of drug that is delivered to the patient.
- The use of a less dense gas, such as a helium-oxygen mixture (heliox), can increase particle deposition.
- Both an MDI and nebulizer can be used effectively in administering inhaled agents to a patient receiving mechanical ventilation.
- To improve aerosol delivery, place a SVN after the humidifier, but as close to the ventilator and away from the circuit Y, instead of between the circuit Y and the ETT.
- VMNs can be placed before the humidifier.
- VMNs and MDIs are effective 6 inches from the circuit Y.
- When using an MDI, timing the actuation of the aerosol device with precise inspiration by the ventilator may increase drug delivery by 30%.
- The application of a breath-hold may provide additional drug delivery.

The use of HFA-MDIs may increase the amount of drug to the intubated patient. Mitchell and colleagues[115] found that the emitted dose of an HFA-MDI was almost 6 times more than that of a CFC-MDI.

BOX 3-11	Summary of Variables Present in Aerosol Delivery to Intubated, Mechanically Ventilated Critical Care Patients

Ventilator
- Nebulizer power system
- Duty cycle (flow, volume, rate)
- Inspiratory flow pattern
- Mode of ventilation
- Breath modifications (PEEP, inflation hold)
- Spontaneous, assisted, or controlled breaths
- Humidification and temperature
- Position of generator in circuit
- Size of endotracheal tube

Aerosol Generator
Small Volume and Vibrating Mesh Nebulizer
- Volume of fill
- Type of solution
- Brand of SVN
- Intraproduct reliability
- Continuous versus intermittent
- Flow rate

Metered Dose Inhaler
- Timing of actuation
- Use and design of reservoir device
- Type of drug used

PEEP, Positive end-expiratory pressure; *SVN,* small volume nebulizer.

? SELF-ASSESSMENT QUESTIONS

Answers can be found in Appendix A.

1. What are the three most common aerosol-generating devices used to deliver inhaled drugs?
2. Describe the inspiratory pattern you would instruct a patient to use with an MDI.
3. What are three advantages offered by a reservoir device used with an MDI?
4. Would a DPI be appropriate for a 3-year-old child with asthma?
5. What is meant by the term *dead volume* in an SVN?
6. What is the optimal filling volume and power gas flow rate to use with an SVN?
7. How does the electrostatic charge affect an MDI when used with a holding chamber?
8. Which device would be better to deliver a β agonist to an adult patient in the emergency department—SVN, MDI, or DPI?

CLINICAL SCENARIO

Answers can be found in Appendix A.

A 17-year-old boy with a history of allergic asthma is given a prescription for MDI albuterol, a bronchodilator used as a rescue agent. The HFA formulation of albuterol (Proventil HFA) is prescribed. After using the MDI a few times, the patient complains to you that he can feel that there is drug in the canister when he shakes it before using, but it feels as if "very little spray" is coming out when he inhales a puff. He believes the MDI is not functioning properly and that he is not getting the regular inhaled dose.

Using the SOAP method, assess this clinical scenario.

REFERENCES

1. Morrow P: An evaluation of the physical properties of monodisperse and heterodisperse aerosols used in the assessment of bronchial function. *Chest* 80:809, 1981.
2. Kohler D, Fleischer W: Established facts in inhalation therapy: a review of aerosol therapy and commonly used drugs. *Lung Respir* 6:1, 1989.
3. Morrow P: Aerosol characterization and deposition. *Am Rev Respir Dis* 110:88, 1974.
4. Lourenco R, Cotromanes E: Clinical aerosols. I. Characterization of aerosols and their diagnostic uses. *Arch Intern Med* 142:2163, 1982.
5. Hiller C, Mazumder M, Wilson D, et al: Aerodynamic size distribution of metered-dose bronchodilator aerosols. *Am Rev Respir Dis* 118:311, 1978.
6. Dolovich M: In vitro measurements of delivery of medications from MDIs and spacer devices. *J Aerosol Med* 9:S49, 1996.
7. Feddah M, Brown K, Gipps E, et al: In-vitro characterisation of metered dose inhaler versus dry powder inhaler glucocorticoid products: influence of inspiratory flow rates. *J Pharm Sci* 3:318, 2000.
8. Heyder J: Deposition of inhaled particles in the human respiratory tract and consequences for regional targeting in respiratory drug delivery. *Proc Am Thorac Soc* 1(4):315, 2004.
9. Yu C, Nicolaides P, Soong T: Effect of random airway sizes on aerosol deposition. *Am Ind Hyg Assoc J* 40(11):999, 1979.
10. Clark A, Gonda I, Newhouse M: Towards meaningful laboratory tests for evaluation of pharmaceutical aerosols. *J Aerosol Med* 11:S1, 1998.
11. Consensus Conference on Aerosol Delivery: Aerosol consensus statement. *Chest* 100:1991.
12. Clay M, Pavia D, Clarke S: Effect of aerosol particle size on bronchodilation with nebulised terbutaline in asthmatic subjects. *Thorax* 41:364, 1986.
13. Johnson M, Newman S, Bloom R, et al: Delivery of albuterol and ipratropium bromide from two nebulizer systems in chronic stable asthma: efficacy and pulmonary deposition. *Chest* 96:6, 1989.
14. Leach CL: The CFC to HFA transition and its impact on pulmonary drug development. *Respir Care* 50:1201, 2005.
15. Barnes P, Basbaum C, Nadel J: Autoradiographic localization of autonomic receptors in airway smooth muscle. *Am Rev Respir Dis* 127:1983.
16. Corkery K, Luce J, Montgomery A: Aerosolized pentamidine for treatment and prophylaxis of Pneumocystis carinii pneumonia: an update. *Respir Care* 33:676, 1988.
17. Newman S: Aerosol deposition considerations in inhalation therapy. *Chest* 88:152S, 1985.
18. Dolovich M: Physical principles underlying aerosol therapy. *J Aerosol Med* 2:171, 1989.
19. Smith G, Hiller C, Mazumder M, et al: Aerodynamic size distribution of cromolyn sodium at ambient and airway humidity. *Am Rev Respir Dis* 121:513, 1980.
20. Hiller F, Mazumder M, Smith G, et al: Physical properties, hygroscopicity and estimated pulmonary retention of various therapeutic aerosols. *Chest* 77:318, 1980.
21. Fuller H, Dolovich M, Chambers C, et al: Aerosol delivery during mechanical ventilation: a predictive in-vitro lung model. *J Aerosol Med* 5:251, 1992.
22. Newman S, Hollingworth A, Clark AR: Effect of different modes of inhalation on drug delivery from a dry powder inhaler. *Int J Pharm* 102:127, 1994.
23. Newman S, Woodman G, Clarke S, et al: Effect of InspirEase on the deposition of metered-dose aerosols in the human respiratory tract. *Chest* 89:551, 1986.
24. Lewis R, Fleming J: Fractional deposition from a jet nebulizer: how it differs from a metered-dose inhaler. *Br J Dis Chest* 79:361, 1985.
25. Fink JB: Aerosol drug therapy. In Kacmarek RM, Stoller JK, Heuer AJ, editors: *Egan's fundamentals of respiratory care*, St Louis, 2013, Mosby, p 844.
26. Fink JB: Humidity and aerosol therapy. In Cairo JM, editor: *Mosby's respiratory care equipment*, St Louis, 2014, Mosby, p 158.
27. Gardenhire DS, Ari A, Hess D, Myers TR: *A guide to aerosol delivery devices for respiratory therapists*, Dallas, TX, 2013, American Association for Respiratory Care.
28. Dennis JH: A review of issues relating to nebulizer standards. *J Aerosol Med* 11(Suppl 1):S73, 1998.
29. Welch MJ: Nebulization therapy for asthma: a practical guide for the busy pediatrician. *Clin Pediatr (Phila)* 47:744, 2008.
30. Rau JL, Ari A, Restrepo RD: Performance comparison of nebulizer designs: constant-output, breath-enhanced, and dosimetric. *Respir Care* 49:174, 2004.
31. Dhand R: Nebulizers that use a vibrating mesh or plate with multiple apertures to generate aerosol. *Respir Care* 47:1406, 2002.
32. Wigley F, Londono J, Wood S, et al: Insulin across respiratory mucosae by aerosol delivery. *Diabetes* 20:552, 1971.
33. Niven R, Ip A, Mittelman S, et al: Some factors associated with the ultrasonic nebulization of proteins. *Pharm Res* 12:53, 1995.
34. Dennis JH: Standardization issues: in vitro assessment of nebulizer performance. *Respir Care* 47:1445, 2002.
35. Hess D, Fisher D, Williams P, et al: Medication nebulizer performance: effects of diluent volume, nebulizer flow, and nebulizer brand. *Chest* 110:498, 1996.
36. Alvine GF, Rodgers P, Fitzsimmons KM, et al: Disposable jet nebulizers: how reliable are they? *Chest* 101:316, 1992.
37. Kradjan W, Lakshminarayan S: Efficiency of air compressor-driven nebulizers. *Chest* 87:512, 1985.
38. Shim C, Williams M: Effect of bronchodilator therapy administered by canister versus jet nebulizer. *J Allergy Clin Immunol* 73:387, 1984.
39. Rau J, Harwood R: Comparison of nebulizer delivery methods through a neonatal endotracheal tube: a bench study. *Respir Care* 37:1233, 1992.
40. Hess DR, Acosta FL, Ritz RH, et al: The effect of heliox on nebulizer function using a beta-agonist bronchodilator. *Chest* 115:184, 1999.
41. Kim IK, Saville AL, Sikes KL, et al: Heliox-driven albuterol nebulization for asthma exacerbations: an overview. *Respir Care* 51:613, 2006.
42. Corcoran TE, Gamard S: Development of aerosol drug delivery with helium oxygen gas mixtures. *J Aerosol Med* 17:299, 2004.
43. Nikander K, Agertoft L, Pedersen S: Breath-synchronized nebulization diminishes the impact of patient-device interfaces (face mask or mouthpiece) on the inhaled mass of nebulized budesonide. *J Asthma* 37:451, 2000.

44. Restrepo RD, Dickson SK, Rau JL, Gardenhire DS: An investigation of nebulized bronchodilator delivery using a pediatric lung model of spontaneous breathing. *Respir Care* 51:56, 2006.

45. O'Callaghan C, Barry PW: The science of nebulised drug delivery. *Thorax* 52(Suppl 2):S31, 1997.

46. Newman S, Pellow P, Clay M, et al: Evaluation of jet nebulisers for use with gentamicin solution. *Thorax* 40:671, 1985.

47. Stopping the spread of germs, Cystic Fibrosis Foundation, 2009.

48. Freedman T: Medihaler therapy for bronchial asthma: a new type of aerosol therapy. *Postgrad Med J* 20:667, 1956.

49. Varvaet C, Byron P: Drug-surfactant-propelled interaction in HFA formulations. *Int J Pharm* 186:13, 1999.

50. Newman SP: Principles of metered-dose inhaler design. *Respir Care* 50:1177, 2005.

51. Leach C: The CFC to HFA transition and its impact on pulmonary drug development. *Respir Care* 50:1201, 2005.

52. Donnell D: Development of a CFC-free glucocorticoid metered-dose aerosol system to optimize drug delivery to the lung. *Pharm Sci Technolo Today* 3:183, 2000.

53. Newman SP, Weisz AW, Talaee N, et al: Improvement of drug delivery with a breath actuated pressurised aerosol for patients with poor inhaler technique. *Thorax* 46:712, 1991.

54. Baum E, Bryant A: The development and laboratory testing of a novel breath-actuated pressurized inhaler. *J Aerosol Med* 1:219, 1988.

55. Gross G, Cohen RM, Guy H: Efficacy response of inhaled HFA-albuterol delivered via the breath-actuated Autohaler inhalation device is comparable to dose in patients with asthma. *J Asthma* 40:487, 2003.

56. Cyr T, Graham S, Li K, et al: Low first-spray drug content in albuterol metered-dose inhalers. *Pharm Res* 8:658, 1991.

57. Everard ML, Devadason SG, Summers QA, et al: Factors affecting total and "respirable" dose delivered by a salbutamol metered dose inhaler. *Thorax* 50:746, 1995.

58. Rubin BK, Durotoye L: How do patients determine that their metered-dose inhaler is empty? *Chest* 126:1134, 2004.

59. Heimer D, Shim C, Williams M: The effect of sequential inhalation of metaproterenol aerosol in asthma. *J Allergy Clin Immunol* 66:75, 1980.

60. Pedersen S: The importance of a pause between the inhalation of two puffs of terbutaline from a pressurised aerosol with a tube spacer. *J Allergy Clin Immunol* 77:505, 1986.

61. Pedersen S, Steffensen G: Simplification of inhalation therapy in asthmatic children: a comparison of two regimes. *Allergy* 41:296, 1986.

62. Schultz RK: Drug delivery characteristics of metered-dose inhalers. *J Allergy Clin Immunol* 96:284, 1995.

63. Ross D, Gabrio B: Advances in metered dose inhaler technology with the development of a chlorofluorocarbon-free drug delivery system. *J Aerosol Med* 12:151, 1999.

64. Niven RW, Kacmarek RM, Brain JD, et al: Small bore nozzle extensions to improve the delivery efficiency of drugs from metered dose inhalers: laboratory evaluation. *Am Rev Respir Dis* 147:1590, 1993.

65. Unzeitig JC, Richards W, Church JA: Administration of metered-dose inhalers: comparison of open- and closed-mouth techniques in childhood asthmatics. *Ann Allergy* 51:571, 1983.

66. Chhabra SK: A comparison of "closed" and "open" mouth techniques of inhalation of a salbutamol metered-dose inhaler. *J Asthma* 31:123, 1994.

67. Dolovich M, Ruffin RE, Roberts R, et al: Optimal delivery of aerosols from metered dose inhalers. *Chest* 80:911, 1981.

68. Lawford P, McKenzie D: Pressurized bronchodilator aerosol technique: influence of breath-holding time and relationship of inhaler to the mouth. *Br J Dis Chest* 76:229, 1982.

69. Dolovich MB, Ahrens RC, Hess DR, et al: Device selection and outcomes of aerosol therapy: evidence-based guidelines. American College of Chest Physicians/American College of Asthma, Allergy, and Immunology. *Chest* 127:335, 2005.

70. Ari A: Optimal delivery of aerosol drugs in the pediatric/neonatal patient populations. *AARC Times* 33:24, 2009.

71. McFadden ER, Jr: Improper patient techniques with metered dose inhalers: clinical consequences and solutions to misuse. *J Allergy Clin Immunol* 96:278, 1995.

72. Dolovich M: Spacer design II: holding chambers and valves. Oral presentation at the International Symposium on Spacer Devices. Horsham, PA: Drug Information Association, 1995.

73. Louca E, Leung K, Coates AL, et al: Comparison of three valved holding chambers for the delivery of fluticasone propionate-HFA to an infant face model. *J Aerosol Med* 19:160, 2006.

74. Rau JL: Practical problems with aerosol therapy in COPD. *Respir Care* 51:158, 2006.

75. Holt S, Holt A, Weatherall M, et al: Metered dose inhalers: a need for dose counters. *Respirology* 10:105, 2005.

76. Ogren R, Baldwin J, Simon R: How patients determine when to replace their metered dose inhalers. *Ann Allergy Asthma Immunol* 75:485, 1995.

77. Rubin B, Durotoye L: How do patients determine their metered-dose inhaler is empty? *Chest* 126:1134, 2004.

78. Sheth K, Wasserman RL, Lincourt WR, et al: Fluticasone propionate/salmeterol hydrofluoroalkane via metered-dose inhaler with integrated dose counter: performance and patient satisfaction. *Int J Clin Pract* 60:1218, 2006.

79. Simmons MS, Nides MA, Kleerup EC, et al: Validation of the Doser, a new device for monitoring metered-dose inhaler use. *J Allergy Clin Immunol* 102:409, 1998.

80. Julius SM, Sherman JM, Hendeles L: Accuracy of three electronic monitors for metered-dose inhalers. *Chest* 121:871, 2002.

81. Williams D: The dose external counting device. *Chest* 116:1499, 1999.

82. Hess DR: Aerosol delivery devices in the treatment of asthma. *Respir Care* 53:699, 2008.

83. Cain WT, Oppenheimer JJ: The misconception of using floating patterns as an accurate means of measuring the contents of metered-dose inhaler devices. *Ann Allergy Asthma Immunol* 87:417, 2001.

84. Brock TP, Wessell AM, Williams DM, et al: Accuracy of float testing for metered-dose inhaler canisters. *J Am Pharm Assoc (Wash)* 42:582, 2002.

85. Rau JL: The inhalation of drugs: advantages and problems. *Respir Care* 50:367, 2005.

86. Fuller R: The Diskus: a new multi-dose powder device-efficacy and comparison with Turbuhaler. *J Aerosol Med* 8:S11, 1995.

87. Ram F, Wright J, Brocklebank D, et al: Systematic review of clinical effectiveness of pressurised metered dose inhalers versus other hand held inhaler devices for delivering β2 agonist bronchodilators in asthma. *BMJ* 323:901, 2001.

88. Chapman K, Friberg K, Balter M, et al: Albuterol via Turbuhaler versus albuterol via pressurized metered-dose inhaler in asthma. *Ann Allergy Asthma Immunol* 78:59, 1997.

89. Hanania N, Wittman R, Kesten S, et al: Medical personnel's knowledge of and ability to use inhaling devices: metered-dose inhalers, spacing chambers, and breath-actuated dry powder inhalers. *Chest* 105:111, 1994.

90. Newman SP, Pavia D, Garland N, Clarke SW: Effects of various inhalation modes on the deposition of radioactive pressurized aerosols. *Eur J Respir Dis Suppl* 119:57, 1982.

91. Leach CL, Davidson PJ, Hasselquist BE, Boudreau RJ: Lung deposition of hydrofluoroalkane-134a beclomethasone is greater than that of chlorofluorocarbon fluticasone and chlorofluorocarbon beclomethasone: A cross over study in healthy volunteers. *Chest* 122:510, 2002.

92. Kim CS, Eldridge MA, Sackner MA: Oropharyngeal deposition and delivery aspects of metered-dose inhaler aerosols. *Am Rev Respir Dis* 135:157, 1987.

93. Lewis RA, Fleming JS: Fractional deposition from a jet nebulizer: how it differs from a metered dose inhaler. *Br J Dis Chest* 79:361, 1985.

94. Newman SP, Busse WW: Evolution of dry powder inhaler design, formulation and performance. *Respir Med* 96:293, 2002.

95. Newman SP, Moren F, Pavia D, et al: Deposition of pressurized suspension aerosols inhaled through extension devices. *Am Rev Respir Dis* 124:317, 1981.

96. Tarala RA, Madsen BW, Paterson JW: Comparative efficacy of salbutamol by pressurized aerosol and wet nebulizer in acute asthma. *Br J Clin Pharmacol* 10:393, 1980.

97. Blake KV, Hoppe M, Harman E, et al: Relative amount of albuterol delivered to lung receptors from a metered-dose inhaler and nebulizer solution. *Chest* 101:309, 1992.

98. Zainudin BM, Biddiscombe M, Tolfree SE, et al: Comparison of bronchodilator responses and deposition patterns of salbutamol inhaled from a pressurised metered dose inhaler, as a dry powder, and as a nebulised solution. *Thorax* 45:469, 1990.

99. Mestitz H, Copland JM, McDonald CF: Comparison of outpatient nebulized vs metered dose inhaler terbutaline in chronic airflow obstruction. *Chest* 96:1237, 1989.

100. Newhouse M, Dolovich M: Aerosol therapy: nebulizer vs metered dose inhaler (editorial). *Chest* 91:799, 1987.

101. Dolovich M: New propellant-free technologies under investigation. *J Aerosol Med* 12(Suppl 1):S9, 1999.

102. Newman SP, Brown J, Steed KP, et al: Lung deposition of fenoterol and flunisolide delivered using a novel device for inhaled medicines: Comparison of RESPIMAT with conventional metered-dose inhaler with and without spacer devices. *Chest* 113:957, 1998.

103. Leach CL, Davidson PJ, Boudreau RJ: Improved airway targeting with the CFC-free HFA-beclomethasone metered-dose inhaler compared with CFC-beclomethasone. *Eur Respir J* 12:1346, 1998.

104. Amirav I, Newhouse MT: Metered-dose inhaler accessory devices in acute asthma: efficacy and comparison with nebulizers: a literature review. *Arch Pediatr Adolesc Med* 151:876, 1997.

105. Turner MO, Patel A, Ginsburg S, et al: Bronchodilator delivery in acute airflow obstruction: a meta-analysis. *Arch Intern Med* 157:1736, 1997.

106. National Asthma Education and Prevention Program, National Heart, Lung, and Blood Institute, National Institutes of Health: *Expert Panel Report 3: Guidelines for the diagnosis and management of asthma*, NIH Publication 08-4051.Bethesda, Md., 2007, National Institutes of Health. Available at: <http://www.nhlbi.nih.gov/guidelines/asthma/asthgdln.htm>. Accessed August 2014.

107. Chester EH, Racz I, Barlow PB, et al: Bronchodilator therapy: comparison of acute response to three methods of administration. *Chest* 62:394, 1972.

108. Dolovich MB, Killian D, Wolff RK, et al: Pulmonary aerosol deposition in chronic bronchitis: intermittent positive pressure breathing versus quiet breathing. *Am Rev Respir Dis* 115:397, 1977.

109. Loren M, Chai H, Miklich D, et al: Comparison between simple nebulization and intermittent positive-pressure in asthmatic children with severe bronchospasm. *Chest* 72:145, 1977.

110. Lin H-L, Restrepo RD, Gardenhire DS: An in vitro investigation of nebulized albuterol delivery by pediatric aerosol facemasks to spontaneously breathing infants. *Respir Care* 50:1551, 2005.

111. Lowenthal D, Kattan M: Facemasks versus mouthpieces for aerosol treatment of asthmatic children. *Pediatr Pulmonol* 14:192, 1992.

112. Rubin BK: Bye-bye, blow-by (editorial). *Respir Care* 52(8):981, 2007.

113. Gardenhire DS: Aerosol delivery for the mechanical ventilation patient. *AARC Times* 37:11, 2013.

114. Duarte A: Inhaled bronchodilator administration during mechanical ventilation. *Respir Care* 49:623, 2004.

115. Mitchell JP, Nagel MW, Wiersema KJ, et al: The delivery of chlorofluorocarbon-propelled versus hydrofluoroalkane-propelled beclomethasone dipropionate aerosol to the mechanically ventilated patient: a laboratory study. *Respir Care* 48:1025, 2003.

116. Fok TF, Lam K, Ng PC, et al: Delivery of salbutamol to nonventilated preterm infants by metered-dose inhaler, jet nebulizer, and ultrasonic nebulizer. *Eur Respir J* 12:159, 1998.

117. Mandelberg A, Tsehori S, Houri S, et al: Is nebulized aerosol treatment necessary in the pediatric emergency department? Comparison with a metal spacer device for metered-dose inhaler. *Chest* 117:1309, 2000.

118. Lin YZ, Hsieh KH: Metered dose inhaler and nebuliser in acute asthma. *Arch Dis Child* 72:214, 1995.

119. Mandelberg A, Chen E, Noviski N, et al: Nebulized wet aerosol treatment in emergency department: is it essential? Comparison with large spacer device for metered-dose inhaler. *Chest* 112:1501, 1997.

CHAPTER **4**

Calculating Drug Doses

Douglas S. Gardenhire

OBJECTIVES

After reading this chapter, the reader will be able to:

1. Define key terms pertaining to calculating drug dose
2. Use the metric system
3. Calculate drug doses using proportions
4. Calculate drug doses using percentage-strength solutions

KEY TERMS AND DEFINITIONS

Percentage Part of the active ingredient that is in a solution containing 100 parts.

Schedule Amount of drug that is needed based on a patient's weight.

Solute Substance or active ingredient that is dissolved in a solution.

Solution Physically homogeneous mixture of two or more substances.

Solvent Substance, usually a liquid, that is used to make a solution.

Strength Amount of solute in a solution; usually expressed as a percentage.

Respiratory therapists are highly skilled health care providers who work in many different areas with other healthcare providers. Demonstrating a general knowledge of drug dosing has positive effects on all patients. Chapter 4 presents calculations of drug doses. Systems of measure are reviewed briefly. Dose calculations from prepared-strength formulations such as liquids, tablets, and capsules are presented with examples. Calculations of doses from solutions whose concentrations are expressed as percentage strength, along with intravenous dose calculations, are presented with examples. Practice problems and answers are included.

SYSTEMS OF MEASURE

Metric System

KEY POINT

Drug calculations use the metric system of measure.

Table 4-1 provides metric units of measures for length, volume, and weight. Primary units in the metric system are:

Length: Meter
Volume: Liter
Mass: Gram

TABLE 4-1	Metric System of Length, Volume, and Mass (Weight)

LENGTH

1 Kilometer (km)	=	10^3 meters	= 1000 meters
1 Hectometer (hm)	=	10^2 meters	= 100 meters
1 Decameter (dam)	=	10^1 meters	= 10 meters
1 Meter (m)		**Base Unit**	**1 meter**
1 Decimeter (dm)	=	10^{-1} meter	= 0.1 meter
1 Centimeter (cm)	=	10^{-2} meter	= 0.01 meter
1 Millimeter (mm)	=	10^{-3} meter	= 0.001 meter
1 Micrometer (µm)	=	10^{-6} meter	= 0.000001 meter

VOLUME (CAPACITY)

1 Kiloliter (kL)	=	10^3 liters	= 1000 liters
1 Hectoliter (hL)	=	10^2 liters	= 100 liters
1 Decaliter (daL)	=	10^1 liters	= 10 liters
1 Liter (L)		**Base Unit**	**1 liter**
1 Deciliter (dL)	=	10^{-1} liter	= 0.1 liter
1 Centiliter (cL)	=	10^{-2} liter	= 0.01 liter
1 Milliliter (mL)	=	10^{-3} liter	= 0.001 liter
1 Microliter (µL)	=	10^{-6} liter	= 0.000001 liter

MASS

1 Kilogram (kg)	=	10^3 grams	= 1000 grams
1 Hectogram (hg)	=	10^2 grams	= 100 grams
1 Decagram (dag)	=	10^1 grams	= 10 grams
1 Gram (g)		**Base Unit**	**1 gram**
1 Decigram (dg)	=	10^{-1} gram	= 0.1 gram
1 Centigram (cg)	=	10^{-2} gram	= 0.01 gram
1 Milligram (mg)	=	10^{-3} gram	= 0.001 gram
1 Microgram (mcg or µg)	=	10^{-6} gram	= 0.000001 gram
1 Nanogram (ng)	=	10^{-9} gram	= 0.000000001 gram
1 Picogram (pg)	=	10^{-12} gram	= 0.000000000001 gram

Fractional parts, or multiples of these primary (base) units, are expressed by adding Latin prefixes for sizes smaller than the primary unit and Greek prefixes for sizes larger than the primary unit. Examples of Latin and Greek prefixes found in Table 4-1 are as follows:

Decreasing prefixes (Latin):

Micro = 1/1,000,000
Milli = 1/1000
Centi = 1/100
Deci = 1/10

Increasing prefixes (Greek):

Deca = 10
Hecto = 100
Kilo = 1000

In calculating drug doses, the metric units for volume and mass (weight) are needed. A commonly encountered unit of volume in respiratory care pharmacology is the milliliter (mL), or 0.001 L. Common units of weight are kilogram (kg), gram (g), milligram (mg), and, with aerosolized drugs, microgram (µg or mcg). Blood levels of drug amounts within the body may be in nanograms per milliliter (ng/

mL). Conversions within the metric system should be familiar, such as converting 1 mg to 0.001 g, 500 mL to 0.5 L, or 0.4 mg to 400 mcg. Familiarity with decimal fractions and with the other basic rules of arithmetic are necessary for drug dose calculations.

A gram is defined as the weight of 1 mL of distilled water at 4° C in vacuo. Under these conditions, 1 g of water and 1 mL of water are equal. This should not be used to convert from weight to volume, however, because, depending on the temperature, pressure, and nature of the substance, 1 g of liquid is not always equal to 1 mL of liquid.

Although three different systems of measure have been used in drug calculations, metric units of measure are currently employed with formulations in the United States. Therefore all the examples in this chapter are based on the metric system.

International System of Units

KEY POINT

Volume and weight measures are commonly encountered in pharmacology.

The International System of Units, or *Système International d'Unités* (SI), was adopted in 1960 and is the modern metric system. The SI system is well presented by Chatburn[1] with conversion factors between older metric units for volume and the English system of measurement units. The SI system is based on the meter-kilogram-second (MKS) system, with volume as a derived unit of length. The primary units of interest in pharmacology calculations are as follows:

Mass: Kilogram (kg)
Volume: Cubic meter (m^3)

Although the base unit of measure in the SI system for volume is the cubic meter (m^3), the liter (L) and its fractions or multiples are currently accepted in measures of liquid volume:

Equivalence: 10^{-3} m^3 = 1 liter (L)

Household Units of Measure

KEY POINT

Household measures (e.g., teaspoon, tablespoon) are also used in administering medication.

In general, the metric system of measure is used for drug amounts. However, household measures such as teaspoons or tablespoons are used for administering medications in the home environment. For example, a cough syrup may have a label giving a usual adult dose as "1 teaspoon every 6 hours." Household measures are inconsistent—a teaspoon may vary from 3 to 5 mL. Although the metric system, which is more exact and consistent with milligrams, micrograms, and milliliters, is recommended in place of household measures, the following equivalences may be helpful. Use of household measures, such as teaspoons, can be very helpful in discussing amounts of substance with a patient.

1 teaspoon = 5 mL = 60 drops
1 tablespoon = 15 mL = 3 teaspoons
1 cup = 240 mL = 8 fluid ounces

CALCULATING DOSES FROM PREPARED-STRENGTH SOLUTIONS

 KEY POINT

The two types of drug calculations include prepared-strength doses and doses from solutions with a concentration expressed as a percentage.

Once the clinician is able to convert freely within the metric system, it is possible to begin calculating drug doses. Calculations generally are of the following two types:

1. Those involving fluids, tablets, or capsules of a given strength (e.g., 5 mg/mL)
2. Those involving solutions of a percentage strength (e.g., 0.5 mL of a 0.5% solution)

Each type of dose calculation is described separately.

Calculating With Proportions

When using a prepared-strength liquid, tablet, or capsule, you need to determine how much liquid or how many tablets or capsules are required to give the amount, or dose, of the drug ordered. For example, if one tablet of a drug contains 5 mg, and you want to give 2.5 mg, half a tablet must be given. The simplest and probably the most accurate, error-free method of calculation when using a vial of a prepared-strength drug (or a tablet or capsule) involves two steps:

1. Convert to consistent units of measure.
2. Set up a straightforward proportion:

$$\frac{\text{Original dose}}{\text{Per amount}} = \frac{\text{Desired dose}}{\text{Per amount}}$$

In step 1, this conversion may be from grams to milligrams within the metric system or from apothecary to metric, if an apothecary dosage strength has been ordered. In step 2, set up the straightforward proportion. Ultimately you will be solving for an unknown, or x.

EXAMPLE 1

You have tablets of a drug, each 250 mg in strength. If the patient needs 0.5 g of the drug, how many tablets should be administered?

Solution: If you need 0.5 g of the drug, either convert 250 mg to 0.25 g or convert 0.5 g to 500 mg (preferred). Once the units are consistent, set up the proportion to find the

unknown—that is, the number of tablets needed to deliver the desired dose to the patient. Using the preceding formula,

Original drug dose = 250 mg
Per amount = per tablet
Desired drug dose = 0.5 g = 500 mg
Per amount = unknown

$$\frac{250 \text{ mg}}{1 \text{ tab}} = \frac{500 \text{ mg}}{x \text{ tab}}$$

$$\frac{250 \times x}{250} = \frac{500 \times 1}{250}$$

$$x \text{ tab} = \frac{500}{250}$$

$$x = 2 \text{ tablets}$$

ANSWER

The amount required is two tablets.

Although this calculation is trivially clear and can be performed mentally, others may require calculation for the sake of accuracy.

EXAMPLE 2

You have 120 mg of a drug in 30 mL of elixir. How many milliliters of elixir will you use to give a 15-mg dose?

Solution:

$$\frac{120 \text{ mg}}{30 \text{ mL}} = \frac{15 \text{ mg}}{x}$$

Cross-multiplying:

$$120 \text{ mg}(x) = 450$$

Divide both sides by 120 to isolate x:

$$\frac{120 x}{120} = \frac{450}{120}$$

$$x \text{ mL} = 3.75 \text{ mL}$$

ANSWER

The amount required is 3.75 mL.

Simplification is possible, such as reducing 120 mg/30 mL to 4 mg/mL. Then, knowing that there are 4 mg in every milliliter, simply divide 4 mg/mL into 15 mg to determine how many milliliters are needed. Reducing a liquid to its dosage strength per 1 mL often allows quick mental computation of the dose. Caution and care should be observed in the initial reduction however. An error at that point causes a subsequent dosage error. *Do not hesitate to write out a calculation:* In a busy clinical setting, a patient's well-being should take precedence over a practitioner's mathematical pride.

Drug Amounts in Units

 KEY POINT

Prepared-strength doses involve calculating how many tablets, capsules, or milliliters of a liquid are needed to administer a given amount of a drug and are most easily calculated using a proportion after units are made consistent as follows:

$$\frac{\text{Original dose}}{\text{Per amount}} = \frac{\text{Desired dose}}{\text{Per amount}}$$

Some drugs are manufactured in units (U) rather than in grams or milligrams. Examples are penicillin, insulin, and heparin. Solving dose problems for these drugs is exactly the same as for the other dosage units previously mentioned.

EXAMPLE 3

A brand of sodium heparin is available as 1000 U/mL. How many milliliters do you need for 500 U of the drug?

Solution: Utilizing (Original dose)/(Per amount) = (desired dose)/(per amount)

$$1000 \text{ U}/1 \text{ mL} = 500 \text{ U}/x \text{ mL}$$

Set up the proportion in the prepared strength formula. By cross-multiplying, we obtain:

$$1000 (x) = 500$$

Divide both sides by 1000 to isolate x:

$$\frac{1000 (x)}{1000} = \frac{500}{1000}$$
$$x \text{ mL} = 0.5 \text{ mL}$$

ANSWER

The amount required for 500 U, given the prepared-strength liquid, is 0.5 mL.

There is no universal equivalence between units as a measure of amount and the metric weight system. Units are used with biologic standardization and are defined for each drug by a standard preparation of that drug when the drug is measured in units. For example, there is a standard preparation of digitalis consisting of dried, powdered digitalis leaves; 100 mg of this preparation equals 1 United States Pharmacopeia (USP) unit of activity. In this way when drugs are extracted from animals, plants, or minerals, there is a standard reference preparation. Note that 100 mg is not 1 U for every drug with units; for example, insulin has a standard preparation of 0.04 mg = 1 U. When a drug is isolated as a pure chemical form, either extracted as the active substance in a natural source or synthesized in the laboratory, biologic standardization based on a standard preparation from the natural source is no longer necessary. The specific chemical amount is given in metric weight or volume measure.

Calculations With a Dosage Schedule

Sometimes the dose of a drug must be obtained from a **schedule**, which may be based on the size of a person. For example, a suggested schedule for albuterol syrup in children 2 to 6 years old is 0.1 mg/kg of body weight. This means that the *dose* must be calculated after the body weight is obtained, and then the amount of the drug preparation needed for treatment can be calculated.

EXAMPLE 4

Using a schedule of 0.1 mg/kg for albuterol syrup and a prepared-strength mixture of 2 mg/5 mL, how much of the syrup is needed for a 20-kg child?

Solution:
Calculate the dose needed:
Dose = 0.1 mg/kg × 20 kg = 2.0 mg
or

$$\frac{0.1 \text{ mg}}{1 \text{ kg}} = \frac{x}{20 \text{ kg}}$$

Next, calculate the amount of the preparation by cross-multiplying and solving for x:

$$\frac{2 \text{ mg}}{5 \text{ mL}} = \frac{2 \text{ mg}}{x \text{ mL}}$$

Simplifying,

$$2(x) = 10$$
$$x \text{ mL} = 5 \text{ mL}$$

ANSWER

This 20-kg child needs 5 mL of albuterol syrup.

Additional Examples: Prepared-Strength Drugs

EXAMPLE 5

An injectable solution of glycopyrrolate with a prepared strength of 0.2 mg/mL is used for nebulization. How many milliliters are needed for a 1.5-mg dose?

Solution:
Original dose per amount: 0.2 mg/mL
Desired dose: 1.5 mg
Amount needed: x mL
Substituting:

$$\frac{0.2 \text{ mg}}{1 \text{ mL}} = \frac{1.5 \text{ mg}}{x \text{ mL}}$$

Using cross-multiplication to simplify:

$$0.2 \text{ mg}(x) = 1.5 \text{ mg}(1 \text{ mL})$$
$$x = \frac{1.5}{0.2}$$
$$x \text{ mL} = 7.5 \text{ mL}$$

ANSWER

An amount of 7.5 mL will contain the desired dose of 1.5 mg, using the prepared strength given.

EXAMPLE 6

You have 1 mg/mL of terbutaline in an ampule for injection. How much do you need to give a 0.25-mg dose subcutaneously?

Solution:

Original dose per amount: 1 mg/mL
Desired dose: 0.25 mg
Amount needed: x mL
Substituting:

$$\frac{1\ mg}{1\ mL} = \frac{0.25\ mg}{x\ mL}$$

Solving for x:

$$1\ mg\,(x\ mL) = 0.25\ mg\,(1\ mL)$$
$$x = 0.25\ mL$$

ANSWER

Give 0.25 mL for the desired dose of 0.25 mg.

EXAMPLE 7

A dosage schedule for a surfactant (see Chapter 10) calls for 5 mL/kg of body weight. If a premature infant weighs 1200 g, how many milliliters are needed?

Solution:

Convert body weight to kilograms:

$$1\ kg/1000\ g \times 1200\ g = 1.2\ kg$$

Multiply the weight in kilograms by the schedule of 5 mL/kg:

$$x\ mL = 1.2\ kg \times 5\ mL/kg = 6\ mL$$

ANSWER

Based on the dosage schedule and weight, 6 mL should be given.

EXAMPLE 8

The prepared strength of a drug is 100 mg/4 mL. The dosage schedule is 100 mg/kg of birth weight. A premature newborn weighs 1100 g. Based on the weight of the newborn, what dose is needed? How many milliliters of the drug should be given to achieve this dose?

Solution: To determine the dose that is needed, perform two steps:

Convert the birth weight to kilograms:

$$1\ kg/1000\ g \times 1100\ g = 1.1\ kg$$

Multiply the birth weight by the dosage schedule to find the dose required:

$$x\ mg = 100\ mg/kg \times 1.1\ kg = 110\ mg$$

The dose needed is 110 mg of drug.

Solution: To find the number of milliliters required to achieve this dose:

Original dose per amount: 100 mg/4 mL
Desired dose: 110 mg
Amount needed: x mL
Substituting:

$$\frac{100\ mg}{4\ mL} = \frac{110\ mg}{x\ mL}$$
$$100\ mg\,(x) = 110\ mg\,(4\ mL)$$
$$x = [110\ mg\,(4\ mL)]/100$$
$$x = 4.4\ mL$$

ANSWER

Based on the dosage schedule, the weight of the newborn, and the prepared strength, 4.4 mL will give the needed dose of 110 mg.

CALCULATING DOSES FROM PERCENTAGE-STRENGTH SOLUTIONS

 KEY POINT

Calculating doses based on a percentage-strength concentration of a solution can be done with the following equation:

$$\text{Percent strength (in decimals)} = \frac{\text{Solute (in grams or cubic centimeters)}}{\text{Total amount (solute and solvent)}}$$

Because an area of expertise for respiratory therapists is solutions for aerosolization, solutions and percentage strengths often are needed to calculate a drug dose. A **solution** contains a **solute**, which is dissolved in a **solvent**, giving a homogeneous mixture. The **strength** of a solution is expressed as the percentage of solute relative to total solvent and solute. **Percentage** means parts of the active ingredient (solute) in a preparation contained in 100 parts of the total preparation (solute *and* solvent).

Types of Percentage Preparations
Weight to Weight

Percent in weight (W/W) expresses the number of grams of a drug or active ingredient in 100 g of a mixture:

W/W: Grams per 100 g of mixture

Weight to Volume

Percent may be expressed as the number of grams of a drug or active ingredient in 100 mL of a mixture:

W/V: Grams per 100 mL of mixture

Volume to Volume

Percent volume in volume (V/V) expresses the number of milliliters of drug or active ingredient in 100 mL of a mixture:

V/V: Milliliters per 100 mL of mixture

Solutions by Ratio

When diluting a medication for use in an aerosol or intermittent positive-pressure breathing (IPPB) treatment, a solute to solvent ratio is frequently given (e.g., epinephrine 1 : 100).

Ratio by Grams to Milliliters

In the preceding example, the following is indicated:

$$1 \text{ g per 200 mL of solution} = \frac{1 \text{ g}}{200 \text{ mL}} = 0.005 \times 100 = 0.5\%$$

(Multiplying by 100 is the same as moving the decimal *two* places to the *right*).

This ratio is what is indicated with traditional examples such as epinephrine 1 : 100, which is a 1% strength solution:

$$\frac{1 \text{ g}}{100 \text{ mL}} = 0.01 \times 100 = 1\%$$

Ratio by Simple Parts

In the following parts-to-parts example, actual parts of medication to parts of solvent are indicated:

$$1 : 8 = 1 \text{ part to 8 parts, which is the same as } \tfrac{1}{4} \text{ cc to 2 cc}$$

Part-to-part ratios do not indicate actual amounts or specific units, although usually milliliters to milliliters is meant. It is assumed you know that $\frac{1}{4}$ or $\frac{1}{2}$ cc of an agent is given as the usual dose and not 1 cc. An order such as 1 : 8 is not precise—without further specifications—about the amount of a drug (e.g., whether 0.25 mL or 0.5 mL) to be given.

Solving Percentage-Strength Solution Problems

For solutions in which the active ingredient itself is pure (undiluted, 100% strength), the following equation can be used:

EQUATION 1

Percent strength (in decimals) =

$$\frac{\text{Solute (in gram or cubic centimeters)}}{\text{Total amount (solute and solvent)}}$$

Alternatively, a ratio format can be used:

EQUATION 2

$$\frac{\text{Amount of solute}}{\text{Total amount}} = \frac{\text{Amount of solute}}{100 \text{ parts (grams or cubic centimeters)}}$$

When the active ingredient, or solute, is already diluted and less than pure, the following equation can be used:

EQUATION 3

Percent strength (in decimals) =

$$\frac{(\text{Dilute solute}) \times (\text{Percent strength of solute})}{\text{Total amount (solution)}}$$

In Equation 3, the solute (active ingredient) multiplied by the percent strength gives the amount of pure active ingredient in the dilute solution. This equation adds only one modification to the formula given in Equation 1: multiplying the dilute solute by its actual percentage strength, with the result indicating the amount of active ingredient at a 100% (pure) strength. For example, 10 mL of 10% solute means you have 1 mL of pure (100%) solute. Put another way, you would need 10 mL of dilute solute to have 1 mL of pure solute (active ingredient). When used in Equation 3, the unknown is usually how much of the dilute solute, or active ingredient, is needed in the total solution to give the desired strength. The preceding equations are illustrated in the following two examples.

 KEY POINT

Move the decimal point to convert easily between grams, percent strength, and milligrams per milliliter. If beginning with percent strength (e.g., 1%), move the decimal *one* place to the *right* to convert to milligrams per milliliter (e.g., 1% = 1.0% = 10 mg/mL). If beginning with percent strength (e.g., 10%), move the decimal *two* places to the *left* to convert to grams (e.g., 10% = 10.0% = 0.10 g).

EXAMPLE 9

Undiluted active ingredient: How many milligrams of active ingredient are there in 2 cc of 1 : 200 isoproterenol?

Solution:

Percent strength: 1 : 200 = 0.5% = 0.005
Total amount of solution: 2 cc
Active ingredient: *x*
Substituting in Equation 1:

$$0.005 = \boldsymbol{x} \textbf{ g}/2 \textbf{ cc}$$
$$\boldsymbol{x} \textbf{ g} = 0.005 \times 2$$
$$\boldsymbol{x} \textbf{ g} = 0.01 \textbf{ g}$$

ANSWER

Converting 0.01 g to milligrams gives 10 mg. In 2 cc of 1:200 solution, there are 10 mg of isoproterenol.

Alternative Solution:

Percent strength: 1:200

$$\frac{1}{200} = 0.005 \text{ g}$$

Move the decimal point *two* places to the *right* (i.e., mathematically multiply by 100) and add a percent sign. At this point, the number changes from grams to a percent solution:

$$0.005 \text{ g} = 000.5 = 0.5\%$$

or

$$0.005 \text{ g} = 0.005 \times 100 = 0.5\%$$

Move the decimal point an additional *one* place (for a total of *three* places, i.e., mathematically multiply by 1000) to convert from percent strength to milligrams per milliliter:

$$0.5\% = 5 = 5 \text{ mg/mL}$$

or

$$0.005 \text{ g} = 0.005 \times 1000 = 5 \text{ mg/mL}$$

The question asks how many milligrams of active ingredients are in 2 cc. If we remember that 1 cc = 1 mL and we know there are 5 mg in every 1 mL, we then multiply by 2 cc to obtain the answer: 10 mg/2 cc. (If you need to set up the equation, refer to the earlier section Calculating With Proportions.)

EXAMPLE 10

Diluted active ingredient: How much 20% acetylcysteine is needed to prepare 5 cc of 10% acetylcysteine?

Solution: Using the equation for dilute active ingredients (here the acetylcysteine is only 20% strength, not pure), the following is obtained:

Desired percent strength (in decimals): 10% = 0.10
Total amount of solution: 5 cc
Percent strength of solute (active ingredient): 20% = 0.20
Dilute solute (i.e., amount of active ingredient needed): x
Substituting in Equation 3:

$$0.10 = x(0.20)/5 \text{ cc}$$

$$x = 5(0.10)/0.20$$

$$x = 2.5 \text{ cc of 20% } \textbf{Mucomyst}$$

ANSWER

The 2.5 cc of 20% acetylcysteine is then mixed with 2.5 cc of normal saline to give a total of 5 cc of solution. This 5 cc will be a 10% strength solution.

Although diluting a 20% solution to a 10% solution is obviously a "half-and-half" procedure and does not require the use of an equation, less intuitive dilutions may need to be calculated. The reader might try diluting 20% acetylcysteine to obtain 5 cc of a 5% strength solution, using the preceding approach.

Alternative Solution: Convert 10% to 100 mg/mL by moving the decimal *one* place to the *right* (think of it as 10.0%, move one place, drop the percent sign and add mg/mL, and it becomes 100 mg/mL; or change the percent to a decimal and multiply by 1000 (10% = 0.10 × 1000 = 100 mg/mL). The question really asks how many milligrams are in 5 cc of 10% acetylcysteine? That is easy: We already know there are 100 mg for every 1 cc of drug, so multiply 100 mg × 5 cc, equaling 500 mg. This is the desired dose, and the original dose is 20%, or 200 mg/mL. Set up the proportions equation (refer to the earlier section, Calculating With Proportions):

Original dose per amount: 200 mg/1 mL
Desired dose: 500 mg
Amount desired: x mL
Substituting:

$$\frac{200 \text{ mg}}{1 \text{ mL}} = \frac{500 \text{ mg}}{x \text{ mL}}$$

Cross-multiply:

$$\frac{200 \text{ mg}(x \text{ mL})}{200 \text{ mg}} = \frac{500 \text{ mg}(1 \text{ mL})}{200 \text{ mg}}$$

$$x = 2.5 \text{ cc of 20% } \textbf{Mucomyst}$$

Answer

The 2.5 cc of the 20% acetylcysteine is then mixed with 2.5 cc of normal saline to give a total solution volume of 5 cc. This 5 cc will be a 10% strength solution. The key is to know the amount of milligrams of drug that is ordered. There is no difference between 5 cc of 10% strength solution and 2.5 cc of 20% solution. They both equal what is ultimately desired—500 mg of the drug.

Summary

Calculations with solutions of drugs, using percentage strengths, can be summarized into four important points:

1. Convert to metric units and decimal expressions.
2. Substitute known entities in the appropriate equation (undilute or dilute active ingredient).
3. Use grams or milliliters in the percentage equation.
4. Express the answer in the units requested.

Quantity Sufficient (qs)

When mixing solutions, determine the amount of active ingredient needed for the percent strength desired and then add enough solvent to "top off" to the total solution amount needed. When ordering a solution, the total needed is indicated by *quantity sufficient (qs)*. For example, to obtain

30 cc of 3% procaine HCl, we calculate 0.9 cc of the active ingredient and add water qs for 30 cc of solution. Do not merely give the difference between solute and total solution (30 cc − 0.9 cc = 29.1 cc), because certain solutes can change volume (e.g., alcohol "shrinks" in water).

Percentage Strengths in Milligrams per Milliliter

The basic definition of percentage strength in solutions involves grams or milliliters. However, the amount of active ingredient in most nebulized drug solutions is in milligrams. A useful and easily remembered clinical reference is to define percentage strengths in terms of milligrams per single milliliter, using a 1% strength reference point. Recall that 1% strength is 1 g/100 mL. Using Equation 1 for percentage strength, you have:

$$0.01 = \frac{1\,g}{100\,mL}$$

For 1 mL of a 1% strength solution, you would have:

$$0.01 = \frac{x\,g}{1\,mL}$$

$$x\,g = 0.01\,g$$

and 0.01 g × 1000 mg/g = 10 mg.

Because 0.01 g equals 10 mg, you have 10 mg/mL in a 1% solution. The 1% strength is an easily learned reference point. Table 4-2 lists some common percentage strengths, giving amounts in milligrams per milliliter, in reference to the 1% concentration.

Note the relationship of 1% to 10%: If there are 10 mg/mL in a 1% solution, there would be 10 times that amount in a 10% solution, or 100 mg/mL. Likewise, a 0.5% solution has one half as much active ingredient as a 1% solution—one half of 10 mg/mL would be 5 mg/mL. This amount of 5 mg/mL could have been used to solve Example 9, an undiluted active ingredient percentage problem. In Example 9, it was found that a 1:200 solution (a 0.5% strength solution) has 10 mg in 2 mL, which is the same as 5 mg in 1 mL.

TABLE 4-2	Drug Amounts in Milligrams per Milliliter for Common Percentage Strengths
PERCENTAGE STRENGTH (%)	**DRUG AMOUNT (mg/mL)**
20	200
10	100
5	50
1	**10**
0.5	5
0.1	1
0.05	0.5

Note: Starting with percentage strength, move the decimal *one* place to the *right* and it becomes a drug amount.

KEY POINT

An easy reference point for the amount of drug contained in a solution, in milligrams per milliliter, is 1% strength, which is 10 mg/mL.

Equations 1 and 3 (above) should be memorized; they represent a more general statement of percentage strengths for solving any problem. However, knowledge of milligrams per milliliter for a 1% solution can be very helpful in many problems to know how many milligrams of the active ingredient are being given. Examples of drug solutions with the strengths listed in Table 4-2 can be given. Albuterol is available as a 0.5% solution or 5 mg/mL, and an ampule of terbutaline (1 mg/cc) is a 0.1% strength solution.

You can easily convert from gram to percent strength to milligrams per milliliter by simply moving the decimal point—no math is needed. *Or,* mathematically, multiply the amount of grams by 1000 to achieve milligrams (0.001 g × 1000 = 1 mg). This math works for any drug expressed as grams, percent strength, or milligrams per milliliter. Using the preceding example:

$$0.001\,g = 0.1\% = 1\,mg/mL$$

Move the decimal point *two* places to the *right* to convert from grams to percent strength. From a percent-strength amount, move the decimal *one* place to the *right* to convert to milligrams per milliliter.

This process can be reversed:

$$50\,mg/mL = 5\% = 0.05\,g$$

If you begin with milligrams per milliliter, move the decimal point *one* place to the *left* to convert to percent strength. From a percent strength, move the decimal point *two* places to the *left* to convert to grams.

Diluents and Drug Doses

A common misconception persists that the amount of diluent added to a liquid drug to be aerosolized by nebulization is intended to "weaken" the dose or strength delivered to the patient. The amount of diluent affects the time required to nebulize a given solution but not the amount of active ingredient in a nebulizer reservoir. Whether it is diluted with 2 cc or 10 cc of normal saline, ½ cc of a 1% drug solution has the same amount (5 mg) of active ingredient. Practicality dictates that 2.5 cc of solution nebulizes in a reasonable time limit of 10 minutes or so, whereas 10 cc may take much longer. The diluent also is needed because disposable nebulizers cannot create an aerosol with less than approximately 1 mL of solution in the reservoir (the dead volume). Theoretically, given a suitable nebulizing device, there is no reason that the original 0.5 cc of 1% drug could not be nebulized undiluted to deliver the dose of 5 mg. The amount of the active ingredient, determined by the percentage strength and quantity in cubic centimeters of the drug, gives a dose amount. Although technically the percentage strength of the resulting solution in the reservoir is weaker, the dose remains unchanged at 5 mg. It is the dose in milligrams that should be of concern to the clinician.

Additional Examples: Solutions

EXAMPLE 11

How many milligrams of active ingredient are in 3 cc of a 2% solution of procaine HCl?

Solution: Use the percentage formula of Equation 1 for a pure-strength ingredient:

$$\text{Percent strength (in decimals)} = \frac{\text{Solute}}{\text{Total amount}}$$

Convert the percentage to decimals and substitute the known values:

$$0.02 = \frac{x \text{ g}}{3 \text{ cc}}$$

$$0.02(3 \text{ cc}) = x \text{ g}$$

$$x \text{ g} = 0.06 \text{ g}$$

In milligrams:

$$0.06 \text{ g} \times 1000 \text{ mg/g} = 60 \text{ mg}$$

ANSWER

In 3 cc of a 2% solution of procaine HCl, there is 60 mg of active ingredient.

Alternative Solution: Moving the decimal can easily convert to milligrams per milliliter. If we think of 2% as 2.0% and move the decimal *one* place to the *right,* we convert the percent to 20 mg/mL. Remember that 1 mL equals 1 cc, so if we need to find how many milligrams of active ingredient are in 3 cc of solution, we simply multiply 3 cc by 20 mg/mL to equal 60 mg. The reader can use the proportions equation to confirm:

$$\frac{20 \text{ mg}}{1 \text{ mL}} = \frac{x}{3 \text{ cc}}$$

Cross-multiply and solve for *x:*

$$x(1 \text{ mL}) = 20 \text{ mg}(3 \text{ cc})$$

$$x = 60 \text{ mg}$$

EXAMPLE 12

A resident wants to dilute 20% acetylcysteine to a strength of 6% for a research study. How many milliliters of 20% drug solution are needed to have 10 mL of 6% strength?

Solution: Use the modified Equation 3 for dilute active ingredient:

Percent strength (decimals) =

$$\frac{\text{(Dilute solution)} \times \text{(Percent strength of solute)}}{\text{Total amount (solution)}}$$

Percent strength desired: 6% = 0.06
Dilute solute: unknown = *x* mL
Percent strength: 20% = 0.20
Total amount of solution: 10 mL
Substituting and solving:

$$0.06 = \frac{(x \text{ mL}) \times (0.20)}{10 \text{ mL}}$$

$$0.06(10 \text{ mL}) = x \text{ mL}(0.20)$$

$$x = 0.06(10)/0.20$$

$$\boldsymbol{x \text{ mL} = 3 \text{ mL}}$$

ANSWER

Draw up 3 mL of the 20% strength and add saline qs for a total of 10 mL. Check your calculation for correctness: 3 mL of 20% strength solution has 600 mg of active ingredient (20% = 200 mg/mL); 600 mg is 0.6 g, and 0.6 g/10 mL (or 6 g/100 mL) is a 6% strength. You obtained the needed amount of drug with 3 mL of the 20% solution.

Alternative Solution: First, we convert the needed amount of drug. The resident asks for 10 mL at 6% strength, so we convert 6% to 60 mg/mL by moving the decimal *one* place to the *right.* If we need 10 mL, then we multiply 10 mL × 60 mg, which equals 600 mg. We now know the resident needs 600 mg of drug. How do we know how much of the 20% strength is needed? We convert 20% to 200 mg/mL and set up the equation as a proportion (original dose/per amount = desired dose/per amount).

$$\frac{200 \text{ mg}}{1 \text{ mL}} = \frac{600 \text{ mg}}{x}$$

Cross-multiply and solve for *x:*

$$\frac{200 \text{ mg}(x)}{200 \text{ mg}} = \frac{600 \text{ mg}(1 \text{ mL})}{200 \text{ mg}}$$

$$x = 3 \text{ mL}$$

EXAMPLE 13

The usual dose of albuterol sulfate is 0.5 mL of a 0.5% strength solution. How many milligrams is this?

Solution: Using Equation 1 for percentage strength:
Percentage in decimals: 0.5% = 0.005
Active ingredient: unknown *(x)*
Total solution: 0.5 mL
Substituting:

$$0.005 = \frac{x \text{ g}}{0.5 \text{ mL}}$$

$$x = 0.005(0.5) = 0.0025 \text{ g}$$

Converting:

$$0.0025 \text{ g} = 2.5 \text{ mg}$$

ANSWER

There is 2.5 mg of active ingredient in the usual dose.
   Alternative Solution: First we need to convert the percent solution to milligrams per milliliter. To do this, move the decimal *one* place to the *right* to convert to milligrams per milliliter (0.5% = 5 mg/mL). If we know that there are 5 mg in 1 mL and we need 0.5 mL, all we need to do is halve 5 mg, which is 2.5 mg.

EXAMPLE 14

Albuterol sulfate is also available as a unit dose of 3 mL at a percentage strength of 0.083%. If the entire amount of 3 mL is given, is this the same as the usual dose of 2.5 mg?
   Solution: Using Equation 1 for percentage strength:
Percent strength (in decimals): 0.083% = 0.00083
Active ingredient: unknown = x
Total amount of solution: 3 mL
Substituting:

$$0.00083 = \frac{x \text{ g}}{3 \text{ mL}}$$

$$x \text{ g} = 3(0.00083) = 0.00249 \text{ g}$$

and 0.00249 g = 2.49 mg

ANSWER

The result is approximately 2.5 mg, the usual dose.
   Alternative Solution: First, we need to convert 0.083% to milligrams per milliliter. To do this, we move the decimal *one* place to the *right* to convert to milligrams per milliliter (0.083% = 0.83 mg/mL). Set up the proportions equation and solve for *x*:

$$\frac{0.83 \text{ mg}}{1 \text{ mL}} = \frac{x}{3 \text{ ml}}$$

$$0.83 (3) = x$$

$$2.49 = x$$

Rounding up, we obtain 2.5 mg.

EXAMPLE 15

Terbutaline sulfate is available as 1 mg per 1 mL of solution. What percentage strength is this?
   Solution: Convert 1 mg to 0.001 g (1 mg × 1 g/1000 mg = 0.001 g). Then,

$$x = \frac{0.001 \text{ g}}{1 \text{ mL}}$$

$$x = 0.001 = 0.1\%$$

ANSWER

The percentage strength is 0.1%.
   Alternative Solution: This is straightforward; all we need to do is remember to move the decimal *one* place to the *left*. This will convert to percent strength (1 mg/mL = 0.1%).

? SELF-ASSESSMENT QUESTIONS

Answers can be found in Appendix A.

Prepared-Strength Dose Calculations

1. A bottle is labeled Demerol (meperidine) 50 mg/cc. How many cubic centimeters are needed to give a 125-mg dose?
2. An agent comes as 500 mg/10 mL. How many milliliters are needed to give a 150-mg dose?
3. Hyaluronidase comes as 150 U/cc. How many cubic centimeters are needed for a 30-U dose?
4. Morphine sulfate 4 mg is ordered; you have a vial with 10 mg/mL. How much do you need?
5. A dosage schedule for the surfactant poractant calls for 2.5 mL/kg birth weight. How much of the drug will you need for an infant weighing 800 g?
6. Diphenhydramine (Benadryl) elixir contains 12.5 mg of diphenhydramine HCl in each 5 mL of elixir. How many milligrams are there in a ½ teaspoonful dose (1 tsp = 5 mL)?
7. A pediatric dose of 100 mg of a syrup is ordered. The dosage form is an oral suspension containing 125 mg/5 cc. How much of the suspension contains a 100-mg dose?
8. How many units of heparin are found in 0.2 mL, if you have 1000 U/mL?
9. Albuterol syrup is available as 2 mg/5 mL. If a dosage schedule of 0.1 mg/kg is used, how much syrup is needed for a 30-kg child? How many teaspoons is this?
10. Terbutaline is available as 2.5-mg tablets. How many tablets do you need for a 5-mg dose?
11. If a cough syrup is available as 120 mg/5 mL, how much of the drug is there in ½ tsp?
12. Theophylline is available as 250 mg/10 mL and is given intravenously at 6 mg/kg body weight. How much solution do you give to a 60-kg woman?
13. Terbutaline sulfate is available as 1 mg/mL in an ampule. How many milliliters are needed for a 0.25-mg dose?
14. A patient is told to take 4 mg of albuterol four times daily. The medication comes in 2-mg tablets. How many tablets are needed for one 4-mg dose?
15. An agent is available as a syrup with 10 mg/5 mL. How many teaspoons should be taken for a 20-mg dose?
16. If an agent is available at 3 mg/mL, how many milliliters are needed for a dose of 9 mg?

Continued

17. If a dosage schedule requires 0.25 mg/kg of body weight, what dose is needed for an 88-kg person?

18. If theophylline is available as 80 mg/15 mL, how much is needed for a 100-mg dose?

19. How much of a drug is needed for a 65-kg adult, using 0.5 mg/kg?

20. The pediatric dosage of an antibiotic is 0.5 g/20 lb body weight, not to exceed 75 mg/kg/24 hr.
    a. What is the dose for a 40-lb child?
    b. If this dose is given twice in 1 day, has the maximal dose been exceeded?

Percentage-Strength Solutions

1. How many grams of calamine are needed to prepare 120 g of an ointment containing 8% calamine?

2. In 147 mL of solution, there is 1 mL of active enzyme. What is the percentage strength of active enzyme in the solution?

3. If theophylline is available in a 250-mg/10 mL solution, what percentage strength is this?

4. You have epinephrine 1:100. How many milliliters of epinephrine would be needed to contain 30 mg of active ingredient?

5. A dose of 0.4 mL of epinephrine HCl 1:100 is ordered. This dose contains how many milligrams of epinephrine HCl (the active ingredient)?

6. If you administer 3 mL of a 0.1% strength solution, how many milligrams of active ingredient have you given?

7. A drug is available as a 1:200 solution and the maximal dose that may be given by aerosol for a particular patient is 3 mg. What is the maximal amount of solution (in milliliters) that may be used?

8. Epinephrine 1:1000 contains how many milligrams of active ingredient per milliliter?

9. How many milligrams per milliliter are there in 0.3 mL of a 5% strength agent?

10. How many milligrams of sodium chloride are needed for 10 mL of a 0.9% solution?

11. If you have lidocaine (Xylocaine) at 5 mg/mL, what percentage strength is it?

12. A 0.5% strength solution contains how many milligrams in 1 mL?

13. Cromolyn sodium contains 20 mg in 2 mL of water. What is the percentage strength?

14. How much active ingredient of acetylcysteine have you given with 4 cc of a 20% solution?

15. You have 20% acetylcysteine; how many milliliters of this do you need to form 4 mL of an 8% solution?

16. The recommended dose of an agent with a percent strength of 5% is 0.3 cc. How many milligrams of solute are there in this amount?

17. Acetylcysteine was marketed as 10% acetylcysteine with 0.05% isoproterenol. How many milligrams of each ingredient were in a 4-cc dose of solution? (Isoproterenol: $0.0005 = x$ g/4 cc; $x = 0.002$ g = 2 mg.)

18. Which contains more drug: ½ cc of a 1% drug solution with 2 mL of saline or ½ cc of a 1% drug solution with 5 mL of saline?

19. How many milligrams per milliliter are in a 20% solution?

 CLINICAL SCENARIO

Answers can be found in Appendix A.

You have a 1 normal (N) solution of saline (NaCl) and you need isotonic saline 0.9%, also called "normal saline," for diluent in a nebulizer solution.

Can you use the 1 N solution as diluent, unchanged?

REFERENCE

1. Chatburn RL: Measurement, physical quantities, and le Système International d'Unités (SI units). *Respir Care* 33:861, 1988.

CHAPTER 5

Central and Peripheral Nervous Systems

Douglas S. Gardenhire

CHAPTER OUTLINE

OBJECTIVES

After reading this chapter, the reader will be able to:

1. Define key terms pertaining to the central and peripheral nervous systems
2. Classify the branches of the nervous system
3. Differentiate among the *central, peripheral,* and *autonomic nervous systems*
4. Discuss the use of *neurotransmitters*
5. Explain in detail the difference between the *parasympathetic* and *sympathetic* branches of the nervous system
6. Differentiate the effects of *cholinergic* and *anticholinergic agents* on the nervous system
7. Differentiate the effects of *adrenergic* and *antiadrenergic agents* on the nervous system
8. Discuss the various receptors in the airways
9. Differentiate among *nonadrenergic, noncholinergic inhibitory,* and *excitatory* nerves

KEY TERMS AND DEFINITIONS

Acetylcholine (Ach) Chemical produced by the body that is used in the transmission of nerve impulses. It is destroyed by the enzyme cholinesterase.

Adrenergic (adrenomimetic) Refers to a drug stimulating a receptor for norepinephrine or epinephrine.

Afferent Signals that are transmitted to the brain and spinal cord.

Antiadrenergic Refers to a drug blocking a receptor for norepinephrine or epinephrine.

Anticholinergic Refers to a drug blocking a receptor for acetylcholine.

Central nervous system (CNS) System that includes the brain and spinal cord; controls voluntary and involuntary acts.

KEY TERMS AND DEFINITIONS—cont'd

Cholinergic (cholinomimetic) Refers to a drug causing stimulation of a receptor for acetylcholine.

Efferent Signals that are transmitted from the brain and spinal cord.

Norepinephrine Naturally occurring catecholamine produced by the adrenal medulla that has properties similar to epinephrine. It is used as a neurotransmitter in most sympathetic terminal nerve sites.

Parasympatholytic Agent blocking or inhibiting the effects of the parasympathetic nervous system.

Parasympathomimetic Agent causing stimulation of the parasympathetic nervous system.

Peripheral nervous system (PNS) Portion of the nervous system outside the CNS, including sensory, sympathetic, and parasympathetic nerves.

Sympatholytic Agent blocking or inhibiting the effect of the sympathetic nervous system.

Sympathomimetic Agent causing stimulation of the sympathetic nervous system.

The goal of Chapter 5 is to provide a clear introduction to and understanding of the peripheral nervous system, its control mechanisms—especially neurotransmitter functions—and its physiologic effects in the body. Understanding of the control mechanisms and physiologic effects forms the basis for a subsequent understanding of drug actions and drug effects, both for agonists and for antagonists that act at various points in the nervous system. This chapter concludes with a summary of autonomic and other neural control mechanisms and their effects in the pulmonary system.

NERVOUS SYSTEM

KEY POINT

One of the major control systems in the body is the *nervous system,* comprising *sensory* afferent nerves; *motor* efferent nerves; and the *autonomic nervous system,* which is divided further into the *sympathetic* and *parasympathetic* branches.

There are two major control systems in the body: the *nervous system* and the *endocrine system.* Both systems of control can be manipulated by drug therapy, which either mimics or blocks the usual action of the control system to produce or inhibit physiologic effects. The endocrine system is considered separately in Chapter 11, which discusses the corticosteroid class of drugs. The nervous system is divided into the **central nervous system (CNS)** and the **peripheral nervous system (PNS)**, both of which offer sites for drug action. The overall organization of the nervous system may be outlined as follows:

I. Central nervous system
  A. Brain
  B. Spinal cord
II. Peripheral nervous system
  A. Sensory (afferent) neurons
  B. Somatic (motor) neurons
  C. Autonomic nervous system
    1. Parasympathetic branch
    2. Sympathetic branch

Figure 5-1 is a functional, but not anatomically accurate, diagram of the CNS and PNS. The *sensory* branch of the nervous system consists of afferent neurons from heat, light, pressure, and pain receptors sending information from the periphery to the CNS. The *somatic* portion (or motor branch) of the nervous system is under voluntary, conscious control and innervates skeletal muscle for motor actions, such as lifting, walking, or breathing. This portion of the nervous system is manipulated by neuromuscular blocking agents that induce paralysis in surgical procedures or during mechanical ventilation. The *autonomic nervous system* is the involuntary, unconscious control mechanism of the body, sometimes said to control vegetative or visceral functions. For example, the autonomic nervous system regulates heart rate, pupillary dilation and contraction, glandular secretion, such as salivation, and smooth muscle contraction in blood vessels and the airway. The autonomic nervous system is divided into the *parasympathetic* and *sympathetic* branches.

AUTONOMIC BRANCHES

Neither motor nor sensory branch neurons have synapses outside the spinal cord before reaching the muscle or sensory receptor site. The motor neuron extends without interruption from the CNS to the skeletal muscle, and its action is mediated by the neurotransmitter **acetylcholine (Ach)**. This is in contrast to the synapses occurring in the sympathetic and parasympathetic divisions of the autonomic system. The multiple synapses of the autonomic system offer potential sites for drug action, as do the terminal neuroeffector sites.

The parasympathetic branch arises from the craniosacral portions of the spinal cord and consists of two types of neurons—a preganglionic fiber leading from the vertebrae to the ganglionic synapse outside the cord and a postganglionic fiber leading from the ganglionic synapse to the gland or smooth muscle being innervated. The parasympathetic branch has good specificity, with the postganglionic fiber arising very near the effector site (e.g., a gland or smooth muscle). As a result, stimulation of a parasympathetic preganglionic neuron causes activity limited to individual effector sites, such as the heart or the eye. Figure 5-2 illustrates the portions of the spinal cord where the parasympathetic and sympathetic nerve fibers originate.

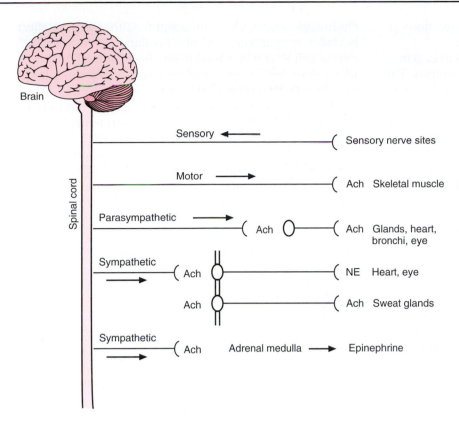

Figure 5-1 Functional diagram of central and peripheral nervous systems, indicating the somatic branches (sensory, motor) and the autonomic branches (sympathetic, parasympathetic), with their neurotransmitters. *Ach,* Acetylcholine; *NE,* norepinephrine.

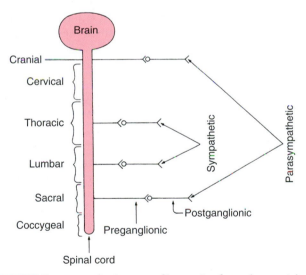

Figure 5-2 Parasympathetic nerve fibers arise from the cranial and sacral portions of the spinal cord, whereas sympathetic fibers leave the cord primarily from the thoracic and lumbar regions.

KEY POINT

Nerve impulses are conducted by electrical and chemical means; the chemical portion of nerve transmission is referred to as a *neurotransmitter.* The neurotransmitter is *acetylcholine (Ach)* at the *myoneural (neuromuscular) junc-tion,* at *ganglia,* and at *parasympathetic end sites.* The neurotransmitter at *sympathetic end sites* is generally *norepinephrine,* except at sweat glands and the adrenal medulla, where *Ach* is the neurotransmitter.

The sympathetic branch arises from the thoracolumbar portion of the spinal cord and consists of short pregangli-onic fibers and long postganglionic fibers. Sympathetic neurons from the spinal cord terminate in ganglia that lie on either side of the vertebral column. In the *ganglia,* or the *ganglionic chain,* the preganglionic fiber makes contact with postganglionic neurons. As a result, when one sympathetic preganglionic neuron is stimulated, the action passes to many or all of the postganglionic fibers. The effect of sym-pathetic activation is widened further because sympathetic fibers innervate the adrenal medulla and cause the release of epinephrine into the general circulation. Circulating epi-nephrine stimulates all receptors responding to **norepi-nephrine,** even if no sympathetic nerves are present. Where the parasympathetic system allows discrete control, the design of the sympathetic system causes a widespread reac-tion in the body.

Parasympathetic and Sympathetic Regulation

There are general differences between the parasympathetic and sympathetic branches of the autonomic nervous system, which can be contrasted. Parasympathetic control is essen-tial to life and is considered a more discrete, finely regulated system than sympathetic control. Parasympathetic effects control the day-to-day body functions of digestion, bladder and rectal discharge, and basal secretion of bronchial mucus. Overstimulation of the parasympathetic branch would render the body incapable of violent action, result-ing in what is termed the *SLUD syndrome:* salivation, lacrimation, *urination*, and *defecation*. These reactions are definitely counterproductive to fleeing or fighting!

By contrast, the sympathetic branch reacts as a general alarm system and does not exercise discrete controls. This is sometimes characterized as a "fight-or-flight" system: heart rate and blood pressure increase, blood flow shifts from the periphery to muscles and the heart, blood sugar increases, and bronchi dilate. The organism prepares for maximal physical exertion. The sympathetic branch is not essential to life; animal models with sympathectomy can survive but are unable to cope with violent stress.

> ### KEY POINT
>
> *Sympathetic effects* are widespread, mediated by norepinephrine at nerve endings and by circulating epinephrine released from the adrenal medulla.

Neurotransmitters

Another general feature of the autonomic nervous system, including the sympathetic and parasympathetic branches, is the mechanism of neurotransmitter control of nerve impulses. Nerve impulse propagation is electrical and chemical (electrochemical). A nerve impulse signal is carried along a nerve fiber by *electrical* action potentials caused by ion exchanges (i.e., sodium and potassium). At gaps in the nerve fiber between neurons (synapses), the electrical transmission is replaced by a chemical neurotransmitter. This is the *chemical* transmission of the electrical impulse, which occurs at the ganglionic synapses and at the end of the nerve fiber, termed the *neuroeffector site.* Identification of the chemical transmitters dates back to Loewi's experiments in 1921 and is fundamental to understanding autonomic drugs and their classifications. The usual neurotransmitters in the PNS, including the ganglionic synapses and terminal sites in the autonomic branches, are shown in Figure 5-1 (Ach and norepinephrine).

Ach is the neurotransmitter conducting the nerve impulse at skeletal muscle sites; this site is referred to as the *neuromuscular junction* or the *myoneural junction.* In the parasympathetic branch, Ach is also the neurotransmitter at both the ganglionic synapse and the terminal nerve site, which is referred to as the *neuroeffector site.* In the sympathetic branch, Ach is the neurotransmitter at the ganglionic synapse; however, norepinephrine is the neurotransmitter at the sympathetic neuroeffector site. There are two exceptions to this pattern, both in the sympathetic branch. Sympathetic fibers to sweat glands release Ach instead of norepinephrine, and preganglionic sympathetic fibers directly innervate the adrenal medulla, where the neurotransmitter is Ach. Sympathetic fibers that have Ach at the neuroeffector sites are *cholinergic* (for Ach) sympathetic fibers.

"Cholinergic sympathetic" would be an apparent contradictory combination of terms if not for the exceptions to the rule of norepinephrine as the sympathetic neurotransmitter. For example, sweating can be caused by giving a cholinergic drug such as pilocarpine, although this effect is under sympathetic control. "Breaking out in a sweat," sweaty palms, and increased heart rate resulting from circulating epinephrine are common effects of stress or fright mediated by sympathetic discharge.

Although it is an oversimplification, an easy way to learn the various neurotransmitters initially is to remember that Ach is the neurotransmitter *everywhere* (skeletal muscle, all ganglionic synapses, and parasympathetic terminal nerve sites) *except* at sympathetic terminal nerve sites, where norepinephrine is the neurotransmitter. The exceptions provided by sympathetic fibers releasing Ach can be remembered as exceptions to the general rule.

Efferent and Afferent Nerve Fibers

> ### KEY POINT
>
> The neurotransmitter Ach is terminated by the enzyme *cholinesterase*, and norepinephrine and sympathetic transmission are terminated by neurotransmitter *reuptake* into the *presynaptic neuron (uptake-1)* and by the enzymes *catechol O-methyltransferase (COMT)* and *monoamine oxidase (MAO).*

The autonomic system is generally considered an **efferent** system—that is, impulses in the sympathetic and parasympathetic branches travel *from* the brain and spinal cord out *to* the various neuroeffector sites, such as the heart, gastrointestinal tract, and lungs. **Afferent** nerves run alongside the sympathetic and parasympathetic efferent fibers and carry impulses *from* the periphery *to* the cord. The afferent fibers convey impulses resulting from visceral stimuli and can form a reflex arc of stimulus input–autonomic output analogous to the well-known somatic reflex arcs, such as the knee-jerk reflex. The mechanism of a vagal reflex arc mediating bronchoconstriction is discussed further in Chapter 7, in conjunction with drugs used to block the parasympathetic impulses.

Terminology of Drugs Affecting the Nervous System

> ### KEY POINT
>
> The terms *cholinergic (cholinoceptor)* and *adrenergic (adrenoceptor)* are used for Ach and norepinephrine/epinephrine receptors in the two autonomic branches.

Terminology of drugs and drug effects on the nervous system can be confusing and may seem inconsistent. The confusion is caused by the fact that drugs and drug effects are derived from the type of nerve fiber (parasympathetic or sympathetic) or, alternatively, the type of neurotransmitter and receptor (Ach or norepinephrine). The following terms are based on the anatomy of the nerve fibers, to describe stimulation or inhibition:

Parasympathomimetic
Parasympatholytic
Sympathomimetic
Sympatholytic

Additional terms are used, based on the type of neurotransmitter and receptor. *Cholinergic* refers to Ach, and *adrenergic* is derived from *adrenaline*, another term for epinephrine, which is similar to norepinephrine and can stimulate sympathetic neuroeffector sites. Because Ach is the neurotransmitter at more sites than just parasympathetic sites, and because receptors exist on smooth muscle or blood cells without any nerve fibers innervating them, these terms denote a wider range of sites than the anatomically based terms such as parasympathomimetic.

Cholinergic can refer to a drug effect at a ganglion, a parasympathetic nerve ending site, or the neuromuscular junction. Adrenergic describes receptors on bronchial smooth muscle or on blood cells, where there are no sympathetic nerves. For this reason, cholinergic and adrenergic are not strictly synonymous with parasympathetic and sympathetic. **Cholinergic (cholinomimetic)** refers to a drug causing stimulation of a receptor for Ach. **Anticholinergic** refers to a drug blocking a receptor for Ach. **Adrenergic (adrenomimetic)** refers to a drug stimulating a receptor for norepinephrine or epinephrine. **Antiadrenergic** refers to a drug blocking a receptor for norepinephrine or epinephrine. *Cholinoceptor* is an alternative term for cholinergic receptor, and *adrenoceptor* is an alternative term for adrenergic receptor.

KEY POINT

Parasympathomimetic = Cholinergic
Parasympatholytic = Anticholinergic
Sympathomimetic = Adrenergic
Sympatholytic = Antiadrenergic

PARASYMPATHETIC BRANCH

Cholinergic Neurotransmitter Function

KEY POINT

Parasympathetic effects on the cardiopulmonary system include decreased heart rate, lower blood pressure, bronchoconstriction, and mucus secretion in the airways.

In the parasympathetic branch, the neurotransmitter *Ach* conducts nerve transmission at the ganglionic site and at the parasympathetic effector site at the end of the postganglionic fiber. This action is illustrated in Figure 5-3. The term *neurohormone* has also been used in place of neurotransmitter. Ach is concentrated in the presynaptic neuron (both at the ganglion and at the effector site). Ach is

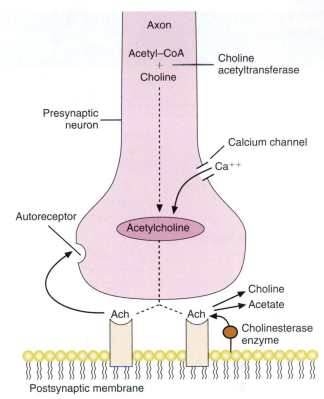

Figure 5-3 *Cholinergic nerve transmission* mediated by the neurotransmitter acetylcholine *(Ach)*. The action of the neurotransmitter is terminated by cholinesterase enzymes; attachment of acetylcholine to presynaptic autoreceptors inhibits further neurotransmitter release. *CoA,* Coenzyme A, used in synthesis; *Ca++,* calcium.

synthesized from acetyl-CoA and choline and catalyzed by the enzyme choline acetyltransferase. Ach is stored in vesicles in quantities of 1000 to 50,000 molecules per vesicle. When a nerve impulse *(action potential)* reaches the presynaptic neuron site, an influx of calcium is triggered into the neuron. Increased calcium in the neuron causes cellular secretion of the Ach-containing vesicles from the end of the nerve fiber. After release, the Ach attaches to receptors on the postsynaptic membrane and initiates an effect in the tissue or organ site.

Ach is inactivated through hydrolysis by cholinesterase enzymes, which split the Ach molecule into choline and acetate, terminating stimulation of the postsynaptic membrane. In effect, the nerve impulse is "shut off." There are also receptors on the presynaptic neuron, termed *autoreceptors,* that can be stimulated by Ach to regulate and inhibit further neurotransmitter release from the neuron. The effects of the parasympathetic branch of the autonomic system on various organs are listed in Table 5-1. Drugs can mimic or block the action of the neurotransmitter Ach to stimulate parasympathetic nerve ending sites (parasympathomimetics) or to block the transmission of such impulses (parasympatholytics). Both categories of drugs affecting the parasympathetic branch are commonly seen clinically. The effects of the parasympathetic system on the heart, bronchial smooth muscle, and exocrine glands should be

TABLE 5-1	Effects of Parasympathetic Stimulation on Selected Organs or Sites	
ORGAN/SITE	**PARASYMPATHETIC (CHOLINERGIC) RESPONSE**
Heart	
SA node	Slowing of rate
Contractility	Decreased atrial force
Conduction velocity	Decreased AV node conduction
Bronchi	
Smooth muscle	Constriction
Mucous glands	Increased secretion
Vascular Smooth Muscle	
Skin and mucosa	No innervation*
Pulmonary	No innervation*
Skeletal muscle	No innervation†
Coronary	No innervation*
Salivary Glands	Increased secretion
Skeletal Muscle	None
Eye	
Iris radial muscle	None
Iris circular muscle	Contraction (miosis)
Ciliary muscle	Contraction for near vision
Gastrointestinal Tract	Increased motility
Gastrointestinal Sphincters	Relaxation
Urinary Bladder	
Detrusor	Contraction
Trigone sphincter	Relaxation
Glycogenolysis	
Skeletal muscle	None
Sweat Glands	None‡
Lipolysis (Multiple Sites)	None
Renin Secretion (Kidney)	None
Insulin Secretion (Pancreas)	Increased

AV, Atrioventricular; *SA*, sinoatrial.

*No direct parasympathetic nerve innervation; response to exogenous cholinergic agonists is dilation.

†Dilation occurs as a result of sympathetic cholinergic discharge or as a response to exogenous cholinergic agonists.

‡Sweat glands are under sympathetic control; receptors are cholinergic, however, and the response to exogenous cholinergic agonists is increased secretion.

mentally reviewed before considering parasympathetic agonists or antagonists (blockers):

- *Heart:* Slows rate (vagus)
- *Bronchial smooth muscle:* Constriction
- *Exocrine glands:* Increased secretion

Muscarinic and Nicotinic Receptors and Effects

Two additional terms are used to refer to stimulation of receptor sites for Ach. They are derived from the action in the body of two substances: the alkaloids *muscarine* and *nicotine*. Receptor sites that are stimulated by these two chemicals are illustrated in Figure 5-4.

Muscarinic Effects

KEY POINT

Muscarinic refers to cholinergic receptors at parasympathetic end sites. Muscarinic receptors are distinguished into subtypes M_1 through M_5; M_2 receptors are in the heart and M_3 receptors are on airway smooth muscle, mediating bronchoconstriction.

Muscarine, a natural product from the mushroom *Amanita muscaria*, stimulates Ach (cholinergic) receptors at the parasympathetic terminal sites: exocrine glands (lacrimal, salivary, and bronchial mucous glands), cardiac muscle, and smooth muscle (gastrointestinal tract). Ach receptors at these sites and the effects of parasympathetic stimulation at these sites are termed *muscarinic*. A muscarinic effect well known to respiratory care clinicians is the increase in airway secretions after administration of Ach-like drugs, such as neostigmine. There is also a decrease in blood pressure caused by slowing of the heart and vasodilation. *In general, a parasympathomimetic effect is the same as a muscarinic effect, and a parasympatholytic effect is referred to as an* antimuscarinic *effect*.

Nicotinic Effects

KEY POINT

The term *nicotinic* refers to cholinergic receptors on ganglia and at the neuromuscular junction.

Nicotine, a substance in tobacco products, stimulates Ach (cholinergic) receptors at autonomic ganglia (parasympathetic and sympathetic) and at skeletal muscle sites. Ach receptors at autonomic ganglia and at the skeletal muscle are termed *nicotinic*, as are the effects on these sites of stimulation. Practical effects of stimulating these nicotinic receptors include an increase in blood pressure resulting from stimulation of sympathetic ganglia, causing vasoconstriction when the postganglionic fibers discharge, and muscle tremor caused by skeletal tissue stimulation.

Subtypes of Muscarinic Receptors

Parasympathetic receptors and cholinergic receptors in general, with or without corresponding nerve fibers, are classified further into subtypes. These differences among cholinergic or muscarinic (M) receptors are based on different responses to different drugs, or recognition through use of DNA probes. Five muscarinic receptor subtypes have been identified: M_1, M_2, M_3, M_4, and M_5. They are all G protein–linked (see Chapter 2). As G protein–linked receptors, these five subtypes of muscarinic receptors share a structural feature common to such receptors—a long, "serpentine" polypeptide chain that crosses the cell membrane seven times (illustrated for G protein receptors in Chapter 2). Table 5-2 summarizes the muscarinic receptor subtypes, including their predominant location and the type of G protein with which they are coupled. Additional details

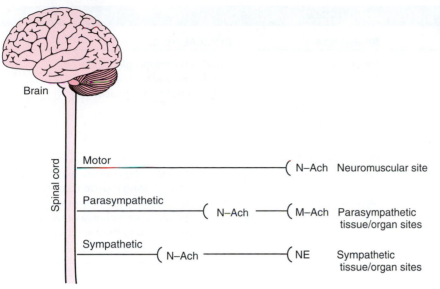

Brain

Spinal cord

Motor ———————————————(N–Ach Neuromuscular site

Parasympathetic ————(N–Ach)————(M–Ach Parasympathetic
tissue/organ sites

Sympathetic ————(N–Ach)————(NE Sympathetic
tissue/organ sites

Figure 5-4 Location of muscarinic and nicotinic receptor sites in the peripheral nervous system. *M-Ach*, Muscarinic site; *N-Ach*, nicotinic site; *NE*, norepinephrine.

TABLE 5-2	Muscarinic Receptor Subtypes, Location, and G-Protein Linkage	
MUSCARINIC RECEPTOR TYPE	**LOCATION**	**G-PROTEIN SUBTYPE**
M_1	Parasympathetic ganglia, nasal submucosal glands	G_q
M_2	Heart, postganglionic parasympathetic nerves	G_i
M_3	Airway smooth muscle, submucosal glands	G_q
M_4	Postganglionic cholinergic nerves, possible effect on CNS, decrease in locomotion	G_i
M_5	Possible effect on CNS	G_q

CNS, Central nervous system.

about muscarinic receptor location and function in the pulmonary system are presented in the final section of this chapter, which summarizes nervous control and receptors in the lung.

CHOLINERGIC AGENTS

Cholinergic drugs mimic the action caused by Ach at receptor sites in the parasympathetic system and neuromuscular junction. Such agents can cause stimulation at the terminal nerve site (neuroeffector junction) by two distinct mechanisms, leading to their classification as direct acting or indirect acting. Table 5-3 lists cholinergic agents, categorized as direct acting or indirect acting, and their clinical uses. The terms *cholinergic, cholinoceptor stimulant,* and *cholinomimetic* are broader than *parasympathomimetic* and denote agents stimulating Ach receptors located in the parasympathetic

system (muscarinic) or other sites such as the neuromuscular junction (nicotinic). A cholinergic drug can activate muscarinic and nicotinic receptors.

Direct-Acting Cholinergic Agents

Direct-acting cholinergic agents are structurally similar to Ach. As shown in Figure 5-3, direct-acting cholinergic agents mimic Ach, binding and activating muscarinic or nicotinic receptors directly. Examples of this group include methacholine, carbachol, bethanechol, and pilocarpine. Methacholine has been used in bronchial challenge tests by inhalation to assess the degree of airway reactivity in asthmatics and others. The parasympathetic effect is bronchoconstriction. Methacholine is a useful diagnostic agent to detect differences in degree of airway reactivity between nonasthmatic individuals and asthmatics with hyperreactive airways.

Indirect-Acting Cholinergic Agents

 KEY POINT

Parasympathomimetic, or cholinergic, agonists are divided into *direct-acting* agents (e.g., methacholine), which resemble Ach and stimulate cholinergic receptors directly, and *indirect-acting* agents (e.g., neostigmine), which inhibit the enzyme cholinesterase and allow increased Ach transmission. A typical *parasympatholytic,* or *anticholinergic,* agent is atropine.

Indirect-acting cholinergic agonists inhibit the cholinesterase enzyme, as seen in Figure 5-3. Because cholinesterase usually inactivates the Ach neurotransmitter, inhibiting this enzyme results in accumulation of endogenous Ach at the neuroeffector junction of parasympathetic nerve endings or the neuromuscular junction. More Ach is made available to attach to receptor sites and to stimulate cholinergic

TABLE 5-3	Examples of Direct-Acting and Indirect-Acting Cholinergic Agents		
CATEGORY	GENERIC NAME	BRAND NAME	CLINICAL USES
Direct Acting	Acetylcholine chloride	Miochol-E	Ophthalmic miotic, glaucoma
	Carbachol	Miostat	Ophthalmic miotic, glaucoma
	Pilocarpine hydrochloride	Pilopine HS, Isopto Carpine, Salagen	Ophthalmic miotic, glaucoma
	Methacholine	Provocholine	Diagnostic, asthma
	Bethanechol	Urecholine	Treatment of urinary retention
Indirect Acting	Echothiophate iodide	Phospholine Iodide	Ophthalmic miotic, glaucoma
	Pyridostigmine	Mestinon, Regonol	Muscle stimulant, myasthenia gravis, reversal of nondepolarizing muscle relaxants
	Ambenonium	Mytelase	Muscle stimulant, myasthenia gravis
	Neostigmine methylsulfate	Bloxiverz	Muscle stimulant, myasthenia gravis, reversal of nondepolarizing muscle relaxants
	Edrophonium	Tensilon, Enlon	Diagnostic, myasthenia gravis

responses. If Ach receptors have been blocked, this increase in neurotransmitter can reverse the blockage by competing with the blocking drug for the receptors. Nerve transmission can then resume, either at the parasympathetic terminal site or at the neuromuscular junction.

The drug echothiophate (Phospholine), listed in Table 5-3, stimulates autonomic muscarinic receptors in the iris sphincter and ciliary muscle of the eye to produce pupillary constriction (miosis) and lens thickening. An increase in the neurotransmitter Ach at the neuromuscular junction makes drugs, such as neostigmine, useful in reversing neuromuscular blockade caused by paralyzing agents, such as pancuronium or doxacurium (see Chapter 18). Neostigmine and edrophonium are also useful in increasing muscle strength in a neuromuscular disease such as myasthenia gravis, in which the cholinergic receptor is blocked by autoantibodies. The drug edrophonium (Tensilon) is used in the Tensilon test to determine whether muscle weakness is caused by overdosing with an indirect-acting cholinergic agent (causing ultimate receptor fatigue and blockade) or undertreatment with an insufficient drug. Because edrophonium is short-acting (5 to 15 minutes, depending on the dose), it is useful as a diagnostic agent, rather than as a maintenance treatment in neuromuscular disease.

When using indirect-acting cholinergic agents such as neostigmine to increase nerve function at the neuromuscular junction, Ach activity at parasympathetic sites such as salivary and nasopharyngeal glands also increases. These undesirable muscarinic effects can be blocked by pretreatment with a parasympatholytic or antimuscarinic drug such as atropine or its derivatives.

Cholinesterase Reactivator (Pralidoxime)

Organophosphates such as parathion and malathion and the drug echothiophate form an irreversible bond with cholinesterase (also called *acetylcholinesterase*). Organophosphates are used as insecticides, and occasionally patients are seen with toxic exposure and absorption. The effects of these agents can be lethal, and because of this, they have also been used as "nerve gas." Because they affect Ach, they

have an effect on neuromuscular function and muscarinic receptors; there is initial stimulation, then blockade if a high enough dosage is absorbed. Muscle weakness and paralysis can result.

The bonding of irreversible inhibitors with cholinesterase is slow, taking up to 24 hours. Once formed, however, the duration is limited only by the body's ability to produce new cholinesterase, which takes 1 to 2 weeks. A drug such as pralidoxime chloride (Protopam Chloride), a cholinesterase reactivator, can be used in the treatment of organophosphate toxicity in the first 24 hours. After this time, the bond of cholinesterase and cholinesterase inhibitors cannot be reversed, but atropine (a parasympatholytic) can be used to block the overly available Ach neurotransmitter at the receptor sites. Support of ventilation and airway maintenance would be required for the duration of the effects.

ANTICHOLINERGIC AGENTS

Anticholinergic agents block Ach receptors and act as cholinergic antagonists. Parasympatholytic (antimuscarinic) agents such as atropine and drug classes such as neuromuscular blockers and ganglionic blockers are anticholinergic because they block Ach at their respective sites. However, a neuromuscular or ganglionic blocking agent would *not* be considered a parasympatholytic or antimuscarinic agent because the site of action is not within the parasympathetic system. Parasympatholytic agents are antimuscarinic because of the limitation to parasympathetic terminal fiber sites.

Atropine as a Prototype Parasympatholytic Agent

Atropine is usually considered the prototype parasympatholytic, and there is renewed interest in the use of aerosolized analogs of atropine in respiratory care; this is discussed more fully in Chapter 7. Atropine occurs naturally as the levo isomer in *Atropa belladonna*, the nightshade plant, and in *Datura stramonium*, or jimsonweed. The drug is referred to as a *belladonna alkaloid*.

Atropine is a *competitive antagonist* to Ach at muscarinic receptor sites (i.e., glands, gastrointestinal tract, heart, and eyes) and can form a reversible bond with these cholinergic receptors. It is nonspecific for muscarinic receptor subtypes and blocks M_1, M_2, and M_3 receptors. Atropine blocks salivary secretion and causes dry mouth. In the respiratory system, atropine decreases secretion by mucous glands and relaxes bronchial smooth muscle by blocking parasympathetically maintained basal tone. Atropine blocks vagal innervation of the heart to produce increased heart rate. There is no effect on blood vessels because these do not have parasympathetic innervation, only the Ach receptors. Vascular resistance would not increase with atropine. If a parasympathomimetic *were* given, atropine would block the dilating effect on blood vessel receptor sites. Pupillary dilation *(mydriasis)* occurs as a result of blockade of the circular iris muscle, and the lens is flattened *(cycloplegia)* by blockade of the ciliary muscle. In the gastrointestinal tract, atropine decreases acid secretion, tone, and mobility. Bladder wall smooth muscle is relaxed, and voiding is slowed. Sweating is inhibited by atropine, which blocks Ach receptors on sweat glands. Sweat glands are innervated by sympathetic cholinergic fibers.

At usual clinical doses, atropine exerts a low level of CNS stimulation, with a slower sedative effect in the brain. Scopolamine, another classic antimuscarinic agent, can produce drowsiness and amnesia. In larger doses, atropine can cause toxic effects in the CNS, including hallucinations.

The anticholinergic (antimuscarinic) effect on the vestibular system can inhibit motion sickness. Scopolamine was used for this, and antihistamine drugs such as dimenhydrinate (Dramamine) that have anticholinergic effects are commonly used to prevent motion sickness. The dry mouth and drowsiness that also occur with a drug such as dimenhydrinate are typical antimuscarinic effects.

Parasympatholytic (Antimuscarinic) Effects

If the basic effects of the parasympathetic system are known, the effects of an antagonist such as atropine can be deduced. For example, if parasympathetic (vagal) stimulation slows the heart rate, parasympatholytic should increase the heart rate by blocking that innervation. Box 5-1 lists the effects and uses of parasympatholytic agents.

SYMPATHETIC BRANCH

KEY POINT

Sympathetic effects on the cardiopulmonary system include increased heart rate and contractile force, increased blood pressure, bronchodilation, and probable increased secretion from mucous glands in the airway.

As noted in the general description of the parasympathetic and sympathetic branches of the autonomic nervous system,

---

BOX 5-1   Uses and Effects of Parasympatholytic (Antimuscarinic) Agents

- Bronchodilation
- Preoperative drying of secretions
- Antidiarrheal agent
- Prevention of bed-wetting in children (increase in urinary retention)
- Treatment of peptic ulcer
- Treatment of organophosphate poisoning
- Treatment of mushroom (*Amanita muscaria*) ingestion
- Treatment of bradycardia

---

sympathetic (adrenergic) effects are mediated both by neurotransmitter release from sympathetic nerves and by the release of circulating catecholamines (i.e., norepinephrine and epinephrine) from the adrenal medulla. Circulating catecholamines stimulate adrenergic receptors throughout the body, not just receptors with nerve fibers present. Sympathetic activation results in stimulation of the heart, increased cardiac output, increased blood pressure, mental stimulation, accelerated metabolism, and bronchodilation in the pulmonary system.

Adrenergic Neurotransmitter Function

In the sympathetic branch of the autonomic nervous system, the usual neurotransmitter at the terminal nerve sites is norepinephrine, with the exceptions described previously (sweat glands and adrenal medulla). Figure 5-5 illustrates neurotransmitter function with norepinephrine. In the presynaptic neuron, tyrosine is converted to dopa and then to dopamine, which is converted by dopamine β-hydroxylase to norepinephrine in the storage vesicles. An action potential in the nerve opens calcium channels, allowing an influx of calcium. Increased intracellular calcium leads to exocytosis of the vesicles containing norepinephrine, which attach to receptors on the postsynaptic membrane. The exact physiologic effect depends on the site of innervation and the type of sympathetic receptor, which can also vary, as described subsequently.

The primary method of terminating the action of norepinephrine at the postsynaptic membrane is through a reuptake process that brings the norepinephrine back into the presynaptic neuron. This is termed *uptake-1*. The neurotransmitter action can be ended by two other mechanisms as well: uptake into tissue sites around the nerve terminal, a process termed *uptake-2* to distinguish it from reuptake into the nerve terminal itself; and diffusion of excess norepinephrine away from the receptor site, to be metabolized in the liver or plasma. In addition, norepinephrine can stimulate *autoreceptors* on the presynaptic neuron, which inhibits further neurotransmitter release. These autoreceptors have been identified as α_2-receptors (discussed later).

The distinction between two types of uptake processes is a result of research published by Iversen in 1965.[1] The uptake-2 process is a mediated uptake of exogenous amines

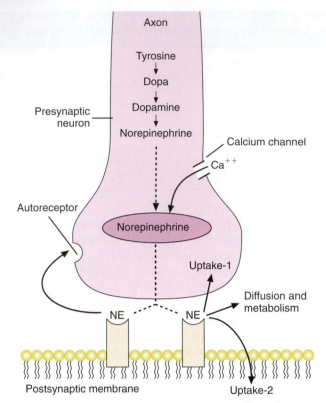

Figure 5-5 Adrenergic nerve transmission mediated by the neurotransmitter norepinephrine *(NE)*. The action of the neurotransmitter is terminated primarily by a reuptake mechanism (uptake-1) and by enzyme metabolism and a second uptake mechanism into tissue sites (uptake-2). Norepinephrine attaches to autoreceptor sites on the presynaptic neuron to inhibit further neurotransmitter release. *Ca++*, Calciumion.)

(chemicals such as norepinephrine) in *nonneuronal* tissues, such as cardiac muscle cells. Iversen and Salt[2] distinguished details of the uptake-2 process:

- It is a mediated transport system.
- It is a low-affinity but high-capacity system.
- It is not as stereochemically specific as uptake-1.
- It is specific to catecholamines.
- The order of affinity for uptake of specific agents, in *decreasing* order, is as follows: isoproterenol > epinephrine > norepinephrine.
- Certain corticosteroids can inhibit the uptake-2 process, potentiating catecholamines.

The last effect of uptake-2 inhibition by corticosteroids is discussed more fully in Chapter 11. Table 5-4 lists the physiologic effects of sympathetic activation. The effects listed in Table 5-4 are given for the same organs as listed in Table 5-1 for the parasympathetic system for comparison.

Enzyme Inactivation

The enzymes that metabolize norepinephrine, epinephrine, and chemicals similar to these neurotransmitters are important for understanding differences in the action of the adrenergic bronchodilator group. Chemicals structurally

TABLE 5-4	Effects of Sympathetic (Adrenergic) Stimulation on Selected Organs or Sites*
ORGAN/SITE	**SYMPATHETIC (ADRENERGIC) RESPONSE**
Heart	
SA node	Increase in rate
Contractility	Increase in force
Conduction velocity	Increased AV node conduction
Bronchi	
Smooth muscle	Relaxation and dilation of airway diameter
Mucous glands	Increased secretion
Vascular Smooth Muscle	
Skin and mucosa	Vasoconstriction
Pulmonary	Dilation/constriction (two types of sympathetic receptors)
Skeletal muscle	Dilation (predominantly)
Coronary	Dilation/constriction (two types of sympathetic receptors)
Salivary Glands	Decreased secretion
Skeletal Muscle	Increased contractility
Eye	
Iris radial muscle	Contraction (mydriasis)
Iris circular muscle	None
Ciliary muscle	Relaxation for far vision†
Gastrointestinal Tract	Decreased motility
Gastrointestinal Sphincters	Contraction
Urinary Bladder	
Detrusor	Relaxation
Trigone sphincter	Contraction
Sweat Glands	Increased secretion‡
Glycogenolysis	
Skeletal muscle	Increased
Lipolysis (Multiple Sites)	Increased
Renin Secretion (Kidney)	Increased
Insulin Secretion (Pancreas)	Decreased

AV, Atrioventricular; *SA*, sinoatrial.
*Effects of sympathetic activation are mediated by direct innervation of nerve fibers and by circulating epinephrine released from the adrenal medulla.
†Relaxes as a result of circulating epinephrine, with sympathetic activation.
‡Innervated by sympathetic nerves with *acetylcholine* neurotransmitter (cholinergic receptors); response to exogenous cholinergic agent is increased sweating.

related to epinephrine are termed *catecholamines,* and their general structure is outlined in Chapter 6 in the discussion of sympathomimetic (adrenergic) bronchodilators. Two enzymes are available that can inactivate catecholamines such as epinephrine: catechol O-methyltransferase (COMT) and monoamine oxidase (MAO). The action of both enzymes on epinephrine (Figure 5-6) is important because COMT is responsible for ending the action of catecholamine bronchodilators.

Sympathetic (Adrenergic) Receptor Types

The effects of adrenergic receptors are mediated by coupling with G proteins, and they are identified as G protein–linked receptors. Adrenergic receptor subtypes, with examples of their location and the type of G protein with which they are coupled, are summarized in Table 5-5.

α and β Receptors

> **! KEY POINT**
>
> Receptors at sympathetic end sites are subdivided into α and β receptors, with α receptors mediating excitatory effects (e.g., vasoconstriction) and β receptors mediating inhibitory effects (e.g., smooth muscle relaxation).

In 1948, Ahlquist[3] distinguished *alpha (α)* and *beta (β)* sympathetic receptors on the basis of differing responses to various adrenergic drugs, all of which were similar to norepinephrine with minor structural differences. These drugs included phenylephrine, norepinephrine, epinephrine, and isoproterenol. The two types of sympathetic receptors were distinguished as follows:

- *α Receptors:* Generally *excite*, with the exception of the intestine and CNS receptors, where inhibition or relaxation occurs
- *β Receptors:* Generally inhibit or *relax*, with the exception of the heart, where stimulation occurs

α-Sympathetic receptors are found on peripheral blood vessels, and stimulation results in vasoconstriction. α-Adrenergic agonists are frequently used for topical vasoconstriction of the nasal mucosa to treat symptoms of nasal congestion caused by the common cold. β-Adrenergic receptors are found on airway smooth muscle and in the heart. Drug activity of adrenergic stimulants (sympathomimetics) ranges along the spectrum seen in Figure 5-7.

As illustrated in Figure 5-7, phenylephrine is one of the purest α stimulants, and isoproterenol is an almost-pure β stimulant. "Pure" reactions do not occur with any drug—that is, even phenylephrine may affect other sites. Epinephrine stimulates α and β sites equally, but norepinephrine has more of an α than β effect.

β₁ and β₂ Receptors

In 1967, Lands and colleagues[4] further differentiated β receptors into β_1 and β_2 subtypes. β_1 Receptors are found in cardiac muscle, and β_2 receptors (which encompass all other β receptors) are found in bronchial, vascular, and skeletal muscle. The distinction among types of β receptors is as follows:

- *β_1 Receptors:* Increases the rate and force of cardiac contraction
- *β_2 Receptors:* Relaxes bronchial smooth muscle and vascular beds of skeletal muscle

TABLE 5-5	**Adrenergic Receptor Subtypes: Location and G-Protein Linkage**	
RECEPTOR TYPE	**LOCATION**	**G-PROTEIN SUBTYPE**
α_1	Peripheral blood vessels	G_q
α_2	Presynaptic sympathetic neurons (autoreceptor), CNS	G_i
β_1	Heart	G_s
β_2	Smooth muscle (including bronchial), cardiac muscle	G_s
β_3	Lipocytes	G_s

CNS, Central nervous system.

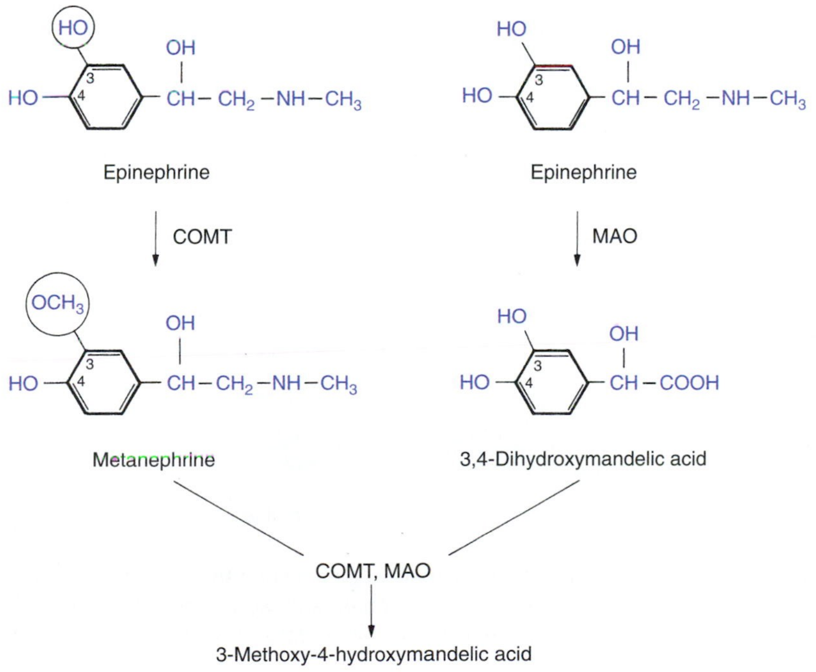

Figure 5-6 Metabolic pathways for the transformation of epinephrine by the enzymes catechol *O*-methyltransferase *(COMT)* and monoamine oxidase *(MAO)* to an inactive form.

Figure 5-7 Spectrum of activity of adrenergic agonists, ranging from excitatory effects to inhibitory effects, by which α and β receptors are distinguished.

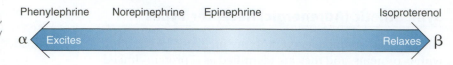

> ## ! KEY POINT
>
> β Receptors are subdivided into β_1 receptors, which are excitatory and found in the heart, and β_2 receptors, which are found elsewhere and mediate inhibitory responses.

β_1 Receptors constitute the exception to the general rule that β receptors cause relaxation. β_2 Receptors form the basis for the class of adrenergic bronchodilators, which act to relax bronchial smooth muscle by stimulation of these receptors. The β receptor, briefly characterized as an example of a G protein–linked receptor in Chapter 2 in the introduction to *pharmacodynamics* (drug-receptor interaction), is discussed in more detail in Chapter 6, which discusses β-adrenergic bronchodilators. A third type of β receptor, the β_3 receptor, has also been distinguished as a β-receptor type found on lipocytes (fat cells) whose stimulation results in lipolysis.

α_1 and α_2 Receptors

> ## ! KEY POINT
>
> α Receptors are subdivided into α_1 receptors, which are excitatory, and α_2 receptors, which are inhibitory and are found on the presynaptic neuron to inhibit further neurotransmitter release.

α Receptors have also been differentiated into α_1 and α_2 receptors. This classification has been made on a *morphologic* basis (location of the receptors) and a *pharmacologic* basis (differences in response to various drugs). The pharmacologic differentiation of α_1 and α_2 receptors is similar to the distinction between α and β receptors (Figure 5-8). This differentiation is based on a response continuum ranging from excitation (α_1) to inhibition (α_2) as different drugs are administered. For example, phenylephrine causes vasoconstriction, as previously mentioned, whereas clonidine

(Catapres) causes a lowering of blood pressure and sympathetic activity. *Both* agents are considered to be α-receptor agonists. Other agents such as prazosin (Minipress) or labetalol (Normodyne) cause a lowering of blood pressure, but yohimbine causes an increase in blood pressure. Yet *all* these agents are considered α-receptor antagonists. Blockade of α_1-excitatory receptors by prazosin would prevent vasoconstriction and decrease blood pressure, whereas blockade of α_2-inhibitory receptors by yohimbine would prevent vasodilation and increase blood pressure.

Because different α agonists can cause opposite effects, and different α blockers do the same, α receptors were subdivided into the two types described. The location-based, or morphologic, differentiation of α_1 and α_2 receptors is more complex. In *peripheral* nerves, α_1 receptors are located on postsynaptic sites, such as vascular smooth muscle, and α_2 receptors are presynaptic (Figure 5-9). Stimulation of these peripheral α_1 receptors causes excitation and vasoconstriction; activation of peripheral (presynaptic) α_2 receptors causes inhibition of further neurotransmitter release. Peripheral α_2 receptors perform a negative feedback control mechanism, referred to as *autoregulation*, which has been shown with sympathetic (adrenergic) neurons; they are referred to as *autoreceptors*[5] (see Figure 5-5). Norepinephrine released from the nerve ending can activate α_1 (postsynaptic) and α_2 (presynaptic) receptors. Postsynaptic stimulation causes a cell response, such as vasoconstriction, but presynaptic stimulation leads to inhibition of further neurotransmitter release. In the CNS, α_2 receptors are generally considered to be on postsynaptic sites; this is the reverse of their location peripherally, where they are presynaptic. These central postsynaptic α_2 receptors are the site of action for antihypertensive agents, such as clonidine (Catapres) or methyldopa (Aldomet). These are discussed further and illustrated in Chapter 22.

To summarize, α_1 and β_1 receptors *excite*, and α_2 and β_2 receptors *inhibit*. This consistency of subscripts for (1) excitation versus (2) inhibition aids in remembering their effects.

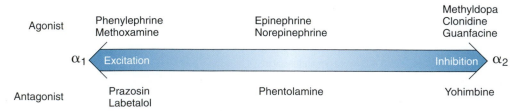

Figure 5-8 Spectrum of activity of α-receptor agonists and antagonists, from excitatory to inhibitory. Epinephrine and norepinephrine can stimulate α_1-receptor and α_2-receptor sites. A drug such as phenylephrine stimulates α_1 receptors and causes vasoconstriction, whereas methyldopa stimulates α_2 receptors and can decrease blood pressure, although both are α-receptor agonists. Prazosin is a selective α_1-blocking agent, and yohimbine is a selective α_2-blocking agent.

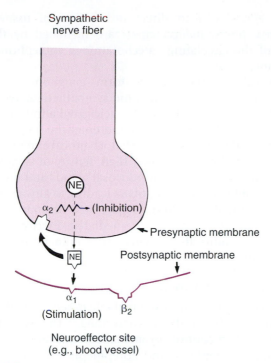

Sympathetic
nerve fiber

NE

α_2 ∿∿∿ (Inhibition)

NE — Presynaptic membrane

NE

Postsynaptic membrane

α_1

(Stimulation) β_2

Neuroeffector site
(e.g., blood vessel)

Figure 5-9 Location and effect of α_2 receptors, also designated *auto-receptors*. Stimulation of α_2 receptors by norepinephrine *(NE)* on the presynaptic neuron inhibits further neurotransmitter release and nerve action.

Dopaminergic Receptors

Other receptors in the CNS (brain) respond to dopamine, a chemical precursor of norepinephrine, and are therefore termed *dopaminergic*. Because dopamine is chemically similar to epinephrine and stimulates α and β receptors, dopaminergic receptors are classified as a type of adrenergic receptor.

SYMPATHOMIMETIC (ADRENERGIC) AND SYMPATHOLYTIC (ANTIADRENERGIC) AGENTS

Drugs that stimulate the sympathetic system and produce adrenergic effects (sympathomimetics) and drugs that block adrenergic effects (sympatholytics) are discussed in greater detail in separate chapters. In this book, emphasis is placed on β-adrenergic agonists used for bronchodilation (see Chapter 6) and on adrenergic agonists used for cardiovascular effects, such as cardiac stimulation (see Chapter 21) or vasoconstriction (see Chapter 22). Adrenergic blocking agents are considered for their antihypertensive and antianginal effects (see Chapter 22. To exemplify both sympathomimetic and sympatholytic agents, Table 5-6 provides selected examples of drugs categorized as agonists or antagonists of the sympathetic system, listing generic names, brand names, and common clinical uses.

NEURAL CONTROL OF LUNG FUNCTION

Both branches of the autonomic nervous system, sympathetic and parasympathetic, exert control of lung function. At present, the two branches form the basis for two classes of respiratory care drugs that modify airway smooth muscle tone: the adrenergic bronchodilator group and the anticholinergic bronchodilator group.

Lung function includes more than just airway smooth muscle tone. Multiple sites and tissues are involved in lung function, as follows:

- Airway smooth muscle
- Submucosal and surface secretory cells
- Bronchial epithelium
- Pulmonary and bronchial blood vessels

TABLE 5-6	Examples of Adrenergic Agonists and Antagonists		
CATEGORY	**GENERIC NAME**	**BRAND NAME**	**USES**
Sympathomimetic	Epinephrine	Adrenalin	Bronchodilator, cardiac stimulant, vasoconstrictor
	Ephedrine	Sudafed, various	Nasal decongestant
	Dextroamphetamine	Dexedrine	CNS stimulant
	Dopamine	Intropin	Vasopressor, shock syndrome
	Albuterol	Proventil, Ventolin, Pro Air	Bronchodilator
	Salmeterol	Serevent	Bronchodilator
Sympatholytic	Phentolamine	Regitine, Oraverse	Vasodilator, pheochromocytoma, reverse effects of local anesthetics on lip and tongue after dental procedures
	Prazosin	Minipress	Antihypertensive
	Labetalol	Generic only	Antihypertensive
	Metoprolol	Lopressor, Toprol-XL	Antihypertensive, antianginal
	Propranolol	Inderal, Innopran-XL	Antihypertensive, antiarrhythmic (PAT)
	Timolol	Betimol, various	Ophthalmic solution, treat increased IOP in patients with glaucoma
	Esmolol	Brevibloc	Antiarrhythmic

CNS, Central nervous system; *IOP,* intraocular pressure; *PAT,* paroxysmal atrial tachycardia.

In addition to autonomic nerve fibers and the receptors associated with them, sites in the lung (smooth muscle, glands, and vascular beds) may be affected by release of mediators from inflammatory cells, such as mast cells and platelets, or by release of epithelial factors, such as a relaxant factor, which can reduce airway contractility in response to spasmogens such as histamine, serotonin, or Ach.[6] Receptors in the lung and airways for mediators released by inflammatory cells include the following:

- *Histamine receptors:* Especially the H_1 type
- *Prostaglandin receptors:* Such as prostacyclin, prostaglandin D_2 (PGD_2), prostaglandin $F_{2\alpha}$ ($PGF_{2\alpha}$), and thromboxane A_2
- *Leukotriene receptors:* Such as LTB_4 and the C_4-D_4-E_4 series that comprise what was formerly termed *slow-reacting substance of anaphylaxis (SRS-A)*
- *Platelet-activating factor (PAF) receptors*
- *Adenosine receptors:* Such as A_1 and A_2
- *Bradykinin receptors*

The mediators of inflammation and their receptors (e.g., histamine and prostaglandins) are discussed in the review of corticosteroids (Chapter 11) and other antiasthmatic drugs (Chapter 12) intended to inhibit or prevent an inflammatory response in the lung.

Sympathetic Innervation and Effects

The sympathetic nervous system exerts its effects by direct and indirect means, as outlined in previous sections.

Direct effects refer to direct innervation of tissue sites by nerve fibers. *Indirect effects* are mediated by the release of the circulating catecholamines epinephrine and norepinephrine.

Sympathetic nerve fibers form ganglionic synapses outside the lung. Postganglionic sympathetic nerve fibers from the cervical and upper thoracic ganglia form plexuses at the hilar region of the lung and enter the lung mingled with parasympathetic nerves. Histochemical and ultrastructural studies show a relatively high density of sympathetic nerve fibers attaching to submucosal glands and bronchial arteries but few or no nerve fibers leading to airway smooth muscle in the human lung.[7] Figure 5-10 illustrates sympathetic innervation and effects mediated directly by nerve action and indirectly by circulating epinephrine in the human lung.

Airway Smooth Muscle

There is little or no direct sympathetic innervation of airway smooth muscle in the human lung.[8] The sympathetic nervous system controls bronchial smooth muscle tone by circulating epinephrine and norepinephrine, which act on α and β receptors on airway smooth muscle. Recall that epinephrine stimulates both α and β receptors, whereas norepinephrine acts primarily on α receptors.

β receptors. β receptors mediate relaxation of airway smooth muscle. This action is mimicked by the class of β-adrenergic bronchodilators, introduced in Chapter 6. β receptors are distributed from the trachea to the terminal bronchioles; the density of these receptors increases as the

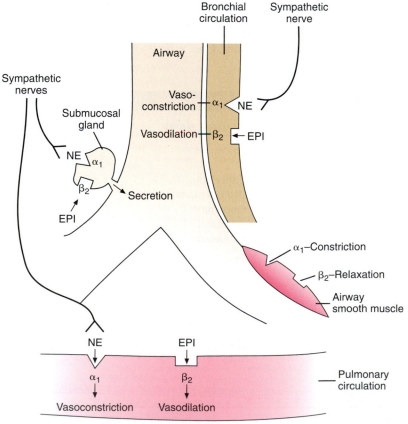

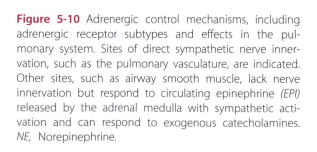

Figure 5-10 Adrenergic control mechanisms, including adrenergic receptor subtypes and effects in the pulmonary system. Sites of direct sympathetic nerve innervation, such as the pulmonary vasculature, are indicated. Other sites, such as airway smooth muscle, lack nerve innervation but respond to circulating epinephrine *(EPI)* released by the adrenal medulla with sympathetic activation and can respond to exogenous catecholamines. *NE,* Norepinephrine.

airway diameter becomes smaller. β agonists can cause relaxation of small airways.

β_2 receptors traditionally have been identified as the β-receptor subtype on the airway smooth muscle; this has been further verified for the human lung by autoradiographic studies and molecular gene studies.[9] There is species variation for the presence of β-receptor subtypes, however, with β_1 and β_2 receptors present in guinea pig and dog airways.

β_1 and β_2 receptors in the lung have also been distinguished as *neuronal* and *hormonal* receptors, respectively. This is based on the concept that β_1 receptors are β receptors for sites where norepinephrine is released from sympathetic nerve terminal fibers (neuronal); β_2 receptors are β receptors responsive to circulating epinephrine (hormonal). Both receptors cause airway smooth muscle relaxation when stimulated, either by sympathetic nerve release of norepinephrine or by circulating epinephrine, in species such as the dog or guinea pig, which have β_1 receptors on airway smooth muscle.[10] In the human lung, which has no sympathetic innervation of the airway smooth muscle, adrenergic receptors are all of the β_2 type; β_1 receptors have been identified by radioligand binding and autoradiographic studies of alveolar walls in the lung periphery.[9] Using this terminology, relaxation of human airway smooth muscle would be accomplished by stimulation of hormonal β receptors via circulating or exogenous catecholamines. β_3 receptors, which have also been identified on lipocytes, have no known function in the human airway.[11]

α receptors. α receptors exist in the human lung in less quantity than β receptors and with no difference in distribution between large and small airways. Norepinephrine stimulates α receptors, but their effect in the airway seems to be minor. Evidence of sympathetic-induced bronchoconstriction has been provided by studies in which lung tissue was treated with a β blocker, or antagonist (e.g., propranolol), and then exposed to epinephrine, which stimulates α and β receptors.[12] Because β receptors were blocked, the epinephrine attached to the free α receptors; the result was contraction of the smooth muscle, providing evidence of the existence of α receptors and showing a contractile effect. The clinical use of α receptor–blocking agents such as dibenamine, thymoxamine, and phentolamine in cases of status asthmaticus has been reported for more than 40 years, lending support to the role of α receptors in bronchial contraction.[13] The role of α receptors in controlling airway smooth muscle remains the subject of investigation.

Lung Blood Vessels

Blood flow in the lung is made up of two different systems: the *pulmonary* and the *bronchial* circulations. The pulmonary circulation receives the body's venous return from the right heart and is critical for gas exchange. The bronchial circulation is an arterial supply and perfuses lung tissue to supply nutrients and remove metabolic byproducts.

The pulmonary circulation is innervated by parasympathetic and sympathetic nerves. Sympathetic nerves release norepinephrine to stimulate α receptors and cause vascular

contraction. β receptors on pulmonary blood vessels cause relaxation and are stimulated by circulating epinephrine. An exogenous catecholamine can cause vasoconstriction, dilation, or no effect, depending on the relative stimulation of receptor types.

The bronchial circulation is innervated predominantly by sympathetic nerves. Activation of sympathetic nerves causes vasoconstriction mediated by α receptors. Stimulation of β receptors by circulating epinephrine causes relaxation and vasodilation of bronchial blood vessels.

Mucous Glands

Human bronchial submucosal glands are innervated by sympathetic and parasympathetic nerves. α and β Receptors are present on tracheal submucosal glands. Stimulation of these receptors causes an increase in secretion of fluid and mucus. Epithelial cells on the airway lining do not have direct sympathetic innervation but do possess β_2 receptors whose stimulation can also increase secretion of fluid. Mucociliary clearance is enhanced, removing trapped particulate matter.[14]

Parasympathetic Innervation and Effects

KEY POINT

In the human lung, glands and blood vessels are innervated by sympathetic nerve fibers, but airway smooth muscle has few, if any, such fibers, responding instead to circulating epinephrine by means of β receptors. Parasympathetic vagal nerves innervate the lung as well, supplying the airway smooth muscle and mucous glands.

The lung is supplied by vagus nerves, with the recurrent laryngeal nerve (part of the thoracic vagus) innervating the trachea; other branches of the vagus enter the lung at the hilum and innervate the intrapulmonary airways. In the trachea and remaining airways, parasympathetic nerves supply airway smooth muscle and glands. The vagus nerves in the lung release Ach and are termed *cholinergic*. Ach couples with muscarinic Ach receptors on airway smooth muscle to cause bronchoconstriction and on submucosal glands to stimulate secretion. The action of Ach is limited by the enzyme acetylcholinesterase, or cholinesterase, which breaks down Ach.

Cholinergic nerve fibers in the lung are densest in the hilar region and decrease in density toward the airway periphery. Cholinergic muscarinic receptors also decrease in density in distal airways. Electrical stimulation of vagus nerves in dog studies caused more contraction in the intermediate bronchi than in the main bronchi or trachea.[15]

Muscarinic Receptors in the Airway

The genes for five subtypes of Ach, or muscarinic, receptors have been identified, designated M_1 through M_5. Only four of these subtypes, M_1 to M_4, have been identified by chemical (ligand)-binding studies pharmacologically. Three of these muscarinic receptor subtypes have been identified in the human lung: M_1, M_2, and M_3. Their locations are illustrated in Figure 5-11, and the function of each is discussed.

M_1 receptors. M_1 receptors are present at the parasympathetic ganglion on the postjunctional membrane. Usually, Ach ganglionic receptors are nicotinic, as described previously. However, the M_1 receptor may facilitate nicotinic receptor activity and nerve transmission, with an overall excitatory effect.

M_2 receptors. M_2 receptors are localized to the presynaptic membrane of postganglionic parasympathetic nerve endings. These receptors are thought to be autoregulatory receptors whose stimulation by Ach inhibits further Ach release from the nerve ending, thereby limiting the cholinergic stimulation. This is analogous to the α_2 receptor inhibiting further release of norepinephrine from sympathetic nerve endings, which identifies it as an autoreceptor as discussed previously (see section on Cholinergic Neurotransmitter Function). Stimulation of prejunctional M_2 receptors in human airways in vitro results in strong inhibition of cholinergic parasympathetic-induced bronchoconstriction. Pilocarpine, a direct-acting cholinergic agonist (parasympathomimetic), is a selective stimulant of M_2 receptors.[16] Inhalation of pilocarpine blocks cholinergic reflex bronchoconstriction caused by sulfur dioxide in nonasthmatic human subjects, verifying that M_2 receptor stimulation can block cholinergic bronchoconstriction.[17]

In asthmatic subjects, pilocarpine does not inhibit bronchoconstriction. This suggests the possibility of M_2 receptor dysfunction in asthma, resulting in increased cholinergic bronchoconstriction. If M_2 receptors fail to provide their normal inhibition of Ach release and bronchial contraction, this may explain why blockade of β receptors can cause such severe bronchoconstriction in asthmatics. The normal balance of Ach inhibition by M_2 receptors is lacking, and β blockade by drugs such as propranolol leaves Ach stimulation of airway smooth muscle unchecked.

M_3 receptors. M_3 receptors are present on submucosal glands and airway smooth muscle and possibly on surface goblet cells. Stimulation of M_3 receptors causes bronchoconstriction of smooth muscle, and exocytosis and glandular secretion from submucosal mucous glands. M_3 receptors may also be present on airway epithelial cells to increase ciliary beat. Antagonism of M_3 receptors is the basis for a class of bronchodilator agents: the anticholinergic bronchodilators (see Chapter 7).

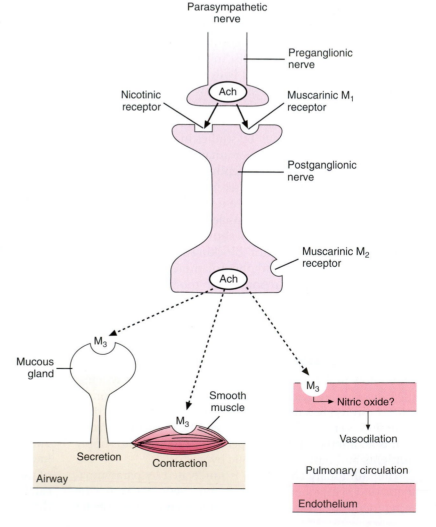

Figure 5-11 Location and effects of muscarinic receptor subtypes in the pulmonary system. *Ach,* Acetylcholine.

Muscarinic Receptors on Blood Vessels

Muscarinic M_3 receptors are located on endothelial cells of both the bronchial and the pulmonary vasculature. Stimulation of M_3 receptors causes release of an endothelium-derived relaxant factor.[18] This relaxant factor, which produces vasodilation and is mediated by an increase in intracellular cyclic guanosine monophosphate (cGMP), has been identified as nitric oxide (NO) or a very similar nitrosocompound.[19]

Nonadrenergic, Noncholinergic Inhibitory Nerves

KEY POINT

In addition to sympathetic and parasympathetic nerves in the lung, there is evidence of a nonadrenergic, noncholinergic (NANC) system. This system has inhibitory and excitatory branches.

There is evidence of a branch of nerves that are neither parasympathetic (cholinergic) nor sympathetic (adrenergic) that can cause relaxation of airway smooth muscle. These nerves have been termed nonadrenergic, noncholinergic (NANC) inhibitory nerves.[20] They are also referred to as simply nonadrenergic inhibitory nerves because adrenergic activity relaxes airway smooth muscle, and this is an additional but nonadrenergic neural method of relaxing such smooth muscle. Evidence of NANC inhibitory nerves is based on the following type of experimentation. When parasympathetic (cholinergic) receptors are blocked with an antagonist, such as atropine, and sympathetic (adrenergic) receptors are also blocked with a β blocker, such as propranolol, electrical field stimulation of the lung produces relaxation of bronchial smooth muscle. Katzung[21] provides a more detailed description and evidence of this methodology. Figure 5-12 illustrates this inhibitory system

that is neither adrenergic nor cholinergic and its possible neurotransmitter substances. A nonadrenergic inhibitory nervous system found in the gastrointestinal tract is primarily responsible for the relaxation of peristalsis and the internal anal sphincter. In the gastrointestinal tract, this system develops in conjunction with the parasympathetic branch. Embryologically, the gastrointestinal and respiratory tracts share a common origin, and the separation of the trachea and gut occurs around the fourth or fifth week of gestation. This common origin adds plausibility to the presence of a nonadrenergic inhibitory system in the lungs similar to that in the gastrointestinal tract.

KEY POINT

Inhibitory effects on airway smooth muscle cause bronchodilation and may be mediated by the neurotransmitter vasoactive intestinal peptide (VIP) or by NO.

The exact neurotransmitter responsible for relaxation responses mediated by NANC inhibitory nerves is under investigation; however, the neurotransmitter vasoactive intestinal peptide (VIP) is the current front-runner.[22] VIP can relax mammalian airway smooth muscle. Another possible neurotransmitter causing airway smooth muscle relaxation is NO. The enzyme responsible for NO synthesis, nitric oxide synthase (NOS), has been found in nerve terminals around airway smooth muscle, and NO produces effects similar to those caused by NANC inhibitory nerve activation. Ricciardolo[23] believed that NANC inhibition is mediated by NO with the help of VIP. An NANC inhibitory neurotransmitter substance has not yet been definitively identified.

Nonadrenergic, Noncholinergic Excitatory Nerves

The existence of NANC excitatory nervous control of airway smooth muscle has also been shown using electrical field

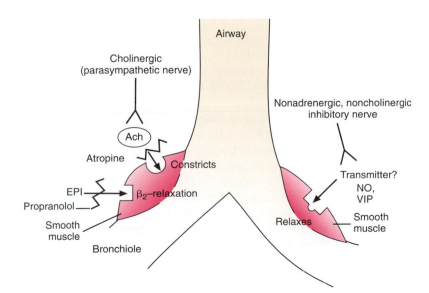

Figure 5-12 Nonadrenergic inhibitory nervous system in the lung, which can cause relaxation of airway smooth muscle. Relaxation of smooth muscle occurs in the presence of cholinergic blockade by atropine and adrenergic blockade by propranolol. *Ach*, Acetylcholine; *EPI*, epinephrine; *NO*, nitric oxide; *VIP*, vasoactive intestinal peptide.

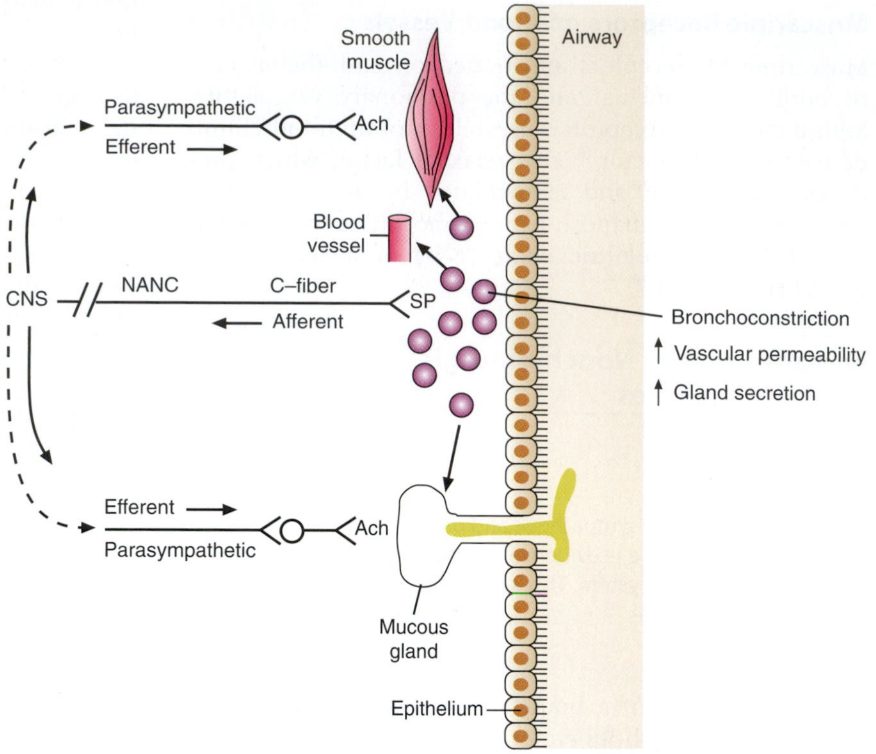

Figure 5-13 Afferent C-fibers making up the nonadrenergic, noncholinergic *(NANC)* excitatory nervous system in the lung. Activation of C-fibers causes an afferent impulse with reflex parasympathetic activity and release of substance P, causing local effects in the airway. *Ach,* Acetylcholine; *CNS,* central nervous system; *SP,* substance P.

stimulation (EFS) techniques. This system is also referred to as simply *noncholinergic excitatory nervous control* because cholinergic activity contracts airway smooth muscle, and this is an additional but noncholinergic neural method of exciting and constricting such smooth muscle. Stimulation of NANC excitatory nerves causes bronchial contraction. Sensory *afferent* nerves termed *C-fibers* are present in the airways, around bronchial blood vessels, around submucosal glands, and within the airway epithelium. These afferent fibers follow vagal nerve tracts into the CNS, as shown in Figure 5-13.

KEY POINT

Excitatory effects such as bronchoconstriction are produced by afferent sensory fibers that have substance P as a neurotransmitter; these effects are caused by local release of substance P and by afferent-efferent reflex arcs involving efferent cholinergic transmission.

Sensory C-fiber nerves contain substance P, which is a tachykinin (a family of small peptide mediators). Substance P is also referred to as a *neuropeptide*. Sensory C-fibers can be stimulated by noxious substances such as capsaicin, found in chili peppers. When stimulated, C-fibers conduct impulses to the CNS that result in reflexes of cough and parasympathetically induced bronchoconstriction. Sensory C-fibers also release their neuropeptides, such as substance P, at the local site of the nerve fiber. Substance P and other tachykinins cause bronchoconstriction in the airways and vasodilation, increased vascular permeability, mucous gland secretion, and enhanced mucociliary activity. The

NANC excitatory C-fiber system has been considered as a possible cause of the hyperreactive airway seen in asthma. The presence of C-fibers is less marked in human airways than in rodent species.

? SELF-ASSESSMENT QUESTIONS

Answers can be found in Appendix A.
1. Which portion of the nervous system is under voluntary control: the autonomic or the skeletal muscle motor nerve portion?
2. What is the neurotransmitter at each of the following sites: neuromuscular junction; autonomic ganglia; and most sympathetic end sites?
3. Where are muscarinic receptors found?
4. What is the effect of cholinergic stimulation on airway smooth muscle?
5. What is the effect of adrenergic stimulation on the heart?
6. Classify the drugs pilocarpine, physostigmine, propranolol, and epinephrine.
7. How do indirect-acting cholinergic agonists (parasympathomimetics) produce their action?
8. What effect would the drug atropine have on the eye and on airway smooth muscle?
9. What is the general difference between α and β receptors in the sympathetic nervous system?
10. What is the primary mechanism for terminating the neurotransmitters acetylcholine and norepinephrine?

11. What is the predominant sympathetic receptor type found on airway smooth muscle?
12. Identify the adrenergic receptor preference for phenylephrine, norepinephrine, and epinephrine.
13. What is the autoregulatory receptor on the sympathetic presynaptic neuron?
14. Classify the following drugs by autonomic class and receptor preference: dopamine, ephedrine, albuterol, phentolamine, propranolol, and prazosin.
15. What is the autoregulatory receptor on the parasympathetic presynaptic neuron at the terminal nerve site?
16. Contrast general α_1-receptor and α_2-receptor effects.
17. What substance may be the neurotransmitter in the NANC inhibitory nervous system in the lung?
18. What substance is the neurotransmitter in the NANC excitatory nervous system in the lung?

 CLINICAL SCENARIO

Answers can be found in Appendix A.

A 42-year-old white woman with a long-standing history of asthma presents to the emergency department (ED) of a local acute care hospital. She states that she has been feeling as if her "heart were racing" today. She currently uses a β-adrenergic bronchodilator (albuterol) as needed and inhales an anticholinergic bronchodilator (ipratropium bromide) before bedtime; both drugs are administered by a metered dose inhaler (MDI).

On admission to the ED, she has the following vital signs: pulse (P) 155 beats/min, regular blood pressure (BP) 146/90 mm Hg, and respiratory rate (RR) 22 breaths/min with mild distress.

Her breath sounds are clear to auscultation, and a chest radiograph (posteroanterior [PA]) shows no abnormalities. A lead II electrocardiogram (ECG) reveals supraventricular tachycardia (SVT). Oxygen saturation as revealed by pulse oximetry (SpO$_2$) is 90%. A resident orders oxygen at 2 L/min by nasal cannula and intravenous propranolol for SVT, which is given. Approximately 5 minutes later, her heart rate is reduced to 110 beats/min, but she begins to wheeze audibly and complains of severe shortness of breath (SOB), and her respiratory pattern is labored at 26 breaths/min. She is anxious, and her SpO$_2$ reading decreases from 92% to 72%.

Using the SOAP method, assess this clinical scenario.

REFERENCES

1. Iversen LL: The uptake of catecholamines at high perfusion concentrations in the rat isolated heart: a novel catecholamine uptake process. *Br J Pharmacol* 25:18, 1965.
2. Iversen LL, Salt PJ: Inhibition of catecholamine uptake 2 by steroids in the isolated rat heart. *Br J Pharmacol* 40:528, 1970.
3. Ahlquist RP: A study of the adrenotropic receptors. *Am J Physiol* 153:586, 1948.
4. Lands AM, Arnold A, McAuliff JP, et al: Differentiation of receptor systems activated by sympathomimetic amines. *Nature* 214:597, 1967.
5. Langer SZ: Presynaptic regulation of the release of catecholamines. *Pharmacol Rev* 32:337, 1980.
6. Barnes PJ: Airway receptors. *Postgrad Med J* 65:532, 1989.
7. Partanen M, Laitinen A, Hervonen A, et al: Catecholamine- and acetylcholinesterase-containing nerves in human lower respiratory tract. *Histochemistry* 76:175, 1982.
8. Barnes PJ: Neural control of human airways in health and disease. *Am Rev Respir Dis* 134:1289, 1986.
9. Carstairs JR, Nimmo AJ, Barnes PJ: Autoradiographic visualization of beta-adrenoceptor subtypes in human lung. *Am Rev Respir Dis* 132:541, 1985.
10. Ariens EJ, Simonis AM: Physiological and pharmacological aspects of adrenergic receptor classification. *Biochem Pharmacol* 32:1539, 1983.
11. Emorine L, Blin N, Strosberg AD: The human 3-adrenoceptor: the search for a physiological function. *Trends Pharmacol Sci* 15:3, 1994.
12. Adolphson RL, Abern SB, Townley RG: Human and guinea pig respiratory smooth muscle: demonstration of alpha adrenergic receptors. *J Allergy* 47:110, 1971 (abstract).
13. Falliers CJ, Tinkelman DG: Alternative drug therapy for asthma. *Clin Chest Med* 7:383, 1986.
14. Biaggioni I, Robertson D: Adrenoceptor agonist and sympathomimetic drugs. In Katzung BG, Masters SB, Trevor AJ, editors: *Basic and clinical pharmacology*, ed 12, New York, 2012, McGraw-Hill Medical.
15. Pappano AJ: Cholinoceptor-activating and cholinesterase-inhibiting drugs. In Katzung BG, Masters SB, Trevor AJ, editors: *Basic and clinical pharmacology*, ed 12, New York, 2012, McGraw-Hill Medical.
16. Barnes PJ: Muscarinic receptor subtypes in airways. *Life Sci* 52:521, 1993.
17. Minette PA, Lammers JW, Dixon CM, et al: A muscarinic agonist inhibits reflex bronchoconstriction in normal but not in asthmatic subjects. *J Appl Physiol* 67:2461, 1989.
18. Cuss FM, Barnes PJ: Epithelial mediators. *Am Rev Respir Dis* 136:S32, 1987.
19. Katzung BG, Chatterjee K: Vasodilators and the treatment of angina pectoris. In Katzung BG, Masters SB, Trevor AJ, editors: *Basic and clinical pharmacology*, ed 12, New York, 2012, McGraw-Hill Medical.
20. Richardson JB, Beland J: Nonadrenergic inhibitory nervous system in human airways. *J Appl Physiol* 41:764, 1976.
21. Katzung BG: Introduction to autonomic nervous system. In Katzung BG, Masters SB, Trevor AJ, editors: *Basic and clinical pharmacology*, ed 12, New York, 2012, McGraw-Hill Medical.
22. Stephens NL: Airway smooth muscle. *Lung* 179:333, 2002.
23. Ricciardolo FLM: Multiple roles of nitric oxide in the airways. *Thorax* 58:175, 2003.

UNIT TWO

Drugs Used to Treat the Respiratory System

CHAPTER 6

Adrenergic (Sympathomimetic) Bronchodilators

Douglas S. Gardenhire

CHAPTER OUTLINE

OBJECTIVES

After reading this chapter, the reader will be able to:

1. Define *sympathomimetic*
2. Define *adrenergic*
3. List all currently available β-adrenergic agents used in respiratory therapy
4. Differentiate between the specific adrenergic agents and formulations
5. Describe the mechanism of action for each specific adrenergic agent and formulation
6. Describe the route of administration available for β agonists
7. Discuss adverse effects of β agonists
8. Clinically assess β-agonist therapy

KEY TERMS AND DEFINITIONS

Adrenergic bronchodilator Agent that stimulates sympathetic nervous fibers, which allow relaxation of smooth muscle in the airway. Also known as sympathomimetic bronchodilator or β_2 agonist.

α-Receptor stimulation Causes vasoconstriction and vasopressor effect; in the upper airway (nasal passages), this can provide decongestion.

Asthma paradox Refers to the increasing incidence of asthma morbidity, and especially asthma mortality, despite advances in

Continued

Chapter 6 presents adrenergic drugs used as inhaled bronchodilators. The specific agents and the clinical indications for this class of drugs are summarized, along with their mechanism of action as mediated by β receptors. Structure-activity relationships of available agents are presented as a basis for their difference in receptor selectivity and duration of action. Differences among routes of administration are discussed, and side effects are reviewed. A brief summary of the debate over possible harmful effects with β agonists is given.

CLINICAL INDICATIONS FOR ADRENERGIC BRONCHODILATORS

KEY POINT

The adrenergic bronchodilator group is used for the treatment of reversible airway obstruction in diseases such as asthma and chronic obstructive pulmonary disease (COPD). These agents produce bronchodilation by stimulating β_2 receptors on airway smooth muscle.

The general indication for use of an **adrenergic bronchodilator** is relaxation of airway smooth muscle in the presence of reversible airflow obstruction associated with acute and chronic asthma (including exercise-induced asthma), bronchitis, emphysema, bronchiectasis, and other obstructive airway diseases. Differences in the rate of onset, peak effect, and duration led to a distinction in use between short-acting and long-acting agents. Various recommendations and guidelines exist for the use of β agonists in chronic obstructive pulmonary disease (COPD) and asthma.

Indication for Short-Acting Agents

Short-acting β_2 agonists such as albuterol, levalbuterol, or metaproterenol are indicated for relief of *acute* reversible airflow obstruction in asthma or other obstructive airway

diseases, such as COPD. Short-acting agents are termed "rescue" agents in the 2007 National Asthma Education and Prevention Program Expert Panel Report 3 (NAEPP EPR 3) guidelines.[1] Short-term acting agents may also be termed "relievers" as discussed in the Global Initiative for Asthma (GINA) guidelines.[2]

Indication for Long-Acting Agents

Long-acting agents such as salmeterol, formoterol, arformoterol, indacaterol, and olodaterol are indicated for the maintenance of bronchodilation and control of **bronchospasm** and nocturnal symptoms in asthma or other obstructive diseases, such as COPD. Salmeterol, formoterol, arformoterol, indacaterol, and olodaterol are long-acting beta agonists (LABA) or "controllers"; the slow time to peak effect makes long-acting agents poor rescue drugs. In asthma, a long-acting bronchodilator is usually combined with anti-inflammatory medication for control of airway inflammation and bronchospasm. Although arformoterol, formoterol, indacaterol, and olodaterol have a rapid onset of action similar to or better than that of albuterol, their slower peak effect and prolonged activity make them a better maintenance drug than an acute reliever or rescue agent.

Indication for Racemic Epinephrine

Racemic epinephrine is often used, either as an inhaled aerosol or by direct lung instillation, for its strong α-adrenergic vasoconstricting effect to reduce airway swelling after extubation; during epiglottitis, croup, or bronchiolitis; and to control airway bleeding during endoscopy.

SPECIFIC ADRENERGIC AGENTS AND FORMULATIONS

Table 6-1 lists adrenergic bronchodilators currently approved for general clinical use in the United States as of the writing of this edition. Practitioners are urged to read package inserts on a drug before administration. These

TABLE 6-1 Inhaled Adrenergic Bronchodilator Agents Currently Available in the United States

DRUG	BRAND NAME	RECEPTOR PREFERENCE	ADULT DOSAGE	TIME COURSE (ONSET, PEAK, DURATION)
Ultra-Short-Acting Adrenergic Bronchodilator Agents				
Racemic epinephrine	Asthmanefrin	α, β	SVN: 2.25% solution, 0.25-0.5 mL (5.63-11.25 mg) qid	*Onset:* 3-5 min *Peak:* 5-20 min *Duration:* 0.5-2 hr
Short-Acting Adrenergic Bronchodilator Agents				
Metaproterenol		β_2	SVN: 0.4%, 0.6% solution, tid, qid Tab: 10 mg and 20 mg, tid, qid Syrup: 10 mg per 5 mL	*Onset:* 1-5 min *Peak:* 60 min *Duration:* 2-6 hr
Albuterol	Proventil HFA, Ventolin HFA, ProAir HFA, AccuNeb, VoSpire ER	β_2	SVN: 0.5% solution, 0.5 mL (2.5 mg), 0.63 mg, 1.25-mg and 2.5-mg unit dose, tid, qid MDI: 90 mcg/puff, 2 puffs tid, qid Tab: 2 mg, 4 mg, and 8 mg, bid, tid, qid Syrup: 2 mg/5 mL, 1-2 tsp tid, qid	*Onset:* 15 min *Peak:* 30-60 min *Duration:* 5-12 hr
Levalbuterol	Xopenex, Xopenex HFA	β_2	SVN: 0.31 mg/3 mL tid, 0.63 mg/3 mL tid, or 1.25 mg/3 mL tid; concentrate 1.25 mg/0.5 mL, tid MDI: 45 mcg/puff, 2 puffs q4-6h	*Onset:* 15 min *Peak:* 30-60 min *Duration:* 5-8 hr
Long-Acting Adrenergic Bronchodilator Agents				
Salmeterol	Serevent Diskus	β_2	DPI: 50 mcg/blister bid	*Onset:* 20 min *Peak:* 3-5 hr *Duration:* 12 hr
Formoterol	Perforomist, Foradil	β_2	SVN: 20 mcg/2-mL unit dose, bid DPI: 12 mcg/inhalation, bid	*Onset:* 15 min *Peak:* 30-60 min *Duration:* 12 hr
Arformoterol	Brovana	β_2	SVN: 15 mcg/2-mL unit dose, bid	*Onset:* 15 min *Peak:* 30-60 min *Duration:* 12 hr
Indacaterol	Arcapta Neohaler	β_2	DPI: 75mcg/inhalation, once daily	*Onset:* 5 min *Peak:* 30 min *Duration:* 24 hr
Olodaterol	Stiverdi Respimat	β_2	DPI: 2.5mcg/actuation, 2 actuations daily	*Onset:* 5 min *Peak:* 30-60 min *Duration:* 24 hr

DPI, Dry powder inhaler; *MDI*, metered dose inhaler; *SVN*, small volume nebulizer.

inserts give details of dosage strengths and frequencies, adverse effects, shelf life, and storage requirements, all of which are needed for safe application. Table 6-1 is not intended to replace more detailed information supplied by the manufacturer on each of the bronchodilator agents. There are three subgroups of adrenergic bronchodilators based on distinct differences in duration of action:

- *Ultra-short-acting* (duration less than 3 hours): Racemic epinephrine
- *Short-acting* (duration 4 to 6 hours): Albuterol, levalbuterol, and metaproterenol
- *Long-acting* (duration 12 to 24 hours): Salmeterol, formoterol, arformoterol, indacaterol, and olodaterol

Catecholamines

The sympathomimetic bronchodilators are all either catecholamines or derivatives of catecholamines. A **catecholamine** is a chemical structure consisting of an aromatic catechol nucleus and a dialiphatic amine side chain. In Figure 6-1, the basic catecholamine structure is seen to be composed of a benzene ring with hydroxyl groups at the third and fourth carbon sites and an amine side chain attached at the first carbon position.

The terminal amine group (NH_2) and the benzene ring are connected by two carbon atoms, designated as α and β, a notation not to be confused with α and β receptors in the sympathetic nervous system. Examples of catecholamines are dopamine, epinephrine, norepinephrine, and isoproterenol. The first three occur naturally in the body. Catecholamines, or **sympathomimetic** amines, mimic the actions of epinephrine more or less precisely, causing tachycardia, elevated blood pressure, smooth muscle relaxation of bronchioles and skeletal muscle blood vessels, glycogenolysis, skeletal muscle tremor, and central nervous system (CNS) stimulation.

Adrenergic Bronchodilators as Stereoisomers

Adrenergic bronchodilators can exist in two different spatial arrangements, producing isomers. Rotation around the β carbon on the ethylamine side chain of the basic molecular structure seen in Figure 6-1 produces two non-superimposable mirror images, termed *enantiomers* or simply *isomers*. Figure 6-2 illustrates epinephrine as a *stereoisomer*, showing the (R)-isomers and (S)-isomers as the mirror image of each other. Enantiomers have similar physical and chemical properties but different physiologic effects. The (R)-isomer, or levo isomer, is active on airway β receptors, producing bronchodilation, and on extrapulmonary adrenergic receptors. The (S)-isomer, or dextro isomer, is not active on adrenergic receptors such as β receptors, and until more recently the (S)-isomer was considered physiologically inert. The two mirror images of the isomers rotate light in opposite directions (see Figure 6-2), providing two isomers and this is the basis for designating them as dextrorotatory (*d*, +) or levorotatory (*l*, −). Using their actual spatial configuration, the levo isomer and dextro isomer are referred to as the *(R)-isomer* (for *rectus*, right) and *(S)-isomer* (for *sinister*, left), respectively. Adrenergic bronchodilators such as epinephrine, albuterol, and salmeterol have been produced synthetically as racemic mixtures, or 50:50 equimolar mixes of the (R)-isomers and (S)-isomers. Natural epinephrine found in the adrenal gland occurs as the (R)-isomer, or levo isomer, only. Levalbuterol, released in 1999, represents the first *synthetic* inhaled solution available as the single (R)-isomer of racemic albuterol. Other bronchodilators such as Formoterol have two or double steriogenic atoms on each side because it is a racemic mixture (50:50). Formoterol will have an RR isomer and a SS isomer; however, arformoterol, the single isomer of formoterol will only have the RR isomer. Structures of the currently available inhaled β agonists to be discussed are shown in Figure 6-3. Only a single isomer form is shown, for simplification and clarity.

Epinephrine. Epinephrine is a potent catecholamine bronchodilator that stimulates α and β receptors. Because epinephrine lacks β2-receptor specificity, there is a high prevalence of side effects, such as tachycardia, blood pressure increase, tremor, headache, and insomnia. Epinephrine occurs naturally in the adrenal medulla and has a rapid onset but a short duration because of metabolism by catechol O-methyltransferase (COMT). It has been administered both by inhalation and by subcutaneous injection to treat patients with asthma exacerbation. It is also used as a cardiac stimulant, based on its strong β1 effects. Self-administered, intramuscular injectable doses of 0.3 mg and 0.15 mg are marketed to control systemic hypersensitivity (anaphylactic) reactions.

This drug is more useful for the management of acute asthma rather than for daily maintenance therapy because of its pharmacokinetics and side effect profile; however, there are better β2 agonists for the treatment of acute asthma. The parenteral form of epinephrine is a natural extract, consisting of only the (R)-isomer, or levo isomer. The synthetic formulation of epinephrine for nebulization, Asthmanefrin, is a racemic mixture of the (R)-isomer, or levo isomer, and (S)-isomer, or dextro isomer. The mechanism of action of racemic epinephrine is the same as with natural epinephrine, giving α and β stimulation. Because only the (R)-isomer is active on adrenergic receptors, a 1:100 strength formulation of natural epinephrine (injectable formulation) has been used for nebulization, whereas a 2.25% strength racemic mixture is used in nebulization. An epinephrine metered dose inhaler (MDI) was sold

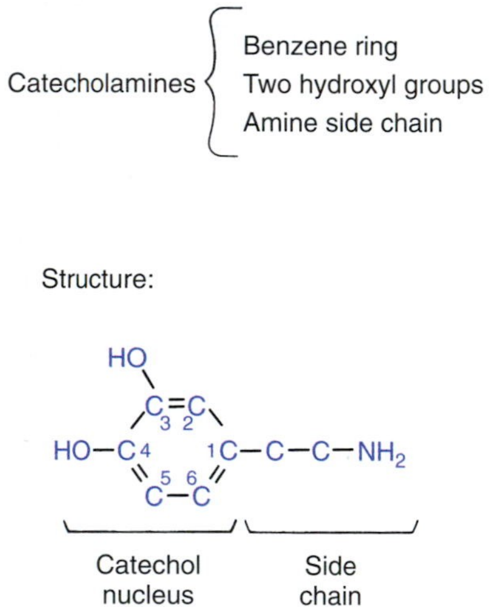

Catecholamines { Benzene ring / Two hydroxyl groups / Amine side chain

Structure:

Figure 6-1 Basic catecholamine structure, showing the catechol nucleus connected to an amine side chain.

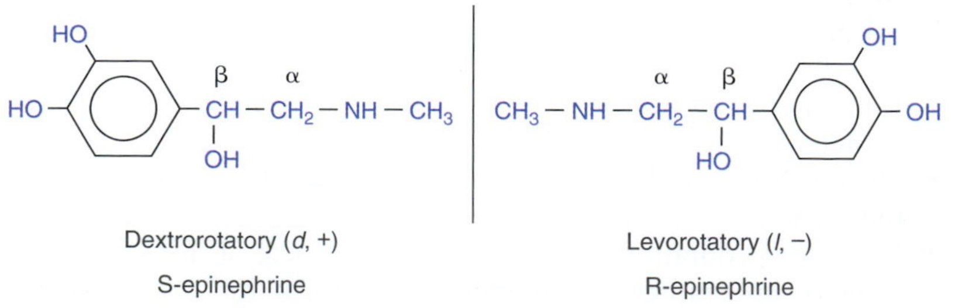

Figure 6-2 Structure of epinephrine, illustrating the (R)-isomer (levo, *l*, −) and (S)-isomer (dextro, *d*, +) as mirror images of each other, termed *enantiomers*. Natural epinephrine is *(R)*-epinephrine. Synthetic formulations for inhalation are racemic (50:50) mixtures of (R)-isomers and (S)-isomers.

Dextrorotatory (*d*, +)

S-epinephrine

Levorotatory (*l*, −)

R-epinephrine

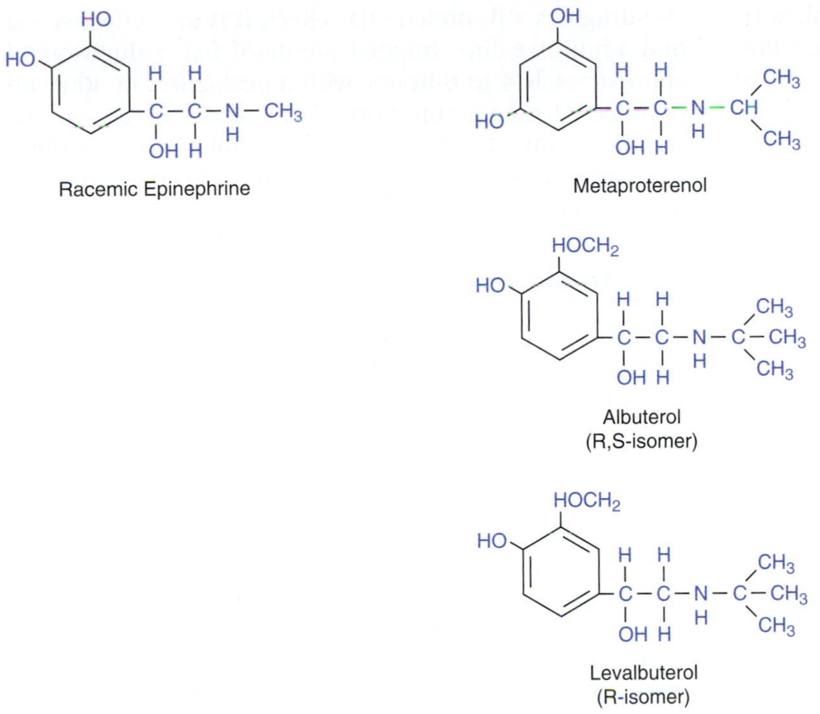

Racemic Epinephrine

Metaproterenol

Albuterol
(R,S-isomer)

Levalbuterol
(R-isomer)

Figure 6-3 Chemical structures of short-acting inhaled adrenergic bronchodilators currently available in the United States. With the exception of natural epinephrine and levalbuterol, all formulations are racemic mixtures and are shown in the same orientation for clarity. The isomers of racemic albuterol and levalbuterol are labeled to indicate the difference between these two drugs. Long-acting agents are illustrated in Figure 6-8. (From Rau JL, *Respir Care* 45:854, 2000.)

over-the-counter as Primatene Mist. The U.S. Food and Drug Administration (FDA) ruled in 2006 that Primatene Mist was not essential, which led to its removal from the market on December 31, 2011.[3] However, Nephron Pharmaceuticals launched Asthmanefrin (racemic epinephrine) over the counter (OTC) in 2012. Asthmanefrin is available as a liquid nebulizer solution and powered by a battery-operated atomizer.

Keyhole Theory of β_2 Specificity

The theory that explains the shift from α activity to β_2 specificity has been termed the *keyhole theory* of β sympathomimetic receptors: The larger the side chain attachment to a catechol base, the greater the β_2 specificity. If the catecholamine structural pattern is understood as a keylike shape, then the larger the "key" (side chain), the more β_2-specific the drug. The increase in side chain substitutions can be seen in the drug structures presented in Figure 6-3

for the three catecholamines described and subsequent β_2-selective agents to be discussed.

Metabolism of Catecholamines

Despite the increase in β_2 specificity with increased side chain bulk, all of the previously mentioned catecholamines are rapidly inactivated by the cytoplasmic enzyme COMT. This enzyme is found in the liver and kidneys and throughout the rest of the body. Figure 6-4, *A*, illustrates the action of COMT as it transfers a methyl group to the carbon-3 position on the catechol nucleus. The resulting compound, metanephrine, is inactive on adrenergic receptors. Because the action of COMT on circulating catecholamines is very efficient, the duration of action of these drugs is severely limited, with a range of 1.5 to at most 3 hours.

Catecholamines are also unsuitable for oral administration because they are inactivated in the gut and liver by conjugation with sulfate or glucuronide at the carbon-4 site.

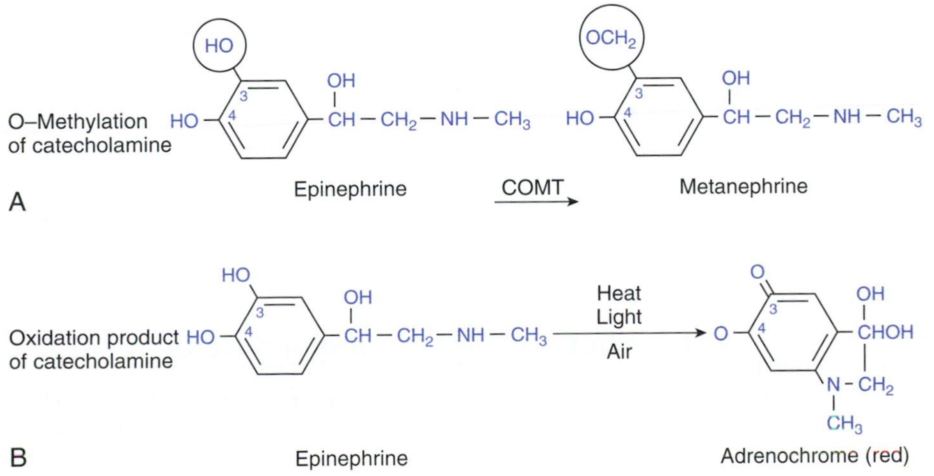

O–Methylation of catecholamine

A   Epinephrine   COMT   Metanephrine

Oxidation product of catecholamine

B   Epinephrine   Heat Light Air   Adrenochrome (red)

Figure 6-4 A, Inactivation of the catecholamine epinephrine by the enzyme catechol *O*-methyltransferase *(COMT)*. **B,** Conversion of a catecholamine such as epinephrine to an adrenochrome.

Because of this action, they have no effect when taken by mouth, limiting their route of administration to inhalation or injection. Catecholamines are also readily inactivated to inert adrenochromes by heat, light, or air (Figure 6-4, *B*). For this reason, racemic epinephrine is stored in an amber-colored bottle or a foil-protected wrapper. Nebulizer *rainout* (i.e., nebulized particles that condense and fall, under the influence of gravity) in the tubing may appear pinkish after treatment, and a patient's sputum may even appear pink-tinged after using aerosols of catecholamines.

Resorcinol Agents

KEY POINT

The basic catecholamine structure, consisting of a catechol ring connected to an amine side chain, directly influences activity. β_2-Receptor specificity is considered to be caused by side chain bulk *(keyhole theory)*. The short duration of action of catecholamines is due to metabolism by the enzyme catechol *O*-methyltransferase (COMT).

Because the limited duration of action with catecholamines is unsuitable for maintenance therapy of bronchospastic airways, drug researchers sought to modify the catechol nucleus, which is so vulnerable to inactivation by COMT. As a result, the hydroxyl attachment at the carbon-4 site was shifted to the carbon-5 position, producing a resorcinol nucleus (see Figure 6-3). This change resulted in *metaproterenol* (named for the 3′,5′-attachments in the meta position). Because metaproterenol is not inactivated by COMT, it has a significantly longer duration of action of 4 to 6 hours compared with the short-acting catecholamine bronchodilators. Metaproterenol can be taken orally because it resists inactivation by sulfatase enzymes in the gastrointestinal tract and liver. For these reasons, the newer generation of resorcinols and other catecholamine derivatives is much better suited for maintenance therapy than the older catecholamine agents. Metaproterenol is slower to reach a peak effect (30 to 60 minutes) than racemic epinephrine. The MDI chlorofluorocarbon (CFC) version of metaproterenol was removed from the market on June 14, 2010.

KEY POINT

Modification of the catecholamine structure produces *noncatecholamines* such as metaproterenol, albuterol, and levalbuterol, which have a 4- to 6-hour duration when inhaled and are β_2 preferential.

Saligenin Agents

A different modification of the catechol nucleus at the carbon-3 site resulted in the saligenin *albuterol*, referred to as *salbutamol* in Europe (see Figure 6-3). Albuterol is available in various pharmaceutical vehicles in the United States, including oral extended-release tablets, syrup, nebulizer solution, and MDI. As with the resorcinol bronchodilators,

this drug has a β_2-preferential effect; it is also effective via oral administration. Inhaled albuterol has a duration of approximately 4 to 6 hours, with a peak effect in 30 to 60 minutes. However, duration of up to 12 hours can be achieved with oral dosing from extended-release tablets. Oral use may lead to greater systemic side effects than its inhaled counterpart.

Pirbuterol

Pirbuterol (Maxair) was an MDI formulation with a breath-actuated inhaler delivery device. The CFC version of pirbuterol was removed from the market in the United States on December 31, 2013.

Prodrug: Bitolterol

Bitolterol (Tornalate) differs from the previous agents discussed in that the administered form must be converted in the body to the active drug. Because of this, bitolterol is referred to as a **prodrug**. The sequence of activation is shown in Figure 6-5.

The bitolterol molecule consists of two toluate ester groups on the aromatic ring at the carbon-3 and carbon-4 positions. These attachments protect the molecule from degradation by COMT. The large *N*-tertiary butyl substituent on the amine side chain prevents oxidation by monoamine oxidase (MAO). Bitolterol is administered as an inhalation solution; once in the body the bitolterol molecule is hydrolyzed by esterase enzymes in the tissue and blood into the active bronchodilator colterol. The process of activation begins when the drug is administered and gradually continues over time, resulting in a prolonged duration or sustained-release effect of up to 8 hours. Onset and peak effect are similar to those of the noncatecholamine agent metaproterenol when administered by inhalation. The active form, colterol, is a catecholamine and is inactivated by COMT similar to any other catecholamine. The speed of this inactivation is offset by the gradual hydrolysis of bitolterol to provide a prolonged duration of activity. The bulky side chain gives a preferential β_2 effect to the active form, colterol.[4]

In animal studies, bitolterol given orally or intravenously selectively distributed to the lungs. The inhalation route in humans seems preferable to treat the lungs locally; the hydrolysis of bitolterol to colterol proceeds faster in the lungs than elsewhere, giving a selective effect and accumulation in the lungs. Colterol is excreted in urine and feces as free and conjugated colterol and as metabolites of colterol. Although interesting from a pharmacologic viewpoint, bitolterol has been removed from market in the United States.

Levalbuterol: (R)-Isomer of Albuterol

Previous inhaled formulations of adrenergic bronchodilators were all synthetic racemic mixtures, containing the (R)-isomer and the (S)-isomer in equal amounts.

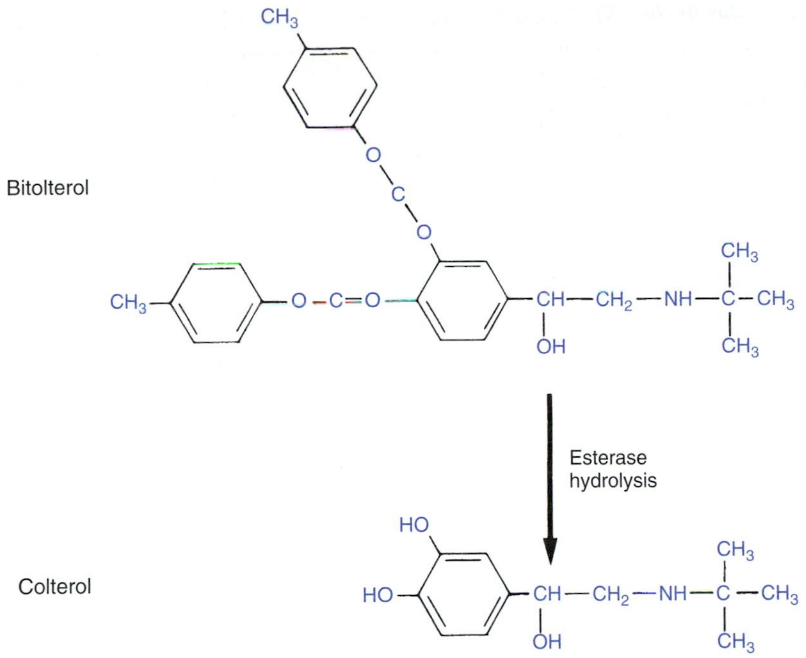

Figure 6-5 Illustration of the structure of bitolterol, showing conversion by esterase enzymes to its active catecholamine form, colterol, a β_2-preferential agonist.

Levalbuterol is the pure (R)-isomer of racemic albuterol. Both stereoisomers of albuterol are shown in Figure 6-6. Although the (S)-isomer is physiologically inactive on adrenergic receptors, there is accumulating evidence that the (S)-isomer is *not* completely inactive. Barnes[5] suggested, however, there is no difference between single isomer levalbuterol and racemic albuterol. Box 6-1 lists some of the physiologic effects of (S)-isomer of albuterol noted in the literature.[6-12] The effects noted would antagonize the bronchodilating effects of the (R)-isomer of an adrenergic drug and promote bronchoconstriction. In addition, the (S)-isomer is more slowly metabolized than the (R)-isomer. Levalbuterol is the single (R)-isomer form of racemic albuterol and is available in an Hydrofluoroalkane (HFA)-propelled MDI, with nebulization solution in three strengths: 0.31-mg, 0.63-mg, and 1.25-mg unit doses. Levalbuterol is also available as a concentrate of 1.25 mg in 0.5 mL. In a study by Nelson and associates,[13] the 0.63-mg dose was found to be comparable to the 2.5-mg racemic albuterol dose in onset and duration (Figure 6-7).

Side effects of tremor and heart rate changes were fewer with the single-isomer formulation. The 1.25-mg levalbuterol dose showed a higher peak effect on forced

---

BOX 6-1 Effects and Characteristics of the (S)-Isomer of Albuterol

- Increases intracellular calcium concentration in vitro[8]
- Activity is blocked by anticholinergic agent atropine[8]
- Does not produce pulmonary or extrapulmonary β_2-mediated effects[9]
- Enhances experimental airway responsiveness in vitro[10]
- Increases contractile response of bronchial tissue to histamine or leukotriene C_4 (LTC_4) in vitro[11]
- Enhances eosinophil superoxide production with interleukin-5 (IL-5) stimulation[12]
- Is metabolized slower than (R)-albuterol in vivo[13]
- Preferentially retained in the lung when inhaled by metered dose inhaler (in vivo)[1]

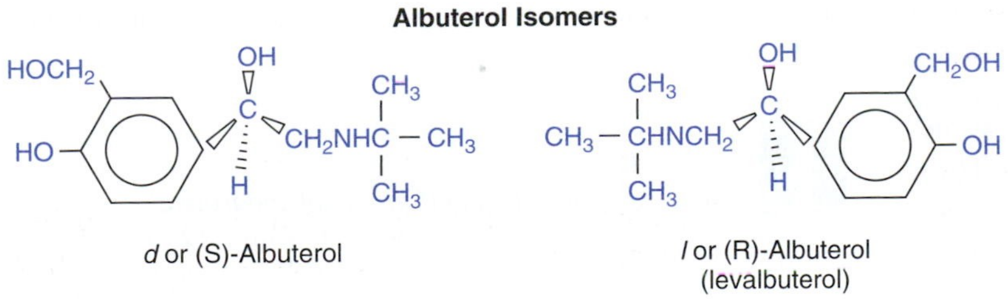

---

expiratory volume in 1 second (FEV_1) with an 8-hour duration compared with racemic albuterol. Side effects with this dose were equivalent to the side effects seen with racemic albuterol. It is significant that an equivalent clinical response was seen with one fourth the racemic dose (0.63 mg) when using the pure isomer, although the racemic mixture contains 1.25 mg of the (R)-isomer (one-half of the total 2.5-mg dose).

Albuterol Isomers

d or (S)-Albuterol

l or (R)-Albuterol
(levalbuterol)

Figure 6-6 The (R)-isomer and (S)-isomer of racemic albuterol. Levalbuterol is the single, (R)-isomer form of racemic albuterol and contains no (S)-isomer.

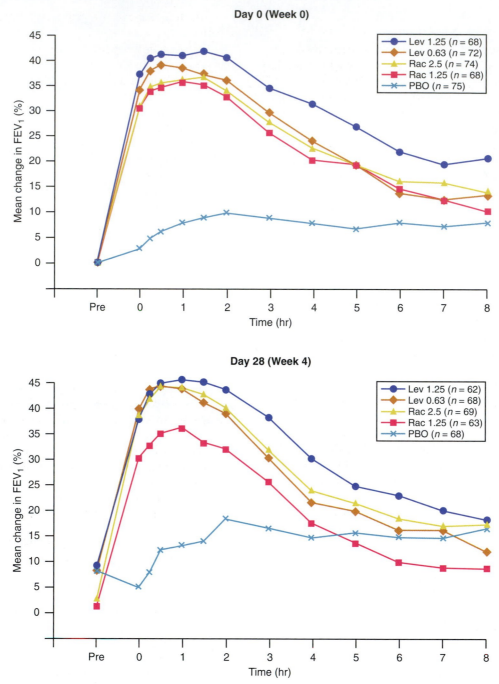

Figure 6-7 Mean percent change in forced expiratory volume in 1 second *(FEV₁)* from baseline (week 0) to the end of treatment (week 4) with various doses of levalbuterol *(Lev)*, racemic albuterol *(Rac)*, and a placebo *(PBO)*. (From Nelson HS, Bensch G, Pleskow WW, et al, *J Allergy Clin Immunol* 102:943, 1998.)

Long-Acting β-Adrenergic Agents

The trend in adrenergic bronchodilators has been toward development from nonspecific, short-acting agents, such as epinephrine, to β_2-specific agents with action lasting 4 to 6 hours, such as albuterol and levalbuterol. Longer-acting agents offer the advantages of less frequent dosing and protection through the night for asthmatic patients. These agents include extended-release albuterol and newer drugs such as salmeterol (Serevent), formoterol (Foradil, Perforomist), arformoterol (Brovana), indacaterol (Arcapta Neohaler), and olodaterol (Striverdi Respimat). Long-acting

bronchodilators are contrasted with short-acting agents. Short-acting agents include albuterol and levalbuterol, although these agents at one time were considered longer acting compared with the ultra-short-acting catecholamines such as racemic epinephrine.

KEY POINT

Salmeterol, formoterol, arformoterol, indacaterol, and *olodaterol* are long-acting β_2 agonists with a 12- to 24-hour duration of action resulting from their unique pharmacodynamics (drug-receptor interaction).

Extended-Release Albuterol

An extended-release form of albuterol is available as VoSpire ER. This is a 4-mg or 8-mg tablet taken orally with extended activity up to 12 hours. The extended activity of VoSpire ER is achieved with a tablet formulation that contains 2 mg of the drug in the coating for immediate release and 2 mg in the core for release after several hours. VoSpire ER uses an osmotic gradient to draw water into the tablet, dissolve the albuterol, and gradually release the active drug through a pinhole in the tablet. The 6-hour duration can be extended for 8 to 12 hours and mimics the effect of taking two doses.

Salmeterol

Salmeterol, a β_2-selective receptor agonist, is available in a dry powder formulation in the Diskus inhaler. Salmeterol xinafoate is a racemic mixture of two enantiomers, with the (R)-isomer containing the predominant β_2 activity.[14]

Bronchodilator effect. Salmeterol represents a new generation of long-acting β_2-specific bronchodilating agents, whose bronchodilation profile differs from the agents previously discussed. The median time to reach a 15% increase in FEV_1 above the baseline (considered the onset of bronchodilation) in asthmatic subjects is longer with salmeterol than albuterol; it has been reported to be approximately 15 minutes.[15] The slower onset of action with salmeterol is significant for its clinical application (discussed subsequently). The time to peak bronchodilating effect is generally 3 to 5 hours, and its duration of action in maintaining an FEV_1 15% above the pretreatment baseline is 12 hours or longer. At each point (onset, peak effect, and duration), salmeterol exhibits slower, longer times for effect compared with shorter-acting bronchodilators such as albuterol.

With inhaled salmeterol xinafoate, an initial peak plasma concentration of 1 to 2 mcg/L is seen 5 minutes after inhalation, with a second peak of 0.07 to 0.2 mcg/L at 45 minutes; the second peak is probably due to absorption of the swallowed dose. The drug is metabolized by hydroxylation, with elimination primarily in the feces.[14] The increased duration of action of salmeterol is due to the increased lipophilicity conferred by the long side chain. The "tail" of the molecule anchors at an exosite in the cell membrane allow continual activation of the β receptor. The mechanism of action is discussed more fully subsequently.

Formoterol

Formoterol is another β_2-selective agonist with a long-acting bronchodilatory effect of 12 hours in duration. Foradil, a racemic mixture of (R,R)-formoterol and (S,S)-formoterol, was approved by the FDA for maintenance treatment of asthma and for acute prevention of exercise-induced bronchospasm in adults and children 5 years or older. Formoterol is also indicated for the treatment of COPD and can be used in conjunction with other inhaled medications, such as inhaled corticosteroids, short-acting β agonists, and theophylline. Racemic formoterol is available as a dry powder aerosol for use with the Aerolizer dry powder inhaler (DPI). The current recommended dosage for adults

and children 5 years or older is 12 mcg twice daily by Aerolizer.

The use of liquid nebulization is still very popular with many patients and is a great alternative to MDI and DPI use. Performomist is available in a liquid nebulization form of 20 mcg/2 mL unit dose and is prescribed twice daily. Currently, it is approved only for use with COPD.

The chemical structure of formoterol is shown in Figure 6-8. As with salmeterol, the extensive side chain, or "tail," makes formoterol more lipophilic than the shorter-acting bronchodilators and is the basis for its longer duration of effect. The increased lipophilicity of salmeterol and formoterol allows the drugs to remain in the lipid cell membrane. Even if a tissue preparation containing the drugs is perfused or washed, the drug activity persists. Salmeterol is more lipophilic than formoterol, and this along with its anchoring capability may explain why salmeterol is less prone to being "washed away" than formoterol.[15]

Bronchodilator effect. Similar to salmeterol, formoterol has a prolonged duration of bronchodilating effect of up to 12 hours. In contrast to salmeterol, the onset of action for formoterol is significantly faster. The time from inhalation to significant bronchodilation is similar to that of albuterol. It has been reported that 1 minute after inhalation of formoterol there is a significant increase in specific airway conductance (SG_{AW}).[16] The onset of bronchodilation is generally considered to be 2 to 3 minutes with formoterol compared with 10 minutes or longer with salmeterol. Figure 6-9 shows the dose-proportional response to inhaled (R,R)-formoterol, the single isomer isolated from the racemic mixture of (R,R)-formoterol and (S,S)-formoterol, compared with inhaled racemic albuterol.[17] A study by van Noord and colleagues[18] compared racemic formoterol, 24 mcg; salmeterol, 50 mcg; and albuterol, 200 mcg. They found the increases in SG_{AW} after 1 minute were 44%, less than 16%, and 44%, respectively. The times to maximal increase in airway conductance were 2 hours, 2 to 4 hours, and 30 minutes; and the maximal increases were 135%, 111%, and 100%.[16,18]

The efficacy of formoterol in relaxing airway smooth muscle—its maximal effect—is greater than that of albuterol, which is greater than that of salmeterol. The lower intrinsic efficacy of salmeterol would make it a better agent than formoterol for patients with cardiovascular disease.[14]

Arformoterol

Arformoterol is one of the latest β_2-selective agonists with a long-acting bronchodilatory effect of 12 hours in duration. Arformoterol is the single, (R,R)-isomer form of racemic formoterol, which is approved by the FDA as Brovana for maintenance treatment of COPD. The current recommended adult dose is 15 mcg twice daily. Brovana is available in 2-mL unit-dose vials and is for nebulization only.

Indacaterol

Indacaterol is an ultra long-acting β agonist approved by the FDA in 2011 as Arcapta Neohaler. In the United States the dose is 75 mcg once daily via a DPI for treatment of

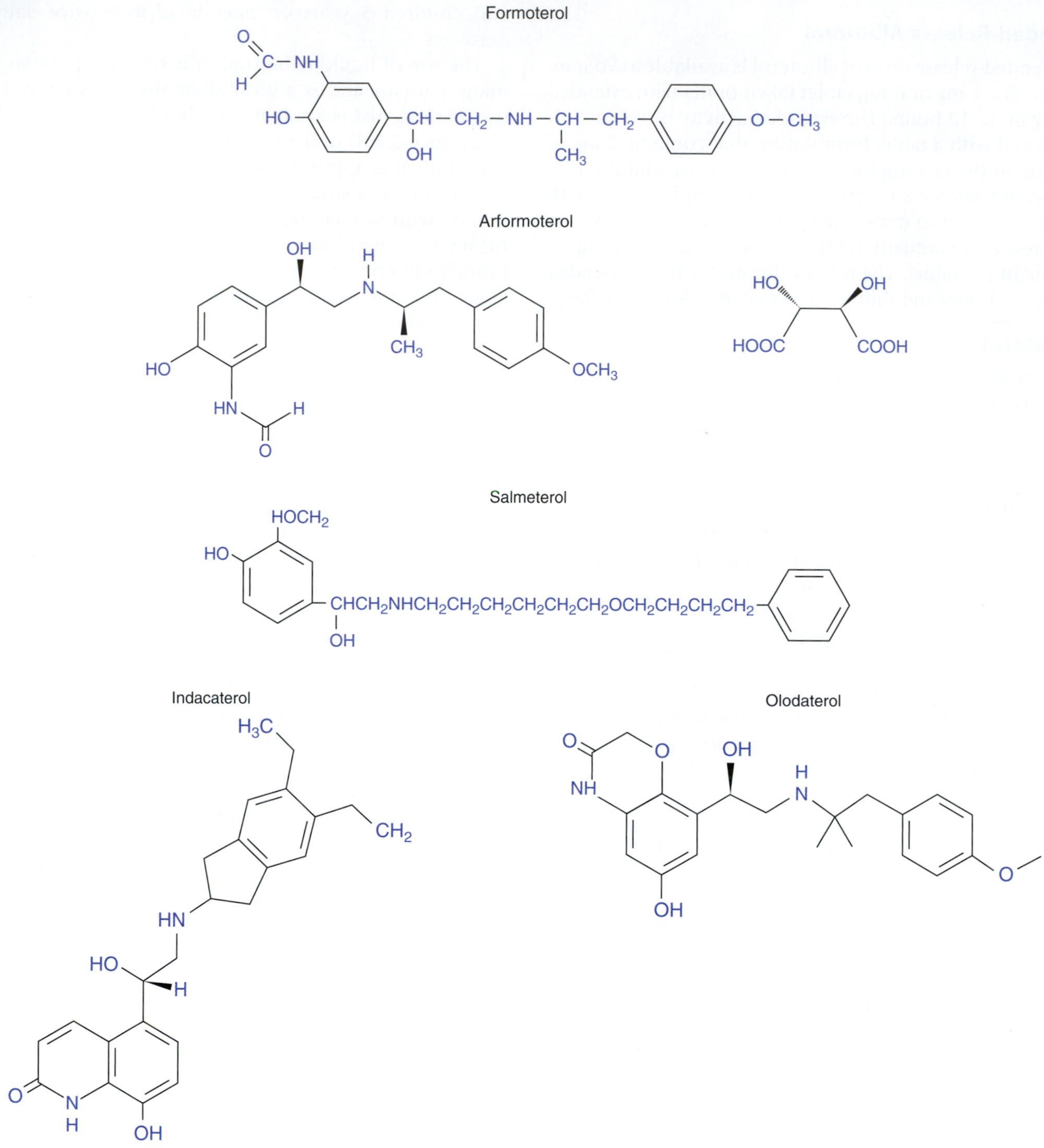

Figure 6-8 Chemical structures of formoletrol, arformoterol, salmeterol, indacaterol, and olodaterol, long-acting β_2 agonists.

COPD; however, in Europe approved doses are as high as 150 mcg and 300 mcg. Indacaterol is similar to formoterol in that it has a quick onset; however, it is even faster at approximately 5 minutes for onset with a duration of 24 hours.[19] Indacaterol is suitable as a first line treatment for COPD. Ribeiro and Chapman[20] found indacaterol appears to be better than bronchodilators used twice daily and just as effective as once-daily tiotropium. Indacaterol is

currently being studied with other anticholinergic agents, which may produce once-daily fixed combination agents.

Olodaterol

Olodaterol (Striverdi Respimat) is an ultra-long-acting β agonist approved by the FDA in 2014. The dose is 5 mcg once daily via the Respimat for treatment of COPD. Olodaterol has a quick onset similar to formoterol and

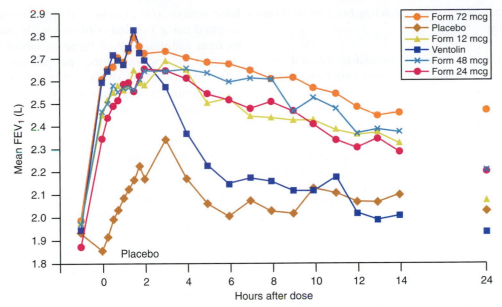

Figure 6-9 Single-dose crossover study of *(R,R)*-formoterol in the treatment of asthmatic adults. Shown are the dose-proportional forced expiratory volume in 1 second *(FEV₁)* responses and duration of action for the single isomer *(R,R)*-formoterol, a long-acting β₂ agonist.

indacaterol. The change in FEV_1 is seen in approximately 5 minutes.[21] Olodaterol exhibited a 24-hour duration in COPD patients.[22] Currently, olodaterol is not FDA approved for asthma, however, it has been shown to be effective as monotherapy and in combination with tiotropium in animal studies.[23]

Vilanterol

Vilanterol is an ultra-long-acting β agonist that is FDA approved in fixed combinations agents with fluticasone (Breo Ellipta) and umeclidinium (Anoro Ellipta). Vilanterol has been studied as monotherapy with effective results in COPD patients.[24] At the time of this edition, vilanterol is not available as monotherapy; it is only found in fixed combinations.

Antiinflammatory Effects

Both the short-acting and the long-acting β agonists show antiinflammatory effects in vitro. β agonists inhibit human mast cell activation and degranulation in vitro, prevent an increase in vascular permeability with inflammatory mediators, and generally diminish the attraction and accumulation of airway inflammatory cells.[15,20-24] Despite these in vitro antiinflammatory effects, they have not been shown to inhibit the accumulation of inflammatory cells in the airway or the increase in inflammatory markers in vivo. Neither drug is considered to have a sufficient effect on airway inflammation in patients with asthma to replace antiinflammatory drugs such as corticosteroids.

Clinical Use

Long-acting β agonists are indicated for maintenance therapy of asthma that is not controlled by regular low-dose inhaled corticosteroids and for COPD needing daily inhaled bronchodilator therapy for reversible airway obstruction. National guidelines recommend the introduction of a long-acting β agonist in step 3 care of asthma (asthma not controlled by lower doses of antiinflammatory medications)[1] and use as deemed necessary for COPD.[25] Use of long-acting β agonists may prevent the need to increase the inhaled dose of corticosteroid. Several points should be noted in the clinical use of long-acting agents because of their differences from shorter-acting β agonists.

- Long-acting β₂ agonists are not recommended for rescue bronchodilation because repeated administration with their longer duration and increased lipophilic property risk accumulation and toxicity.[15]
- A shorter-acting β₂ agonist, such as albuterol or other agents previously discussed, should be prescribed and available for asthmatics for treatment of breakthrough symptoms if additional bronchodilator therapy is needed between scheduled doses of a long-acting β₂ agonist; asthmatics must be well educated in the appropriate use of the two types of β agonists (shorter-acting versus long-acting).
- Although they have antiinflammatory effects, short-acting or long-acting β agonists are not a substitute for inhaled corticosteroids in asthma maintenance or for other antiinflammatory medications if such are required.
- The difference in rate of onset between salmeterol and formoterol, indacaterol, or olodaterol may require classifying β₂ agonists as "fast" and "slow" in addition to "short" and "long" acting, with salmeterol classified as a slow and long-acting bronchodilator versus formoterol as a fast and long-acting bronchodilator.[25] We may also see the classification for agents such as indacaterol and

olodaterol be termed "ultra"-long-acting because of their 24-hour duration.

The addition of a long-acting β_2 agonist to inhaled corticosteroids can lead to improved lung function and a decrease in symptoms.[24-27] A combination product of salmeterol and fluticasone in a Diskus inhaler (Advair Diskus) showed superior asthma control and better lung function than either drug taken alone.[28-31] Because of their prolonged bronchodilation, long-acting β_2 agonists taken twice daily have a greater area under the FEV_1 curve compared with short-acting agents taken four times daily. However, once-daily long-acting β_2 agonists are demonstrating better area under the curve than those agents taken BID.[19-24] Figure 6-10 illustrates dose-response curves for albuterol and salmeterol. In contrast to albuterol, which tends to return to baseline in 4 to 6 hours, salmeterol provides a more sustained level of bronchodilation, giving a higher baseline of lung function.[32-33] The same effect has been found in comparing twice-daily salmeterol with four-times-daily inhaled ipratropium bromide,[33] a shorter-acting anticholinergic bronchodilator that is discussed in Chapter 7.

Salpeter and associates,[34] in a meta-analysis, reported that long-acting β_2 agonists increased the risk of asthma hospitalizations and deaths compared with a placebo. Nelson and colleagues[33] also described an increase in death rate among patients using salmeterol; their findings reported the highest death rate among African Americans. These studies did not take into account the severity of asthma or whether the participants used other medications. Asthma in some participants may have been worse than in others. Concerning co-treatments, the studies could not account for other medications participants may have been taking or with what regularity they were taking them. The latter could

have serious consequences if, for example, a participant stopped using inhaled corticosteroids that were prescribed to treat asthma. Any of these variables—asthma severity, presence of co-treatments, and patient adherence—could affect interpretation of data. Nevertheless, the labeling of these agents has been changed to warn that death can occur.

Because of the ongoing concerns about the safety of long-acting β_2 agonists, the FDA is now requiring changes on how long-acting β_2 agonists are used in the treatment of asthma. As of June 2, 2010, the FDA now requires the following:

- Long-acting β_2 agonists are not to be used without a controller medication (i.e., corticosteroid).
- Long-acting β_2 agonists should not be used by patients who are controlled on low-dose or medium-dose inhaled corticosteroids.
- Long-acting β_2 agonists should be used only if patients are not controlled with agents such as inhaled corticosteroids.
- Long-acting β_2 agonists should be for short-term use only. Once asthma is controlled, the long-acting β_2 agonist should be discontinued.
- Children should use a long-acting β_2 agonist only in conjunction with a corticosteroid. The use of a combination product is needed to increase adherence.

MECHANISM OF ACTION

The bronchodilating action of the adrenergic drugs is due to stimulation of β_2 receptors located on bronchial smooth muscle. In addition to β_2 receptors, some adrenergic bronchodilators can stimulate α and β_1 receptors, with the following clinical effects.

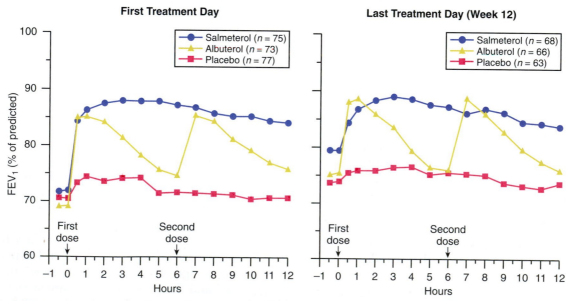

Figure 6-10 Mean forced expiratory volume in 1 second (*FEV₁*) response and duration of effect for inhaled salmeterol, 42 mcg twice daily; albuterol, 180 mcg four times daily; and a placebo. (Modified from Pearlman DS, Chervinsky P, LaForce C, et al, *N Engl J Med* 327:1420, © 1992 Massachusetts Medical Society. All rights reserved.)

- **α-Receptor stimulation:** Causes vasoconstriction (i.e., a *vasopressor* effect); in the upper airway (nasal passages), this can provide decongestion
- **β_1-Receptor stimulation:** Causes increased myocardial conductivity, heart rate, and contractile force
- **β_2-Receptor stimulation:** Causes relaxation of bronchial smooth muscle, with some inhibition of inflammatory mediator release and stimulation of mucociliary clearance

Both α and β receptors are examples of G protein–linked receptors. Table 6-2 lists each of the adrenergic receptor types, along with its particular type of G protein, effector system, second messenger, and an example of cell response in the lungs. As described in Chapter 2, the G protein is a heterotrimer whose α subunit differentiates the type of G protein. The G protein couples the adrenergic receptor to the effector enzyme, which initiates the cell response by means of a particular intracellular second messenger. The mechanism of action with β-receptor, α_2-receptor, and α_1-receptor stimulation is described for each.

β-Receptor and α_2-Receptor Activation

The mechanism of action of β agonists and the β receptors has been well characterized, although the activity of α receptors is not as well understood. The mechanism of action for relaxation of airway smooth muscle when a β_2 receptor is stimulated is illustrated in Figure 6-11. Adrenergic agonists, such as albuterol or epinephrine, attach to β receptors, which are polypeptide chains that traverse the cell membrane seven times and have an extracellular NH_2 terminus and an intracellular carboxy (COOH) terminus. This attachment causes activation of the stimulatory G protein, designated Gs. The actual binding site of a β agonist is within the cell membrane, inside the "barrel" or circle formed by the transmembrane loops of the receptor chain. The β agonist forms bonds with elements of the third, fifth, and sixth transmembrane loops. When stimulated by a β agonist, the receptor undergoes a conformational change that reduces the affinity of the α subunit of the G protein for guanosine diphosphate (GDP). The GDP is replaced by guanosine triphosphate (GTP), and the α subunit dissociates from the receptor and the β-γ portion of the G protein to link with the effector system. The effector system for the β receptor is adenylyl cyclase, a membrane-bound enzyme. Activation of adenylyl cyclase by the α subunit of the G_s protein causes increased synthesis of the second messenger, **cyclic adenosine 3′,5′-monophosphate (cAMP)**. cAMP may cause smooth muscle relaxation by increasing the inactivation of myosin light chain kinase, an enzyme that initiates myosin-actin interaction and subsequent smooth muscle contraction. An increase in cAMP also leads to a decrease in intracellular calcium.

A similar sequence of events is responsible for the action of α_2-receptor stimulation, which can inhibit further

TABLE 6-2	Adrenergic Receptor Types: G Proteins, Effector Systems, Second Messengers, and Examples of Cell Responses			
RECEPTOR	**G PROTEIN**	**EFFECTOR**	**SECOND MESSENGER**	**RESPONSE**
α_1	G_q	Phospholipase C (PLC)	Inositol triphosphate (IP_3), diacylglycerol (DAG)	Vasoconstriction
α_2	G_i	Adenylyl cyclase (inhibits)	cAMP (inhibits)	Inhibition of neurotransmitter release
β (β_1, β_2, β_3)	G_s	Adenylyl cyclase (stimulates)	cAMP (increases)	Smooth muscle relaxation

cAMP, Cyclic adenosine 3′,5′-monophosphate.

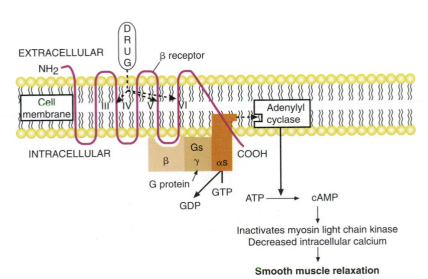

Figure 6-11 Diagram illustrating mechanism of action by which stimulation of the G protein–linked β receptor by a β agonist causes smooth muscle relaxation. *ATP,* Adenosine triphosphate; *cAMP,* cyclic adenosine 3′,5′-monophosphate; *COOH,* carboxy; *NH₂,* amine group; *GDP,* guanosine diphosphate; *GTP,* guanosine triphosphate.

neurotransmitter release from the presynaptic neuron when stimulated by norepinephrine in a feedback, autoregulatory fashion (see Chapter 5). However, stimulation of α_2 receptors (not shown in Figure 6-11) results in activation of an inhibitory G protein, designated Gi, whose α subunit serves to inhibit the enzyme adenylyl cyclase, lowering the rate of synthesis for intracellular cAMP.

α_1-Receptor Activation

Stimulation of an α_1 receptor by an agonist such as phenylephrine or epinephrine (which has affinity for both α and β receptors) results in vasoconstriction of peripheral blood vessels, including vessels in the airway. The mechanism of action for this effect as mediated by the G protein–linked α_1 receptor is illustrated in Figure 6-12. Stimulation of the α_1 receptor causes a conformational change in the receptor, which activates the G protein designated Gq. With activation, GDP dissociates from the G protein; GTP binds to the α subunit of the G protein; and the α subunit dissociates from the β-γ dimer, to activate the effector phospholipase C (PLC). Activation of the effector, PLC, leads to the conversion of membrane phosphoinositides into inositol 1,4,5-trisphosphate (IP$_3$) and diacylglycerol (DAG). IP$_3$ stimulates release of intracellular stores of calcium into the cytoplasm of the cell, and DAG activates protein kinase C. Contraction of vascular smooth muscle results.

Long-Acting β Agonists: Mechanism of Action

The mechanism of action for long-acting β agonists in providing sustained protection from bronchoconstriction differs to a degree from that of the previously described adrenergic bronchodilators. The difference in pharmacodynamics of long-acting β agonist is reflected in its pharmacokinetics with a slower onset and time to peak effect and a longer duration of action compared with previous adrenergic agents.

The structures of long-acting agents are shown in Figure 6-8 for comparison. The agents are a modification of the saligenin albuterol, with a long nonpolar (i.e., *lipophilic*) N-substituted side chain. For example, salmeterol consists of a polar, or *hydrophilic*, phenyl ethanolamine "head" with a large lipophilic "tail" or side chain. As a result of this structure, salmeterol is lipophilic, in contrast to most short-acting β agonists, which are hydrophilic and approach the β receptor directly from the aqueous extracellular space. In contrast, salmeterol, as a lipophilic molecule, diffuses into the cell membrane phospholipid bilayer and approaches the β receptor laterally, as shown in Figure 6-13. The lipophilic nonpolar side chain binds to an area of the β receptor referred to as the *exosite*, a hydrophobic region. With the side chain ("tail") anchored in the exosite, the active saligenin "head" binds to and activates the β receptor at the same location as albuterol.

The binding properties of long-acting β agonists differ from those of albuterol and other short-acting β agonists. Because the side chain of long-acting agents is anchored at the exosite, the active "head" portion continually attaches to and detaches from the receptor site. This activity provides ongoing stimulation of the β receptor and is the basis for the persistent duration of action of long-acting agents. This model of activity is supported by studies of the effect of β antagonists on the β-agonist action of long-acting agents and molecular binding. If albuterol is attached to the β receptor, the smooth muscle relaxation can be fully reversed by a β-blocking agent such as propranolol or sotalol, indicating a competitive blockade. When the β-blocking agent is removed, there is no further relaxation of smooth muscle. The albuterol has been displaced, and the action of the drug is terminated. If long-acting β agonists stimulates a receptor, a β antagonist such as propranolol would also reverse the effect of relaxation. However, when the propranolol is removed from the tissue, the relaxant effect of the long-acting β agonists is reestablished. This indicates that the long-acting β agonists remain anchored in the receptor and

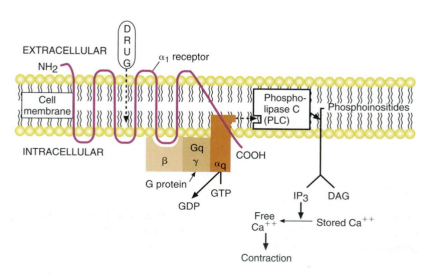

Figure 6-12 Diagram illustrating mechanism of action by which stimulation of the G protein–linked α_1 receptor by an α agonist causes smooth muscle contraction, which can result in vasoconstriction of blood vessels. *ATP*, Adenosine triphosphate; *Ca^{++}*, calcium ion; *COOH*, carboxy; *DAG*, diacylglycerol; *IP$_3$*, inositol 1,4,5-trisphosphate; *NH$_2$*, amine group; *GDP*, guanosine diphosphate; *GTP*, guanosine triphosphate.

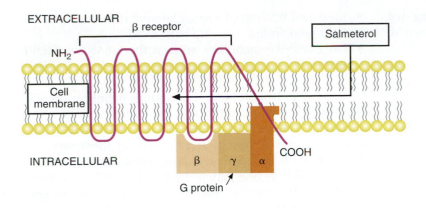

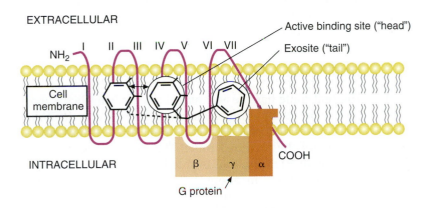

Figure 6-13 Illustration of mechanism of action by which salmeterol, a long-acting β_2-specific bronchodilator, interacts with the β receptor via an exosite anchor, that is, its lipophilic side chain (the "tail"), allowing continual stimulation of the receptor via its active binding site (the "head"). *COOH*, Carboxy; *NH₂*, amine group.

are available to stimulate the β receptor continually after the blocking agent is removed.[15,19-24]

ROUTES OF ADMINISTRATION

β-Adrenergic bronchodilators are currently available for inhalation (MDI, nebulizer solution, DPI, Respimat), oral administration (tablets or syrup), and parenteral administration (injection), although not all agents are found in each form. Regardless of the route of administration, there are three general patterns to the time course of bronchodilation with drugs in this group. The *catecholamines* show a rapid onset of 1 to 3 minutes, a peak effect at about 15 to 20 minutes, and a rapid decline in effect after 1 hour. The *noncatecholamines* (resorcinols and saligenins), with the exception of salmeterol, show an onset of 5 to 15 minutes, a peak effect at 30 to 60 minutes, and a duration of 4 to 6 hours. Salmeterol differs significantly, with a slower onset (more than 20 minutes) and peak effect (at about 3 hours) and a 12-hour duration. Formoterol and arformoterol are similar in duration to salmeterol but with an onset as rapid as that of albuterol. Indacaterol, olodaterol, and vilanterol all have a duration of at least 24 hours. Aside from these general patterns, which depend on the type of drug used, the route of administration further affects the time course of a drug. Inhaled and injected adrenergic bronchodilators have a quicker onset than orally administered agents.

> **KEY POINT**
>
> Routes of administration for β agonists include inhalation (aerosol), oral, and parenteral; minimal side effects are seen with inhalation.

Inhalation Route

All of the β-adrenergic bronchodilators marketed in the United States are available for inhalation delivery using an MDI, a nebulizer (including intermittent positive-pressure breathing nebulization), a DPI, or Respimat. Catecholamines must be given by inhalation because they are ineffective orally. Inhalation is the preferred route for administering β-adrenergic drugs for the following reasons:

- Onset is rapid.
- Smaller doses are needed compared with doses for oral use.
- Side effects such as tremor and tachycardia are reduced.
- Drug is delivered directly to the target organ (i.e., lung).
- Inhalation is painless and safe.

The use of aerosol delivery *during* an acute attack of airway obstruction has been questioned. However, several studies have failed to show substantial differences between inhaled and parenteral β-adrenergic agents in acute severe asthma.[36,37] There is no reason to avoid these bronchodilators as inhaled aerosols during acute episodes.[38] The inhalation route targets the lung directly. Combining oral delivery with additional inhalation has been shown to produce good additive effects with albuterol.[39]

The major difficulties with aerosol administration are the time needed for nebulization (5 to 10 minutes), the possible embarrassment of using an MDI in public or at school, and inability to use an MDI correctly. Difficulty in correctly using an MDI can be remedied by using spacer devices or, alternatively, by using a gas-powered handheld nebulizer. A DPI can eliminate problems associated with nebulizers and MDIs.

Continuous Nebulization

Administration of inhaled adrenergic agents by continuous nebulization has been used to manage severe asthma, in an effort to avoid respiratory failure, intubation, and mechanical ventilation. The *Guidelines for the Diagnosis and Management of Asthma* released by NAEPP EPR 3 recommend 2.5 to 5 mg of albuterol by nebulizer every 20 minutes for three doses and 10 to 15 mg/hr by continuous nebulization.[1] Because a nebulizer treatment takes approximately 10 minutes, giving three treatments every 20 minutes requires repeated therapist attendance. Continuous administration by nebulizer may simplify such frequent treatments. The use of continuous nebulization of β-agonist bronchodilators was reviewed by Fink and Dhand,[40] who presented a summary of studies, including dosages used. With continuous nebulization, there are no general standards for dosages other than the recommendation from NAEPP EPR 3; in the studies cited by Fink and Dhand,[40] dosages vary from 2.5 to 15 mg/hr and include schedules based on milligrams per kilogram per hour.

The effect and optimal use of continuous nebulization versus intermittent nebulization are unclear. In the five randomized controlled trials cited by Fink and Dhand,[40] there was similar improvement between continuous versus intermittent nebulization. One study by Lin and associates[41] showed faster improvement using continuous nebulization in patients with FEV$_1$ less than 50% of predicted. A study by Shrestha and colleagues[42] compared a high dose (7.5 mg) and low dose (2.5 mg) of albuterol with both continuous and intermittent nebulization. FEV$_1$ improved more with continuous than intermittent nebulization, and the low dose of 2.5 mg was as effective as the higher dose of 7.5 mg with continuous administration. These and other results suggest that there is a benefit to continuous nebulization in severe airflow obstruction, but a dosage less than 10 to 15 mg/hr may be effective, with less toxicity. Less clinician time is required for the administration of continuous nebulization. Fink and Dhand[40] suggested that for emergency department patients with severe airway obstruction who do not respond sufficiently after 1 hour of intermittent nebulization of β agonists, continuous nebulization offers a practical approach to optimal dosing in a cost-effective manner.

Delivery methods. Several delivery methods to accomplish continuous nebulization have been tried and reported, including the following.

- Measured refilling of a small volume nebulizer (SVN)
- Volumetric infusion pump with SVN[43]
- Large-reservoir nebulizer, such as the HEART or HOPE nebulizer

Toxicity and monitoring. Continuous nebulization of β$_2$ agonists is not standard therapy, and patients receiving this treatment have serious airflow obstruction. Potential complications include cardiac arrhythmias, hypokalemia, and hyperglycemia. Unifocal premature ventricular contractions were reported in one patient by Portnoy and associates.[44] Significant tremor may also occur. Subsensitivity to continuous therapy was not observed by Portnoy and associates. Close monitoring of patients receiving continuous β agonists is necessary and includes observation and cardiac and electrolyte monitoring. Selective β$_2$ agonists, such as albuterol, should be used to reduce side effects.

Oral Route

The oral route has the advantages of ease, simplicity, short time required for administration, and exact reproducibility and control of dosage. However, in terms of clinical effects, this is not the preferred route. The time course of oral β agonists differs from that of inhaled β agonists. The onset of action begins in about 1.5 hours, with a peak effect reached after 1 to 2 hours, and a duration of action between 3 and 6 hours.[45] Larger doses are required than with inhalation, and the frequency and degree of unwanted side effects increases substantially. Catecholamines are ineffective by mouth, as previously discussed. Noncatecholamine bronchodilators in the adrenergic group seem to lose their β$_2$ specificity with oral use, possibly because of the reduction of the side chain bulk in a first pass through the liver.[46] Patient compliance on a three- or four-times-daily schedule may be better than with a nebulizer. If this is the case with an individual patient and the side effects are tolerable, oral use may be indicated for bronchodilator therapy. The introduction of an oral tablet of albuterol with extended action properties (Vospire ER) offers the possibility of protection from bronchoconstriction for up to 12 hours. However, inhaled salmeterol, formoterol, and arformoterol offer 12-hour duration. Now agents such as indacaterol and olodaterol can provide 24-hour duration in one dose. Either the extended-release tablet or a long-acting β agonist is advantageous in preventing nocturnal asthma and deterioration of flow rates in the morning.

Parenteral Route

β-Adrenergic bronchodilators have been given subcutaneously and intravenously, usually in the emergency management of acute asthma. Subcutaneously, epinephrine 0.3 mg (0.3 mL of 1:1000 strength), every 15 to 20 minutes up to 1 mg in 2 hours, and terbutaline, 0.25 mg (0.25 mL of a 1-mg/mL solution) repeated every 15 to 30 minutes, not exceeding 0.5 mg in 4 hours, have been used. Shim[47] suggested that for practical purposes both aerosolized and subcutaneous routes should be used to manage acute obstruction, although there may be little difference in effect with using the two routes. No difference in effect between epinephrine and terbutaline has been found when given subcutaneously.

The intravenous route has been used most commonly with isoproterenol and with albuterol. Intravenous administration of these agents was thought to be useful during severe obstruction because these agents would be distributed throughout the lungs, whereas aerosol delivery would not allow them to penetrate the periphery. This assumption is questionable for both subcutaneous and intravenous bronchodilator therapy because aerosols do exert an effect with obstruction. Intravenous isoproterenol is not clearly advantageous as a bronchodilator, although this route is used for cardiac stimulation in shock and bradycardia. The dose-limiting factor is tachycardia. Intravenous therapy is a last resort and requires an infusion pump, cardiac monitor, and close attention. Pediatric dosages range from 0.1 to 0.8 mcg/kg/min, and adult dosages range from 0.03 to 0.2 mcg/kg/min, until bronchial relaxation or side effects occur.[47] The combination of myocardial stimulation and hypoxia can cause serious arrhythmias; intravenous isoproterenol should be avoided in acute asthma, in favor of β_2-specific agents. Albuterol has been given intravenously as a bolus of 100 to 500 mcg or by infusion of 4 to 25 mcg/min.[48] Although albuterol is more β_2 specific by aerosol than isoproterenol, the usefulness of intravenous administration compared with oral, aerosol, or subcutaneous administration is not clearly established.

ADVERSE SIDE EFFECTS

Just as adrenergic bronchodilators exert a therapeutic effect by stimulation of α-adrenergic, β_1-adrenergic, or β_2-adrenergic receptors, they can likewise cause unwanted effects as a result of stimulation of these receptors. Generally, the term *side effect* indicates any effect other than the intended therapeutic effect. The most common clinically observed side effects of adrenergic bronchodilators are listed in Box 6-2 and are briefly discussed. The number and severity of these side effects vary among patients; not every side effect is seen with each patient. The later adrenergic agents (albuterol, levalbuterol, salmeterol, formoterol, arformoterol, indacaterol, olodaterol, and vilanterol) are much more β_2 specific than previous agents such as ephedrine, epinephrine, or isoproterenol, and because of this, there is a greater likelihood of cardiac stimulation causing tachycardia and blood pressure increases with the last three agents than with the newer drugs. The more recent agents are safe, and the side effects listed are more of a nuisance than a danger and are easily monitored by clinicians. The introduction of single-isomer β agonists such as levalbuterol may show a further specificity and decrease in side effects, which are potentially caused by the detrimental effects of the (S)-isomer of β agonists.

BOX 6-2   Side Effects Seen With β-Agonist Use

- Tremor
- Palpitations and tachycardia
- Headache
- Insomnia
- Increase in blood pressure
- Nervousness
- Dizziness
- Nausea
- Tolerance to bronchodilator effect
- Loss of bronchoprotection
- Worsening ventilation-perfusion ratio (resulting in decreased arterial oxygen pressure [PaO$_2$])
- Hypokalemia
- Bronchoconstrictor reaction to solution additives (small volume nebulizer [SVN]) and propellants (metered dose inhaler [MDI])

KEY POINT

Adverse side effects can occur with β agonists and include tremor (very common), headache, insomnia, bronchospasm (with metered dose inhaler [MDI] use), palpitations, and some tolerance.

Tremor

The annoying effect of muscle tremor with β agonists is due to stimulation of β_2 receptors in skeletal muscle. It is dose related and is the dose-limiting side effect of the β_2-specific agents, especially with oral administration. The adrenergic receptors mediating muscle tremor have been shown to be of the β_2 type.[49,50] As shown previously, this side effect is much more noticeable with oral delivery, which provides a rationale for aerosol administration of these agents. Tolerance to the side effect of tremor usually develops after days to weeks with the oral route, and patients should be reassured of this when beginning to use these drugs.

Cardiac Effects

The older adrenergic agents with strong β_1-stimulating and α-stimulating effects were considered dangerous in the presence of congestive heart failure. The dose-limiting side effect with these agents is tachycardia. They increase cardiac output and oxygen consumption by stimulating β_1 receptors, leading to a decrease in cardiac efficiency, which is the work relative to oxygen consumption. Newer agents have a preferential β_2 effect to minimize cardiac stimulation. However, tachycardia may also follow use of the newer agents, and there is evidence that this is due to the presence of β_2 receptors even in the heart.[51] β_2 agonists cause vasodilation, and this can cause a reflex tachycardia. Despite this effect, agents such as terbutaline or albuterol can actually improve cardiac performance. Albuterol and terbutaline can cause peripheral vasodilation and increase myocardial contractility without increasing oxygen demand by the

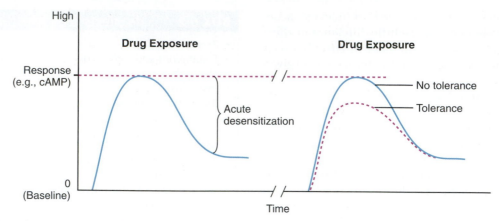

Figure 6-14 Graphic representation of acute and long-term desensitization of the β-receptor response to β agonists. Cell response during actual receptor stimulation by agonist immediately declines *(left side)*; subsequent exposure to drug would produce a lower peak initial response if tolerance or long-term desensitization occurs *(right side)*. *cAMP,* Cyclic adenosine 3′,5′-monophosphate.

heart.[34] The net effect is to reduce afterload and improve cardiac output with no oxygen cost. These agents are therefore attractive for use with airway obstruction combined with congestive heart failure.

Seider and colleagues[52] reported that neither heart rate nor frequency of premature beats was significantly affected by inhaled terbutaline or ipratropium bromide (an anticholinergic bronchodilator) in 14 patients with COPD and ischemic heart disease. Although there are no written standards, most healthcare practitioners accept no more than a 20% change in pretreatment pulse after bronchodilator therapy has been initiated. This is why it is important to check the pulse rate before, during, and after bronchodilator therapy to evaluate cardiac response. If the pulse rate has increased more than 20% relative to the pretreatment pulse, stopping treatment with referral to the prescribing healthcare practitioner may be warranted to prevent unwanted cardiac effects.

Tolerance to Bronchodilator Effect

Adaptation to a drug with repeated use is a concern because use of the drug is actually reducing its effectiveness. With β agonists, there is in vitro evidence of an acute desensitization of the β receptor within minutes of exposure to a β agonist, as well as a longer term desensitization. Figure 6-14 shows both an acute decrease in response during sustained exposure of the receptor to the agonist and a long-term decrease in maximal response with subsequent drug exposure. This decrease in bronchodilator response has been observed with short-acting and long-acting β agonists.

Exposure of cells with β receptors to isoproterenol causes a short-term, acute reduction in adenylyl cyclase activity and production of cAMP. The immediate desensitization is caused by an "uncoupling" of the receptor and the effector enzyme adenylyl cyclase.[53] A model for desensitization of the β receptor is diagrammed in Figure 6-15. When stimulated by a β agonist, the β receptor goes into a low-affinity binding state (i.e., has reduced affinity for binding with a β agonist). Simultaneously, the β agonist causes an increase

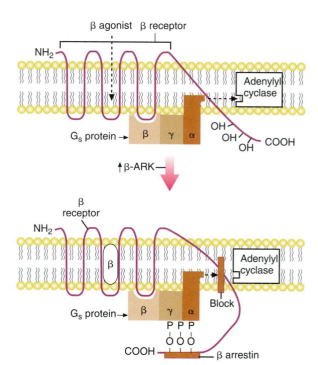

Figure 6-15 Model for β-receptor desensitization through phosphorylation of the β receptor at the carboxy-terminal site by β-adrenergic receptor kinase *(β-ARK),* blocking the action of the α₂ subunit on the effector enzyme adenylyl cyclase. *COOH,* Carboxy; *NH₂,* amine group; *O,* oxygen; *OH,* hydroxyl groups; *P,* phosphate groups.

in cAMP, which increases protein kinase A, also referred to as *β-adrenergic receptor kinase (β-ARK).* β-ARK causes phosphorylation (transfer of phosphate groups [P]) of the hydroxyl groups (OH) on the carboxy-terminal portion of the β receptor. This phosphorylation induces binding of a protein named β-arrestin, which prevents the receptor from interacting with Gₛ and disrupts the coupling of Gₛ with the effector enzyme adenylyl cyclase. Removal of the β agonist allows the dissociation of β-arrestin and the phosphate groups from the receptor, and the receptor returns to a fully active state.

Long-term desensitization is considered to be caused by a reduction in the number of β receptors; this is termed **downregulation**. Both norepinephrine and albuterol have caused a reduction of almost 50% in vitro in the number of β-adrenergic receptors in airway smooth muscle of guinea pigs.[53] Exposure of isolated human bronchus to isoproterenol or terbutaline produces similar desensitization.[54] Long-term desensitization is also illustrated in Figure 6-14, as indicated by the lower peak response to subsequent administration of an adrenergic agonist.

Although use of an inhaled β agonist does cause a reduction in peak effect, the bronchodilator response is still significant and stabilizes within several weeks with continued use.[18] Such tolerance is not generally considered clinically important and does not contraindicate the use of these agents. The same phenomenon of tolerance is also responsible for diminished side effects, such as muscle tremor, among patients regularly using inhaled β-agonist bronchodilators.

In addition to loss of receptors (downregulation) by exposure to a β agonist, altered β-receptor function may be caused secondary to inflammation. Increased levels of phospholipase A_2 (PLA_2) may destabilize membrane support of the β receptor, changing its function. Cytokines such as interleukin-1β (IL-1β) may cause desensitization, and platelet-activating factor (PAF) inhibits the relaxing effect of isoproterenol on human tracheal tissue.

Corticosteroids can reverse the desensitization of β receptors and are said to be able to potentiate the response to β agonists.[55] Corticosteroids have the following effects in relation to β-agonist and β-receptor function:

- Corticosteroids increase the proportion of β receptors expressed on the cell membrane (upregulation).
- Corticosteroids increase the proportion of β receptors in the high-affinity binding state.
- Corticosteroids inhibit the release and action of inflammatory mediators such as PLA_2, cytokines, and PAF.

β agonists may have a positive effect on corticosteroid function and activity. A review by Anderson[25] explored possible mechanisms for the beneficial interaction of β agonists and corticosteroids.

Loss of Bronchoprotection

A distinction was found by Ahrens and colleagues[56] to exist between the *bronchodilating effect* and the *bronchoprotective effect* of β agonists. The bronchodilating effect of a β agonist can be measured on the basis of airflow change, as indicated by a change in FEV_1 or peak expiratory flow rate (PEFR). The bronchoprotective effect refers to the reaction of the airways to challenge by provocative stimuli such as allergens or irritants and is measured with doses of histamine, methacholine, or cold air. Ahrens and colleagues[54] found that the protective effect with agonists such as metaproterenol or albuterol declines more rapidly than the bronchodilating effect. Not only is there a difference in time between these effects, but also it was found that tolerance occurs

with the bronchoprotective effect of a β agonist, just as with the bronchodilating effect. Results from a study by O'Connor and associates[57] are shown in Figure 6-16. The difference in dose of adenosine (AMP) and methacholine required to induce a 20% decline in FEV_1 (PC_{20}) after the inhalation of terbutaline compared with a placebo is seen before and after 7 days of steady treatment with terbutaline. Airway response to challenge is seen to occur with a significantly lower dose of either AMP or methacholine in subjects with mild asthma *after* 7 days of β-agonist exposure, showing tolerance to the protective effect of terbutaline. The development of tolerance to the bronchoprotective effect of the long-acting β agonist salmeterol was shown to occur both in the absence of corticosteroid therapy (Bhagat and colleagues[58]) and with concomitant inhaled corticosteroid treatment (Kalra and associates[59]). In a study by Rosenthal and associates,[60] after the first 4 weeks of regular treatment with salmeterol, there was no increase in bronchial hyperresponsiveness or loss of bronchoprotection. Sustained improvements were seen in pulmonary function and asthma symptom control.[60]

The mechanism underlying the increase in bronchial hyperresponsiveness with use of β agonists is unclear. Evidence accumulating on the effects of the (S)-isomer of β agonists suggests a possible cause.[61] The same effects could conceivably be implicated in the reduction in maximal bronchodilator effect with repeated use.

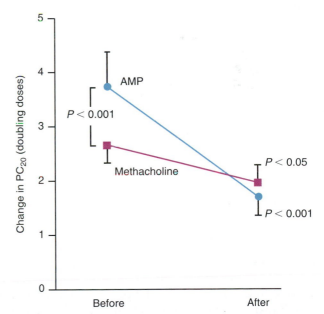

Figure 6-16 Data of O'Connor and colleagues[55] showing decrease in the challenge dose of adenosine (AMP) and methacholine after inhaling 500 mcg of terbutaline compared with a placebo, before and after a 7-day treatment period with terbutaline, indicating a loss of protection against airway stimuli with regular terbutaline use, especially with the inflammatory agent AMP. The higher the number of doubling doses needed for bronchoconstriction, the lower the airway responsiveness—that is, the greater the airway protection. (From O'Connor BJ, Aikman SL, Barnes PJ, *N Engl J Med* 327:1204, © 1992 Massachusetts Medical Society. All rights reserved.)

Central Nervous System Effects

Commonly reported side effects of the adrenergic bronchodilators include headache, nervousness, irritability, anxiety, and insomnia, which are caused by CNS stimulation. Feelings of nervousness or anxiety may be due to the muscle tremor seen with these drugs, rather than to direct CNS stimulation. Excessive stimulation of the CNS, or at least symptoms of such, should be noted by clinicians and can warrant evaluation of the dosage used.

Fall in Arterial Oxygen Pressure

A decrease in arterial oxygen pressure (PaO_2) has been noted with isoproterenol administration during asthmatic bronchospasm when ventilation improves and the exacerbation is relieved. The same effect has subsequently been noted with newer β agonists such as albuterol and salmeterol.[62] The mechanism seems to be an increase in perfusion (i.e., blood flow) of poorly ventilated portions of the lung. It is known that regional alveolar hypoxia produces regional pulmonary vasoconstriction in an effort to shunt perfusion to lung areas of higher oxygen tension. This vasoconstriction is probably accomplished by α-sympathetic receptors.[63]

Administration of inhaled β agonists may reverse hypoxic pulmonary vasoconstriction by $β_2$ stimulation, which increases perfusion to underventilated lung regions.[64] Preferential delivery of the inhaled aerosol to better-ventilated lung regions increases the ventilation-perfusion mismatch. It has been noted that such decreases in PaO_2 are statistically significant but physiologically may be negligible.[62,65] Oxygen tension decreases most in subjects with the highest initial PaO_2. Decreases in PaO_2 rarely exceed 10 mm Hg, and the PaO_2 values tend to be on the flat portion of the oxyhemoglobin curve so that decreases in arterial oxygen saturation (SaO_2) are minimized. Oxygen tensions usually return to baseline within 30 minutes.

Metabolic Disturbances

Adrenergic bronchodilators can increase blood glucose and insulin levels and decrease serum potassium levels. This is a normal effect of sympathomimetics. In diabetic patients, clinicians should be aware of a possible effect on glucose and insulin levels. Hypokalemia has also been reported after parenteral administration of albuterol and epinephrine.[66] The clinical importance of this side effect is controversial, and it would be of concern mainly for patients with cardiac disease or in interpreting serum potassium levels obtained shortly after use of adrenergic bronchodilators. The mechanism of the effect on potassium is probably activation of the sodium-potassium pump by the β receptor, with enhanced transport of potassium from the extracellular to the intracellular compartment. Such metabolic effects are minimized with inhaled aerosols of β-adrenergic agents because plasma levels of the drug remain low. However, the use of large inhaled doses and of multiple doses, such as utilizing short- and long-acting sympathomimetics together, should warrant monitoring of potassium.

Propellant Toxicity and Paradoxic Bronchospasm

The use of MDIs powered by CFC (e.g., Freon) did cause bronchospasm of hyperreactive airways. This reaction to the propellant was shown by Yarbrough and colleagues.[67] They found that 7% of 175 subjects who used an MDI with a placebo and propellant experienced a decrease of 10% or more in FEV_1. The incidence was about 4% when using an MDI with metaproterenol and propellant, probably because the bronchodilating effect overcame the propellant effect. In most cases, bronchospasms last less than 3 minutes. There is apparently no noticeable difference in adverse reactions among patients using a CFC MDI and patients using an HFA MDI.[68] A dry powder formulation is an ideal alternative formulation to an MDI if sensitivity to propellants exists, assuming drug availability and adequate inspiratory flow rate. Use of a nebulizer instead of an MDI may also be considered if bronchospasm occurs in a patient. Finally, the oral route offers an alternative to the inhalation route of administration. Cocchetto and associates[69] reviewed the literature on paradoxic bronchospasm with use of inhalation aerosols.

Sensitivity to Additives

An increasingly publicized problem for individuals with hyperreactive airways is sensitivity to sulfite preservatives, with resulting bronchospasm. Sulfites are used as preservatives for food and are used as antioxidants for bronchodilator solutions to prevent degradation and inactivation. Sulfites include sodium or potassium sulfite, bisulfite, and metabisulfite. When a sulfite is placed in solution, at warm temperature in an acid pH such as saliva, it converts to sulfurous acid and sulfur dioxide. Sulfur dioxide is known to cause bronchoconstriction in asthmatic patients. A solution of racemic epinephrine is known to contain sulfites as preservatives. There have been reports of coughing and wheezing and pruritus after use of sulfite-containing bronchodilators.

Other additives and preservatives that can potentially have an effect on airway smooth muscle include benzalkonium chloride (BAC), ethylenediamine tetraacetic acid (EDTA), and hydrochloric or sulfuric acid to adjust pH of the solution. Asmus and colleagues[70] recommended that only additive-free, sterile-filled unit-dose bronchodilator solutions be used for nebulizer treatment of acute airflow obstruction, especially if doses are given hourly or continuously. Clinicians should check aerosol formulations for BAC or EDTA, and if symptoms of bronchoconstriction occur, consider these as a possible cause.

COMPATIBILITY OF OTHER AGENTS WITH BRONCHODILATORS

Respiratory therapists often mix multiple agents into the liquid medication cup of nebulizer. However, most, if not all, agents are not FDA approved to be mixed with other agents.

Several studies have tested the compatibility of common bronchodilators with other agents used in respiratory care. Kamin and associates[71] found no chemical changes when they mixed albuterol with ipratropium, cromolyn, budesonide, tobramycin, or colistin. However, when antibiotics are to be administered in a nebulizer, it is best to separate the antibiotics and administer in the nebulizer individually. Bonasia and colleagues[72] reported that levalbuterol is compatible with ipratropium, cromolyn, acetylcysteine, and budesonide for at least 30 minutes at room temperature. Akapo and coworkers[73] discovered that formoterol nebulizer solution was compatible with ipratropium, cromolyn, acetylcysteine, and budesonide.

Mixing solutions is a common practice, and the literature supports the mixing of many common agents used in respiratory care. Mixing of agents should be done with caution, however. Special attention should be directed to the nebulizer in use and its function.

β-AGONIST CONTROVERSY

The **asthma paradox** is a descriptive phrase for the increasing incidence of asthma morbidity, and especially asthma mortality, despite advances in the understanding of asthma and availability of improved drugs to treat asthma. Many studies have implicated the use of short-acting β agonists in asthma near-death emergencies and deaths,[74,75] worsening clinical outcomes,[76,77] and increased hyperreactivity.[78,79] The events described in these studies may have been related to lack of corticosteroid use, leaving uncontrolled asthma symptoms to be treated only with short-acting β agonists.

Short-acting drugs, such as albuterol, and long-acting agents, such as salmeterol, have not in general been associated with a significant worsening of asthma.[80] However, more recent evidence has indicated that long-acting β agonists may have a potential to increase asthma hospitalization or cause death.[34,35] It has been noted that regular use of fenoterol and isoproterenol, but not other β agonists, may lead to worsening asthma control.[61] Tolerance to the bronchodilator effect does occur with the use of β agonists, although this stabilizes and does not progress. There is an increase in bronchial hyperreactivity after institution of regular β-agonist therapy, which is not well explained. Evidence suggests that this

effect may be caused or enhanced by the (S)-enantiomer of β agonists, which has a range of proinflammatory effects.

Asthma Morbidity and Mortality

 KEY POINT

The β agonists have been questioned as a possible factor in the increase in asthma mortality, leading to the "β-agonist controversy."

A complete analysis of the relationship between β agonists and worsening asthma based on the literature seems to indicate that there is *not* a class effect of these drugs causing deterioration of asthma.[61] Although it is unclear that β-agonist use increases risk of morbidity or death from asthma, asthma mortality is reported to be increasing in the United States and worldwide, despite more available treatment options, including $β_2$-specific and longer-acting adrenergic bronchodilators.[81] There are several causes, not all involving β-agonist therapy, that may potentially lead to worsening asthma severity:

- Use of β agonists may allow allergic individuals to expose themselves to allergens and stimuli, with no immediate symptoms to warn them but with development of progressive airway inflammation and increasing bronchial hyperresponsiveness.
- Repeated self-administration of β agonists gives temporary relief of asthma symptoms through bronchodilation, which may cause underestimation of severity and delay in seeking medical help. β Agonists do not block progressive airway inflammation, which can lead to death from lethal airway obstruction and hypoxia.
- Use of β agonists to alleviate symptoms of wheezing and resistance may lead to insufficient use—through poor patient education, poor patient compliance, or both—of antiinflammatory therapy to control the basic inflammatory nature of asthma.
- Accumulation of the (S)-isomer with racemic β agonists could exert a detrimental effect on asthma control.
- There is increased airway irritation with environmental pollution and lifestyle changes.[82]

Discussion of the relationship of β-agonist use to asthma morbidity and mortality should review the use of β agonists in the context of the NAEPP guidelines. The 1991, 1997, 2002, and 2007 documents all stress that asthma is a disease of chronic airway inflammation. Treatment with regular β-agonist therapy in severe asthma (asthma requiring step 2 care or greater) does not address the underlying inflammatory process. In evaluating β-agonist therapy in asthma, one must evaluate concomitant antiinflammatory therapy (or the lack of it) and environmental management of the asthma.

RESPIRATORY CARE ASSESSMENT OF β-AGONIST THERAPY

Before Treatment

- Assess the effectiveness of drug therapy on the basis of indication for the aerosol agent: Presence of reversible airflow resulting from primary bronchospasm or obstruction secondary to an inflammatory response or secretions, either acute or chronic.
- Monitor flow rates with bedside peak flow meters, by portable spirometry, or on the basis of laboratory reports of pulmonary function before and after bronchodilator studies to assess reversibility of airflow obstruction.
- Perform respiratory assessment of breathing rate and pattern and breath sounds by auscultation, before and after treatment.
- Assess pulse before, during, and after treatment; a 20% increase from baseline may constitute changing medication or discontinuing therapy.

During Treatment and Short Term

- Assess the patient's subjective reaction to treatment for any change in breathing effort or pattern.
- Assess arterial blood gases or pulse oximeter saturation, as needed, for acute states with asthma or COPD, to monitor changes in ventilation and gas exchange (oxygenation).
- Note the effect of β agonists on blood glucose (increase) and potassium (decrease) laboratory values, if high doses, such as with continuous nebulization or emergency department treatment, are used.

Long Term

- Monitor pulmonary function studies of lung volumes, capacities, and flows.
- Instruct asthmatic patients in the use and interpretation of disposable peak flow meters to assess the severity of asthmatic episodes and to ensure there is an action plan for treatment modification.
- Patient education should emphasize that β agonists do not treat underlying inflammation or prevent progression of asthma, and additional antiinflammatory treatment or more aggressive medical therapy may be needed if there is a poor response to the rescue β agonist.
- Instruct and then verify correct use of the aerosol delivery device (SVN, MDI, reservoir, DPI).
- Instruct patients in the use, assembly, and especially cleaning of aerosol inhalation devices.

For Long-Acting β Agonists

- Assess ongoing lung function, including predose FEV_1 over time and variability in peak expiratory flows.
- Assess amount of rescue β-agonist use and nocturnal symptoms.

- Assess number of exacerbations, unscheduled clinic visits, and hospitalizations.
- Assess days of absence resulting from symptoms.
- Assess ability to reduce the dose of concomitant inhaled corticosteroids.

General Contraindications

- Bronchodilators are generally safe. However, regular, long-term use of short- and long-acting bronchodilators is not recommended.
- Use of bronchodilator therapy in patients with cardiac problems should be closely monitored.
- Patients with chronic disease (cystic fibrosis, COPD, and asthma) may be less responsive to bronchodilator therapy, possibly because of side effects from long-term use.

? SELF-ASSESSMENT QUESTIONS

Answers can be found in Appendix A.

1. Identify an adrenergic bronchodilator used clinically that is a catecholamine.
2. Which catecholamine has been used as a bronchodilator and is commonly given to treat allergic reaction by self-injection?
3. What is the duration of action of the catecholamine bronchodilators?
4. Identify two advantages introduced with the modifications of the catecholamine structure in adrenergic bronchodilators.
5. Identify the usual dose by aerosol for an SVN for levalbuterol and albuterol.
6. What is an extremely common side effect with $β_2$-adrenergic bronchodilators?
7. Identify the approximate duration of action for racemic epinephrine, albuterol, salmeterol, and olodaterol.
8. Identify the generic drug for each of the following brand names: Brovana, Arcapta, Serevent Diskus, and Ventolin HFA.
9. Which route of administration is more likely to have greater severity of side effects with a β-agonist oral or inhaled aerosol?
10. You notice a pinkish tinge to aerosol rainout in the large-bore tubing connecting a patient's mouthpiece to a nebulizer after a treatment with racemic epinephrine; what has caused this?
11. A patient exhibits paradoxic bronchoconstriction from the propellant when using an HFA MDI. Suggest an alternative for the patient.
12. If you are working with an asthmatic with occasional symptoms of wheezing and chest tightness, which respond well to an inhaled β agonist, would you suggest using salmeterol?
13. Suggest a β agonist that would be appropriate for the patient in Question 12.

CLINICAL SCENARIO

A 24-year-old white man moved to the metropolitan Atlanta area in the fall of the previous year. He presents to your outpatient clinic with a complaint of difficulty in breathing. He has no history of asthma or other previous pulmonary disease. He is an accountant with a medium-size firm. He noticed a few "chest colds" from October through January, but these resolved with over-the-counter (OTC) cold medications such as decongestants and cough suppressants. It is now late May, and during a round of golf he had difficulty breathing. On interview, he described a tightness in his chest and the sound of wheezing. The golf course had recently been mown. The pollen count was quite high at the time, and there was an increased ozone concentration, leading to a smog alert on the day of his round. He also complained of waking up several times during the night with mild shortness of breath.

His respiratory rate (RR) is 14 breaths/min, with no obvious distress at rest; blood pressure (BP) is 128/74 mm Hg; heart rate (HR) is 76 beats/min; and temperature (T) is within normal limits. His oxygen saturation by pulse oximetry (SpO$_2$) is 93% on room air. You detect mild expiratory wheezing bilaterally on auscultation.

Using the SOAP method, assess this clinical scenario.

REFERENCES

1. National Asthma Education and Prevention Program, National Heart, Lung, and Blood Institute, National Institutes of Health: *Expert Panel Report 3: Guidelines for the Diagnosis and Management of Asthma*, Bethesda, MD, 2007, National Institutes of Health. Available at: <http://www.nhlbi.nih.gov/guidelines/asthma/asthgdln.htm>. Accessed August 2014. NIH Publication No. 08-4051.

2. Global Initiative for Asthma (GINA): *Global strategy for asthma management and prevention*, 2014, National Heart, Lung, and Blood Institute (Bethesda, MD) and World Health Organization (Geneva, Switzerland). Available at: <http://www.ginasthma.org/local/uploads/files/GINA_Report_2014_Jun11.pdf>. Accessed August 2014.

3. *Drug Facts and Comparisons*, St Louis, 2014, Facts & Comparisons, Wolters Kluwer Health.

4. Orgel HA, Kemp JP, Tinkelman DG, et al: Bitolterol and albuterol metered-dose aerosols: comparison of two long-acting beta-2 adrenergic bronchodilators for treatment of asthma. *J Allergy Clin Immunol* 75:55, 1985.

5. Barnes PJ: Treatment with (R)-albuterol has no advantage over racemic albuterol. *Am J Respir Crit Care Med* 174:969–972, 2006.

6. Mitra S, Ugur M, Ugur O, et al: S)-Albuterol increases intracellular free calcium by muscarinic receptor activation and a phospholipase C-dependent mechanism in airway smooth muscle. *Mol Pharmacol* 53:347, 1998.

7. Lipworth BJ, Clark DJ, Koch P, et al: Pharmacokinetics and extrapulmonary β$_2$ adrenoceptor activity of nebulised racemic salbutamol and its R and S isomers in healthy volunteers. *Thorax* 52:849, 1997.

8. Johansson FJ, Rydberg I, Aberg G, et al: Effects of albuterol enantiomers on in vitro bronchial reactivity. *Clin Rev Allergy Immunol* 14:57, 1996.

9. Templeton AG, Chapman ID, Chilvers ER, et al: Effects of S-salbutamol on human isolated bronchus. *Pulm Pharmacol Ther* 11:1, 1998.

10. Volcheck GW, Gleich GJ, Kita H: Pro- and anti-inflammatory effects of beta adrenergic agonists on eosinophil response to IL-5. *J Allergy Clin Immunol* 101:S35, 1998.

11. Schmekel B, Rydberg I, Norlander B, et al: Stereoselective pharmacokinetics of S-salbutamol after administration of the racemate in healthy volunteers. *Eur Respir J* 13:1230, 1999.

12. Dhand R, Goode M, Reid R, et al: Preferential pulmonary retention of (S)-albuterol after inhalation of racemic albuterol. *Am J Respir Crit Care Med* 160:1136, 1999.

13. Nelson HS, Bensch G, Pleskow WW, et al: Improved bronchodilation with levalbuterol compared with racemic albuterol in patients with asthma. *J Allergy Clin Immunol* 102:943, 1998.

14. Cazzola M, Testi R, Matera MG: Clinical Pharmacokinetics of Salmeterol. *J Clin Pharmacokinet* 40(1):19–30, 2002.

15. Moore RH, Khan A, Dickey BF: Long-acting inhaled β$_2$-agonists in asthma therapy. *Chest* 113:1095, 1998.

16. Bartow RA, Brogden RN: Formoterol: an update of its pharmacological properties and therapeutic efficacy in the management of asthma. *Drugs* 56:303, 1998.

17. Vaickus L, Claus R: (R,R)-Formoterol: rapid onset and 24 hour duration of response after a single dose. *Am J Respir Crit Care Med* 161:A191, 2000. (abstract).

18. van Noord JA, Smeets JJ, Raaijmakers JA, et al: Salmeterol versus formoterol in patients with moderately severe asthma: dose and duration of action. *Eur Respir J* 9:1684, 1996.

19. Cazzola M, Bardaro F, Stirpe E: The role of indacaterol for chronic obstructive pulmonary disease (COPD). *J Thorac Dis* 5(4):559–566, 2013.

20. Ribeiro M, Chapman KR: Comparative efficacy of indacaterol in chronic obstructive pulmonary disease. *Int J Chron Obstruct Pulmon Dis* 7:145–152, 2012.

21. Gibb A, Yang LPH: Olodaterol: First global approval. *Drugs* 73:1841–1846, 2013.

22. van Noord JA, Smeets JJ, Drenth BM, et al: 24-hour bronchodilation following a single dose of the novel β$_2$-agonist olodaterol in COPD. *Pulm Pharmacol Ther* 24(6):666–672, 2011.

23. Smit M, Zuidhof AB, Bos SIT, et al: Bronchoprotection by olodaterol is synergistically enhanced by tiotropium in a guinea pig model of allergic asthma. *J Pharmacol Exp Ther* 348:303–310, 2013.

24. Hanania NA, Feldman G, Zachgo W, et al: The efficacy and safety of the novel long-acting β$_2$ agonist vilanterol in COPD patients: a randomized placebo-controlled trial. *Chest* 142(1):119–127, 2012.

25. Global Initiative for Chronic Obstructive Lung Disease: *Global strategy for the diagnosis, management, and prevention of COPD*, 2014, National Heart, Lung, and Blood Institute (Bethesda, MD) and World Health Organization (Geneva, Switzerland). Available at: <http://www.goldcopd.org/uploads/users/files/GOLD_Report_2014_Jun11.pdf>. Accessed August 2014.

26. Politiek MJ, Boorsma M, Aalbers R: Comparison of formoterol, salbutamol and salmeterol in methacholine-induced severe bronchoconstriction. *Eur Respir J* 13:988, 1999.

27. Anderson GP: Interactions between corticosteroids and β-adrenergic agonists in asthma disease induction, progression, and exacerbation. *Am J Respir Crit Care Med* 161:S188, 2000.

28. Walters JA, Wood-Baker R, Walters EH: Long-acting β$_2$-agonists in asthma: an overview of Cochrane systematic reviews. *Respir Med* 99:384, 2005.

29. Castle W, Fuller R, Hall J, et al: Serevent nationwide surveillance study: comparison of salmeterol with salbutamol in asthmatic patients who require regular bronchodilator treatment. *BMJ* 306:1034, 1993.

30. Bateman ED, Boushey HA, Bousquet J, et al: GOAL Investigators Group: can guideline-defined asthma control be achieved? The

Gaining Optimal Asthma controL study. *Am J Respir Crit Care Med* 170:836, 2004.

31. Shapiro G, Lumry W, Wolfe J, et al: Combined salmeterol 50 mcg and fluticasone propionate 250 mcg in the Diskus device for the treatment of asthma. *Am J Respir Crit Care Med* 161:527, 2000.

32. Pearlman DS, Chervinsky P, LaForce C, et al: A comparison of salmeterol with albuterol in the treatment of mild-to-moderate asthma. *N Engl J Med* 327:1420, 1992.

33. Mahler DA, Donohue JF, Barbee RA, et al: Efficacy of salmeterol xinafoate in the treatment of COPD. *Chest* 115:957, 1999.

34. Salpeter SR, Buckley NS, Ormiston TM, et al: Meta-analysis: effect of long-acting β-agonists on severe asthma exacerbations and asthma-related deaths. *Ann Intern Med* 144:904, 2006.

35. Nelson HS, Weiss ST, Bleecker ER, et al: SMART Study Group: The Salmeterol Multicenter Asthma Research Trial: a comparison of usual pharmacotherapy for asthma or usual pharmacotherapy plus salmeterol. *Chest* 129:15, 2006.

36. McFadden ER, Jr: Clinical use of β-adrenergic agonists. *J Allergy Clin Immunol* 76:352, 1985.

37. Robertson C, Levison H: Bronchodilators in asthma. *Chest* 87:64S, 1985.

38. Tinkelman DG, Vanderpool GE, Carroll MS, et al: Comparison of nebulized terbutaline and subcutaneous epinephrine in the treatment of acute asthma. *Ann Allergy* 50:398, 1983.

39. Fernandez E: Beta-adrenergic agonists. *Semin Respir Med* 8:353, 1987.

40. Fink J, Dhand R: Bronchodilator resuscitation in the emergency department. II. Dosing strategies. *Respir Care* 45:497, 2000.

41. Lin RY, Sauter D, Newman T, et al: Continuous versus intermittent albuterol nebulization in the treatment of acute asthma. *Ann Emerg Med* 22:1993, 1847.

42. Shrestha M, Bidadi K, Gourlay S, et al: Continuous vs intermittent albuterol, at high and low doses, in the treatment of severe acute asthma in adults. *Chest* 110:42, 1996.

43. Moler F, Hurwitz M, Custer J: Improvement of clinical asthma scores and PaCO$_2$ in children with severe asthma treated with continuously nebulized terbutaline. *J Allergy Clin Immunol* 81:1101, 1988.

44. Portnoy J, Nadel G, Amado M, et al: Continuous nebulization for status asthmaticus. *Ann Allergy* 69:71, 1992.

45. Popa V: Beta-adrenergic drugs. *Clin Chest Med* 7:313, 1986.

46. Leifer KN, Wittig HJ: The β$_2$ sympathomimetic aerosols in the treatment of asthma. *Ann Allergy* 35:69, 1975.

47. Shim C: Adrenergic agonists and bronchodilator aerosol therapy in asthma. *Clin Chest Med* 5:659, 1984.

48. Popa V: Clinical pharmacology of adrenergic drugs. *J Asthma* 21:183, 1984.

49. Larsson S, Svedmyr N: Studies of muscle tremor induced by β-adrenostimulating drugs. *Scand J Respir Dis* 88(Suppl):54, 1974.

50. Marsden CD, Foley TH, Owen DA, et al: Peripheral β-adrenergic receptors concerned with tremor. *Clin Sci* 33:53, 1967.

51. Brown JE, McLeod AA, Shand DG: Evidence for cardiac adrenoreceptors in man. *Clin Pharmacol Ther* 33:424, 1983.

52. Seider N, Abinader EG, Oliven A: Cardiac arrhythmias after inhaled bronchodilators in patients with COPD and ischemic heart disease. *Chest* 104:1070, 1993.

53. Jenne JW: β$_2$-adrenergic receptor-agonist interaction. In Leff AR, editor: *Pulmonary and critical care pharmacology and therapeutics,* New York, 1996, McGraw-Hill.

54. Avner BP, Jenne JW: Desensitization of isolated human bronchial smooth muscle to beta receptor agonists. *J Allergy Clin Immunol* 68:51, 1981.

55. Svedmyr N: Action of corticosteroids on β-adrenergic receptors: clinical aspects. *Am Rev Respir Dis* 141:S31, 1990.

56. Ahrens RC, Harris JB, Milavetz G, et al: Use of bronchial provocation with histamine to compare the pharmacodynamics

of inhaled albuterol and metaproterenol in patients with asthma. *J Allergy Clin Immunol* 79:876, 1987.

57. O'Connor BJ, Aikman SL, Barnes PJ: Tolerance to the nonbronchodilator effects of inhaled β$_2$-agonists in asthma. *N Engl J Med* 327:1204, 1992.

58. Bhagat R, Kalra S, Swystun VA, et al: Rapid onset of tolerance to the bronchoprotective effect of salmeterol. *Chest* 108:1235, 1995.

59. Kalra S, Swystun VA, Bhagat R, et al: Inhaled corticosteroids do not prevent the development of tolerance to the bronchoprotective effect of salmeterol. *Chest* 109: 953, 1996.

60. Rosenthal RR, Busse WW, Kemp JP, et al: Effect of long-term salmeterol therapy compared with as-needed albuterol use on airway hyperresponsiveness. *Chest* 116:595, 1999.

61. Beasley R, Pearce N, Crane J, et al: β-agonists: what is the evidence that their use increases the risk of asthma morbidity and mortality? *J Allergy Clin Immunol* 104:S18, 1999.

62. Khoukaz G, Gross NJ: Effects of salmeterol on arterial blood gases in patients with stable chronic obstructive pulmonary disease: comparison with albuterol and ipratropium. *Am J Respir Crit Care Med* 160:1028, 1999.

63. Hales CA, Kazemi H: Hypoxic vascular response of the lung: effect of aminophylline and epinephrine. *Am Rev Respir Dis* 110:126, 1974.

64. Chick TW, Nicholson DP: Effects of bronchodilators on the distribution of ventilation and perfusion in asthma. *Chest* 63:11S, 1973.

65. Sharp JT: Workshop No. 2: bronchodilator therapy and arterial blood gases. *Chest* 3(Suppl):980, 1978.

66. Kung M: Parenteral adrenergic bronchodilators and potassium. *Chest* 89:322, 1986.

67. Yarbrough J, Mansfield LE, Ting S: Metered dose inhaler induced bronchospasm in asthmatic patients. *Ann Allergy* 55:25, 1985.

68. Huchon G, Hofbauer P, Cannizzaro G, et al: Comparison of the safety of drug delivery via HFA- and CFC-metered dose inhalers in CAO. *Eur Respir J* 15:663, 2000.

69. Cocchetto DM, Sykes RS, Spector S: Paradoxical bronchospasm after use of inhalation aerosols: a review of the literature. *J Asthma* 28:49, 1991.

70. Asmus MJ, Sherman J, Hendeles L: Bronchoconstrictor additives in bronchodilator solutions. *J Allergy Clin Immunol* 104:S53, 1999.

71. Kamin W, Schwabe A, Kramer I: Inhalation solutions: which ones are allowed to be mixed? Physico-chemical compatibility of drug solution in nebulizers. *J Cyst Fibros* 5:205–213, 2006.

72. Bonasia PJ, McVicar WK, Bill W, et al: Chemical and physical compatibility of levalbuterol inhalation solution concentrate mixed with budesonide, ipratropium bromide, cromolyn sodium, or acetylcysteine sodium. *Respir Care* 53:1716–1722, 2008.

73. Akapo S, Gupta J, Martinez E, et al: Compatibility and aerosol characteristics of formoterol fumarate mixed with other nebulizing solutions. *Ann Pharmacother* 42:1416–1424, 2008.

74. Crane J, Pearce N, Flatt A, et al: Prescribed fenoterol and death from asthma in New Zealand, 1981-1983: case-control study. *Lancet* 1:917, 1989.

75. Pearce N, Grainger J, Atkinson M, et al: Case-control study of prescribed fenoterol and death from asthma in New Zealand 1977-81. *Thorax* 45:170, 1990.

76. van Schayck CP, Dompeling E, van Herwarden CLA, et al: Bronchodilator treatment in moderate asthma or chronic bronchitis: continuous or on demand? A randomized controlled study. *BMJ* 303:1426, 1991.

77. Sears MR, Taylor DR, Print CG, et al: Regular inhaled β-agonist treatment in bronchial asthma. *Lancet* 336:1391, 1990.

78. Cockcroft DW, McParland CP, Britto SA: Regular inhaled salbutamol and airway responsiveness to allergen. *Lancet* 342:833–837, 1993.

79. Wong S, Wahedna I, Pavord ID, et al: Effect of regular terbutaline and budesonide on bronchial reactivity to allergen challenge. *Am J Respir Crit Care Med* 150:1268, 1994.

80. Williams C, Crossland L, Finnerty J, et al: A case-control study of salmeterol and near fatal attacks of asthma. *Thorax* 53:7, 1998.

81. Sears MR: Worldwide trends in asthma mortality. *Bull Int Union Tuberc Lung Dis* 66:79, 1991.

82. Platts-Mills TA, Woodfolk JA, Chapman MD, et al: Changing concepts of allergic disease: the attempt to keep up with real changes in lifestyles. *J Allergy Clin Immunol* 98:S297, 1996.

CHAPTER 7

Anticholinergic (Parasympatholytic) Bronchodilators

Douglas S. Gardenhire

CHAPTER OUTLINE

OBJECTIVES

After reading this chapter, the reader will be able to:

1. Define terms that pertain to anticholinergic bronchodilators
2. Differentiate between *parasympathomimetic* and *parasympatholytic*
3. Differentiate between *cholinergic* and *anticholinergic*
4. Differentiate between *muscarinic* and *antimuscarinic*
5. List all available anticholinergic agents used in respiratory therapy
6. Discuss the indication for anticholinergic agents
7. Explain the mode of action for anticholinergic agents
8. Identify the route of administration available for anticholinergic agents
9. Discuss adverse effects for anticholinergic agents
10. Discuss the clinical application for anticholinergic agents

KEY TERMS AND DEFINITIONS

Anticholinergic bronchodilator Agent that blocks parasympathetic nervous fibers, which allow relaxation of smooth muscle in the airway.

Antimuscarinic bronchodilator Same as anticholinergic bronchodilator—agent that blocks the effect of acetylcholine (Ach) at the cholinergic site.

Cholinergic Agent that produces the effect of Ach.

Muscarinic Same as cholinergic—agent that produces the effect of Ach or an agent that mimics Ach.

Parasympatholytic Blocking parasympathetic nervous fibers.

Parasympathomimetic Producing effects similar to the parasympathetic nervous system.

Chapter 7 discusses a second class of bronchodilators: anticholinergic agents. Anticholinergic drugs given by inhaled aerosol can block cholinergic-induced airway constriction. The chapter reviews their mode of action and their pharmacologic effects, based on their structural differences. Specific agents are profiled, and their clinical effect in chronic obstructive pulmonary disease (COPD) and asthma is discussed.

CLINICAL INDICATIONS FOR USE

 KEY POINT

Anticholinergic agents given by inhalation are a second class of *bronchodilating agents.*

Indication for Anticholinergic Bronchodilators

Ipratropium, tiotropium, aclidinium, and umeclidinium are indicated as bronchodilators for maintenance treatment in COPD, including chronic bronchitis and emphysema. Ipratropium is used and may be indicated in some individuals with asthma.

Indication for Combined Anticholinergic and β-Agonist Bronchodilators

A combination anticholinergic and β agonist, such as ipratropium and albuterol (Combivent, DuoNeb) and umeclidinium and vilanterol (Anoro Ellipta), is indicated for use in patients receiving maintenance treatment for COPD who require additional bronchodilation for relief of airflow obstruction. Ipratropium is also commonly used in addition to β agonists in severe asthma, especially bronchoconstriction that does not respond well to β-agonist therapy.

Anticholinergic Nasal Spray

A nasal spray formulation is indicated for symptomatic relief of allergic and nonallergic perennial rhinitis and the common cold.

SPECIFIC ANTICHOLINERGIC (PARASYMPATHOLYTIC) AGENTS

Parasympatholytic (anticholinergic, or antimuscarinic) agents that are given by aerosol include ipratropium, a combination of ipratropium and albuterol, tiotropium, aclidinium, umeclidinium, and a combination of umeclidinium and vilanterol. Table 7-1 provides dosage and administration information for each agent.

Atropine sulfate had been administered as a nebulized solution, using either the injectable solution or, preferably, solutions marketed for aerosolization; however, this agent is no longer aerosolized. Duration of bronchodilation and the incidence of side effects are dose dependent. Dosages for children based on dose-response curves had been given

TABLE 7-1	Inhaled Anticholinergic Bronchodilator Agents*		
DRUG	**BRAND NAME**	**ADULT DOSAGE**	**TIME COURSE (ONSET, PEAK, DURATION)**
Ipratropium bromide	Atrovent HFA	HFA MDI: 17 mcg/puff; 2 puffs qid SVN: 0.02% solution (0.2 mg/mL), 500 mcg tid, qid Nasal spray: 21 mcg; 42 mcg; 2 sprays per nostril 2-4 times daily (dosage varies)	*Onset:* 15-30 min *Peak:* 1-2 hr *Duration:* 6 hr
Ipratropium bromide and albuterol	Combivent Respimat	SMI: ipratropium 20 mcg/puff and albuterol 100 mcg/puff, 1 inhalation qid	*Onset:* 15 min *Peak:* 1-2 hr *Duration:* 6 hr
	DuoNeb	SVN: ipratropium 0.5 mg and albuterol 2.5 mg	
Aclidinium bromide	Tudorza Pressair	DPI: 400 mcg/inhalation, 1 inhalation bid	*Onset:* 10 min *Peak:* 2 hr *Duration:* 12
Tiotropium bromide	Spiriva	DPI: 18 mcg/inhalation, 1 inhalation once daily (one capsule)	*Onset:* 30 min *Peak:* 1-3 hr *Duration:* 24 hr
	Spiriva Respimat	SMI: 2.5 mcg/inhalation, 2 inhalations once daily	
Tiotropium bromide and olodaterol	Stiolto Respimat	SMI: tiotropium 2.5 mcg/inhalation and olodaterol 2.5 mcg/inhalation, 2 inhalations once daily	*Onset:* 15 min *Peak:* 1-2 hr *Duration:* 24 hr
Umeclidinium bromide	Incruse Ellipta	DPI: 62.5 mcg/inhalation, 1 inhalation daily	*Onset:* 5-15 min *Peak:* 1-3 hr *Duration:* 24 hr
Umeclidinium bromide and vilanterol	Anoro Ellipta	DPI: umeclidinium 62.5 mcg/inhalation and vilanterol 25 mcg/inhalation, 1 inhalation daily	*Onset:* 5-15 min *Peak:* 1-3 hr *Duration:* 24 hr

DPI, Dry powder inhaler; *HFA,* hydrofluoroalkane; *MDI,* metered dose inhaler; *SMI,* soft-mist inhaler; *SVN,* small volume nebulizer.
*A holding chamber is recommended with MDI administration to prevent accidental eye exposure.

as 0.05 mg/kg three or four times daily.[1] Dosages for adults are based on a schedule of 0.025 mg/kg three or four times daily.[2] Although greater bronchodilation and duration were seen with dosage schedules of 0.05 or 0.1 mg/kg for adults, the side effects of dry mouth, blurred vision, and tachycardia became unacceptable. Because it is a tertiary ammonium compound and not fully ionized, atropine is readily absorbed from the gastrointestinal tract and respiratory mucosa. Systemic side effects (which are discussed subsequently) were seen in doses required for effective bronchodilation when given as an inhaled aerosol. The drug is not recommended for inhalation as a bronchodilator because of its widespread distribution in the body and the availability of the approved agents ipratropium and tiotropium.

Ipratropium bromide (Atrovent) is a nonselective antagonist of M_1, M_2, and M_3 receptors (for a discussion of muscarinic receptors, see Chapter 5). Ipratropium is currently available in two formulations for bronchodilator use: as a hydrofluoroalkane (HFA)-propelled metered dose inhaler (MDI) with 17 mcg/puff and as a nebulizer solution of 0.02% concentration in a 2.5-mL vial, giving a 500-mcg dose per treatment. One other option for the delivery of ipratropium in combination with albuterol is the soft-mist, propellant-free Respimat inhaler. As a quaternary ammonium derivative of atropine, ipratropium is fully ionized and does not distribute well across lipid membranes, limiting its distribution mostly to the lung when inhaled. Ipratropium is approved specifically for the maintenance treatment of airflow obstruction in COPD.

Ipratropium is poorly absorbed into the circulation from both the nasal mucosa, when given by nasal spray, and the airway, when inhaled orally by aerosol. Approximately 20% of the nasal dose and the MDI dose is absorbed, with only 2% of the larger nebulizer solution absorbed into the bloodstream. Ipratropium is partially metabolized by ester hydrolysis into inactive products. It is minimally bound to plasma proteins such as albumin (less than 9%), and the elimination half-life is about 1.6 hours.

The profile of clinical effect for ipratropium differs from that of inhaled β-adrenergic agonists. The onset of bronchodilation begins within minutes but proceeds more slowly to a peak effect 1 to 2 hours after inhalation. β agonists can peak between 20 and 30 minutes depending on the agent. In asthma, the duration of bronchodilator effect is about the same for ipratropium as for β agonists. In COPD, the duration is longer by 1 to 2 hours.[3]

Ipratropium bromide (Atrovent nasal spray) is also available for treatment of rhinopathies and rhinorrhea, including nonallergic perennial rhinitis, viral infectious rhinitis (colds), and allergic rhinitis, if intranasal corticosteroids fail to control symptoms.[4] The nasal spray is available in two strengths, with a 0.03% solution delivering 21 mcg/spray and the 0.06% solution delivering 42 mcg/spray. The 0.03% strength is given as two sprays per nostril two or three times daily, and the 0.06% strength is given as two sprays per nostril three or four times daily. Optimal dosage varies. Intranasal ipratropium has been shown to significantly reduce the volume of nasal secretions and symptoms in

patients with allergic rhinitis and in patients with nonallergic rhinitis.[4] Side effects with the nasal spray are largely local and have included nasal dryness, itching, and epistaxis in a few patients. Dry mouth and dry throat have also occurred. Systemic symptoms such as blurred vision or urinary hesitancy are rare.

Ipratropium and albuterol (Combivent Respimat) is a combination utilizing a soft-mist inhaler known as the Respimat (see Chapter 3), providing 20 mcg/puff of ipratropium and 100 mcg/puff of albuterol. The combination therapy has been shown to be more effective in stable COPD than either agent alone.[5] The chlorofluorocarbon (CFC) version of Combivent was removed from market on December 31, 2013. Another agent, DuoNeb, is available as a combination of ipratropium (0.5 mg) and an albuterol base (2.5 mg).

Glycopyrrolate is a quaternary ammonium derivative of atropine that, similar to ipratropium, does not distribute well across lipid membranes in the body. It is usually administered parenterally as an antimuscarinic agent during reversal of neuromuscular blockade as an alternative to atropine; it has fewer ocular or central nervous system (CNS) side effects. The injectable solution has been nebulized in a 1-mg dose for bronchodilation. Gal and colleagues[6] reported a comparison of glycopyrrolate with atropine and established dose-response curves. Glycopyrrolate has an onset of action of approximately 15 to 30 minutes, a peak effect at 0.5 to 1 hour, and a duration of approximately 6 hours. Although the injectable formulation of glycopyrrolate is used as a less expensive alternative to the Atrovent brand of ipratropium, it is not approved for inhalation. More recently in new research of asthma and COPD, glycopyrrolate as an inhaled agent currently under investigation (NVA-237) has found favor. In a small study Hansel and coworkers[7] found superiority over ipratropium in the protection of bronchospasm from methacholine.

Tiotropium bromide (Spiriva), a muscarinic receptor antagonist, is a long-acting bronchodilator. It is a quaternary ammonium compound structurally related to ipratropium. Similar to ipratropium, tiotropium is poorly absorbed after inhalation. Inhalation of a single dose gives a peak plasma level within 5 minutes with a rapid decline to very low levels within 1 hour.[8,9] Tiotropium exhibits receptor subtype selectivity for M_1 and M_3 receptors. The drug binds to all three muscarinic receptors (M_1, M_2, and M_3) but dissociates much more slowly than ipratropium from the M_1 and M_3 receptors. This results in a selectivity of action on M_1 and M_3 receptors. Atropine and ipratropium block all three types of muscarinic receptors. The M_2 receptor is an autoreceptor inhibiting further release of acetylcholine (Ach), so that blockade can increase Ach release and may offset the bronchodilating effect of atropine or ipratropium.[8] In patients with COPD, tiotropium gives a bronchodilating effect for up to 24 hours with an adequate dose. The effect of tiotropium can be seen for 32 hours; however, it dips between 16 and 24 hours owing to circadian rhythm. The drug also gives a prolonged, dose-dependent protection against inhaled methacholine challenge.[10]

KEY POINT

Anticholinergic bronchodilators are specifically *parasympatholytic*, that is, *antimuscarinic* agents, blocking the effect of Ach at the cholinergic (muscarinic) receptors on bronchial smooth muscle.

Several studies have examined the bronchodilating effect of various doses of tiotropium compared with placebo and ipratropium.[10-12] A single dose of 18 mcg inhaled once daily from the HandiHaler, a dry powder inhaler (DPI),[13] provided significant bronchodilation for up to 24 hours with a low side effect profile. An increase of 15% from baseline forced expiratory volume in 1 second (FEV_1) occurred 30 minutes after inhalation, with a peak effect at about 3 hours. Improvement in FEV_1 was greater 3 hours after inhalation for tiotropium than for ipratropium. After a dose of tiotropium, the trough, or lowest, value for FEV_1 remained above that of ipratropium because of the prolonged action of tiotropium. Ipratropium had a more rapid onset of action than tiotropium, but after the initial dosing this difference loses relevance because tiotropium maintains a higher level of baseline bronchodilation. In a meta-analysis, Barr and associates[14] found that tiotropium reduces COPD exacerbations and hospitalizations, improves quality-of-life symptoms, and may slow the decline in a patient's FEV_1.

In the United States, tiotropium is available as a DPI and as a soft-mist, propellant-free Respimat inhaler. Spiriva Respimat, approved in September 2014 provides 2.5 mcg per actuation. The recommended dose is two actuations once daily. *Aclidinium bromide* (Tudorza Pressair) is a long-acting, inhaled anticholinergic developed by Forest Laboratories and approved by the FDA in July 2012 as a maintenance treatment for COPD.[15] This agent is a potent antagonism of all muscarinic receptors, dissociating slowly at M_3 and in a shorter time at M_2, indicating the potential to provide sustained bronchodilation that is similar in action to tiotropium.[16] Aclidinium is rapidly hydrolyzed in human plasma in contrast to ipratropium and tiotropium.[16,17] This rapid hydrolysis results in very low and transient systemic exposure, suggesting a reduced potential for systemic side effects.[16,17]

Early clinical studies in healthy subjects have confirmed the low systemic bioavailability and favorable safety profile of single and multiple doses of aclidinium.[18,19] In a subsequent study, which included patients with moderate to severe COPD, aclidinium displayed long-lasting bronchodilation and was well tolerated.[20]

Tiotropium bromide and olodaterol (Stiolto Respimat) is a combination agent providing 2.5 mcg of tiopropium and 2.5 mcg of olodaterol—a long-acting anticholinergic and β agonist used to treat airflow limitations in COPD—once daily. Stiolto Respimat, approved in May 2015, should not be used to treat asthma or acute deterioration of COPD. The recommended dosage is two actuations once daily.

Umeclidinium (Incruse Ellipta) is a long-acting anticholinergic developed by Theravance and GlaxoSmithKline and approved by the FDA in May 2014 for once-daily maintenance treatment of airflow obstruction in patients with COPD. Incruse Ellipta is a DPI that should be used daily at the same time each day. Umeclidinium bromide has activity across multiple muscarinic receptors and exerts its bronchodilatory activity by competitively inhibiting the binding of Ach with muscarinic cholinergic receptors on airway smooth muscle (M_3). It demonstrates slow reversibility at the M_3 receptor, providing long duration of bronchodilation in the lungs.[21]

Umeclidinium bromide and vilanterol (Anoro Ellipta) is a combination agent providing 62.5 mcg of umeclidinium and 25 mcg of vilanterol—a long-acting anticholinergic and β agonist used to treat airflow limitations in COPD once daily. In a randomized, double-blind, placebo-controlled, parallel-controlled study of almost 1500 patients Anoro Ellipta provided greater improvements in lung function, health status, and dyspnea scores compared with the individual use of the drugs in the combination.[22] Although the use of combination agents in respiratory care is common, not all patients need combination agents. The use of β agonists (see Chapter 6) and inhaled glucocorticoids (see Chapter 11) do present risks.

KEY POINT

The only approved anticholinergic agents for inhalation as an aerosol at this time are *ipratropium* (Atrovent), which is available as an MDI, an SVN solution, and an intranasal spray; *tiotropium* (Spiriva) as an MDI and Respimat, *aclidinium* (Tudorza Pressair), and *umeclidinium* (Incruse Ellipta), which are both available only in DPI form.

CLINICAL PHARMACOLOGY

Structure-Activity Relationships

Chemical structures of the two naturally occurring belladonna alkaloids, atropine and scopolamine (also called hyoscine), are illustrated in Figure 7-1. Atropine, including its sulfate (atropine sulfate), and scopolamine are tertiary ammonium compounds that differ from each other only by an oxygen bridging the carbon-6 and carbon-7 positions. Quaternary ammonium derivatives of atropine include atropine, ipratropium, and tiotropium. Another quaternary atropine derivative, which has been administered experimentally as a bronchodilator by aerosol, is glycopyrrolate (Robinul) (not shown in Figure 7-1).

Tertiary ammonium forms, such as atropine sulfate or scopolamine, are easily absorbed into the bloodstream, distribute throughout the body, and in particular cross the blood-brain barrier to cause CNS changes. Quaternary ammonium forms (e.g., ipratropium, tiotropium, and glycopyrrolate) are fully ionized and poorly absorbed into the bloodstream or CNS. As a result, the systemic side effects seen with aerosol administration of the tertiary ammonium atropine sulfate do not occur or are minimal with a quaternary ammonium such as ipratropium. Quaternary ammonium agents given by inhalation generally are poorly absorbed from the lung. They are not rapidly removed from the aerosol deposition site and do not cross the blood-brain

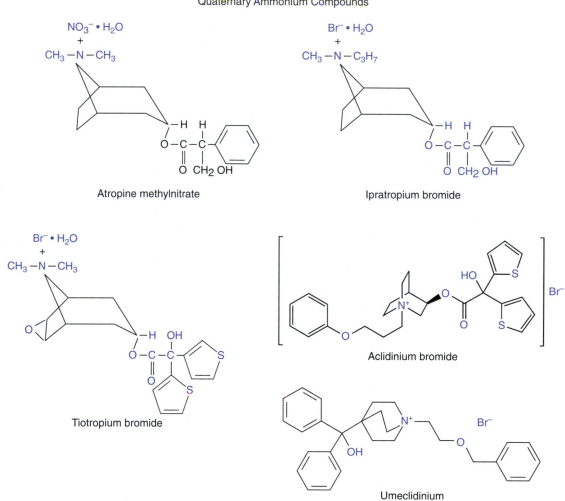

Figure 7-1 Chemical structures of anticholinergic (parasympatholytic) agents: tertiary compounds, such as atropine and scopolamine, and quaternary compounds, such as ipratropium, tiotropium, aclidinium, and umeclidinium.

barrier as atropine sulfate does, giving them a wider therapeutic margin in relation to side effects.

Pharmacologic Effects of Anticholinergic (Antimuscarinic) Agents

The general effects of **cholinergic (muscarinic)** stimulation and the corresponding effects produced by anticholinergic (antimuscarinic) action are listed in Table 7-2. Specific

effects differ for tertiary and quaternary ammonium compounds because of their absorption differences as previously outlined for their structure-activity relationships. These effects and their differences are summarized in Table 7-3 and discussed subsequently.

Tertiary Ammonium Compounds

Tertiary compounds include atropine sulfate, scopolamine, and hyoscyamine sulfate. They are well absorbed across

TABLE 7-2	Comparison of Cholinergic Antagonism (Antimuscarinic Effects) with Cholinergic Effects (Muscarinic Effects)

CHOLINERGIC EFFECT	ANTICHOLINERGIC EFFECT
Decreased heart rate	Increased heart rate
Miosis (contraction of iris, eye)	Mydriasis (pupil dilation)
Contraction (thickening) of lens, eye	Cycloplegia (lens flattened)
Salivation	Drying of upper airway
Lacrimation	Inhibition of tear formation
Urination	Urinary retention
Defecation	Antidiarrheal or constipation
Secretion of mucus	Mucociliary slowing
Bronchoconstriction	Inhibition of constriction

TABLE 7-3	Pharmacologic Effects of Tertiary versus Quaternary Anticholinergic Agents Given by Inhaled Aerosol

	TERTIARY (ATROPINE)	QUATERNARY (IPRATROPIUM AND TIOTROPIUM)
Respiratory tract	Bronchodilation	Bronchodilation
	Decreased mucociliary clearance	Little or no change in mucociliary clearance
	Blockage of hypersecretion	Blockage of nasal hypersecretion
CNS	Altered CNS function (dose related)	No effect
Eye	Mydriasis	Usually no effect*
	Cycloplegia	
	Increased intraocular pressure	
Cardiac	Minor slowing of heart rate (small dose); increased heart rate (larger dose)	No effect
Gastrointestinal	Dry mouth, dysphagia; slows motility	Dry mouth
Genitourinary	Urinary retention	Usually no effect†

CNS, Central nervous system.
*Assumes aerosol is not sprayed into eye; use with caution in glaucoma.
†Use with caution in prostatic enlargement or urinary retention.

mucosal surfaces and their effects increase with the size of the dose. Effects are summarized for these agents for the organ systems.

Respiratory tract effects. Atropine sulfate, a prototype tertiary compound, inhibits and reduces mucociliary clearance, as shown by Groth and associates.[23] Atropine seems to block hypersecretion stimulated by cholinergic agonists in both the lower airway and the nose (upper airway) more than basal secretion.[24] Atropine relaxes airway smooth muscle, which is the basis for its use in asthma.

Central nervous system effects. Tertiary compounds cross the blood-brain barrier and produce dose-related effects. Small doses of 0.5 to 1.0 mg can cause effects that include restlessness, irritability, drowsiness, fatigue, or, alternatively, mild excitement. Increased doses can cause disorientation, hallucinations, or coma. Inhaled atropine has been reported to cause an acute psychotic reaction.[25,26]

Eye effects. Tertiary anticholinergic compounds given by inhalation distribute through the bloodstream and can affect vision. They block contraction of the iris to cause pupil dilation and paralyze the ciliary muscle of the lens to prevent thickening of the lens for near sight accommodation, causing blurred vision. These effects can increase intraocular pressure in glaucoma. Atropine-like agents are contraindicated in narrow-angle glaucoma.

Cardiac effects. Atropine in small doses causes minor slowing of heart rate; larger doses increase heart rate through vagal blockade.

Gastrointestinal effects. Anticholinergic agents generally cause dryness of the mouth as a result of inhibition of salivary gland secretions, and atropine is used for this effect to reduce upper airway secretions before surgery and anesthesia or when reversing neuromuscular blockade (see Chapter 18). Larger doses can cause dysphagia. Gastrointestinal motility is slowed, an effect that is the basis for the inclusion of atropine in Lomotil, an antidiarrheal. Inhibition of gastrointestinal motility and emptying has been noted with normal doses of atropine given by aerosol to asthmatics.[27]

Genitourinary effects. Atropine-like agents can inhibit parasympathetic-controlled relaxation of the urinary sphincter. In men with prostate gland enlargement, this can produce acute urinary retention. Atropine-like drugs can predispose male patients to impotency because penile erection is also under parasympathetic control. Ejaculation is a sympathetic function.

Quaternary Ammonium Compounds

Quaternary compounds include the approved aerosol agent ipratropium, tiotropium, and glycopyrrolate. The following effects are discussed primarily for ipratropium, which is well known as an inhaled bronchodilator. Generally, quaternary ammonium compounds do not cross lipid membranes easily and do not distribute throughout the body when inhaled. Agents such as ipratropium produce an anticholinergic effect at the site of delivery; with inhalation, this would be the nose or mouth and the upper and lower airway.

Respiratory tract effects. Ipratropium has minimal or no effect on mucociliary clearance or mucus viscosity, despite the fact that the aerosol is delivered topically to the airways. The drug causes bronchodilation by blocking cholinergic contractile action. In the nasal passages, however, ipratropium reduces hypersecretion, which is the basis for its use in rhinitis.

Central nervous system effects. Because quaternary compounds do not cross the blood-brain barrier, they do not cause CNS effects as the tertiary agents do.

Eye effects. As long as ipratropium and other quaternary agents are not sprayed directly in the eye, there are no effects on intraocular pressure, pupil size, or lens accommodation when inhaled as an aerosol. Topical delivery to the eye can cause pupillary dilation (mydriasis) and lens paralysis (cycloplegia). Subjects using quaternary ammonium **antimuscarinic bronchodilators** (an agent that blocks effects of Ach) must be cautioned to protect their eyes from the aerosol drug.

Cardiac effects. Ipratropium has minimal effects on heart rate or blood pressure when given by inhaled aerosol. However, several meta-analyses have suggested that ipratropium and tiotropium may cause an increase in cardiovascular events. When other meta-analyses were conducted and reexamined, no incidence of cardiovascular involvement from inhaled anticholinergics was found. Currently, no information has been conclusive in showing that these agents have any adverse effects on the cardiovascular system.[28]

Gastrointestinal effects. In most patients, inhaled ipratropium has little effect on gastrointestinal motility. A portion of the aerosol dose is swallowed, however, allowing exposure of the gastrointestinal tract to the drug. There has been a report of meconium ileus in an adult with cystic fibrosis receiving nebulized ipratropium.[29] Use of a reservoir device with MDI administration can reduce oropharyngeal impaction and the amount of swallowed drug.

Genitourinary effects. When tested in men 50 to 70 years of age, ipratropium had no effect on urinary ability.[30]

KEY POINT

Quaternary compounds, such as ipratropium, are fully ionized and less absorbed into body tissues than *tertiary compounds,* such as atropine sulfate. Consequently, side effects with quaternary compounds are localized to the site of drug exposure.

MODE OF ACTION

In Chapter 5, the autonomic innervation of the airway is outlined; this consists of the traditional sympathetic and parasympathetic branches and nonadrenergic, noncholinergic (NANC) inhibitory and excitatory branches. The sympathetic branch does not actually extend its fibers beyond the peribronchial ganglia or plexuses to the airway, although adrenergic receptors are present throughout the airway, especially in the periphery. Parasympathetic nerves enter the lung at the hila, deriving from the vagus, and travel along the airways. Parasympathetic postganglionic fibers terminate on or near the airway epithelium, submucosal mucous glands, smooth muscle, and probably mast cells. Parasympathetic innervation and muscarinic receptors are concentrated in the larger airways, although they are present from the trachea to the respiratory bronchioles.

In the normal airway, a basal level of bronchomotor tone is caused by parasympathetic activity. This basal level of tone can be abolished by anticholinergic agents such as atropine, indicating it is mediated by Ach. Administration of **parasympathomimetic** (cholinergic) agents such as methacholine (e.g., in bronchial provocation testing) can intensify the level of bronchial tone to the point of constriction in healthy subjects and more so in asthmatic patients.

Cholinergic stimulation of muscarinic receptors on airway smooth muscle and submucosal glands causes contraction and release of mucus. Anticholinergic agents, such as atropine or ipratropium, are antimuscarinic; they competitively block the action of Ach at parasympathetic postganglionic effector cell receptors. Because of this action, anticholinergic agents block cholinergic-induced bronchoconstriction, as shown in Figure 7-2.

An important point to realize with use of a blocking agent, such as an **anticholinergic bronchodilator**, is that the effect seen depends on the degree of tone present that can be blocked. In healthy subjects, there is minimal airway dilation with an anticholinergic agent because there is only a basal or resting level of tone to be blocked. Variation in the clinical effect of such drugs is partially due to variation in the degree of parasympathetic activity. One particular mechanism for parasympathetic activity in the lung is vagally mediated reflex bronchoconstriction, which is discussed in the next section.

KEY POINT

The anticholinergic agents ipratropium, tiotropium, aclidinium, and umeclidinium are indicated for the treatment of airflow obstruction in COPD.

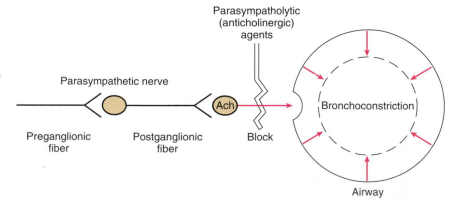

Figure 7-2 Conceptual overview of the action of anticholinergic (parasympatholytic) bronchodilating agents in preventing cholinergic-induced bronchoconstriction. *Ach,* Acetylcholine.

Vagally Mediated Reflex Bronchoconstriction

A portion of the bronchoconstriction seen in COPD may be due to a mechanism of vagally mediated reflex innervation of airway smooth muscle (Figure 7-3). Sensory C-fiber nerves respond to various stimuli, such as irritant aerosols (hypotonic or hypertonic), cold air and high airflow rates, cigarette smoke, noxious fumes, and mediators of inflammation such as histamine. When activated, they produce an afferent nerve impulse to the CNS, which results in a reflex cholinergic efferent impulse to cause constriction of airway smooth muscle and release of secretion from mucous glands, as well as a cough.

Because atropine and its derivatives are competitive inhibitors of Ach at the neuroeffector junction, such antagonists should block parasympathetic reflex bronchoconstriction. Atropine has been shown to inhibit exercise-induced asthma and psychogenic bronchospasm and bronchoconstriction caused by β blockade or cholinergic agents. Application of a topical anesthetic, such as 4% lidocaine by aerosol, to the large airways has also inhibited reflex bronchoconstriction by blocking the sensory irritant receptors in the epithelial lining.

Changes in the airway may also sensitize the subepithelial cough receptors, making them more responsive to lower thresholds of stimulation. This sensitization is often seen during colds that involve lung congestion. Lung inflation during a deep breath stimulates the cough receptors, resulting not only in coughing but also increased bronchomotor tone. It has been suggested that greater bronchial reactivity in asthmatic patients or patients with COPD may be caused by mucosal edema and deformation of airway tissue, which increases the sensitivity of these receptors in response to

irritants. Several reviews of cholinergic mechanisms of airway obstruction have been published.[31-35]

Muscarinic Receptor Subtypes

Anticholinergic agents cause bronchodilation by blocking M_1 receptors at the parasympathetic ganglia, which facilitate cholinergic neurotransmission and bronchoconstriction, and M_3 receptors on airway smooth muscle, which cause bronchoconstriction. Muscarinic receptor subtypes are reviewed in Chapter 5 and are illustrated for the lung in Figure 7-4. M_1 receptors on the postganglionic parasympathetic neuron facilitate cholinergic nerve transmission, leading to release of Ach. Ach stimulates M_3 receptor subtypes on airway smooth muscle and submucosal glands, causing contraction of smooth muscle and exocytosis of secretion from the mucous gland. Additionally, the M_2 receptor subtype at cholinergic nerve endings inhibits further Ach release from the postganglionic neuron.

M_3 receptors are G protein–linked receptors (see Chapters 2 and 5). Table 7-4 lists the various muscarinic receptor subtypes and their G proteins, along with their effector enzymes. Stimulation of the M_3 receptor subtype activates a Gq protein, which activates phospholipase C (PLC). PLC causes the breakdown of phosphoinositides into inositol

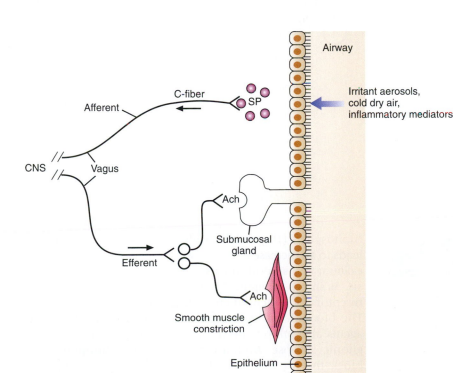

Figure 7-3 Mechanism of vagally mediated reflex bronchoconstriction induced by nonspecific stimuli on sensory C-fibers. *Ach,* Acetylcholine; *CNS,* central nervous system; *SP,* substance P.

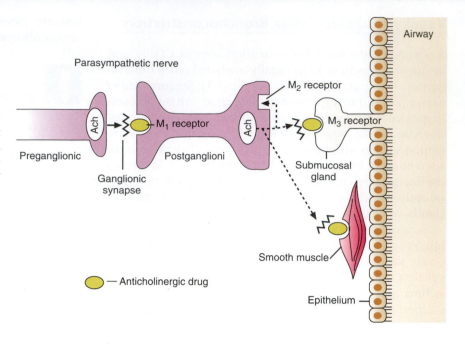

Figure 7-4 Identification and location of muscarinic receptor subtypes M_1, M_2, and M_3 in the vagal nerve, submucosal gland, and bronchial smooth muscle in the airway, showing nonspecific blockade by anticholinergic drugs such as ipratropium. *Ach,* Acetylcholine.

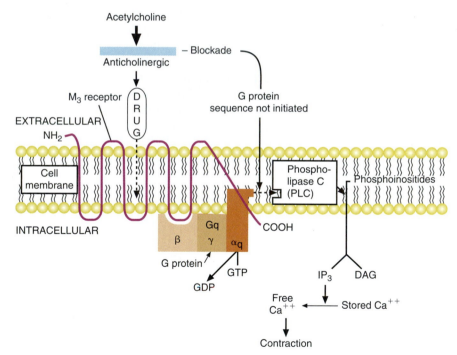

Figure 7-5 Illustration of the M_3 receptor as a G protein–linked receptor, showing the Gq protein; its effector system, phospholipase C (PLC); and the mechanism of smooth muscle constriction, which is blocked by an anticholinergic agent preventing stimulation of the M_3 receptor. *DAG,* Diacylglycerol; *IP_3,* inositol triphosphate; *GDP,* guanosine diphosphate; *GTP,* guanosine triphosphate.

TABLE 7-4	Muscarinic Receptor Subtypes: G Proteins and Effector Systems	

RECEPTOR	G PROTEIN	EFFECTOR
M_1	Gq	Phospholipase C
M_2	Gi	Adenylyl cyclase (decreases)
M_3	Gq	Phospholipase C
M_4	Gi	Adenylyl cyclase (decreases)
M_5	Gq	Phospholipase C leads to an increase

triphosphate (IP_3) and diacylglycerol (DAG); this ultimately leads to an increase in the cytoplasmic concentration of free calcium and smooth muscle contraction or gland exocytosis. As shown in Figure 7-5, the competitive blockade of M_3 receptors by anticholinergic agents prevents this sequence. The blockade of M_1 receptor subtypes by anticholinergic agents also inhibits nerve transmission by Ach at the ganglionic synapse. Both ipratropium and tiotropium also block the M_2 receptor. This receptor inhibits continued release of Ach. As a result, blockade of the M_2 receptor can enhance Ach release, possibly counteracting the bronchodilator effect of M_3 receptor blockade. As noted in the discussion of ipratropium and tiotropium, tiotropium has selective affinity for M_1 and M_3 receptors because it dissociates much more rapidly from the M_2 receptor and remains bound to the M_1 and M_3 subtypes.

The use of agents such as ipratropium for allergic and nonallergic rhinitis is based on the parasympathetic control of submucosal glands in the nasal mucosa. Ach stimulates muscarinic receptors in the nose, where approximately 55% are M_3 receptors and the rest are M_1 receptors.[36] M_2 receptors were not identified in human nasal mucosa in an autoradiographic study by Okayama and associates.[37] Blockade of muscarinic M_1 and M_3 receptors on submucosal nasal glands by ipratropium given as a nasal spray prevents gland secretion and rhinitis.

KEY POINT

The anticholinergic bronchodilators are *nonspecific blockers of muscarinic receptor subtypes* (M_1, M_2, and M_3) in the airway. Blockade of the M_3 receptor subtype on bronchial smooth muscle prevents activation of the linking Gq protein and its effector system phospholipase C (PLC), subsequently increasing free calcium with bronchoconstriction or gland exocytosis.

KEY POINT

Blockade of M_1 and M_3 receptors in the nasal passages prevents gland secretion and rhinitis.

ADVERSE EFFECTS

It has been stated that the safety profile of quaternary ammonium antimuscarinic bronchodilators (e.g., ipratropium and tiotropium) is superior to that of β agonists, particularly with regard to cardiovascular effects.[9] Changes in electrocardiogram, blood pressure, or heart rate are not usually seen. There is no worsening of ventilation-perfusion abnormalities in COPD, which would otherwise cause an increase in hypoxemia. A tolerance to bronchodilation and loss of bronchial protection have not been observed. The lack of these effects is due to the poor absorption and systemic distribution of quaternary compounds, such as ipratropium. Cugell[38] provided a detailed review of the clinical pharmacology and toxicology of ipratropium.

The side effects seen with the MDI and small volume nebulizer (SVN) formulations of ipratropium, the agent with the most clinical experience, are primarily related to the local, topical delivery to the upper and lower airway with inhalation. Similar side effects would be expected with other antimuscarinic agents, such as tiotropium. The most common side effect seen with this class of bronchodilator is dry mouth. Possible side effects are listed in Box 7-1. The SVN solution has also been associated with additional side effects in a few patients, including pharyngitis, dyspnea, flulike symptoms, bronchitis, and upper respiratory infection. The amount of drug in the nebulizer dose is more than

BOX 7-1 Side Effects Seen With Anticholinergic Aerosol Ipratropium*

MDI and SVN (Common)
- Dry mouth
- Cough

MDI (Occasional)
- Nervousness
- Irritation
- Dizziness
- Headache
- Palpitation
- Rash

SVN (Occasional)
- Pharyngitis
- Dyspnea
- Flulike symptoms
- Bronchitis
- Upper respiratory infections
- Nausea
- Occasional bronchoconstriction
- Eye pain
- Urinary retention (less than 3%)

MDI, Metered dose inhaler; *SVN*, small volume nebulizer.
Precautions: Use with caution in patients with narrow-angle glaucoma, prostatic hypertrophy, bladder neck obstruction, constipation, bowel obstruction, or tachycardia.

*Side effects were reported in a small percentage (less than 3% to 5%) of patients.

10 times greater than in the MDI dose (500 mcg versus 40 mcg). If the patient receives approximately 10% of an inhaled aerosol to the lung, a much larger dose is given with an SVN. The orally swallowed portion would be proportionately higher also. Systemic side effects such as tachycardia, palpitations, urinary hesitancy, constipation, blurred vision, and increased ocular pressure are less likely with quaternary agents, such as ipratropium, tiotropium, aclidinium, or umeclidinium, than with tertiary agents, such as atropine. Although ipratropium is not contraindicated in subjects with prostatic hypertrophy, urinary retention, or glaucoma, the drug should be used with caution and adequate evaluation for possible systemic side effects in these subjects.

The eye must be protected from aerosol drug exposure resulting from accidental spraying or during nebulizer delivery. Blockade of muscarinic receptors causes mydriasis by blocking the sphincter muscle of the iris and inhibits the ciliary muscle of the lens, preventing lens thickening (accommodation). As the iris dilates outward and the lens remains flattened, drainage of intraocular aqueous humor is reduced. In patients with narrow-angle glaucoma, intraocular pressure can increase. Because many patients with COPD are older, narrow-angle glaucoma may be present more commonly. Subjects using quaternary ammonium antimuscarinic bronchodilators must be informed of this hazard and should use proper aerosol inhalation technique. A holding chamber should be used with MDI administration. With nebulizer delivery, the mouthpiece should be kept in the mouth and a reservoir tube attached to the expiratory side of the T mouthpiece to vent aerosol away from the face. The ideal nebulizer would be a dosimetric device with no ambient exposure from the device on exhalation. If the nebulizer solution is delivered by facemask (which is not recommended), the eyes should be closed or covered to prevent drug exposure. Because of the greater risk of eye exposure with a nebulizer, especially disposable, constant-output devices, an MDI with a holding chamber is recommended for delivery of this class of bronchodilator.

KEY POINT

The most common side effects with quaternary ammonium antimuscarinic bronchodilators are dry mouth and perhaps a cough caused by the aerosol particles.

KEY POINT

Direct spraying in the eye must be avoided to prevent ocular effects. Patients with COPD can show a greater response in reversibility of airflow obstruction with an anticholinergic agent than a β agonist.

CLINICAL APPLICATION

Anticholinergic (antimuscarinic) aerosols have been investigated for use with asthma and with COPD. Table 7-5 compares the general effects seen with anticholinergic bronchodilators and β-adrenergic bronchodilators.

Use in Chronic Obstructive Pulmonary Disease

Antimuscarinic agents were found to be more potent bronchodilators than β-adrenergic agents in bronchitis/emphysema, and this is likely to be their primary clinical application. This difference is illustrated in Figure 7-6 with data from Tashkin and colleagues.[39] In the 90-day,

multicenter study, the investigation compared 40 mcg of ipratropium with 1.5 mg of metaproterenol, both given by MDI, in a population of patients with COPD. Explanations for the superiority of anticholinergic action in COPD are debated but may relate to the complicated, inflammatory, noncholinergic pathways seen in asthma, especially owing to stimuli mentioned previously in the section on vagally mediated reflex bronchoconstriction. Conversely, the pathology of COPD may reveal the reason for the superior effect of anticholinergic over β-adrenergic drugs. Ipratropium has been approved by the FDA specifically for use in the treatment of COPD, although the drug is also prescribed for treatment of asthma.

Rennard and associates[40] analyzed data from the clinical trials of ipratropium compared with a β agonist. Their analysis showed that use of ipratropium over the 90-day interval tested was associated with improved baseline lung function and response to acute bronchodilator use. Subjects using β agonists over the same period had little change in baseline lung function and a small decrease in airway response to acute bronchodilator treatment.

Tiotropium, an antimuscarinic bronchodilator, offers a prolonged duration of action of 24 hours with a single daily inhalation. In dose-ranging trials, an inhaled dose of 18 mcg once per day has been found to give significant bronchodilation in patients with COPD with few side effects.[10,12] Figure 7-7 illustrates the effect on FEV_1 with single inhaled doses of tiotropium of various strengths compared with a placebo.[9] There is also prolonged dose-dependent protection against inhaled methacholine challenge. Both the bronchodilating and the bronchoprotective effect can be compared with the 6-hour effect of ipratropium. Perhaps one of the more important effects of a long-acting drug such as tiotropium is the elevation in baseline, predose FEV_1. In contrast to ipratropium, lung function is maintained more consistently at a higher level throughout

TABLE 7-5	Comparison of Effects for Anticholinergic and β-Adrenergic Bronchodilators	
	ANTICHOLINERGIC	**β AGONIST**
Onset	Slightly slower	Faster
Time to peak effect	Slower	Faster
Duration	Longer	Shorter
Tremor	None	Yes
Decrease in PaO_2	None	Yes
Tolerance	None	Yes
Site of action	Larger, central airways	Central and peripheral airways

PaO_2, Arterial oxygen pressure.

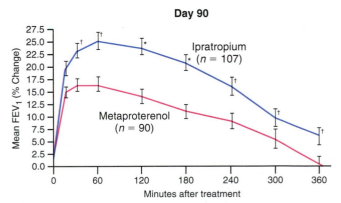

Figure 7-6 Effect of the β agonist metaproterenol and the anticholinergic ipratropium on forced expiratory volume in 1 second (*FEV₁*) in patients with chronic obstructive pulmonary disease (COPD) after 90 days of treatment (*P less than 0.01; †P less than 0.05). (From Tashkin DP, Ashutosh K, Bleecker ER, et al: Comparison of the anticholinergic bronchodilator ipratropium bromide with metaproterenol in chronic obstructive pulmonary disease: a 90-day multi-center study, *Am J Med* 81[suppl 5A]:59, 1986. From Excerpta Medica, Inc.)

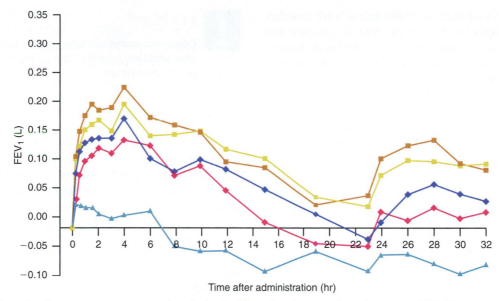

Figure 7-7 Bronchodilator responses measured on the basis of forced expiratory volume in 1 second (FEV₁) in patients with chronic obstructive pulmonary disease (COPD) given single doses of tiotropium, a long-acting antimuscarinic bronchodilator. *Orange*, 80 mcg; *yellow*, 40 mcg; *navy blue*, 20 mcg; *red*, 10 mcg; *light blue*, placebo. (Data from Maesen FP, Smeets JJ, Sledsens TJ, et al: Tiotropium bromide, a new long-acting antimuscarinic bronchodilator: a pharmacodynamic study in patients with chronic obstructive pulmonary disease [COPD], *Eur Respir J* 8:1506, 1995.)

the day with tiotropium. This effect may be significant in relation to quality of life and reduction of breathlessness in patients with COPD. Beeh and colleagues[41] reported that an inhaled dose of 18 mcg once per day improved lung function and reduced exacerbations in patients with COPD of different severities. Adams and associates[42] also found improvement in lung function and dyspnea in patients with COPD. The prolonged effect may also be useful in controlling nocturnal asthma symptoms, where cholinergic mechanisms seem to increase airway tone.[43]

Current COPD guidelines do not dictate the use of any one specific bronchodilator.[44,45] It is noted, however, that the use of a short-term β₂ agonist and an anticholinergic, such as ipratropium, improves the FEV₁ in patients with COPD.[45] The use of a long-term anticholinergic, such as tiotropium,[45] aclidinium, or umeclidinium, improves the health of patients with COPD. The use of a single agent or combination is dictated by the patient's response.

Use in Asthma

Anticholinergic (antimuscarinic) agents, such as ipratropium, do not have a labeled indication for asthma in the United States. Current asthma guidelines state that ipratropium may have some additive benefit when given with inhaled β agonists.[46,47] Antimuscarinic bronchodilators are not clearly superior to β-adrenergic agents in treating asthma. Antimuscarinic and β-adrenergic agents have an approximately equal effect on flow rates in many patients. These agents may be especially useful in the following applications when prescribed for asthmatic patients[48]:

- Nocturnal asthma, in which the slightly longer duration of action may protect against nocturnal deterioration of flow rates[49]

- Psychogenic asthma, which may be mediated through vagal parasympathetic fibers
- Asthmatic patients with glaucoma, angina, or hypertension who require treatment with β-blocking agents
- As an alternative to theophylline in patients with notable side effects from that drug
- Acute, severe episodes of asthma not responding well to β agonists

A large, randomized controlled study by Qureshi and colleagues[50] in 434 children 2 to 8 years old with acute moderate to severe asthma found that the overall rate of hospitalization was reduced with the addition of inhaled ipratropium to nebulized albuterol. However, the most striking effect on admission was seen in children with severe asthma (peak expiratory flow less than 50% predicted). A meta-analysis of the addition of anticholinergic bronchodilators to β agonists in children and adolescents, conducted by Plotnick and Ducharme,[51] concluded that adding multiple doses of anticholinergic (antimuscarinic) bronchodilators to β₂ agonists was safe, improved lung function, and may avoid hospital admission in 1 of 11 treated patients. Multiple doses should be preferred to single doses of antimuscarinic agents.

Combination Therapy: β-Adrenergic and Anticholinergic Agents in Chronic Obstructive Pulmonary Disease

Theoretically, a combination of β-adrenergic and anticholinergic agents should offer advantages in the treatment of COPD (and asthma as well), based on the following considerations.

- Complementarity of sites of action exists, with anticholinergic effect seen in the more central airways and β-agonist effect in the smaller, more peripheral airways.
- Mechanisms of action from anticholinergic and β-adrenergic agents are separate and complementary.

Pharmacokinetics of shorter-acting agents (albuterol or ipratropium) in the two classes of bronchodilator are complementary; β agonists peak sooner but also terminate sooner, whereas anticholinergics tend to peak more slowly and last longer. This consideration is irrelevant, however, with longer-acting agents in both classes, such as salmeterol, formoterol, arformoterol, indacaterol, tiotropium, aclidinium, and umeclidinium.

Additive Effect of β Agonists and Anticholinergic Agents

Conflicting results have been found regarding the question of whether the bronchodilator effect of β agonists is increased by adding an anticholinergic agent, in either COPD or asthma.[52-56] However, a large study—the Combivent Inhalation Aerosol Study Group,[5] a well-controlled study conducted over 85 days with 462 patients at 24 centers on patients with stable COPD—showed superior efficacy of the combination therapy of ipratropium and albuterol compared with either agent alone. Figure 7-8 compares this study of ipratropium plus albuterol versus albuterol or ipratropium alone on the percentage change in FEV_1. The mean *peak* increases in FEV_1 were 31% to 33% for combined drug therapy compared with 24% to 25% for ipratropium alone and 24% to 27% for albuterol alone. Flow rates were significantly better on all test days. Symptom scores did not differ among the three groups, however. As a large, well-designed study, these results support combination anticholinergic and β-agonist therapy in COPD.

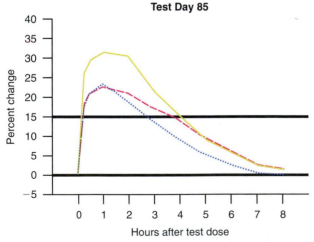

Test Day 85

Figure 7-8 Percentage change in forced expiratory volume in 1 second (FEV_1) on test day 85, for combined ipratropium and albuterol compared with either drug alone, in patients with chronic obstructive pulmonary disease (COPD). *Dotted line,* Albuterol; *dashed line,* ipratropium; *solid line,* ipratropium plus albuterol. (From COMBIVENT Inhalation Aerosol Study Group: In chronic obstructive pulmonary disease, a combination of ipratropium and albuterol is more effective than either agent alone: an 85-day multicenter trial, *Chest* 105:1411, 1994.)

 KEY POINT

Combined anticholinergic and β-agonist therapy may give additive bronchodilating results in COPD and in severe, acute asthma.

Sequence of Administration

The order in which a $β_2$ agonist and an anticholinergic are administered via an MDI has been debated. Because an anticholinergic bronchodilator acts in the central, larger airways, some practitioners argue that it should be given *before* the $β_2$ agonist. No data have been published to support this sequence, however. The $β_2$ agonist is often given first, and this can be rationalized for two reasons: (1) a $β_2$ agonist has a more rapid onset of action than an anticholinergic bronchodilator, and (2) $β_2$ receptors are distributed in large and small airways. The order of administration is probably not important. Combination products such as Combivent and DuoNeb (ipratropium and albuterol) make order of administration a moot point.

Most discussion and clinical use of $β_2$ agonists and anticholinergics have centered on agents with shorter duration. Other combination agents have included long-acting $β_2$ agonists and inhaled corticosteroids. The use of long-acting $β_2$ agonists and long-acting anticholinergics may be as effective as shorter-acting agents. In a study of tiotropium and formoterol, it was found that lung function improved with the combination compared with the agents given as monotherapy in patients with stable COPD.[57] Another study of moderate to severe COPD patients found that receiving a combination of tiotropium and formoterol increased forced vital capacity (FVC) and FEV_1 more than delivering the agents alone.[58]

Two of the largest, long-term drug trials for COPD—Towards a Revolution in COPD Health (TORCH) and Understanding Potential Long-Term Impacts on Function with Tiotropium (UPLIFT)—have provided insight into the prescribing practice of medications used to treat COPD. Miravitlles and Anzueto[59] reviewed both studies. The main conclusion concerning combination agents is that long-term agents tiotropium and salmeterol, with the addition of an inhaled corticosteroid, improve lung function and may reduce the progression of COPD. The use of these agents is being termed "triple therapy," suggesting improvement when all three are used in combination.[60-62]

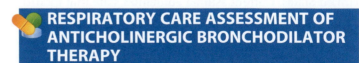

RESPIRATORY CARE ASSESSMENT OF ANTICHOLINERGIC BRONCHODILATOR THERAPY

Before Treatment

- Assess effectiveness of drug therapy based on the indication for the aerosol agent: Presence of reversible airflow resulting from primary bronchospasm or obstruction secondary to an inflammatory response or secretions, either acute or chronic.

- Monitor flow rates using bedside peak flow meters, portable spirometry, or laboratory reports of pulmonary function. Before-and-after bronchodilator studies performed with a β agonist may not reliably predict response to an anticholinergic (antimuscarinic) agent such as ipratropium.
- Perform respiratory assessment: Breathing rate and pattern and breath sounds by auscultation, before and after treatment.
- Assess pulse before, during, and after treatment.

During Treatment and Short Term

- Assess patient's subjective reaction to treatment for any change (positive or negative) in breathing effort or pattern.
- Assess arterial blood gases or pulse oximeter saturation as needed for acute states with COPD or asthma to monitor changes in ventilation and gas exchange (oxygenation).

Long Term

- Monitor pulmonary function studies of lung volumes, capacities, and flows.
- Instruct and then verify correct use of aerosol delivery device (SVN, MDI, reservoir, DPI). Emphasize that the eye must be protected from aerosol sprays. Instruct patients in use, assembly, and especially cleaning of aerosol inhalation devices.
- For long-acting antimuscarinic bronchodilators:
  - Assess ongoing lung function, including predose FEV_1, over time.
  - Assess amount of concomitant β-agonist use and nocturnal symptoms.
  - Assess number of exacerbations, unscheduled clinic visits, and hospitalizations.
  - Assess days of absence because of symptoms.

General Contraindications

- Anticholinergic bronchodilators generally are safe. However, regular, long-term use of short-acting and long-acting agents should be regularly assessed, especially if agents are used in combination with other agents.
- Use of anticholinergic bronchodilator therapy in patients with vision problems such as glaucoma should be closely monitored.

SELF-ASSESSMENT QUESTIONS

Answers can be found in Appendix A.

1. What was the first FDA-approved anticholinergic bronchodilator for aerosol inhalation?
2. What is currently the only FDA-approved long-acting anticholinergic combination product(s) on the market?
3. What is the usual recommended dose of ipratropium by MDI and by SVN?
4. Identify a long-acting anticholinergic bronchodilator and give its duration of action.
5. What is the usual clinical indication for use of an anticholinergic bronchodilator such as ipratropium?
6. Which disease state, asthma or COPD, may show greater response to an anticholinergic bronchodilator rather than a β agonist?
7. With which type of anticholinergic agent are you more likely to observe systemic side effects: the tertiary ammonium or quaternary ammonium compounds?
8. What are the most common side effects seen with inhaled ipratropium and tiotropium?
9. Can ipratropium be used with subjects who have glaucoma?
10. Can ipratropium be alternated with or combined with a β agonist in the treatment of COPD and asthma?
11. What precautions should you observe if administering ipratropium by SVN?
12. What is the clinical indication for the use of an anticholinergic intranasal spray?

 CLINICAL SCENARIO

Answers can be found in Appendix A.

Logan O'Connor is a 66-year-old retired, well-educated middle-level manager for a major film company. He is referred to a pulmonologist for his complaint of shortness of breath. On interview, he states that he has increasingly noticed exertional dyspnea with mild physical activity over the past few months. With questioning, he admits to occasional social alcohol intake of either one or two beers or a couple of mixed drinks several times a week. He has been happily married to the same woman since he was 24. He also admits to regular cigarette smoking of about one pack a day since he was 20 years old. He leads a sedentary life with no physical exercise. He states that he does have a chronic cough, which is worse in the morning, although he denies much productivity. He appears to be well nourished, is articulate, and his color is good. No cyanosis or use of accessory muscles is noted at rest.

Physical examination reveals very mild digital clubbing, a slightly increased anteroposterior (AP) diameter, diminished and distant breath sounds bilaterally with some rhonchi, mildly hyperresonant percussion notes, no jugular venous distention upright or supine, and no peripheral edema. His vital signs are as follows: blood pressure (BP) 146/90 mm Hg, temperature (T) 37.2° C, pulse (P) 88 beats/min, respiratory rate (RR) 16 breaths/min with no laboring. His arterial blood gas (room air) results are as follows: pH 7.40, arterial carbon dioxide

Continued

pressure (PaCO$_2$) 42.5 mm Hg, arterial oxygen pressure (PaO$_2$) 62 mm Hg, base excess 1.9 mEq/L, and hemoglobin (Hgb) 14.5 g/dL.

His pulmonary function results are as follows:

Observed	% Predicted
Forced vital capacity (FVC), 2.98 L	74
Forced expiratory volume in 1 second (FEV$_1$), 1.94 L	60
FEV$_1$/FVC	65 (Calculated)
Residual volume/total lung capacity (RV/TLC)	42 (Calculated)
Diffusing capacity of the lung for carbon monoxide (DLCO), 18.4 (mL/min/mm Hg)	70

Mr. O'Connor's chest radiograph (posterior-anterior lateral) shows some loss of lung markings, mild flattening of the hemidiaphragms, and increased AP diameter. His electrolytes and white blood cell count are normal.

His chief complaint, smoking history, physical findings, and laboratory results all indicate early manifestations of COPD. He is mildly hypoxemic at rest (PaO$_2$, 62 mm Hg), but his acid-base status is normal. Moderate airflow obstruction is present as evidenced by the FEV$_1$ of 1.94 L, FEV$_1$/FVC of 65%, and increased RV/TLC ratio. Gas exchange is impaired, as seen in the below-normal DLCO. There is no evidence of cardiac failure or acute exacerbation at this time. His diagnosis is COPD with mixed bronchitis and emphysema.

Using the SOAP method, assess this clinical scenario.

REFERENCES

1. Cavanaugh MJ, Cooper DM: Inhaled atropine sulfate: dose response characteristics. *Am Rev Respir Dis* 114:517, 1976.
2. Pak CC, Kradjan WA, Lakshminarayan S, et al: Inhaled atropine sulfate: dose-response characteristics in adult patients with chronic airflow obstruction. *Am Rev Respir Dis* 125:331, 1982.
3. Gross NJ: Anticholinergic agents: clinical application. In Leff AR, editor: *Pulmonary and critical care pharmacology and therapeutics,* New York, 1996, McGraw-Hill.
4. Meltzer EO: Intranasal anticholinergic therapy of rhinorrhea. *J Allergy Clin Immunol* 90:1055, 1992.
5. COMBIVENT Inhalation Aerosol Study Group: In chronic obstructive pulmonary disease, a combination of ipratropium and albuterol is more effective than either agent alone: an 85-day multicenter trial. *Chest* 105:1411, 1994.
6. Gal TJ, Suratt PM, Lu J: Glycopyrrolate and atropine inhalation: comparative effects on normal airway function. *Am Rev Respir Dis* 129:871, 1984.
7. Hansel TT, Neighbour H, Erin EM, et al: Glycopyrrolate causes prolonged bronchoprotection and bronchodilation in patients with asthma. *Chest* 128:1974–1979, 2005.
8. Witek TJ, Jr: Anticholinergic bronchodilators. *Respir Care Clin N Am* 5:521, 1999.
9. Barnes PJ: The pharmacological properties of tiotropium. *Chest* 117:63S, 2000.
10. Maesen FP, Smeets JJ, Sledsens TJ, et al: Tiotropium bromide, a new long-acting antimuscarinic bronchodilator: a pharmacodynamic study in patients with chronic obstructive pulmonary disease (COPD). *Eur Respir J* 8:1506, 1995.
11. Van Noord JA, Bantje TA, Eland ME, et al: Dutch Tiotropium Study Group: A randomised controlled comparison of tiotropium and ipratropium in the treatment of chronic obstructive pulmonary disease. *Thorax* 55:289, 2000.
12. Littner MR, Ilowite JS, Tashkin DP, et al: Long-acting bronchodilation with once-daily dosing of tiotropium (Spiriva) in stable chronic obstructive pulmonary disease. *Am J Respir Crit Care Med* 161:1136, 2000.
13. Chodosh S, Flanders J, Serby CW, et al: Effective use of HandiHaler dry powder inhalation system over a broad range of COPD disease severity. *Am J Respir Crit Care Med* 159:A524, 1999. (abstract).
14. Barr RG, Bourbeau J, Camargo CA, Jr, et al: Tiotropium for stable chronic obstructive pulmonary disease: a meta-analysis. *Thorax* 61:854, 2006.
15. Pisano M, Mazzola N: Aclidinium bromide inhalation powder (Tudorza): A long-acting anticholinergic for the management of chronic obstructive pulmonary disease. *P T* 38(7):393, 2013.
16. Gavaldà A, Miralpeix M, Ramos I, et al: Aclidinium bromide, a novel muscarinic receptor antagonist combining long residence at M$_3$ receptors and rapid plasma clearance. *Eur Respir J* 30(Suppl 51):209S–210S, 2007.
17. Gavaldà A, Sentellas S, Alberti J, et al: Aclidinium bromide, a novel long-acting anticholinergic, is rapidly inactivated in plasma. *Am J Respir Crit Care Med* 177:A-654, 2008.
18. Janset JM, Lamarca R, Garcia Gil E, et al: Safety and pharmacokinetics of single doses of aclidinium bromide, a novel long-acting, inhaled antimuscarinic, in healthy subjects. *Int J Clin Pharmacol Ther* 47:460–468, 2009.
19. Janset JM, Lamarca R, de Miquel G, et al: Safety and pharmacokinetics of multiple doses of aclidinium bromide, a novel long-acting muscarinic antagonist for the treatment of chronic obstructive pulmonary disease, in healthy participants. *J Clin Pharmacol* 49:1239–1246, 2009.
20. Chanez P, Burge PS, Dahl R, et al: Aclidinium bromide provides long-acting bronchodilation in patients with COPD. *Pulm Pharmacol Ther* 23:15–21, 2010.
21. Decramer M, et al: Bronchodilation of umeclidinium, a new long-acting muscarinic antagonist, in COPD patients. *Respir Physiol Neurobiol* 185(2):393–399, 2013.
22. Celli B, et al: Once-daily umeclidinium/vilanterol 125/25 µg therapy in COPD: a randomized, controlled study. *Chest* 145(5):981–991, 2014.
23. Groth ML, Langenback EG, Foster WM: Influence of inhaled atropine on lung mucociliary function in humans. *Am Rev Respir Dis* 144:1042, 1991.
24. Wanner A: Effect of ipratropium bromide on airway mucociliary function. *Am J Med* 81(Suppl 5A):32, 1986.
25. Bergman KR, Pearson C, Waltz GW, et al: Atropine-induced psychosis, an unusual complication of therapy with inhaled atropine sulfate. *Chest* 78:891, 1980.
26. Herschman ZL, Silverstein J, Blumberg G, et al: Central nervous system toxicity from nebulized atropine sulfate. *J Toxicol Clin Toxicol* 29:273, 1991.
27. Botts LD, Pingleton SK, Schroeder CE, et al: Prolongation of gastric emptying by aerosolized atropine. *Am Rev Respir Dis* 131:725, 1985.
28. Salpeter SR: Do inhaled anticholinergics increase or decrease the risk of major cardiovascular event? A synthesis of the available evidence. *Drugs* 69:2025–2033, 2009.
29. Mulherin D, Fitzgerald MX: Meconium ileus equivalent in association with nebulized ipratropium bromide in cystic fibrosis. *Lancet* 335:552, 1990.
30. Molkenboer JFWM, Lardenoye JG: The effect of Atrovent on micturition function, double-blind cross-over study. *Scand J Respir Dis* 103(Suppl):154, 1979.
31. Barnes PJ: Autonomic control of airway function in asthma. *Chest* 91(Suppl):45S, 1987.
32. Bleecker ER: Cholinergic and neurogenic mechanisms in obstructive airways disease. *Am J Med* 81(Suppl 5A):2, 1986.

33. Hogg JC: The pathophysiology of asthma. *Chest* 82(Suppl):8S, 1982.

34. Leff A: Pathophysiology of asthmatic bronchoconstriction. *Chest* 82(Suppl):13S, 1982.

35. Simonsson BG, Jacobs FM, Nadel JA: Role of autonomic nervous system and the cough reflex in the increased responsiveness of airways in patients with obstructive airway disease. *J Clin Invest* 46:1812, 1967.

36. Baraniuk JN: Muscarinic receptors. In Leff AR, editor: *Pulmonary and critical care pharmacology and therapeutics*, New York, 1996, McGraw-Hill.

37. Okayama M, Baraniuk JN, Hausfeld JN, et al: Autoradiographic localization of muscarinic receptor subtypes in human nasal mucosa. *J Allergy Clin Immunol* 89:1144, 1992.

38. Cugell DW: Clinical pharmacology and toxicology of ipratropium bromide. *Am J Med* 81(Suppl 5A):18, 1986.

39. Tashkin DP, Ashutosh K, Bleecker ER, et al: Comparison of the anticholinergic bronchodilator ipratropium bromide with metaproterenol in chronic obstructive pulmonary disease: a 90-day multi-center study. *Am J Med* 81(Suppl 5A):59, 1986.

40. Rennard SI, Serby CW, Ghafouri M, et al: Extended therapy with ipratropium is associated with improved lung function in patients with COPD: a retrospective analysis of data from seven clinical trials. *Chest* 110:62, 1996.

41. Beeh KM, Beier J, Buhl R, et al: ATEM-Studiengruppe: Efficacy of tiotropium bromide in patients with COPD of different severities. *Pneumologie* 60:341, 2006.

42. Adams SG, Anzueto A, Briggs DD, et al: Tiotropium in COPD patients not previously receiving maintenance respiratory medication. *Respir Med* 100:1495, 2006.

43. Morrison JFJ, Pearson SB, Dean HG: Parasympathetic nervous system in nocturnal asthma. *BMJ* 296:1427, 1988.

44. Celli BR, MacNee W: ATS/ERS Task Force: Standards for the diagnosis and treatment of patients with COPD: a summary of the ATS/ERS position paper. *Eur Respir J* 23:932, 2004.

45. Global Initiative for Chronic Obstructive Lung Disease: *Global strategy for the diagnosis, management, and prevention of COPD*, 2014, National Heart, Lung, and Blood Institute (Bethesda, MD) and World Health Organization (Geneva, Switzerland). Retrieved from http://www.goldcopd.org/uploads/users/files/GOLD_Report_2014_Jun11.pdf.

46. National Asthma Education and Prevention Program, National Heart, Lung, and Blood Institute, National Institutes of Health: *Expert Panel Report 3: Guidelines for the Diagnosis and Management of Asthma*, NIH Publication 08-4051, Bethesda, MD, 2007, National Institutes of Health. Retrieved from http://www.nhlbi.nih.gov/guidelines/asthma/asthgdln.htm.

47. Global Initiative for Asthma (GINA): *Global strategy for asthma management and prevention*, 2014, National Heart, Lung, and Blood Institute (Bethesda, MD) and World Health Organization (Geneva, Switzerland). Retrieved from http://www.ginasthma.org/local/uploads/files/GINA_Report_2014_Jun11.pdf.

48. Weber RW: Role of anticholinergics in asthma. *Ann Allergy* 65:348, 1990. (editorial).

49. Cox ID, Hughes DTD, McDonnell KA: Ipratropium bromide in patients with nocturnal asthma. *Postgrad Med J* 60:526, 1984.

50. Qureshi F, Pestian J, Davis P, et al: Effect of nebulized ipratropium on the hospitalization rates of children with asthma. *N Engl J Med* 339:1030, 1998.

51. Plotnick LH, Ducharme FM: Should inhaled anticholinergics be added to β_2 agonists for treating acute childhood and adolescent asthma? A systematic review. *BMJ* 317:971, 1998.

52. Rebuck AS, Chapman KR, Abboud R, et al: Nebulized anticholinergic and sympathomimetic treatment of asthma and chronic obstructive airways disease in the emergency room. *Am J Med* 82:59, 1987.

53. Owens MW, George RB: Nebulized atropine sulfate in the treatment of acute asthma. *Chest* 99:1084, 1991.

54. Karpel JP: Bronchodilator responses to anticholinergic and β-adrenergic agents in acute and stable asthma. *Chest* 99:871, 1991.

55. Lightbody IM, Ingram CG, Legge JS, et al: Ipratropium bromide, salbutamol and prednisolone in bronchial asthma and chronic bronchitis. *Br J Dis Chest* 72:181, 1978.

56. Petrie GR, Palmer KNV: Comparison of aerosol ipratropium bromide and salbutamol in chronic bronchitis and asthma. *BMJ* 1:430, 1975.

57. Cazzola M, Di Marco F, Santus P, et al: The pharmacodynamic effects of single inhaled doses of formoterol, tiotropium and their combination in patients with COPD. *Pulm Pharmacol Ther* 17:35–39, 2004.

58. Van Noord JA, Aumann JL, Janssens E, et al: Comparison of tiotropium once daily, formoterol twice daily and both combined once daily in patients with COPD. *Eur Respir J* 26:214–222, 2005.

59. Miravitlles M, Anzueto A: Insights into interventions in managing COPD patients: lessons from the TORCH and UPLIFT studies. *Int J Chron Obstruct Pulmon Dis* 4:185–201, 2009.

60. Perng DW, Wu CC, Su KC, et al: Additive benefits of tiotropium in COPD patients treated with long-acting beta agonists and corticosteroids. *Respirology* 11:598–602, 2006.

61. Singh D, Brooks J, Hagan G, et al: Superiority of "triple" therapy with salmeterol/fluticasone propionate and tiotropium bromide versus individual components in moderate to severe COPD. *Thorax* 63:592–598, 2008.

62. Aaron SD, Vandemheen KL, Fergusson D, et al: Canadian Thoracic Society/Canadian Respiratory Clinical Research Consortium: Tiotropium in combination with placebo, salmeterol, or fluticasone-salmeterol for treatment of chronic obstructive pulmonary disease: a randomized trial. *Ann Intern Med* 146:545–555, 2007.

CHAPTER **8**

Xanthines

Douglas S. Gardenhire

OBJECTIVES

After reading this chapter, the reader will be able to:

1. Define *xanthine*
2. List all available xanthines used in respiratory therapy
3. Differentiate between the clinical indications of xanthines

4. Differentiate between the uses of xanthines
5. Discuss the proposed theories of activity for xanthines
6. Discuss adverse effects and toxicity of xanthines
7. Be able to assess xanthine therapy clinically

KEY TERMS AND DEFINITIONS

Alkaloids Group of alkaline substances taken from plants, which react with acids to form salts (e.g., theophylline).

Methylxanthines Chemical group of drugs derived from xanthines. There are three methylated (CH_3) xanthines: caffeine, theophylline, and theobromine.

Phosphodiesterase (PDE) Group of enzymes that change intracellular signaling.

Chapter 8 reviews the pharmacology of the xanthine drugs, such as theophylline. Theophylline traditionally has been used to treat patients with asthma and chronic obstructive pulmonary disease (COPD) in stable and acute phases. The mechanism of action of xanthines is unclear, and their clinical use in asthma and COPD has been relegated to second- or third-line agents, although this remains an issue of debate.

KEY POINT

Theophylline, and its salt, *aminophylline,* are members of the *methylxanthine* group of drugs, which also includes *dyphylline.*

CLINICAL INDICATIONS FOR THE USE OF XANTHINES

 KEY POINT

Clinical uses of theophylline include the management of asthma, chronic obstructive pulmonary disease (COPD), and apnea of prematurity in neonates.

Theophylline has traditionally been used in the management of asthma and COPD. Theophylline and caffeine have been used to treat apnea of prematurity. A now-obsolete use of theophylline was as a diuretic. Although theophylline is usually classified as a bronchodilator, it has a relatively weak bronchodilating effect compared with β_2 agonists. Its therapeutic action in asthma and COPD may occur by other means, such as stimulation of the ventilatory drive or direct strengthening of the diaphragm. Any of these actions could result in the clinical outcome of improved ventilatory flow rates; this is discussed later in the section on Clinical Uses of Theophylline.

Use in Asthma

Sustained-release theophylline is indicated as an alternative for maintenance (step 2) therapy of mild, persistent asthma and higher in patients older than 5 years of age and is listed as an alternative in step 3 and higher for patients older than 5 years of age in combination with an inhaled corticosteroid (ICS). Sustained-release theophylline is considered a less-preferred alternative to low-dose ICS, cromolyn-like agents, or antileukotrienes as second-line maintenance drug therapy in stable asthma. Theophylline is not recommended in the guidelines for children younger than 5 years or for any person with acute exacerbation of asthma.[1]

Use in Chronic Obstructive Pulmonary Disease

Current guidelines for the treatment of stable COPD state that bronchodilators are central to symptom management. The Global Initiative for Chronic Obstructive Lung Disease (GOLD) states that inhaled bronchodilators are preferred when available. Theophylline is considered effective in COPD but, because of potential toxicity, is recommended as an alternative to inhaled bronchodilators such as β_2 agonists or anticholinergic agents.[2] Barr and associates[3] conducted a meta-analysis on the use of xanthines for the treatment of COPD exacerbations. Their findings suggest that xanthines should not be used in the treatment of COPD exacerbations. In randomized controlled trials, intravenous aminophylline has not shown any significant benefit over β_2 agonists and anticholinergic therapy for COPD patients.[4,5]

Use in Apnea of Prematurity

If pharmacologic therapy is needed to stimulate breathing in apnea of prematurity, methylxanthines are considered the first-line agents of choice. Theophylline has been used most extensively, but Bhatia[6] suggested that caffeine citrate may be the agent of choice. Caffeine citrate penetrates the cerebrospinal fluid better and has a higher therapeutic index with fewer side effects compared with theophylline. Caffeine citrate (Cafcit) has been approved for administration either intravenously or orally.

SPECIFIC XANTHINE AGENTS

Theophylline is related chemically to the natural metabolite xanthine, which is a precursor of uric acid. Figure 8-1 shows the general xanthine structure and the structures of theophylline (1,3-dimethylxanthine) and caffeine (1,3,7-trimethylxanthine). Because of their methyl attachments, these agents are often referred to as **methylxanthines**. Another xanthine is theobromine. All three agents are found as **alkaloids** in plant species. Caffeine is found in coffee beans and kola nuts. Caffeine and theophylline are contained in tea leaves, and caffeine and theobromine are in cocoa seeds or beans. Historically, these natural plant substances have been used as brews for their stimulant effect.

There are several synthetic modifications to the naturally occurring methylxanthines, including dyphylline (7-[2,3-dihydroxypropyl]theophylline), proxyphylline (7-[2-hydroxypropyl]theophylline), and enprofylline (3-propylxanthine). Table 8-1 lists xanthine derivatives, brand names, and available formulations. Theophylline is available in a variety of formulations, including sustained-release oral forms, as aminophylline for oral or intravenous administration, and rectal suppository forms.

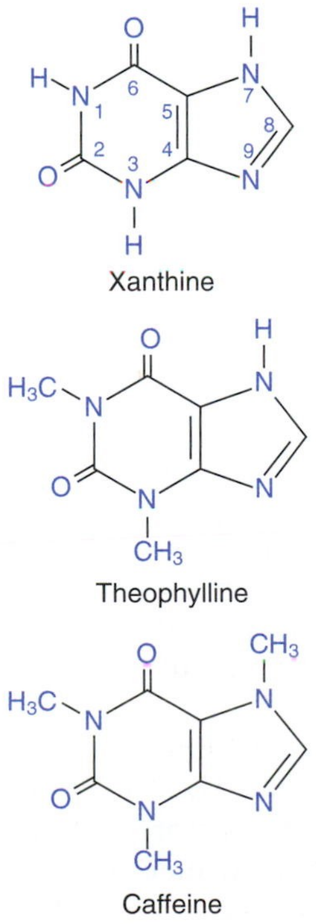

Figure 8-1 Chemical structure of xanthine and its methylated derivatives theophylline and caffeine.

TABLE 8-1	Xanthine Derivatives Used as Bronchodilators in Obstructive Airways Diseases, With Selected Brand Names and Available Formulations	
XANTHINE DERIVATIVE	**BRAND NAMES**	**FORMULATIONS**
Theophylline	Theochron, Elixophyllin, Theo-24	Tablets, capsules, syrup, elixir, extended-release tablets, capsules, injection
Oxtriphylline	Choledyl SA	Tablets, syrup, elixir, sustained-release tablets
Aminophylline	Aminophylline	Tablets, oral liquid, injection, suppositories
Dyphylline	Lufyllin	Tablets, elixir

TABLE 8-2	Differences in Intensity of Effects for Caffeine and Theophylline	
EFFECT	**CAFFEINE**	**THEOPHYLLINE**
Central nervous system stimulation	+++	++
Cardiac stimulation	+	+++
Smooth muscle relaxation	+	+++
Skeletal muscle stimulation	+++	++
Diuresis	+	+++

GENERAL PHARMACOLOGIC PROPERTIES

KEY POINT

Xanthines generally have *stimulant* properties, exemplified by the xanthine caffeine. Other effects of this class of drug include diuresis and smooth muscle relaxation (e.g., bronchodilation).

The xanthine group has the following general physiologic effects in humans:

- Central nervous system (CNS) stimulation
- Cardiac muscle stimulation
- Diuresis
- Bronchial, uterine, and vascular smooth muscle relaxation
- Peripheral and coronary vasodilation
- Cerebral vasoconstriction

Some of the effects seen with xanthines are well known to individuals who drink caffeinated beverages (e.g., coffee, colas, and tea). Coffee in particular can be used for the CNS stimulatory effect to remain awake. The diuretic effect after drinking coffee or cola is also well known. Caffeine or theophylline can also cause tachycardia, and the cerebral vasoconstricting effect has been used to treat migraine headaches. A special agent intended for this use is Cafergot, each tablet of which contains 100 mg of caffeine and 1 mg of ergotamine tartrate.

Caffeine and theophylline differ in the intensity of the effects listed previously. These differences are summarized in Table 8-2. Caffeine has more CNS-stimulating effect than theophylline, and this includes ventilatory stimulation. In clinical use, theophylline is generally classified as a bronchodilator because of the relaxing effect on bronchial smooth muscle.

Structure-Activity Relationships

Figure 8-2 illustrates the general xanthine structure and the effect of attachments at various sites on the molecule. Also, the chemical structure of theophylline is shown in comparison with the theophylline derivatives dyphylline and enprofylline. The methyl attachments at the nitrogen-1 and nitrogen-3 positions for theophylline enhance its bronchodilating effect and its toxic side effects, which are discussed later in this chapter. In contrast, the structure of caffeine (see Figure 8-1) has an additional methyl group at the nitrogen-7 position, decreasing its bronchodilator effect in relation to theophylline. Dyphylline has the same methyl attachments at the nitrogen-1 and nitrogen-3 positions as theophylline but also has a large attachment at the nitrogen-7 position that decreases its bronchodilator potential. Enprofylline, which is not clinically available in the United States at this time, has potent bronchodilating effects, probably because of the large substitution at the nitrogen-3 position.

KEY POINT

The exact *mechanism of action* of xanthines is unclear; antagonism of adenosine receptors may occur, perhaps as a partial mechanism for the effects of drugs such as theophylline.

Proposed Theories of Activity

The exact mechanism of action of xanthines, and theophylline in particular, is unknown.[7] It was originally thought that xanthines caused smooth muscle relaxation by inhibition of **phosphodiesterase (PDE)**, leading to an increase in intracellular cyclic adenosine 3′,5′-monophosphate (cAMP). An increase in cAMP causes relaxation of bronchial smooth muscle. The effect of increased cAMP is described in Chapter 6 in the discussion of β-adrenergic agents. Use of this explanation to account for therapeutic xanthine actions has been questioned, however. Several alternative theories concerning the action of xanthines have been proposed in addition to PDE inhibition. Each of the proposed theories of activity for xanthines is briefly described and commented on in the following sections.

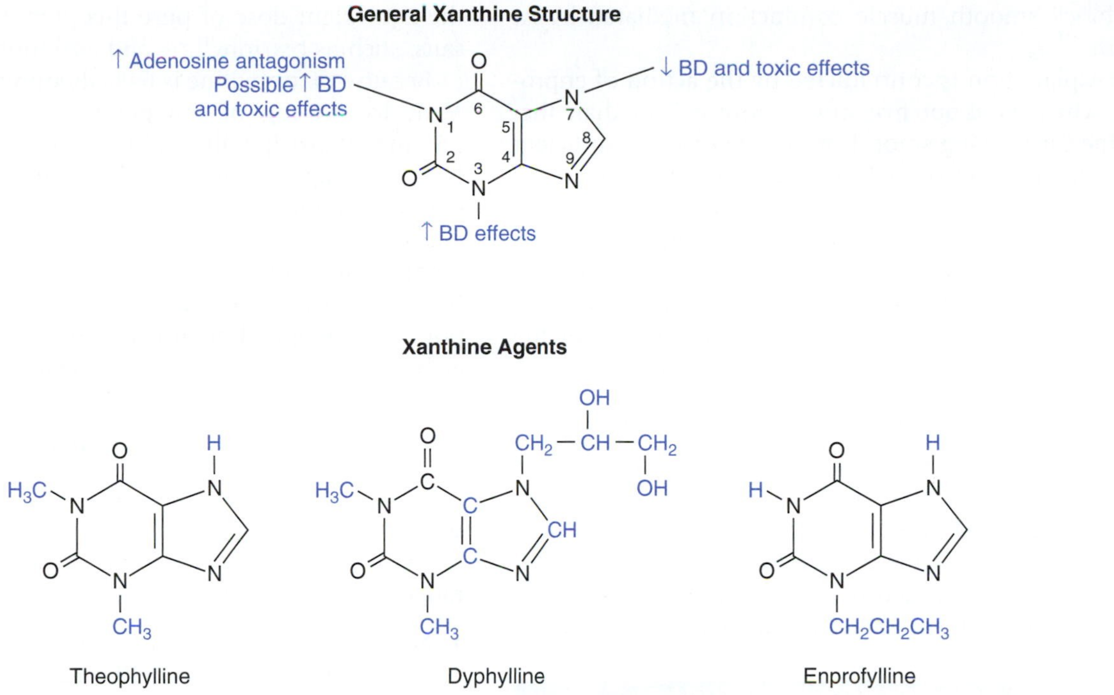

General Xanthine Structure

↑ Adenosine antagonism
Possible ↑ BD
and toxic effects

↓ BD and toxic effects

↑ BD effects

Xanthine Agents

Theophylline

Dyphylline

Enprofylline

Figure 8-2 Effect of attachments at various sites on the xanthine molecule and comparative illustration of the structures of theophylline, dyphylline, and enprofylline. *BD*, Bronchodilation.

Inhibition of Phosphodiesterase

Theophylline is a weak and nonselective inhibitor of cAMP-specific PDE. The pathway by which this inhibition can lead to an increase in intracellular cAMP, with consequent bronchial relaxation or antiinflammatory effects, is illustrated in Figure 8-3, *A*. However, at the dosage levels used clinically in humans, theophylline is a poor inhibitor of the enzyme.[8] As a result, this may not be the best theory on how xanthines exert a therapeutic effect. *PDE* is a generic term referring to at least 11 distinct families that have been identified as hydrolyzing cAMP or cyclic guanosine 3',5'-monophosphate (cGMP) and that have unique tissue and subcellular distributions. The various PDE families differ in substrate specificity, inhibitor sensitivity, and cofactor requirements.[7] There are two cAMP-hydrolyzing PDEs, referred to as *PDE3* and *PDE4*, that may play a role in asthma. PDE 3 is expressed in regulating heart muscle, vascular smooth muscle, and platelet aggregation. PDE3 inhibitors have been developed to treat heart failure and cardiogenic shock. PDE4 is expressed in airway smooth muscle, pulmonary nerves, and many proinflammatory and immune cells. PDE4 inhibitors suppress processes thought to contribute to asthma inflammation by blocking the degradation of cAMP in target cells and tissue. The antiinflammatory effect of theophylline and xanthines is reviewed in the discussion of the clinical application of these drugs in COPD and asthma.

Antagonism of Adenosine

An alternative explanation of bronchodilation is that theophylline acts by blocking the action of adenosine. This

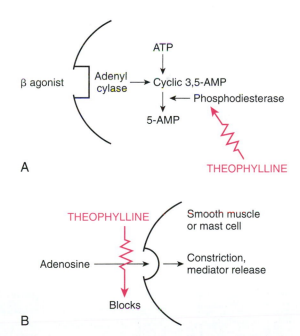

Figure 8-3 Two proposed mechanisms of action by which theophylline and xanthines reverse airway obstruction. **A,** Inhibition of phosphodiesterase. **B,** Blockade of adenosine receptors. *AMP,* Adenosine monophosphate; *ATP,* adenosine triphosphate.

mechanism is illustrated in Figure 8-3, *B*. Adenosine is a purine nucleoside that can stimulate A_1 and A_2 receptors. A_1-receptor stimulation inhibits cAMP, whereas A_2-receptor stimulation increases cAMP. Inhaled adenosine has produced bronchoconstriction in asthmatic patients. Theophylline is a potent inhibitor of both A_1 and A_2 receptors and could block smooth muscle contraction mediated by A_1 receptors.

This explanation is contradicted by the action of enprofylline, which is about five times more potent than theophylline for relaxing smooth muscle yet lacks a sufficient attachment at the nitrogen-1 position to provide adenosine antagonism.[9] This can be seen in Figure 8-2 by comparing the structures of theophylline and enprofylline. In addition, A_1 receptors are sparse in smooth muscle, and isolated animal tissue preparations have shown smooth muscle relaxation through adenosine stimulation of the A_2 receptors.

Catecholamine Release

A third explanation of xanthine action is that these agents cause the production and release of endogenous catecholamines, which could cause muscle tremor, tachycardia, and bronchial relaxation. Studies on plasma levels of catecholamines such as epinephrine have reported conflicting results, with both an increase and no change reported.[10]

TITRATING THEOPHYLLINE DOSES

In the past, clinical use of the xanthine theophylline, in its many forms, was questioned because of wide variability in its therapeutic effect. It was subsequently found that individuals metabolize theophylline at differing rates, which makes it difficult to determine therapeutic doses. This situation is complicated further by the fact that different forms of the drug are not always equivalent.

Equivalent Doses of Theophylline Salts

The standard with which salts of theophylline are compared is anhydrous theophylline. Anhydrous theophylline is 100% theophylline. By contrast, salts of theophylline such as oxtriphylline (Choledyl SA) are not pure theophylline by weight. A 400-mg dose of Choledyl SA contains approximately 256 mg of theophylline, whereas Theo-24 (a brand of theophylline) is 100% anhydrous theophylline. A 200-mg dose of Choledyl SA does not give the same amount of theophylline as a 200-mg dose of Theo-24. Table 8-3 lists

TABLE 8-3	Theophylline Content of Salts of Theophylline, With Amount Needed for Equivalence to 100% Anhydrous Theophylline

THEOPHYLLINE SALT	THEOPHYLLINE (%)	EQUIVALENT DOSE (mg)
Theophylline anhydrous	100	100
Theophylline monohydrate	91	110
Aminophylline anhydrous	86	116
Aminophylline dihydrate	79	127
Oxtriphylline	64	156

the equivalent dose of pure theophylline provided by the salts, such as oxtriphylline and aminophylline.

Because oxtriphylline is 64% theophylline, a dose equivalent to 100 mg of theophylline anhydrous would be 156 mg of oxtriphylline (100 mg/0.64 = 156 mg). Similarly, 127 mg of aminophylline dihydrate (theophylline ethylenediamine) would be required for equivalency to 100 mg of theophylline anhydrous. Dyphylline is not a theophylline but a derivative of theophylline. It does not form theophylline in the body and is about one-tenth as potent as theophylline; this is consistent with its structure-activity relationship, described previously.

Serum Levels of Theophylline

In 1972, Jenne and colleagues[11] indicated that the optimal serum theophylline level for maximal bronchodilation in adults was 10 to 20 mcg/mL. The effects associated with a range of serum levels are as follows:

- No effects seen: Less than 5 mcg/mL
- Therapeutic range: 10 to 20 mcg/mL
- Nausea: Greater than 20 mcg/mL
- Cardiac arrhythmias: Greater than 30 mcg/mL
- Seizures: 40 to 45 mcg/mL

KEY POINT

Because individuals vary in the rate at which theophylline is metabolized, dosage must be titrated to clinical effectiveness, avoidance of side effects, and, most precisely, a *therapeutic serum level* of 5 to 10 mcg/mL in COPD management and 5 to 15 mcg/mL in asthma management.

Since the originally proposed serum levels of 10 to 20 mcg/mL, the recommended range has been changed to a more conservative 5 to 15 mcg/mL for the management of asthma.[12] GOLD recommendations for the use of theophylline in COPD suggest a target serum level of 5 to 10 mcg/mL.[2] Both of these ranges seek maximal therapeutic effect with minimal toxicity and side effects. It is stressed that the ranges listed for toxic effects are general. It is possible for an individual to bypass the nauseous phase of toxicity and immediately enter the seizure phase.

Although there is a dose-related response to higher serum levels of theophylline, there is evidence that the response does not continue at the same rate of increase as levels increase. The improvement in forced expiratory volume in 1 second (FEV_1) tends to flatten above a serum level of 10 to 12 mcg/mL, whereas the toxic effects of theophylline (discussed subsequently) tend to increase even within the therapeutic range of 10 to 20 mcg/mL.[13]

Dosage Schedules

Because of the variability in the rate at which individuals metabolize theophylline and the other factors that affect theophylline metabolism and clearance rates, dosage schedules are used to titrate the drug. These schedules are found in the product literature, references such as *Drug Facts and Comparisons* and *Physicians' Desk Reference*, and general pharmacology texts.

For rapid theophyllinization, the patient may be given an oral loading dose of 5 mg/kg, *provided* that the patient was not previously receiving theophylline. This dose is based on anhydrous theophylline. Ideal body weight should be used in calculating theophylline doses because theophylline does not distribute into fatty tissue. In titrating the dose, each 0.5-mg/kg dose of theophylline given as a loading dose results in a serum level of approximately 1 mcg/mL. If theophylline was taken previously by the patient, a serum theophylline level should be measured if possible.

For long-term therapy, a slow titration is helpful, with an initial dose of 16 mg/kg/24 hr or 400 mg/24 hr, whichever is less. These dosages may need to be modified in the presence of factors such as age (younger children versus the elderly), congestive heart disease, or liver disease. The effects of these factors on serum theophylline levels and on dosage are discussed subsequently. The dosage guidelines given have been obtained from theophylline product information.

Dosage of theophylline can be guided by the clinical reaction of the patient or, better, by measurement of serum drug levels. Without a serum drug level, the dose of theophylline should be based on the benefit provided and should be reduced if the patient experiences toxic side effects. When monitoring serum theophylline levels, the sample should be taken at the time of peak absorption of the drug—1 to 2 hours after administration for immediate-release forms and 5 to 9 hours after the morning dose for sustained-release forms.

The previous examples of dosage schedules are not complete for all situations; they are intended only as an example of such schedules and of the complexity involved in treating patients with theophylline. Complete tables for different ages and clinical applications should be consulted when administering theophylline.

Theophylline Toxicity and Side Effects

KEY POINT

Theophylline has a *narrow therapeutic margin*, and side effects such as gastric upset, headache, insomnia, nervousness, palpitations, and diuresis occur frequently, even within the therapeutic range of dosing. Blood levels of theophylline are affected by many factors, which can either increase or decrease the amount of drug in the body.

An important problem with the use of theophylline is its narrow therapeutic margin; there is very little difference between the dose and serum level that give therapeutic benefit and that cause toxic side effects. Even within the therapeutic serum levels of 10 to 20 mcg/mL, distressing

BOX 8-1	Adverse Reactions Seen With Theophylline Treatment, Organized by Organ System*

Central Nervous System
- Headache
- Anxiety
- Restlessness
- Insomnia
- Tremor
- Convulsions

Gastrointestinal System
- Nausea
- Vomiting
- Anorexia
- Abdominal pain
- Diarrhea
- Hematemesis
- Gastroesophageal reflux

Respiratory System
- Tachypnea

Cardiovascular System
- Palpitations
- Supraventricular tachycardia
- Ventricular arrhythmias
- Hypotension

Renal System
- Diuresis

*Effects are not listed in order of severity or progression.

side effects can be experienced. Inhaled theophylline is being studied to research possible reduced side effects.[14] The most common adverse reactions usually seen with theophylline are listed in Box 8-1.

Gastric upset, headache, anxiety, and nervousness are not unusual as less-toxic side effects of theophylline and can result in loss of school time or workdays. The diuretic effect should be noted in patients with excess airway secretions (e.g., patients with bronchitis or cystic fibrosis), with adequate fluid replacement when necessary to prevent dehydration and thickening of secretions.

Reactions to levels of theophylline also can be unpredictable from patient to patient. Studies are cited in which reported serum levels of 78.5 mcg/mL and 104.8 mcg/mL caused only gastrointestinal symptoms, whereas mean levels of 35 mcg/mL caused cardiac arrhythmias or seizures.[13] Also, minor side effects may provide little warning before serious toxic effects such as arrhythmias or seizures occur.

Factors Affecting Theophylline Activity

Theophylline is metabolized in the liver and eliminated by the kidneys. Any condition that affects these organs can affect theophylline levels in the body. Interactions between other drugs and theophylline can affect serum levels of the

Data from Weinberger M, Hendeles L, *Am J Respir Crit Care Med* 152:S77, 1995.
IV, Intravenous.
*+, Increase in theophylline level; –, decrease in theophylline level.

BOX 8-2	Factors That Can Increase or Decrease Blood Levels of Theophylline and Affect Dosage Requirements

Increase
- Alcohol (0.9 g/kg)
- β-Blocking agents
- Calcium channel blockers
- Cimetidine, ranitidine
- Corticosteroids
- Disulfiram
- Influenza virus vaccine
- Interferon
- Ephedrine
- Estrogen
- Macrolide antibiotics (e.g., clarithromycin)
- Mexiletine
- Methotrexate
- Pentoxifylline
- Quinolones, oral contraceptives
- Tacrine
- Ticlopidine
- Troleandomycin
- Zileuton
- Cirrhosis
- Congestive heart failure
- Hepatitis
- Pneumonia
- Renal failure

Decrease
- β Agonists
- Aminoglutethimide
- Barbiturates
- Carbamazepine
- Cigarette smoking
- Isoniazid (+ or –)*
- Isoproterenol (IV)
- Ketoconazole
- Loop diuretics (+ or –)*
- Moricizine
- Phenytoin
- Rifampin
- Sulfinpyrazone

drug. Some common drugs and conditions that increase or decrease theophylline levels are listed in Box 8-2.

Viral hepatitis or left ventricular failure can cause elevated serum levels of theophylline for a given dose because of decreased liver metabolism of the drug. An opposite effect—decreased serum levels—is caused by cigarette smoking, which stimulates the production of liver enzymes that inactivate methylxanthines[15]; this necessitates higher theophylline doses. Some drugs used for the treatment of tuberculosis, such as isoniazid, and the loop diuretics, such as furosemide (Lasix) or bumetanide (Bumex), are unpredictable in their effect and may either increase or decrease theophylline levels. Measurement of serum levels is extremely important when using these agents with theophylline.

β Agonists and theophylline have an additive effect and are often combined when treating patients with asthma or COPD. Theophylline may antagonize the sedative effect of benzodiazepines (e.g., Valium). Theophylline can also reverse the paralyzing effect of nondepolarizing neuromuscular blocking agents (pancuronium and atracurium) in a dose-dependent manner. This is important to realize when paralyzing patients with severe asthma to facilitate ventilatory support and when intravenous administration of aminophylline is used.

Clinical Uses of Theophylline

More recent guidelines for the pharmacologic management of asthma and COPD do not indicate theophylline as first-line therapy.[1,2] The disadvantages of theophylline are its narrow therapeutic margin, toxic effects, unpredictable blood levels and need for individual dosing, and numerous drug-drug and drug-condition interactions. The use of theophylline in asthma and COPD is described in the following sections.

Use in Asthma

 KEY POINT

Theophylline has been relegated to the level of a second- or third-line drug in treating *asthma* and is considered only if β agonists and antiinflammatory therapy fail to control symptoms.

The role of theophylline preparations in the management of acute and stable asthma and COPD has been debated.[16,17] In the treatment of asthma, theophylline is suggested for use after reliever agents, such as a β_2 agonist, other controller agents, such as ICS, or mediator antagonists (cromolyn-like drugs) targeting the underlying inflammation.[1,2]

Adachi and colleagues[18] compared a combination of salmeterol and fluticasone propionate with a combination of fluticasone and sustained-release theophylline. Results favored the salmeterol/fluticasone combination in the treatment of moderate asthmatics.

Use in Chronic Obstructive Pulmonary Disease

 KEY POINT

In COPD, the *nonbronchodilating effects* of theophylline, such as ventilatory drive stimulation, and enhanced respiratory muscle function are of value, although use of theophylline in COPD is debated.

Use as a maintenance agent in COPD is indicated if anticholinergics and β_2 agonists fail to provide adequate control. Development of long-acting β_2 agonists, such as salmeterol, formoterol, and arformoterol, offers an additional drug choice to preserve lung function in COPD before using theophylline, especially if theophylline was used to prevent nocturnal symptoms. The increased FEV_1 with salmeterol gives more consistent improvement in lung function on a 12-hour basis and maintains a higher baseline of lung function.[19] Theophylline and its salt, aminophylline, are listed as bronchoactive agents for managing an acute exacerbation of COPD in the GOLD guidelines; however, use of other bronchodilators is preferred.[2]

 KEY POINT

COPD guidelines suggest the use of inhaled β agonists (e.g., albuterol) and anticholinergics (e.g., ipratropium) over the use of theophylline because of its side effects.

Because of side effects in the gastrointestinal system, xanthines are contraindicated in subjects with active peptic ulcers or acute gastritis. Suppositories should not be used if the rectum or lower colon is irritated. If stomach upset occurs with theophylline, the drug may be taken with food. Ingestion of large amounts of caffeine from sources such as tea or coffee may precipitate side effects when taking theophylline.

Nonbronchodilating Effects of Theophylline

Although theophylline is classified as a bronchodilator, it has a relatively weak bronchodilating action. The efficacy of theophylline in obstructive lung disease may be due to its nonbronchodilating effects on ventilation. This concept of the effectiveness of theophylline is consistent with the finding of significant clinical improvement despite little increase in expiratory flow rates in asthmatic patients.[20] Mahler and colleagues[21] documented the effect of theophylline in reducing dyspnea in patients with COPD when there was no reversibility of obstruction and no objective improvement in lung function, gas exchange, or exercise performance capability. The nonbronchodilating effects of theophylline are listed with a brief commentary.

Respiratory Muscle Strength

Theophylline can increase the force of respiratory muscle contractility, and this effect is thought to inhibit or reverse muscle fatigue and subsequent ventilatory failure. Theophylline can have the same effect on skeletal limb muscle. Aubier and associates[22] showed increased diaphragmatic strength and transdiaphragmatic pressure generation by using electromyographic stimuli before and after theophylline administration.

Respiratory Muscle Endurance

Methylxanthines also show evidence of increasing respiratory muscle endurance and strength. Fatigue of the respiratory muscles can be prevented, especially with increased resistance. Xanthines have been shown to increase the time that an external inspiratory load could be sustained.[20]

Central Ventilatory Drive

Methylxanthines have also been shown to increase ventilatory drive at the level of the CNS. In particular, theophylline can increase phrenic nerve activity for a given level of chemical stimulus.[21] This effect on ventilatory drive seems to occur at the level of the midbrain and may involve the neurotransmitter dopamine.

Cardiovascular Effects

Theophylline use may have nonbronchodilating advantages in patients with COPD who also have cardiac disease or cor pulmonale. Theophylline can increase cardiac output, decrease pulmonary vascular resistance, and improve myocardial muscle perfusion in ischemic regions.[23]

Antiinflammatory Effects

Theophylline also has some antiinflammatory effects that may explain its efficacy despite the fact that the drug is a relatively weak bronchodilator.[16,24] Evidence indicates that theophylline can produce some degree of immunomodula-

tion and an antiinflammatory and bronchoprotective effect through inhibition of cAMP-specific PDE enzymes, particularly PDE3 and PDE4, in proinflammatory cells and tissues. Theophylline has been shown to cause the following (see references for detailed antiinflammatory effects of theophylline[16,24-28]):

- Decreased migration of activated eosinophils into bronchial mucosa with allergen stimuli and reduced eosinophil survival
- Reduced T-cell proliferation and accumulation in atopic asthma with corresponding improvement in pulmonary function
- Inhibition of proinflammatory cytokines, such as interleukin (IL)-1β, tumor necrosis factor-α, and interferon-γ, and increased production of the antiinflammatory cytokine IL-10
- Attenuation of the late phase response to histamine in patients with allergic asthma
- Reduced airway responsiveness to stimuli such as histamine, methacholine, allergens, sulfur dioxide, distilled water, cyanates, and adenosine
- Increased activation of a group of enzymes, histone deacetylase, also known as lysine deacetylase, which are used by corticosteroids to reduce inflammatory response.

The antiinflammatory and immunomodulating effects of theophylline occur at lower plasma concentrations such as 9 to 10 mcg/mL, in contrast to the concentrations usually recommended for bronchodilation, and may result in a steroid-sparing effect.[25] Inhibitors of PDE4, with more selectivity than theophylline and reduced toxic effect profiles, may offer a new class of antiinflammatory agents.[7]

Use in Apnea of Prematurity

When nonpharmacologic methods are unsuccessful in apnea of prematurity, xanthines such as theophylline and caffeine are still considered a first-line choice of drug therapy, as stated in the indications for this class of drug. Theophylline is biotransformed to caffeine in neonates.[29] However, caffeine is preferable to theophylline for various pharmacologic reasons, as follows[6]:

- Caffeine penetrates more readily than theophylline into cerebrospinal fluid and can be effective in infants refractory to theophylline therapy.
- Caffeine is a more potent stimulant of the CNS and the respiratory system than theophylline.
- Dosing regimens are simpler and give more predictable results with caffeine than with theophylline, most likely because of smaller plasma fluctuations with caffeine.
- Caffeine has a wider therapeutic margin with fewer side effects than theophylline.

A standard preparation of caffeine, caffeine citrate (Cafcit), is available, which can be administered either orally or intravenously. The recommended loading dose is 20 mg/kg of caffeine citrate (equivalent to 10 mg/kg of caffeine); this is followed 24 to 48 hours later by a single daily maintenance dose of 5 mg/kg of caffeine citrate (2.5 mg/kg of caffeine).

RESPIRATORY CARE ASSESSMENT OF XANTHINES

Before Treatment

- Assess the effectiveness of drug therapy on the basis of indications for the aerosol agent: Presence of reversible airflow resulting from primary bronchospasm or obstruction secondary to an inflammatory response or secretions, either acute or chronic.
- Monitor flow rates with bedside peak flow meters, by portable spirometry, or on the basis of laboratory reports of pulmonary function before and after bronchodilator studies, to assess reversibility of airflow obstruction.
- Perform respiratory assessment: Breathing rate and pattern and breath sounds by auscultation, before and after treatment.
- Assess serum blood levels of agent.

During Treatment and Short Term

- Assess the patient's subjective reaction to treatment for any change in breathing effort or pattern.
- Assess arterial blood gases or pulse oximeter saturation as needed for acute states with asthma or COPD to monitor changes in ventilation and gas exchange (oxygenation).

Long Term

- Monitor pulmonary function studies of lung volumes, capacities, and flows.
- Instruct asthmatic patients in the use and interpretation of disposable peak flow meters to assess the severity of asthmatic episodes and to ensure there is an action plan for treatment modification.
- Patient education should emphasize that xanthines do not treat underlying inflammation or prevent progression of asthma or COPD, and additional antiinflammatory treatment or more aggressive medical therapy may be needed if there is a poor response to the agent.
- Because the agent is systemic, assess ongoing function of all body systems.
- Assess serum blood levels of agent.

General Contraindications

- Xanthines have a narrow therapeutic index margin. Overdosing is possible and should be monitored.
- Because of different body systems being affected, all patients should be closely monitored.

- Patients with chronic disease (cystic fibrosis, COPD, and asthma) may consider using other agents with better safety profiles, such as corticosteroids.

 SELF-ASSESSMENT QUESTIONS

Answers can be found in Appendix A.

1. What drug in the xanthine group is used most often therapeutically?
2. What is the difference between aminophylline and theophylline?
3. What is the recommended therapeutic plasma level for theophylline in asthma and COPD?
4. How do you know whether a given dose of theophylline would produce a satisfactory treatment effect in an asthmatic?
5. Identify at least three adverse side effects seen with theophylline.
6. What is meant by a "narrow therapeutic margin"?
7. Although theophylline is a weak bronchodilator, what other effects make it useful in treating chronic airflow obstruction?
8. True or False: Theophylline causes bronchodilation and improved airflow solely by inhibiting PDE, which breaks down cAMP.

CLINICAL SCENARIO

Answers can be found in Appendix A.

A 70-year-old white man arrived at the emergency department. He was severely short of breath (SOB) and could take only a few steps before complaining of dyspnea. He reported coughing up thick, greenish sputum with some tinges of blood in the last few days. He appeared oriented, coherent, and malnourished, with thin arms. On interview, he admitted to smoking two packs of cigarettes a day since age 18, stopping about 2 years ago. He has had six hospitalizations within the last 2 years. Current medications include ipratropium bromide by MDI, 2 puffs four times daily, with a β_2 agonist by MDI as needed, 1 to 3 puffs. He has been using the β_2-agonist MDI regularly during the last month, at least four times daily.

On physical examination, he was very SOB, even at rest, and used accessory muscles with a respiratory rate (RR) of 22 breaths/min. There was little discernible chest expansion. His breath sounds were distant in all areas, with expiratory wheezes, and air movement appeared poor. He was afebrile, pulse (P) was 120 beats/min, and blood pressure (BP) was 170/112 mm Hg.

Laboratory values on admission showed normal electrolyte levels, but his white blood cell count (WBC) was 15.2×10^3/cc, and his hemoglobin was 10.6 g/dL. Arterial blood gas values on room air were as follows: pH 7.40, arterial carbon dioxide pressure ($PaCO_2$) 42.4 mm Hg, arterial oxygen pressure (PaO_2) 64 mm Hg, base excess +1.9 mEq/L, and arterial oxygen saturation (SaO_2) 90%.

A posteroanterior chest radiograph shows hyperinflation of the lung fields, with flattened diaphragms.

Using the SOAP method, assess this clinical scenario.

REFERENCES

1. National Asthma Education and Prevention Program, National Heart, Lung, and Blood Institute, National Institutes of Health: *Expert Panel Report 3: Guidelines for the Diagnosis and Management of Asthma*, NIH Publication No. 08-4051, Bethesda, MD, 2007, National Institutes of Health. Retrieved from http://www.nhlbi.nih.gov/guidelines/asthma/asthgdln.htm.

2. Global Initiative for Chronic Obstructive Lung Disease: *Global strategy for the diagnosis, management, and prevention of COPD*, 2014, National Heart, Lung, and Blood Institute (Bethesda, MD) and World Health Organization (Geneva, Switzerland). Retrieved from http://www.goldcopd.org/uploads/users/files/GOLD_Report_2014_Jun11.pdf.

3. Barr RG, Rowe BH, Camargo CA: Methylxanthines for exacerbations of chronic obstructive pulmonary disease. *Cochrane Database Syst Rev* (2):CD002168, 2003.

4. Rice KL, Leatherman JW, Duane PG, et al: Aminophylline for acute exacerbations of chronic obstructive pulmonary disease: a controlled trial. *Ann Intern Med* 107:305–309, 1987.

5. Duffy N, Walker P, Diamantea F, et al: Intravenous aminophylline in patients admitted to hospital with non-acidotic exacerbations of chronic obstructive pulmonary disease: a prospective randomized trial. *Thorax* 60:713–717, 2005.

6. Bhatia J: Current options in the management of apnea of prematurity. *Clin Pediatr* 39:327, 2000.

7. Giembycz MA: Phosphodiesterase 4 inhibitors and the treatment of asthma. *Drugs* 59:193, 2000.

8. Jenne JW: Physiology and pharmacodynamics of the xanthines. In Jenne JW, Murphy S, editors: *Drug therapy for asthma: research and clinical practice*, New York, 1987, Marcel Dekker.

9. Persson CGA, Karlsson J: In vitro responses to bronchodilator drugs. In Jenne JW, Murphy S, editors: *Drug therapy for asthma: research and clinical practice*, New York, 1987, Marcel Dekker.

10. Svedmyr N: Theophylline. *Am Rev Respir Dis* 136(Suppl):568, 1987.

11. Jenne JW, Wyze MS, Rood FS, et al: Pharmacokinetics of theophylline: application to adjustment of the clinical dose of aminophylline. *Clin Pharmacol Ther* 13:349, 1972.

12. Kaliner M: Goals of asthma therapy. *Ann Allergy Asthma Immunol* 75:169, 1995.

13. Kelly HW: Theophylline toxicity. In Jenne JW, Murphy S, editors: *Drug therapy for asthma: research and clinical practice*, New York, 1987, Marcel Dekker.

14. Momeni A, Mohammadi MH: Respiratory delivery of theophylline by size-targeted starch microspheres for treatment of asthma. *J Microencapsul* 1–10, 2009.

15. Powell JR, Vozeh S, Hopewell P, et al: Theophylline disposition in acutely ill hospitalized patients: the effect of smoking, heart failure, severe airway obstruction and pneumonia. *Am Rev Respir Dis* 118:229, 1978.

16. Weinberger M, Hendeles L: Theophylline in asthma. *N Engl J Med* 334:1380, 1996.

17. Lam A, Newhouse MT: Management of asthma and chronic airflow limitation: are methylxanthines obsolete? *Chest* 98:44, 1990.

18. Adachi M, Aizawa H, Ishihara K, et al: Comparison of salmeterol/fluticasone propionate combination with fluticasone propionate + sustained release theophylline in moderate asthma patients. *Respir Med* 102:1055–1064, 2008.

19. Mahler DA, Donohue JF, Barbee RA, et al: Efficacy of salmeterol xinafoate in the treatment of COPD. *Chest* 115:957, 1999.

20. Supinski GS: Effects of methylxanthines on respiratory skeletal muscle and neural drive. In Jenne JW, Murphy S, editors: *Drug therapy for asthma: research and clinical practice*, New York, 1987, Marcel Dekker.

21. Mahler DA, Matthay RA, Snyder PE, et al: Sustained-release theophylline reduces dyspnea in nonreversible obstructive airway disease. *Am Rev Respir Dis* 131:22, 1985.

22. Aubier M, De Troyer A, Sampson M, et al: Aminophylline improves diaphragmatic contractility. *N Engl J Med* 305:249, 1981.

23. Ziment I: Pharmacologic therapy of obstructive airway disease. *Clin Chest Med* 11:461, 1990.

24. Sullivan P, Bekir S, Jaffar Z, et al: Antiinflammatory effects of low-dose oral theophylline in atopic asthma. *Lancet* 343:1006, 1994.

25. Page CP: Recent advances in our understanding of the use of theophylline in the treatment of asthma. *J Clin Pharmacol* 39:237, 1999.

26. Markham A, Faulds D: Theophylline: a review of its potential steroid sparing effects in asthma. *Drugs* 56:1081, 1998.

27. Spears M, Donnelly I, Jolly L, et al: Effect of low-dose theophylline plus beclomethasone on lung function in smokers with asthma: a pilot study. *Eur Respir J* 33:1010–1017, 2009.

28. Ito K, Yamamura S, Essilfie-Quaye S, et al: Histone deacetylase 2–mediated deacetylation of the glucocorticoid receptor enables NF-kappaB suppression. *J Exp Med* 203:7–13, 2006.

29. Cuzzolin L: Drug metabolizing enzymes in the perinatal and neonatal period: differences in the expression and activity. *Curr Drug Metab* 14:167–173, 2013.

CHAPTER 9

Mucus-Controlling Drug Therapy

Bruce K. Rubin, Markus Henke

OBJECTIVES

After reading this chapter, the reader will be able to:

1. Define terms that pertain to mucus-controlling drug therapy
2. Interpret the physiology and mechanisms of mucus secretion and clearance
3. Name the types of mucoactive medications and their presumed modes of action
4. Describe the medications approved for the therapy of mucus clearance disorders and their approved indications
5. Identify the contraindications to the use of mucoactive medications
6. Explain the interaction between airway clearance devices or physical therapy and mucoactive medications

KEY TERMS AND DEFINITIONS

Abhesives Substances that reduce adhesion.

Elasticity Rheologic property characteristic of solids; it is represented by the storage modulus G' (energy storage).

Expectorants Medications meant to increase the volume or hydration of airway secretions.

Gel Macromolecular description of pseudoplastic material having both viscosity and elasticity.

Glycoproteins Proteins with attached oligosaccharide (sugar) units.

Mucins The principal constituents of mucus and a high-molecular-weight glycoprotein that gives mucus its physical properties, such as viscoelasticity.

Mucoactive agent Term connoting any medication or drug that has an effect on mucus secretion; may include mucolytic, expectorant, mucospissic, mucoregulatory, or mucokinetic agents.

Mucokinetic agents Medications that increase cough or ciliary clearance of respiratory secretions.

Mucolytic agent Medications that degrades polymers in secretions. Classic mucolytics degrade mucin, and peptide mucolytics break pathologic filaments of DNA or actin in sputum.

Mucoregulatory agents Drugs that reduce the volume of airway mucus secretion and appear to be especially effective in

hypersecretory states, such as bronchorrhea, diffuse panbronchiolitis (DPB), and some forms of asthma.

Mucospissic agents Medications that increase viscosity of secretions and may be effective in the therapy of bronchorrhea.

Mucus Secretion from surface goblet cells and submucosal glands composed of water, proteins, and glycosylated mucins. The glycoprotein portion of the secretion is termed mucin. Mucus (noun) is the secretion; mucous (adjective) is the cell or gland type.

Oligosaccharide Sugar that is the individual carbohydrate unit of glycoproteins.

Phlegm Purulent material in the airways. From the Greek word for inflammation. When expectorated, phlegm is called sputum.

Rheology Study of the deformation and flow of matter in response to an applied stress.

Sol Also called the periciliary layer; it is the weak gel containing attached mucins that bathes the beating cilia and usually separates that mucus layer from the epithelial surface.

Sputum Expectorated phlegm that contains respiratory tract, oropharyngeal, and nasopharyngeal secretions, bacteria, and products of inflammation, including polymeric DNA and actin.

Viscosity Resistance of liquid to sheer forces or energy loss with applied stress; a rheologic property characteristic of liquids and represented by the loss modulus G'.

Chapter 9 presents an in-depth review of the mucociliary system and the nature of mucus as a basis for discussing pharmacologic agents used in the treatment of respiratory secretions. The drugs currently used in North America by aerosol administration—*N*-acetylcysteine (NAC; Mucomyst), dornase alfa (Pulmozyme), and hyperosmolar saline (Hypersal)—are discussed, along with investigational agents, and future directions for mucoactive drug therapy are outlined.

DRUG CONTROL OF MUCUS: A PERSPECTIVE

KEY POINT

Mucoactive therapy should be considered after therapy to decrease infection and inflammation.

The self-renewing, self-cleansing mucociliary escalator is a major defense mechanism of the lung. Failure of this system results in mechanical obstruction of the airway, often with thickened, adhesive secretions. A slowing of mucus transport is reported in many diseases associated with abnormal mucociliary function.[1,2] Whether such slowing is due to changes in the physical properties of mucus, decreased ciliary activity, or both is not always clear. Mucus is found in many areas of the body exposed to the outside environment, including the airways, gastrointestinal tract, eyes, and genitourinary tract. Regardless of its location, mucus is protective, lubricating, and waterproofing, and it protects against osmotic or inflammatory changes. The mucus barrier can also entrap microorganisms, inhibiting chronic bacterial infection and biofilm formation.

Historically in respiratory care, drug therapy for secretions has been aimed at liquefying thick mucus to a watery state (called *mucolysis*). Because mucus is a **gel** with physical properties of viscosity and elasticity, drug therapy for mucus clearance disorders should affect the physical properties of the mucus gel to improve cough or mucociliary clearance. Thinning of secretions, or mucolysis, can decease secretion clearance, thus the term **mucolytic agent** is better replaced with **mucoactive agent**. A review of mucus physiology presents the concepts necessary for discussing the current and possible future pharmacologic management of retained secretions.

Clinical Indication for Use

 KEY POINT

Mucus lubricates, waterproofs, and protects against osmotic or inflammatory changes. The normal mucus barrier can entrap microorganisms, inhibiting chronic bacterial infection and biofilm formation.

The general indication for mucoactive therapy is to reduce the accumulation of airway secretions, improving pulmonary function and gas exchange and preventing repeated infection and airway damage. Diseases in which mucoactive therapy is indicated are those with hypersecretion or poor clearance of airway secretions, including chronic bronchitis (CB), cystic fibrosis (CF), diffuse panbronchiolitis (DPB), asthma, and bronchiectasis. Not all patients with mucus retention benefit from mucoactive drug therapy; those who have strong expiratory airflow and cough usually have a better response. The use of mucoactive therapy to promote secretion clearance should be considered after therapy to decrease infection and inflammation and after minimizing or removing irritants to the airway, including tobacco smoke.[3]

Classification of Mucoactive Medications

Table 9-1 presents general information about mucoactive agents that are approved, available, or commonly administered as inhaled aerosols in the United States. Greater detail is given on indications, dosage and administration, hazards and side effects, and assessment of drug therapy in discussions of individual agents.[4]

Mucoactive medications differ in their mechanisms of action. Secretion properties that impair airway clearance also differ among different diseases and at different times

in the course of a disease. The source and properties of airway secretions and the mechanisms of action for the mucoactive agents are the basis for clinical use of these drugs.

PHYSIOLOGY OF THE MUCOCILIARY SYSTEM

Source of Airway Secretions

The conducting airways in the lung and the nasal cavity to the oropharynx are lined by a mucociliary system, illustrated diagrammatically in Figure 9-1. The secretion lining the surface of the airway is called **mucus** and has been described as having two phases: (1) A gel layer (0.5 to 20 μm) is propelled toward the larynx by the cilia and lies atop (2) a weak gel periciliary layer about the height of a fully extended cilium.[3] Cells responsible for secretion in the airway and the source of components found in respiratory mucus have been summarized by Voynow and Rubin.[5] Although there are many cell types in the mammalian airway, the essential secretory structures of the mucociliary system are the following:

- Surface epithelial cells
  - Pseudostratified, columnar, ciliated epithelial cells
  - Surface goblet (or mucous) cells
  - Club cells (formerly called Clara cells) in the distal airway
- Submucosal glands, with serous and mucous cells

Submucosal glands are found in cartilaginous airways. These mucus-producing glands are not found beyond the distal airways. Mucus secreted by surface epithelial cells and glands in the airway provides for basic protection of the respiratory tract, including humidification and warming of inspired gas, mucociliary transport of debris, waterproofing and insulation, and antibacterial activity.[3]

Terminology: Mucus, Phlegm, and Sputum

There has been confusion regarding the nomenclature used to classify mucoactive medications. Although some have used "mucolytic" as a generic term, most of these medications are thought to mobilize secretions by mechanisms

TABLE 9-1	Mucoactive Agents Available for Aerosol Administration		
DRUG	**BRAND NAME**	**ADULT DOSAGE**	**USE**
N-Acetylcysteine L-cysteine (NAC)	10% Mucomyst, 20% Mucomyst	SVN: 3-5 mL	Efficacy has not been demonstrated with any dose of NAC for any lung disease
Dornase alfa	Pulmozyme	SVN: 2.5 mg/ampule, one ampule daily*	Cystic fibrosis (CF) only
Aqueous water, saline	—	SVN: 3-5 mL, as ordered	Sputum induction
Hyperosmolar 7% saline	Hyper-Sal	SVN: 4 mL	Airway clearance (mucokinetics) for
Dry powder mannitol	Bronchitol		therapy of CF (7% saline and Mannitol)
3% hyperosmolar saline			3% saline used for infantile bronchiolitis

SVN, Small volume nebulizer
*Use recommended nebulizer system—see package insert.

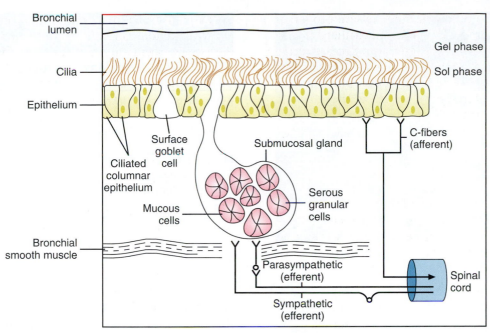

Figure 9-1 Principal components and innervation of the mucociliary system in the respiratory tract.

other than by the direct "thinning" of mucus. For example, although the mucociliary transportability of sputum may be improved by reducing sputum viscosity while preserving elasticity, the ability to clear secretions via cough is greater with *increased* sputum viscosity and decreased adhesivity. Knowledge of mucus properties has given us tools to better understand the mechanisms of airway disease and muco-active therapy. The currently accepted terminology is defined in the *Key Terms and Definitions* list at the start of this chapter. For more details on current terminology and its evolution, see Reid and Clamp,[6] Basbaum,[7] Voynow and Rubin,[5] and King and Rubin.[8]

Surface Epithelial Cells

The surface of the trachea and bronchi primarily includes ciliated and goblet cells, at a ratio of approximately 5:1. There are more than 6000 goblet cells per square millimeter of normal airway mucosa. Goblet cells do not seem to be directly innervated in the human lung, although they respond to irritants and inflammatory mediators and peptides by increasing the production of mucus and are, themselves, immune effector cells. Figures 9-2 and 9-3 show scanning electron micrographs of the mucus lining[9] (Figure 9-2) and of the bronchiolar surface with the mucus stripped away[9] (Figure 9-3). In addition to ciliated and goblet cells, microvilli, which may have absorptive and sensory functions, can be seen in Figure 9-3.

Submucosal Mucous Glands

Submucosal glands below the epithelial surface are thought to provide much of the mucin on the airway surface. The submucosal gland is under parasympathetic (vagal) control and responds to cholinergic stimulation by increasing the amount of mucus secreted. Evidence also suggests that

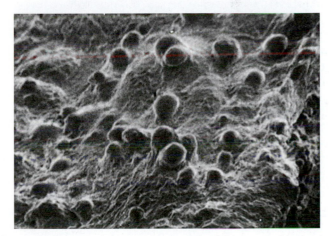

Figure 9-2 Scanning electron micrograph of the mucus blanket in a bronchiole, prepared from hamster lung. (From Nowell JA, Tyler WS. Scanning electron microscopy of the surface morphology of mammalian lungs. *Am Rev.Respir Dis.* 1971;103[3]:313-328.)

submucosal glands in the respiratory tract are innervated by sympathetic axons and the peptidergic nerve system.

Two types of cells, mucous and serous, are found in the glands. Figure 9-4 shows a section of ferret airway stained for mucin, with the surface mucous (goblet) cells and the submucosal gland's serous and mucous cells identified. Secretions from the serous and mucous cells mix in the submucosal gland and are transported through a ciliated duct onto the airway lumen.

Ciliary System

 KEY POINT

The airway secretion consists of a *mucus layer*, where *mucin glycoprotein* is secreted, and a weak gel *periciliary layer*.

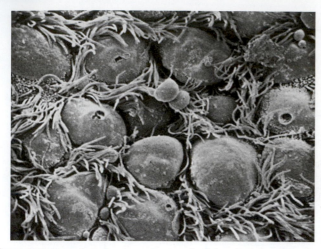

Figure 9-3 Scanning electron micrograph of the airway surface shows epithelial cells with cilia, possible surface goblet cells dehiscing, and some microvilli. (From Nowell JA, Tyler WS. Scanning electron microscopy of the surface morphology of mammalian lungs. *Am Rev.Respir Dis.* 1971;103[3]:313-328.)

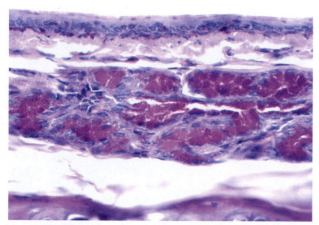

Figure 9-4 Light microscopy showing immunohistochemical staining of ferret airway, using horseradish peroxidase–conjugated *Dolichos biflorus* agglutinin *(DBA)*. Tracheal section shows the mucociliary apparatus, including surface mucous (goblet) cells, ciliated epithelial cells, and serous and mucous glands.

Droplets of mucus from the secretory cells form plaques in the distal, nonciliated airway, and these coalesce into a continuous layer in the more proximal ciliated airway. Mucociliary transport results from the movement of the mucus gel by the beating cilia. There are approximately 200 cilia on each ciliated cell. Cilia are about 7 μm in length in larger airways and shorten to 5 μm or less in smaller bronchioles. Luk and Dulfano[10] examined the ciliary beat frequency on biopsy samples from various tracheobronchial regions and found rates of 8 to 18 Hertz (Hz) (Hz = 1 cycle/sec) at 37° C. A ciliary beat is composed of an *effective* (power) stroke and a *recovery* stroke with about a 1:2 ratio. In the effective stroke, the cilium moves in an upright position through a full forward arc to contact the underside of the mucus layer and propel it forward. In the recovery stroke, the cilium swings back around to the starting point near the cell surface to avoid pulling secretions back. Cilia

TABLE 9-2	Effects of Various Drug Groups on Mucociliary Clearance		
DRUG GROUP	**CILIARY BEAT**	**MUCUS PRODUCTION**	**TRANSPORT**
β-Adrenergic agents	Increase	Increase*	±
Cholinergic agents	Increase	Increase†	Increase
Methylxanthines	Increase	Increase†	±
Corticosteroids	None	None†	None
Anticholinergics	None	None	None

*Data from Wanner A: *Am J Respir Dis* 116:73, 1977.
†Data from Iravani J, Melville GN: *Respiration* 32:305, 1975.

beat in a coordinated, or metachronal wave of motion to propel airway secretions.[11] A functional surfactant layer lies at the tips of the cilia and separates the periciliary fluid from the mucus gel. This layer allows the cilia to transmit kinetic energy effectively to the mucus without becoming entangled. This layer also facilitates mucus spreading as a continuous layer and prevents water loss from the periciliary fluid.

Factors Affecting Mucociliary Transport

Mucociliary transport velocity varies in the normal lung and has been estimated at about 1.5 mm/min in peripheral airways and 20 mm/min in the trachea. Transport rates are slower in the presence of the following conditions or substances, many of which are associated with airway damage:

- Chronic obstructive pulmonary disease (COPD) and CF
- Airway drying (e.g., with the use of dry gas for mechanical ventilation)
- Narcotics
- Endotracheal suctioning, airway trauma, and tracheostomy
- Tobacco smoke and tobacco smoke extract
- Atmospheric pollutants (SO_2, NO_2, ozone) and allergens may increase transport, especially at low concentration, but at higher, toxic concentrations or with prolonged exposure, these decrease transport rates
- Hyperoxia and hypoxia

Table 9-2 summarizes the effects of drug groups commonly used in respiratory care on ciliary beat, mucus output, and overall transport.

Food Intake and Mucus Production

A common belief is that drinking dairy milk increases the production of mucus and congestion in the respiratory tract. Respiratory care personnel may be asked for advice on withholding milk from children with colds, respiratory infections, or chronic respiratory conditions such as CF.[12] In a study of 60 healthy subjects with experimentally induced rhinovirus respiratory infections, milk intake ranged from 0 to 11 glasses a day. There was no association between milk or dairy product intake and respiratory tract symptoms of congestion or nasal secretion weight. None of the subjects were allergic to cow's milk. The investigators concluded that the data do not support the withholding of milk or the belief that milk increases respiratory tract congestion.

Secretory Hyperresponsiveness and Mucus Hypersecretion

The term "secretory hyperresponsiveness" is used for increased mucus secretion either intrinsically or in response to bronchoprovocation. Certain groups of patients appear to have greater mucus secretory response, including those with middle lobe syndrome, cough-dominant ("cough-variant") asthma, and severe asthma. Secretory hyperresponsiveness also is a component of forms of lung cancer associated with bronchorrhea. An extreme form of secretory hyperresponsiveness may lead to plastic bronchitis, a disease characterized by rigid branching mucus casts that obstruct the airway. Secretory hyperresponsiveness and mucus hypersecretion appear to be related to activation of the extracellular regulated kinase (ERK ½), signaling through the epidermal growth factor receptor (EGFR) or secretory phospholipases A2 (sPLA2).

NATURE OF MUCUS SECRETION

A healthy person is thought to produce about 100 mL of mucus every 24 hours that is clear, viscoelastic, and sticky. Most of this secretion is reabsorbed in the bronchial mucosa or swallowed with saliva. The individual rarely notices this. During disease, the volume of secretions can increase dramatically and secretion clearance can be decreased so that secretions are expectorated or swallowed. A primary function of respiratory tract mucus is thought to be transporting and removing trapped inhaled particles, cellular debris, and dead and aging cells.

Structure and Composition of Mucus

The structure and major constituents of the mucus secreted by submucosal glands and surface goblet cells are pictured in Figure 9-5 and have been reviewed elsewhere.[5,7,13-16] Airway mucus forms a protective barrier between the respiratory tract epithelium and the environment. Mucus is composed mainly of water and ions, with approximately 5% of the content from proteins secreted by airway cells and lipids.[17-19] In health, the mucin **glycoproteins** are the major macromolecular component of the mucus gel. **Mucins** are responsible for the protective and clearance properties of mucus.[20-22] Data suggest that the transportability of the mucus layer is dependent on the concentration of mucins in the mucus layer as a function of the mucin concentration to the power of 2.5.[23]

There are two major classes of mucins: the secreted and the membrane-tethered mucins.[24,25] Four secreted mucins (MUC2, MUC5AC, MUC5B, and MUC6) have genes that are clustered on chromosome 11p15 and contain domains with significant homology to the von Willebrand factor D domains that are sites for oligomerization.[26] In sputum, MUC5AC and MUC5B are the major oligomeric gel-forming mucins.[27] MUC5AC apparently is produced primarily by the goblet cells in the tracheobronchial surface epithelium, whereas MUC5B is secreted primarily by the submucosal glands; although the goblet cell is also capable of secreting MUC5B.[28] The membrane-tethered mucins, MUC1, MUC3, MUC4, MUC12, and MUC13, contain a transmembrane domain and a short cytoplasmic domain.[26] At least 12 mucin genes (*MUC1, MUC2, MUC4, MUC5AC, MUC5B, MUC7, MUC8, MUC11, MUC13, MUC15, MUC19, and MUC20*) have been observed at the mRNA level in tissues of the lower respiratory tract from healthy individuals.[24,26,29-35]

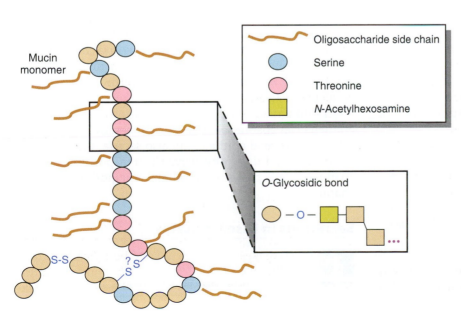

Figure 9-5 Basic structure and constituents of the mucus macromolecule. *S–S–*, Disulfide bonds.

Mucus is a complex, high-molecular-weight macromolecule consisting of a mucin protein backbone to which carbohydrate (**oligosaccharide**) side chains are attached. The airway mucus gel-forming mucins are primarily MUC5AC and MUC5B; the periciliary layer contains tethered mucins including MUC1 (a signaling mucin also found in some cancers that is able to regulate inflammation) and MUC4.[23,30] The carbohydrate content is 80% or more of the total weight of the macromolecule. This structure is similar to a bottlebrush in appearance. This general structure of protein and attached oligosaccharide side chains is termed a *glycoprotein.* Mucin forms a flexible, threadlike strand 200 nm to 6 µm in length[36] that is linearly cross-linked with disulfide bonds bridging adjacent cysteine residues. Strands may also be linked with each other by hydrogen bonding and van der Waals forces. The result is a gel that consists of a high water content (90%-95%) organized around the structural elements and that is intensely hydrophilic and spongelike.[37,38]

Under normal circumstances, bonding within mucus produces low viscosity but moderate elasticity. Although mucus incorporates water during its formation, a gel acts like both a liquid and a solid. For example, cooking gelatin is mostly water but organizes into a semisolid by its chemical structure as the liquid gels. It is important clinically that sufficient water must be available to form mucus with normal physical properties, but once formed, mucus does not readily incorporate additional water.[39] Phospholipids are also present in the serous cell granules of the submucosal glands. When released onto the airway surface, phospholipids serve as lubricants affecting the surface-active and adhesive properties of mucus, both of which can affect mucociliary transport.[3]

In addition to the mucus gel secreted in the airway, bronchial secretions contain serum and secreted proteins, lipids, and electrolytes. Antibacterial defense in the airway is provided by mucin, secretory Immunoglobulin A (IgA), Immunoglobulin G (IgG), lysozyme, lactoferrin, defensins, and peroxidase and serine proteases. Bronchial secretions control the potentially destructive action of protease enzymes with two major antiproteases: α_1-protease inhibitor and secretory leukoprotease inhibitor (sLPI), a cationic protein found in serous secretory glandular cells.[3] In healthy airways, antiproteases are present in higher quantities than protease enzymes and provide a protease screen.[40] These antiproteases also prevent abnormal mucin degradation in vitro as reported in CF and in CB.[41,42]

Epithelial Ion and Water Transport

KEY POINT

Epithelial ion exchange in the airway surface liquid maintains normal periciliary fluid depth.

The composition and volume of the periciliary fluid layer is regulated in part by ion transport across the epithelial cells lining the airway lumen. If the periciliary layer is not approximately the height of an extended cilium, mucus

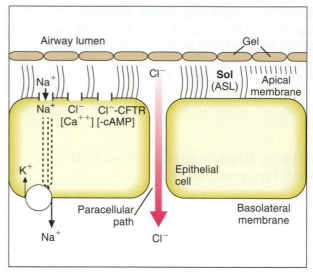

Figure 9-6 Illustration of ion-exchange mechanisms across normal airway epithelium controlling absorption and secretion for the periciliary airway surface liquid *(ASL).* Under basal conditions, sodium (Na⁺) is absorbed along with liquid, with no net chloride (Cl⁻) secretion from the cell into the liquid layer. *cAMP,* Cyclic adenosine 3′,5′-monophosphate; *CFTR,* cystic fibrosis transmembrane ion conductance regulator; *K⁺,* potassium ion.

movement is less effective.[43] Defective ion transport may contribute to the cycle of retained secretions and infection seen in CF.[44,45] Normal airway epithelial ion transport is illustrated in Figure 9-6.

In the basal, unstimulated state, sodium (Na⁺) absorption into the epithelial cell is the dominant ion exchange that absorbs liquid from the airway periciliary layer. Na⁺ absorption occurs as an active transport process through Na⁺ channels (the epithelial Na⁺ channel [ENaC]) on the apical or airway side of the cell. Na⁺ in the epithelial cell is pumped from the cell, driven by a sodium/potassium-ATPase pump on the basolateral membrane of the epithelial cell, as shown in Figure 9-6. When Na⁺ is absorbed from the airway surface liquid, there is an accompanying absorption of chloride (Cl⁻) ions and water.[46] Cl⁻ secretion can occur through at least two different types of Cl⁻ channel in the cell apex. One channel is dependent on cyclic adenosine 3′,5′-monophosphate (cAMP), the CF transmembrane ion-conductance regulator (CFTR) channel; the other channel is calcium activated.

To summarize, under normal conditions, healthy airway epithelia can absorb salt and water driven by an active Na⁺ transport. Normal epithelia can also secrete liquid into the periciliary fluid driven by active Cl⁻ transport through ion channels and passively through aquaporins or water channels.

Secretions in Disease States

KEY POINT

Mucus or mucociliary clearance can be abnormal in pulmonary diseases such as chronic bronchitis (CB), asthma, or cystic fibrosis (CF).

The normal clearance of airway mucus can be altered by changes in the volume, hydration, or composition of the secretion, as well as by changes in ciliary function. The composition of respiratory mucus is undergoing investigation based on structural analysis techniques.[47,48]

Knowledge of these features of respiratory mucus may lead to a better understanding of diseases characterized by an abnormal production of mucus, such as CB and asthma, in which there is mucus hypersecretion, and CF, in which there is a decrease of intact mucin but an increase of pathologic DNA-actin polymers. Although it had been hypothesized that patients with CF hypersecrete viscous mucus, leading to airway obstruction, it has been shown that tenacious (but not viscous) secretions that characterize CF airway disease are composed almost entirely of DNA—rich with characteristics most similar to pus rather than to normal airway mucus.[49] Secreted CF mucins are rapidly degraded by serene proteases (including bacterial proteases) in the airway. This also occurs during exacerbations of CB. Airway damage may predispose patients to bacterial infections in CB because of impaired clearance of mucus.

Sputum, or expectorated phlegm, is composed of mucus mixed with inflammatory cells, cellular debris, polymers of DNA and filamentous (F)-actin, and bacteria. Mucus is usually cleared by airflow and ciliary movement, and sputum is cleared by cough.[50] Purulent, green **phlegm** is caused by the neutrophil-derived enzyme myeloperoxidase, indicating neutrophil activation; this sputum contains very little mucin and can be considered pus.[51] Bronchial obstruction by secretions, either mucus or pus, can increase airflow resistance and lead to complete airway obstruction and atelectasis.[14] Regardless of whether the airway is full of mucus or phlegm, effective airway clearance is important for airway hygiene.

Chronic Bronchitis

CB is defined clinically as daily sputum expectoration for 3 months of the year for at least 2 consecutive years, usually in a tobacco smoker or ex-smoker. In the airway of a subject with CB, there is hyperplasia of submucosal glands and goblet cells. The number of goblet cells increases and there is hypertrophy of the submucosal glands, as measured by the Reid Index of gland-to-airway wall thickness ratio.[52] When studied in vitro, it was found that submucosal glands from subjects with CB produce excessive amounts of mucus.[53] Tobacco smoke is considered the most important predisposing factor to airway irritation and mucus hypersecretion, but other factors can include viral infections, pollutants, and genetic predisposition.[14,54] It has been reported that chronic sputum expectoration is associated with a more rapid decline in lung function and, for persons with COPD, more frequent admissions to the hospital.[55]

Asthma

Mucus hypersecretion can occur during an acute asthmatic episode or can be a chronic feature of asthma, accompanying airway inflammation. It has been reported[56] that as many as 80% of patients with asthma report increased sputum expectoration.

In acute severe and fatal asthma, there is profound hypersecretion of highly viscous and rigid mucus, leading to complete airway obstruction.[57] Because most of these patients have received large amounts of β-agonist bronchodilators, sometimes even by the intravenous route, it is likely that β receptors are fully saturated. β Agonists may induce the secretion of viscous mucus and may contribute to airway obstruction.[58]

Bronchorrhea

Bronchorrhea is defined as the production of large volumes of watery sputum. This occurs in about 9% of adults with chronic asthma.[59] Some of these patients respond well to antiinflammatory therapy such as corticosteroids,[60] indomethacin by aerosol,[61] anticholinergic medications, or macrolide antibiotics.[62] These are considered mucoregulatory medications and are most effective when bronchorrhea is associated with airway inflammation. Patients with congenital fucosidosis also have a form of bronchorrhea caused by the inability of mucins to polymerize. This form of bronchorrhea does not respond to mucoregulatory therapy.[63]

Plastic Bronchitis

Plastic bronchitis is a rare disease characterized by the formation of large gelatinous or rigid branching airway casts.[64] This is dramatically different from the mucus or sputum plugs expectorated by patients with purulent airway diseases like CF because the plastic bronchitis casts repeat airway branching. Plastic bronchitis has not been shown to occur as a result of CF. Casts are often too thick to be easily suctioned through a bronchoscope and too friable to be grasped and removed with forceps. Some patients are able to expectorate even large casts spontaneously. Not all patients expectorate casts, and this may delay the diagnosis.

The prevalence of plastic bronchitis is unknown. This disease may also overlap with diseases such as asthma and with the severe mucus plugging sometimes seen in bronchopulmonary *aspergillosis* or middle lobe syndrome. Differentiating between severe asthma with mucus plugging and plastic bronchitis can be difficult.

The mortality rate among patients with plastic bronchitis has been estimated as 6% to 50% for patients with "inflammatory" casts, 28% to 60% for patients with asthma, and there have been no reported deaths in patients with plastic bronchitis with acute chest syndrome in sickle cell disease. Patients who die usually have respiratory failure related to central airway obstruction.

There is only anecdotal evidence that any specific therapy is beneficial, and this evidence has generally been provided only by single case reports. If chylous casts are present, dietary modification or thoracic duct ligation may help. Selective embolization of aberrant intrapulmonary thoracic duct channels has also been reported to be effective in decreasing symptoms of plastic bronchitis in patients who have congenital heart disease with single ventricle (Fontan) physiology.[65] In patients with asthma or atopy, therapy should be directed toward treating underlying inflammation. The 14- and 15-member macrolide antibiotics are immunomodulatory and mucoregulatory drugs. We have had success using macrolides as immunomodulating agents in two patients with eosinophilic plastic bronchitis (unpublished data). Macrolides have been successfully used in other disorders, primarily DPB and CF. There is clear evidence that these effects are not related to the antimicrobial activity of the macrolide.[64,66] There is some evidence that these casts may form, in part, by fibrin polymerization. Aerosol tissue plasminogen activator (tPA) has been shown to help some patients with active cast formation, but this medication is irritating and its use has been associated with airway bleeding. It has not been shown that aerosol tPA will inhibit cast formation when used chronically. Aerosol heparin decreases cast formation in some patents with congenital heart disease and plastic bronchitis, either by acting as an antiinflammatory medication or as an inhibitor of tissue factor.

Cystic Fibrosis

CF is a hereditary disease characterized by impaired function of the CFTR protein. There is chronic airway infection, often with *Pseudomonas* and other gram-negative organisms. There is also chronic airway inflammation; infection and inflammation together lead to bronchiectasis, progressive pulmonary function decline, and eventually death. Although there may be mucus hypersecretion in CF, it is now known that with established CF bronchiectasis, the airway secretions contain very little intact mucin and obstruction appears to be due to DNA-actin polymers. The airways in CF are almost entirely filled with pus derived from neutrophil degradation and neutrophil extracellular traps. The decreased mucin in CF sputum may be related to chronic bacterial infection by *Pseudomonas aeruginosa* and breakdown of mucins by proteases derived from neutrophils or bacteria.[49,67]

It is unclear how abnormal CFTR function leads to chronic infection and inflammation. Airway epithelia in CF have excessive absorption of Na^+ compared with normal epithelia. There is a limited ability for the epithelial cells to secrete Cl^- through the Cl^- CFTR channels (see Figure 9-6) stimulated by cAMP. The result of excessive Na^+ absorption and limited Cl^- secretion may lead to decreased water and increased reabsorption of the periciliary fluid.[46] Abnormal phospholipids and surfactant degradation in CF secretions may also increase sputum adhesion and stickiness by altering surface properties of the secretion.[3] CF sputum is biophysically similar to bronchiectasis sputum.[68]

PHYSICAL PROPERTIES OF MUCUS

The biochemical composition and structure of mucus determine its physical properties, which influence the effectiveness of mucus transport.

KEY POINT

Physical properties of mucus include *viscosity, elasticity, cohesivity,* and *adhesivity.*

Surface Forces

Adhesion refers to forces between unlike molecules. In the airway, adhesive forces refer to the attractive forces between the mucus and airway surface. Adhesion reduces the ability to clear secretions by airflow (cough).[69] Mucokinetic agents are either **abhesives**, such as surfactant, which reduces the adhesivity of secretions, or agents that increase the power of airflow and cough. Mucolytics may work, in part, by severing the bonding of mucus to the epithelium, reducing inertial (frictional) adhesion.

Viscoelasticity and Cohesivity

Cohesion refers to forces between like molecules. Cohesive forces result from the elongation of the mucus macromolecule. A property of spinnability has been described as a surrogate measure of cohesivity.

Rheology or Viscoelasticity

Rheology is the study of the dynamic deformation and flow of matter. The rheologic behavior of mucus describes the way it responds to applied force (stress). Viscosity is a property of liquids and describes the energy loss from the applied stress by deforming the liquid. Elasticity is a property of solids and describes energy stored by the solid with applied stress. It is important to understand that viscosity and elasticity are not constant measurements, but vary with the rate and intensity of the applied stress. Thus we describe either a range of viscosity measurements, or more commonly, quasistatic viscosity at a controlled stress. A gel, like airway mucus, has both viscous (liquid) and elastic (solid) properties. There is no single measurement that can be called "viscoelasticity."

Viscosity, or loss modulus, is the resistance of a fluid to flow. The viscous properties of an ideal or Newtonian liquid can be described by the loss modulus G''. **Elasticity**, or storage modulus, is the ability of a deformed material to return to its original shape. Ideal or Hookean solids store energy during deformation, and this energy is available when the force is removed. The properties of an ideal solid can be described by the storage modulus G'. The complex modulus (G^*) is the vectorial sum of viscosity and elasticity. Figure 9-7 illustrates the concept of viscosity and of elasticity.[70-72]

Mucus as a Viscoelastic Material

The mucus gel is a viscoelastic material and responds to an applied stress as a fluid and as a solid. As a solid, a gel has elastic deformation, storing energy with applied force (e.g., ciliary beating), and as a liquid, a gel flows under applied force (e.g., extrusion from submucosal glands). As the tips of the cilia contact the gel during the forward power stroke, the gel is stretched, and its elastic recovery causes it to snap forward. At the same time, the mucus gel flows forward as a liquid under the forward beat of the cilia.

This model of gel transport is seen in Figure 9-8, using unvulcanized rubber as an example of a viscoelastic

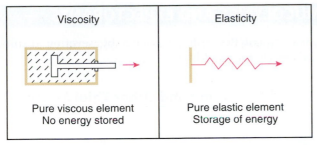

Viscosity: Resistance to flow.

Elasticity: Property of deforming under force, resuming shape.

Figure 9-7 Illustration of concepts of viscosity and elasticity.

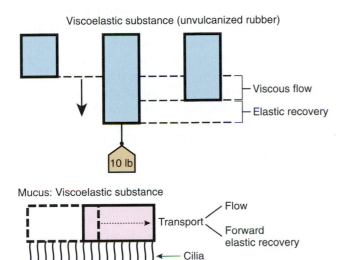

Figure 9-8 Illustration of viscous and elastic properties affecting the movement of viscoelastic substances, such as unvulcanized rubber and mucus.

substance. If such a rubber strip is loaded on one end with a weight and allowed to hang, it would initially stretch as an elastic solid. If the applied force remains, the strip would slowly elongate because of its viscosity (i.e., the rubber would "flow"). After removing the weight, the rubber recovers most of the elastic elongation because of stored energy, but it would not recover the entire length because of flow. Mucus behaves similarly. Mucociliary transport results from flow and forward elastic recovery. For this reason, the physical properties of viscosity and elasticity are important for efficient transport of respiratory secretions. Normal mucus generally has a relatively low viscosity, and its elasticity is high enough to provide forward propulsive energy.

Spinnability (Cohesivity) of Mucus

The ability of mucus to be drawn out into threads was initially identified for cervical mucus; it was termed *spinnability* and described in the German literature as *Spinnbarkeit*. The property of spinnability was subsequently studied by Puchelle and colleagues[73] for respiratory mucus. They used a device to stretch mucus vertically at a constant rate and measured the spinnability of a mucus thread as the maximal length to which the thread could be drawn before breaking. In general, there was a significant and positive correlation between spinnability of mucus and its mucociliary transport rate. Spinnability was found to increase with increasing elasticity. Spinnability varied widely, however, with low viscosities, and mucus with high spinnability showed normal ciliary transport even though viscosity and elasticity were abnormally low. Spinnability and mucus transport were also found to decrease as the purulence of sputum from CB patients increased.

Spinnability gives information about internal cohesion forces in mucus. *Cohesivity* is defined as interfacial tension multiplied by the new area created after a test substance is pulled apart and can be approximated by measuring spinnability. *Tenacity* is defined as the product of cohesivity and adhesive work. Tenacity is one of the strongest determinants of the ability of sputum to be cleared by cough. The greater the tenacity of sputum, the poorer the cough clearability.

Non-Newtonian Nature of Mucus

Evaluation of mucus properties is complicated by the fact that mucus exhibits non-Newtonian rheology. A non-Newtonian gel, such as mucus, has changing viscosity with varying applied force (shear rate). As the shear rate increases, the apparent viscosity of mucus usually decreases. Some mucus exhibits a sudden collapse of viscous behavior at high applied stress; this is called *apparent yield stress*. Sputum that yields may be more easily cleared by cough.[74] These changes in viscosity are consistent with rupture or change of the macromolecular chains and cross-linking network of the gel. Mucus can also be *thixotropic*—stable at rest but becoming more fluid with applied force and then thickening again when stress is removed. A common thixotropic gel is house paint.

Because of its non-Newtonian behavior, evaluation of the properties of mucus and of the effect of drugs on those properties is complicated and must be performed under standardized conditions of dynamic shear rate and across the linear portion of the stress-strain curve. Otherwise, interpretation of research findings on mucus viscosity is inaccurate.[48,75] Many review articles and compendia are devoted to the physiology of mucus secretion in the lung and the nature of mucus.*

MUCOACTIVE AGENTS

 KEY POINT

Three drugs are currently used in the United States to modify airway secretions: *N-acetylcysteine (NAC), dornase alfa,* and *hypertonic saline.*

*References 7, 10, 14, 18, 50, 76-79.

TABLE 9-3	Drugs Used or Under Investigation as Aerosol Mucoactive Medications
DRUG	**DESCRIPTION**
Dornase alfa	Peptide mucolytic
Hyperosmolar saline	Expectorant
Dry powder mannitol	Expectorant
Thymosin β_4	Peptide mucolytic
Surfactants	Abhesive, mucokinetic
β Agonists	Secretagogues; potentially mucokinetic if airflow increases
Anticholinergic agents	Mucoregulatory
Corticosteroids	Mucoregulatory
Dapsone	Mucoregulatory

At the time of this edition, three drugs have been used in the United States as an aerosol, to treat abnormal pulmonary secretions: NAC, dornase alfa, and 7% saline. The first two of these drugs are considered mucolytic in action, disrupting disulfide bonds in mucus (NAC) or enzymatically breaking down DNA in airway secretions (dornase), although there is no evidence that NAC is mucolytic in vivo or that it is therapeutically effective. Inhalation of 7% hypertonic saline as an aerosol is now recommended as part of the treatment regimen for CF. Bicarbonate solutions for aerosol instillation are not approved for use and are irritating to the airway. Table 9-3 summarizes the spectrum of agents in current use with the potential to improve mucus clearance.

Mucolysis and Mucociliary Clearance

Mucolytic agents decrease the elasticity and viscosity of mucus. Because elasticity is crucial for mucociliary transport, mucolytics have the potential for a negative effect on normal physiologic mucus clearance. Reduction of mucus gel to a more liquid state *may* facilitate aspiration of secretions with the use of suction catheters.[80] The status of mucolytic agents in pulmonary disease has been reviewed at several conferences on the scientific basis of respiratory care.[81-83]

The therapeutic options for controlling mucus hypersecretion are outlined as follows:

1. Remove causative factors where possible
   a. Treat infections
   b. *Avoid all tobacco smoke exposure*
   c. Avoid pollution and allergens
2. Improve tracheobronchial clearance
   a. Use bronchodilators if these are able to increase expiratory airflow (i.e., in asthma)
   b. Use bronchial hygiene measures
      (1) Cough, deep breathing
      (2) Chest physical therapy (CPT)
      (3) Other airway clearance devices and maneuvers
   c. Improve airflow by exercise and nutrition rehabilitation
3. Use mucoactive agents when indicated

MUCOLYTICS AND EXPECTORANTS

Classic mucolytics reduce mucins by severing disulfide bonds or charge shielding.

N-Acetyl-L-Cysteine and Other Thiol Mucolytics
Indications for Use

KEY POINT

Acetylcysteine does *not* improve mucus clearance when given as an aerosol or when given orally and should not be used as a mucoactive medication.

As a mucolytic, NAC has been used in conditions associated with viscous mucus secretions. A second use of NAC is as an antioxidant antidote to reduce hepatic injury with acetaminophen overdose.[84] The drug is given orally for this use. Despite in vitro mucolytic activity and a long history of use, there are no data showing that aerosolized NAC is effective therapy for any lung disease,[85] and its use may be harmful. This harm may be due, in part, to NAC selectively depolymerizing the essential mucin polymer structure and leaving the pathologic polymers of DNA and F-actin intact. Because there are no data that show NAC to be effective for lung disease and because of the risk of side effects, we do not recommend its use.

Mode of Action

NAC disrupts the structure of the mucus polymer by substituting free thiol (sulfhydryl) groups for the disulfide bonds connecting mucin proteins. The substituted sulfhydryl group in mucus does not provide a bond or cross-linking between strands. When in physical contact with mucus, NAC begins to reduce viscosity, and mucolytic activity increases with a higher pH of 7 to 9. The solution of NAC contains a chelating agent, ethylene dia-minetetraacetic acid (EDTA). A light purple solution indicates metal ion removal. It is suggested that opened vials of the drug be stored in a refrigerator and discarded after 96 hours to prevent contamination. Additional details in the manufacturer's package insert should be reviewed.

Hazards

The most serious potential complication with NAC is bronchospasm caused by its acidity (pKa 2.2). Bronchospasm is more likely in asthmatic patients. Other complications include stomatitis, nausea, and rhinorrhea. Mechanical obstruction of the airway can occur, and suction should be available with artificial airways. The disagreeable odor of NAC is due to the release of hydrogen sulfide, and this may provoke nausea or vomiting. In prolonged nebulization, the manufacturer suggests that after three-fourths of the solution is nebulized, the remaining one-fourth should be diluted with an equal volume of sterile water to prevent the formation of a highly concentrated residue that could irritate the airway. An aerosol of NAC may leave a sticky film on the hands or face.

Incompatibility with Antibiotics in Mixture

NAC is incompatible in mixture with the following antibiotics:

- Sodium ampicillin
- Amphotericin B
- Erythromycin lactobionate
- Tetracyclines (tetracycline, oxytetracycline)
- Aminoglycosides

Incompatibility is taken to mean the formation of a precipitate; a change in color, clarity, or odor; or other physical or chemical change. NAC is reactive with numerous substances, including rubber, copper, iron, and cork. A complete list of incompatibilities for NAC can be found in the manufacturer's literature.

Dornase alfa (Pulmozyme)

KEY POINT

Dornase alfa is indicated only for clearance of purulent secretions in *cystic fibrosis (CF)*.

Peptide mucolytics reduce extracellular DNA and F-actin polymers. Dornase alfa is a recombinant form of the human DNase I enzyme, which digests extracellular DNA. In February 1994, the U.S. Food and Drug Administration (FDA) approved dornase alfa for general use in treating the abnormally tenacious DNA-containing sputum of CF.

Dornase alfa was the first approved mucoactive agent for the treatment of CF. Dornase alfa is safe and effective in patients with more severe pulmonary disease, defined as a forced vital capacity (FVC) less than 40% of the predicted value.[86] Efficacy has not been shown for therapy of acute exacerbations of CF lung disease or for the treatment of other chronic airway diseases.[87] A phase 1 study showed no efficacy in non-CF bronchiectasis, and the use of dornase appeared to decrease pulmonary function in adults with non-CF bronchiectasis.[88] Dornase has also not been shown to improve pulmonary function but does increase the risk of death when given to adults with COPD This worsening of disease may be due to the fact that secretions in COPD are composed primarily of mucin and related proteins,[89] whereas CF airway secretions primarily contain neutrophil-derived pus.[49]

Indication and Use in Cystic Fibrosis

Dornase alfa is indicated for the management of CF to reduce the frequency of respiratory infections and to improve or preserve pulmonary function in CF patients. The bulk and surface properties of respiratory secretions in CF are due to the presence of DNA from dying neutrophils or neutrophil extracellular nets present during chronic respiratory infections, and to surfactant phospholipid hydrolysis by products of inflammation. In the presence of infection, neutrophils move into to the airways and release DNA.[90,91] DNA in secretions may also contribute to reduced effectiveness of aminoglycoside antibiotics, perhaps by binding the antibiotic to the polyvalent anions of the DNA.

Mode of Action

Dornase alfa reduces the viscosity and adhesivity of infected respiratory secretions when given by aerosol (Figure 9-9).

When mixed with purulent sputum from subjects with CF, dornase alfa reduced the viscosity and adhesivity of the sputum.[86] This reduction was associated with a decrease in the size of the DNA polymers in the sputum. The change in sputum viscosity with the addition of dornase alfa is dose-dependent, with greater reduction occurring at higher concentrations of the drug.

Dose and Administration

The aerosol product of dornase alfa is available as single-use ampoule, with 2.5 mg of drug in 2.5 mL of clear, colorless solution. The solution should be refrigerated and protected

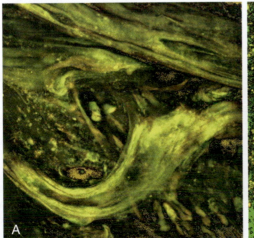
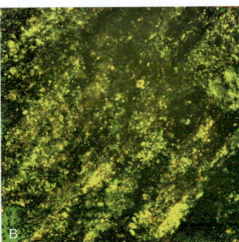

Figure 9-9 Illustration of the mode of action of dornase alfa in reducing DNA polymers in CF sputum. Confocal micrograph showing CF sputum stained (with YOYO-1) for DNA before **(A)** and after **(B)** treatment with dornase alfa in vitro. The long DNA polymers are degraded after dornase treatment.

from light. The usual dosage is 2.5 mg daily, delivered by one of the following approved nebulizers: Hudson RCI UP-DRAFT II OPTI-NEB nebulizer with tee (Teleflex Medical, Research Triangle Park, North Carolina) or the Acorn II nebulizer (Vital Signs, Totowa, New Jersey) with a DeVilbiss Pulmo-Aide compressor (Sunrise Medical, Carlsbad, California), or the PARI LC PLUS nebulizer (PARI Respiratory Equipment, Midlothian, Virginia) with PARI Inhaler Boy compressor.[92] Although other nebulizer systems may perform suitably in nebulizing dornase alfa, this should not be assumed without testing. Optimal delivery of the enzyme requires a nebulizer system capable of suitable aerosol generation (i.e., particle size and quantity). This is especially important when administering expensive drugs or aerosol medications with a narrow therapeutic index.

Adverse Effects

Side effects of dornase alfa differed little from those of a placebo in CF clinical trials, and the discontinuation rate was similar for dornase alfa (3%) and the placebo (2%). Common side effects with use of the drug have included voice alteration, pharyngitis, laryngitis, rash, chest pain, and conjunctivitis. Other, less common side effects reported include respiratory symptoms (cough increase, dyspnea, pneumothorax, hemoptysis, rhinitis, and sinusitis), flu syndrome and malaise, gastrointestinal obstruction, hypoxia, and weight loss. Contraindications include hypersensitivity to the medication. On the other hand, inhaled dornase has not been shown to be effective for treating any other lung disease and may be harmful when used to treat pneumonia, severe CB, or non-CF bronchiectasis.

Clinical Application and Evaluation

The intent of treatment with dornase alfa is to preserve or improve lung function in CF while reducing the frequency and severity of respiratory infections by improving secretion clearance. A reduction in use of intravenous antibiotic therapy and the need for hospitalizations has also been reported. Evaluation of drug treatment is based not only on lung function but also on a reduction in the number and severity of infectious exacerbations and the need for antibiotics and hospitalization.[93]

Filamentous Actin-Depolymerizing Drugs: Thymosin β₄

Chronic inflammation is characterized by inflammatory cell necrosis and release of polymeric DNA, F-actin, and intracellular enzymes from neutrophils. These inflammatory products are present in the sputum from patients with CF. DNA and F-actin in the sputum copolymerize to form a rigid network that is entangled in the mucin gel. Peptide mucolytics degrade these filaments, although they leave the glycoprotein network relatively intact. Gelsolin, an 85-kDa actin-severing peptide, decreases the viscosity of CF sputum in a dose-dependent manner. However, clinical trials of this drug failed to show any benefit, most likely because of the

large size and rigidity of the protein, which makes it susceptible to degeneration with aerosolization. Thymosin β₄, a much smaller peptide, decreases sputum cohesivity and viscosity in a dose-dependent and time-dependent manner.[94,95] In vitro studies have shown that administration of F-actin-depolymerizing agents along with dornase alfa results in greater reduction in sputum cohesivity and viscoelasticity than administration of either agent alone.[96,97] Actin-depolymerizing agents destabilize the actin-DNA filament network and increase the depolymerizing activity of dornase alfa on the DNA filaments.

Expectorants

KEY POINT

Potassium iodide and glycerol guaiacolate are considered *expectorants*, rather than mucolytics, but these drugs have not been shown to be effective for treating acute or chronic airway disease.

Iodide-Containing Agents

Iodide-containing agents (e.g., supersaturated potassium iodide [SSKI]) are generally considered to be **expectorants**. They are thought to stimulate the secretion of airway fluid. Iodopropylidene glycerol (IPG) may acutely increase tracheobronchial clearance as measured by radiolabeled aerosol in patients with CB.[98] However, in a double-blinded cross-over study in subjects with stable CB, therapy with IPG failed to show any improvement in pulmonary function, gas trapping, or sputum properties and this medication has subsequently been taken off the market.[99]

Sodium Bicarbonate

Sodium bicarbonate (2%) is a base that has occasionally been used for direct tracheal irrigation or as an aerosol. The inflammation caused by bicarbonate is thought to draw water into secretions, but this has not been shown clinically. Local bronchial irritation may occur with a bronchial pH greater than 8.0. Sodium bicarbonate has not been shown to improve airway mucus clearance.

Guaifenesin

Guaifenesin is usually considered to be an expectorant rather than a mucolytic. It can be ciliotoxic when applied directly to the respiratory epithelium.[100] It is thought that the expectorant action of guaifenesin is mediated by stimulation of the gastrointestinal tract and not by systemic exposure to the drug.[101]

Guaifenesin has been approved as an expectorant by the FDA in a bilayer extended-release tablet (Mucinex, Reckitt Benckiser). A large study of this drug in adults with acute infectious bronchitis failed to show any significant differences in sputum volume, sputum properties, or symptom resolution compared with a placebo.[102] One study suggested that, as an adjunctive therapy for patients taking antibiotics with upper airway infections, guaifenesin/

pseudoephedrine shortened time to relief and improved symptoms for nasal congestion and sinus headache better than a placebo.[103] Guaifenesin may cause nephrolithiasis.[104]

Dissociating Solvents

Urea is a dissociating agent that can break ionic and hydrogen bonds. In mucin gels, urea disrupts the hydrogen bonds between the oligosaccharide side chains of the neighboring mucus molecules, with subsequent decrease in the physical entanglements between the molecules and decreased viscosity of the mucus. Urea may also decrease the interaction between DNA molecules. Because the mucolytic action of urea occurs only at very high concentrations of urea (3 to 8 mol/L),[105,106] it is inappropriate for human use.

Oligosaccharides

Oligosaccharide side chains constitute about 80% of the mucin structure. These hydrogen bonds are weak and can be disrupted by agents such as dextran, mannitol, and lactose. The lower molecular weight fractions of dextran are primarily responsible for the mucoactive effects of dextran. Furthermore, an osmotic effect of dextran with increased hydration of the mucus could possibly improve clearance of secretions. Dextran administration via aerosol has been shown to improve tracheal mucus velocity in dogs.[107]

Mannitol administered by dry powder inhaler (DPI) (Bronchitol) has been approved in Australia and Europe for treatment of CF and non-CF bronchiectasis. Clinical studies have shown Bronchitol to be safe and well tolerated for treating patients with CF or bronchiectasis. However, because some children with CF have acute decrease in pulmonary function (bronchial hyperreactivity) with inhaled mannitol, similar to hyperosmolar saline,[108] it is important to pretreat with a short-acting bronchodilator before use.

The charged oligosaccharide heparin has a greater mucolytic and mucokinetic capacity compared with the neutral oligosaccharide dextran. Heparin may cause hydrogen bond disruption and improved ionic interactions. Aerosolized low-molecular-weight heparin shows promise in the treatment of asthma, presumably by interfering with antigen-receptor binding.[109] Aerosolized heparin has also been used effectively to prevent airway cast formation in persons with plastic bronchitis.

P2Y₂ Agonists

Cl^- conductance through the Ca^{2+}-dependent Cl^- channels is preserved in the CF airway. The tricyclic nucleotides UTP and ATP regulate ion transport through $P2Y_2$ purinergic receptors, which increase intracellular calcium. UTP aerosol, alone or in combination with amiloride, increases the transepithelial potential difference and the clearance of inhaled radioaerosol.[110] Denufosol is an agent that stimulates this Cl^- secretion pathway; however, clinical trials of denufosol for the therapy of CF failed to meet the primary objective (lung function) end points and the drug has been withdrawn from further clinical study.

Mucokinetic agents increase cough clearance by increasing expiratory airflow or by reducing sputum adhesivity and tenacity.

Bronchodilators

Beta agonists increase ciliary beat frequency, but this has no significant effect on mucus clearance. Of greater importance is that these medications can increase expiratory airflow in individuals with an asthmatic component of airway disease.[111] However, airway muscle relaxation can also decrease expiratory airflow by producing dynamic airway collapse in persons with "floppy airways," such as those with bronchomalacia or tracheomalacia. Beta agonists are also mucus secretagogues and therefore can *potentially* increase mucus plugging if they increase dynamic collapse and decrease expiratory airflow.

Surface-Active Phospholipids

Surfactant is produced in the conducting airways and in the alveoli and is important for mucociliary and cough clearance. A surfactant sheet between the periciliary fluid and the mucus gel prevents airway dehydration, permits mucus spreading on extrusion from glands, and allows efficient ciliary coupling with mucus and, more importantly, ciliary release from mucus once kinetic energy is transmitted. With airway inflammation, surfactant can be degraded by phospholipases, and inflammatory peptides can inhibit surfactant function further. In the absence of surfactant, mucus sticks to the epithelium, rendering cough less effective. There is severe loss of surfactant in the inflamed airway of patients with CB or CF.[112,113]

It has been reported in a randomized, multicenter study that surfactant aerosol improves pulmonary function and sputum transportability in patients with CB and that this effect is dose-dependent. No significant side effects were attributable to the surfactant therapy.[114] As a wetting and spreading agent, surfactant also has the ability to increase the lower airway deposition of other aerosol medications, such as dornase alfa or gene therapy vectors, and may increase small particle translocation through the mucus layer.[115]

MUCOREGULATORY MEDICATIONS

Another approach to reducing the burden of airway secretions is to decrease hypersecretion by goblet cells and submucosal glands. Medications that decrease mucus hypersecretion are referred to as **mucoregulatory agents**. These medications include antiinflammatory drugs such as corticosteroids, which are effective at decreasing the inflammatory stimulus that leads to mucus hypersecretion. Aerosolized indomethacin has also been used in Japan to treat patients with mucus hypersecretion.[61]

Anticholinergic medications are also used as mucoregulatory medications. Atropine is routinely given perioperatively to prevent laryngospasm and to decrease mucus secretion associated with endotracheal intubation. Atropine and its derivatives are mucoregulatory medications because they do not "dry" secretions or increase viscosity, but they do decrease hypersecretion that is mediated through muscarinic cholinergic stimulation. The quaternary ammonium derivatives of atropine, including ipratropium bromide and tiotropium, do not significantly cross the blood-airway barrier, and, as such, their use is not associated with systemic effects of anticholinergic medications, such as flushing or tachycardia. Studies have also shown that the use of ipratropium is associated with a reduction in the volume of mucus secretion in patients with CB.[116] Tiotropium is now widely used in patients with CB and there is increasing evidence that it is also effective in patients with asthma.[117]

The mucoregulatory medications include the macrolide antibiotics. These antibiotics were discovered nearly 60 years ago, and derivatives of erythromycin A have been widely used for the treatment of bacterial infection. Since the mid-1960s, data have been accumulating showing that these medications also have immunomodulatory properties; they decrease hyperimmunity or inflammation to more normal and beneficial levels. The mechanism for these properties is different from that of corticosteroids.

The immunomodulatory and mucoregulatory properties of macrolide antibiotics have been exploited for the treatment of DPB, a chronic inflammatory airway disease with great morbidity and mortality when untreated. DPB has primarily been described in East Asia. The etiology is unknown, but the disease results in chronic sinobronchitis with mucus hypersecretion and debilitation. Antibiotics and corticosteroids are ineffective for the treatment of DPB. By virtue of their immunomodulatory and mucoregulatory properties, the macrolide antibiotics have been shown to be the most effective agents for the treatment of DPB.[118] The 15-member azilide, but not the 14- or 16-member macrolides, is also highly effective for the therapy of CF airway disease.[119,120] Macrolide mucoregulatory properties are now thought to be due to inhibition of ERK $\frac{1}{2}$,[121] which is also in the common mucus secretory pathways from surface activation of the innate immunity toll-like receptor 4 or the EGFR.[122]

OTHER MUCOACTIVE AGENTS

Antiproteases

Patients with CF have increased activity of serine proteases on the respiratory epithelial surface. Neutrophils, when activated or degenerating, release proteases, such as elastase, that can directly damage epithelial cells and impair airway clearance. Neutrophil proteases cause a secretory response from submucosal glands with an increase in mucus production.[123]

Intravenous administration or inhalation of α_1-antitrypsin suppresses the activity of neutrophil elastase and restores the bacteria-killing capacity of neutrophils. Recombinant secretory leukocyte protease inhibitor (rsLPI), when given to a small number of CF patients at a dosage of 100 mg bid for 1 week, decreased neutrophil elastase and interleukin-8 in airway fluid. No significant side effects were reported.[124] It has also been reported that heparin has significant antiprotease activity, as well as activity against the important inflammatory peptide high-mobility group protein B1 (HMGB1).[125] These qualities may account for heparin's antiinflammatory properties and suggest that forms of heparin that do increase the risk of bleeding may be effective for treating diseases like CF or plastic bronchitis.

Hyperosmolar Saline and Mannitol

For many years, sputum induction by hyperosmolar saline inhalation has been used to obtain specimens for the diagnosis of pneumonia. Hypertonic saline has been used as an irritant to induce cough. Hypertonic saline (7%) can improve mucociliary transport and lung function, thought to be largely due to the acute effects of inducing cough and hydrating airway surface fluid.[126,127] In a pilot study, 58 CF subjects were randomly assigned to receive 10 mL of either 0.9% normal saline or 6% hypertonic saline twice daily by ultrasonic nebulization.[128] Spirometry was performed before treatment, at the end of 2 weeks of treatment, and 2 weeks after treatment. At the end of treatment, there was a significant increase in FEV_1 in the hypertonic saline group, with a return to baseline by 28 days. Despite pretreatment with 600 mcg of inhaled salbutamol (albuterol), several patients had an acute decrease in FEV_1 after inhaling hypertonic saline. Similarly, hyperosmolar dry powder mannitol (Bronchital, Pharmaxis) improves quality of life and pulmonary function in adult subjects with non-CF bronchiectasis and significantly improves the surface adhesivity and cough clearability of expectorated sputum.[129]

Studies summarized in the *Cochrane Database of Systematic Reviews* confirm that the long-term use of inhaled hyperosmolar saline improves pulmonary function in patients with CF,[126,130,131] and inhaled hyperosmolar saline or mannitol is beneficial in bronchiectasis.[132] Although this therapy is readily available and inexpensive, it has been reported that hypertonic saline aerosol is not as effective as dornase alfa in the therapy of CF lung disease.[133] In CF, hyperosmolar saline promotes mucus clearance with improvement in pulmonary function and a decrease in respiratory tract exacerbations.[126,130] It is now recommended as part of the treatment regimen for this disease. It is important to note that in a study of COPD patients, there was no clinical improvement using hypertonic saline, but cough or bronchospasm occurred more frequently than in controls.[134]

GENE THERAPY

Gene transfer therapy represents a novel use for aerosols. Efforts in this arena have centered largely on complementary DNA transfer of the normal *CFTR* gene in CF patients. Gene transfer was first attempted by inserting the normal *CFTR* gene into a replication-defective adenovirus vector by bolus bronchoscopic delivery of the vector. An unanticipated host immune response to the vector led to reevaluation of this strategy.[135]

For gene transfer to be effective, the vector and its package must be nonimmunogenic, stable to shear forces during aerosolization, and safe for transfected cells. The vector should not increase cell turnover. It should either stably integrate into the progenitor (basal) cell genome or be safe and effective with repeated administration, and should be able to reach the cellular target of relevance. Part of the difficulty with CF is that its cellular target has not been clearly identified as the epithelial cell, goblet cell, submucous gland, or all of these. The amount of gene and vector and persistence in the airway must also be determined for each vector and delivery system.[136,137]

Viral vectors that have been studied include *adenoviruses*, the *adeno-associated virus (AAV)*, and the *lentivirus*. Adenoviruses naturally target the airway epithelium. AAVs are very small organisms that require a "helper" virus to replicate. These viruses are capable of site-directed insertion into DNA, reducing the risk of insertional mutagenesis (initiating cancer by activation of an oncogene or inactivation of an oncogene suppressor).[138] Lentiviruses are retroviruses, such as human immunodeficiency virus (HIV). They are able to transfect cells that are not terminally differentiated, such as the basal or airway progenitor cell, but insertional mutagenesis is a risk.[139]

The primary nonviral vectors studied to date have been cationic *liposomes*. These lipid capsules are able to form complexes with DNA and then enter cells. With the first generation of liposome vectors, the efficiency of gene transfer was poor; however, this has improved with newer systems.[140,141]

USING MUCOACTIVE THERAPY WITH PHYSIOTHERAPY AND AIRWAY CLEARANCE DEVICES

A guideline for airway clearance therapies (ACT) in CF has been published recommending ACT for all CF patients for sputum clearance, maintaining lung function, and improving quality of life.[142] Although none of the therapies used has been shown to be superior,[143] there may be advantages of particular therapies for individual patients. Patient preference should be considered with the anticipation that this will be associated with greater adherence to therapy.[142]

Many physical factors affect secretion clearance. Cephalad airflow bias is responsible for the movement of mucus in airways during normal breathing.[144-147] The narrowing of airways on exhalation increases the velocity and shearing forces in the airway, creating a cephalad airflow bias with tidal breathing. This bias is amplified during coughing, when increased transmural pressure causes the airways to fold and constrict, increasing airflow velocity further.[147]

In acute airway diseases leading to ciliary dysfunction, mucus hypersecretion, or both, cough is the primary mechanism for secretion clearance from the central airways, and cephalad airflow contributes increasingly to peripheral airway clearance. Cough is one of the most common respiratory complaints of patients seeking medical attention.[148] During a normal cough, the expiratory airflow increases to a maximum along with narrowing of the intrathoracic airways. The narrowing of the airways is a product of high airflows and pressure differentials across the lung. Airflow velocity varies inversely with the cross-sectional area of the airways, creating high linear velocity, increased turbulence, high shearing forces within the airway, and high kinetic energy. These forces shear secretions and debris from the airway walls, propelling them toward the central and upper airway, where they are expectorated or swallowed. In COPD, narrowing airways may close prematurely, trapping gas, reducing expiratory flow, and limiting the effectiveness of the cough. Directed cough or huff (forced expiration with the glottis open) is a primary maneuver in these patients to improve secretion clearance.

Conventional CPT, consisting of chest percussion and directed cough produces greater expectoration than no treatment in patients with CF.[149] There is no evidence that postural or gravity assisted drainage contributes to the effectiveness of airway clearance with CPT and there is a risk of increased gastroesophageal reflux when postural drainage is used.[150] Alternative methods of airway clearance (e.g., positive expiratory pressure [PEP], high-frequency chest wall compression [HFCWC]) all seem to work as well as CPT as long as they include directed cough. The choice between CPT and alternative methods mainly depends on patient preference and the response of the individual patient to treatment.[150]

Insufflation-Exsufflation; Cough Assist

An insufflation-exsufflation device inflates the lungs with positive pressure followed by a negative pressure to simulate a cough.[151] The cycle begins with an inspiratory pressure of 20 to 40 cm H_2O for 1 to 2 seconds, followed by an expiratory pressure of 30 to 40 cm H_2O for 1 to 2 seconds. It can be used with an oronasal mask or attached to an artificial airway. Its primary application has been in patients with muscular weakness unable to cough unassisted. Although anecdotal reports suggest that routine use can decrease the frequency of pneumonia in patients with weak cough, there are no published randomized controlled clinical trials confirming this impression. Early work in COPD suggested benefits, but more recent evidence is lacking.[152]

Active Cycle of Breathing and Forced Expiratory Technique Maneuver

The active cycle of breathing (ACB) technique involves a combination of breathing control, thoracic expansion control (deep breaths), and forced exhalation from progressively increasing lung volumes. Although sometimes used by patients with CF, there are no controlled studies documenting benefits from this mode of airway clearance.[153]

Forced expiratory technique (FET) consists of a breath taken in to mid-lung volume and air quickly exhaled by contracting the chest wall and abdominal muscles with the mouth and glottis kept open. The huff should not be a violent or explosive exhalation.[154,155]

Autogenic Drainage

Autogenic drainage (AD) attempts to progressively increase airflow to move secretions without forced exhalation.[156,157] This technique incorporates staged breathing, starting with small tidal breaths from expiratory reserve volume and repeating until secretions "collect" in the central airways. Patients are instructed to suppress cough. A larger volume of air is taken for a series of 10 to 20 breaths, followed by a series of even larger (approaching vital capacity) breaths, followed by several huff coughs. This technique requires a great deal of patient cooperation and is used only for patients older than 8 years of age and patients who have a good sense of their own breathing. AD can be difficult to teach and administer; application varies in different CF centers, and there are no randomized, controller, clinical trials demonstrating the effectiveness of AD.

Exercise

Exercise causes increased sputum production likely because of increased expiratory flow.[158,159] Exercise seems to augment bronchial hygiene and should be encouraged.

Positive Airway Pressure

Positive airway pressure (PAP) techniques can be effective alternatives to CPT in expanding the lungs and mobilizing secretions. Evidence suggests that PAP therapy is more effective than incentive spirometry or intermittent positive pressure breathing (IPPB) in the management of postoperative atelectasis[160,161] and more effective than HFCWC in treating CF.[162] Cough, FET, and other airway clearance techniques are components of PAP therapy.[163]

Pursed-lip breathing is a procedure that can be used to relieve air trapping caused by collapse of unstable airways during expiration. The resistance at the mouth during a pursed-lip exhalation transmits back pressure to splint the airways open, preventing compression and premature closure (similar to a fixed orifice resistor). Pursed-lip breathing represents a functional predecessor to modern device-based strategies of applying PEP to the airway. Expiratory positive airway pressure (EPAP) is produced as expired air passes through a fixed orifice or threshold resistor. However continuous positive airway pressure (CPAP) has not been shown to improve mucus clearance.[164] By preventing expiratory airway collapse, PAP increases expiratory flow and may improve the distribution of ventilation throughout the lungs, via collateral intrabronchiolar channels.[165-167]

High-Frequency Chest Wall Compression

HFCWC has been shown to enhance secretion clearance. Shearing at the air-mucus interface could enhance tracheal mucus clearance during HFCWC, although there is no demonstrable effect on secretion rheology.[168] Pilot studies suggest that dornase alfa is more effective for CF when given during HFCWC therapy than when given before or after therapy.[169] Although there are now four HFCWC devices available in the U.S. market, differences among these devices appear to be minimal and there are no studies demonstrating superior effectiveness of one device over another. Furthermore, none of these devices has been shown to be effective for therapy of any other airway disease but CF.

Oscillatory Positive Expiratory Pressure

The Flutter mucus clearance device (Aptalis Pharma, Bridgewater, Connecticut) combines the techniques of PEP with high-frequency oscillations at the airway opening. The weight of the ball serves as a PEP device (approximately 10 cm H_2O) and the internal shape of the bowl allows the ball to flutter, generating oscillations of about 2 to 32 Hz, varying with the position of the device. The proposed mechanism of effect includes shearing of mucus from the airway wall by oscillatory action; stabilization of airways, preventing early airway closure; and facilitation of cephalad flow of mucus.

Although the Flutter has been available for 20 years, little has been published on its efficacy.[163] In a small acute intervention study,[170] the amount of sputum expectorated by subjects with CF was greater than the amount expectorated with either voluntary cough or postural drainage. Another study reported that Flutter therapy was an acceptable alternative to conventional CPT in hospitalized patients with CF.[171] However, these results have not been confirmed by other studies, the relevance of expectorated sputum volume to clinical effectiveness is unproven, and most of the more recent studies of the Flutter have not shown it to be effective for airway clearance.[172-176] Device performance varies with changes in expiratory flow and angle of inclination.[177] This lack of efficacy under "real life" conditions may be due to the Flutter device being tiring to use correctly, which results in poor adherence. Similar devices such as the Acapella (Smiths Medical, St. Paul, Minnesota) and the Frequencer (Dymedso, Inc., Boisbriand, Quebec, Canada) may have less technique-dependent performance, but to date any improvement has yet to be reported. We generally do not recommend the use of these devices.

Intrapulmonary percussive ventilation (IPV) of the lungs involves the use of a pneumatic device called a

Percussionator (Percussionaire Corp, Sandpoint, Idaho) with an aim to enhance the mobilization and clearance of retained secretions, and deliver nebulized medications to the distal airways.[178] With IPV, the patient breathes through a mouthpiece that delivers high-flow minibursts at rates exceeding 200 cycles/min. During these percussive bursts of gas into the airway, continuous airway pressure is maintained while the pulsatile percussive intra-airway pressure progressively increases. Each percussive cycle is programmed by holding a thumb button for 5 to 10 seconds for the percussive inspiratory cycle and releasing the button for exhalation. Treatments of approximately 20 minutes are recommended by the manufacturer. Impaction pressures of 25 to 40 pounds-force per square-inch gauge (psig) are delivered at a frequency ranging from less than 100 up to 225 percussive cycles/min at 40 psig. Some small studies have reported comparable results with IPV and standard CPT[179-181] but there are no published long-term randomized controlled studies showing benefits.

Chest Wall Compression

HFCWC was first shown to improve mucus clearance more than 30 years ago and there are now different HFCWC systems on the market; these are similar in operation, and probably in effectiveness. Although this technique is sometimes called high-frequency chest wall *oscillation*, this term is inaccurate and should not be used. These devices consist of a large-volume, variable-frequency air pulse delivery system attached to an inflatable vest that is worn by the patient so that it extends over the entire torso. Pressure pulses that fill the vest and vibrate the chest wall are controlled by the patient and applied during exhalation or throughout the respiratory cycle. Pulse frequency is adjustable from 5 to 25 Hz, with pressure varying from 28 mm Hg at 5 Hz to 39 mm Hg at 25 Hz. However, the compressions can be held at a single frequency between 10 and 15 Hz for the duration of therapy. Theoretically, rapid compression of the chest wall causes transient increases in airflow in the lungs to augment the movement of mucus. The frequency of compression (cycles per second) and flow bias (inspiratory versus expiratory) may influence effectiveness.[182,183] The Vest has been shown to be effective for secretion clearance in patients with CF[184-186] but there are no randomized controlled studies showing effectiveness in other patients, and there may risks to using this device when patients have a weak or ineffective cough.[187]

KEY POINT

Patients with long-term problems of secretion management should be taught as many of these techniques as they can master for adoption in their therapeutic routines.[188]

FUTURE MUCUS-CONTROLLING AGENTS

In the past, mucolytics were targeted only at reducing the viscosity of mucus. In the context of the normal physiology

of ciliary movement, logic suggests that thicker mucus would be moved more efficiently by ciliary contact and elastic recovery than would thin, low-viscosity solutions. The conceptual analogy is that of raking water—little transport occurs. This assumes mucus clearance is being optimized *physiologically*. Endotracheal aspiration of secretions by suction would be easier with low-viscosity mucus. Research supports the theory that elasticity is important for mucus transport.[75,180]

It has been suggested that the treatment of bronchial hypersecretion would be better aimed at *normalizing* the rheologic properties of mucus to improve transport, rather than at simply lysing or liquefying bronchial secretions as is traditionally done. Indeed, cough clearance is enhanced by a cohesive and more viscous secretion that does not stick to the airway wall. In this sense, it can be considered easier to shoot a solid pea from a pea shooter than it would be to shoot pea soup.

Purulent sputum has high elasticity *and* viscosity, and mucolytic agents such as dornase alfa might restore normal transport properties by reducing tenacity, viscosity, and elasticity. With low viscoelasticity (e.g., bronchorrhea), restructuring or cross-linking agents would increase viscosity and elasticity to improve transport. Such agents have been termed **mucospissic agents**.[181,183] Drugs with mucospissic activity include tetracycline.[180] The thickening effect of tetracycline can occur with oral and aerosol administration, although more so with direct aerosol. Tetracycline may bind to mucus proteins to increase viscosity and elasticity, although exact binding sites remain unclear. With adhesive sputum, mucokinetic agents that decrease tenacity and preserve viscoelasticity might be useful.

At present, no drugs are available in the United States as mucus-controlling agents that selectively modify viscosity or elasticity. Further investigation may produce clinically useful agents tailored to specific secretion problems, as illustrated in Figure 9-10. A better understanding of adhesivity and cohesivity, the components of tenacity, has focused attention on control of the abnormal surface properties of mucus and sputum and their role in cough clearance.

RESPIRATORY CARE ASSESSMENT OF MUCOACTIVE DRUG THERAPY

Assessment of drug therapy for respiratory secretions is difficult. FEV_1 is relatively insensitive to changes in mucociliary clearance. Change in gas trapping or the rate of change in lung function over time may be a better way to assess effectiveness. In addition, during maintenance therapy the volume of sputum expectorated is variable from day to day and does not reflect effective therapy. Therefore the following assessments should be performed.

Before Treatment

• Assess patient's adequacy of cough and level of consciousness to determine the need for mechanical

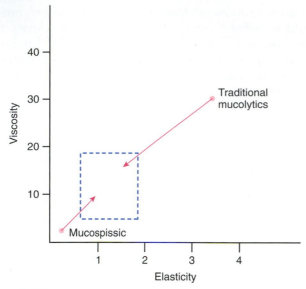

Figure 9-10 Conceptual representation of an optimal range of viscosity and elasticity of mucus for mucociliary transport.

suctioning or need for adjunct bronchial hygiene to clear airway with treatment, or whether treatment is contraindicated.

During Treatment and Short Term

- Instruct and then verify correct use of aerosol nebulization system, including cleaning.
- Assess therapy based on indication for the drug or device.
- Monitor airflow changes for adverse effects, such as a decrease in FEV_1.
- Assess breathing pattern and rate.
- Assess patient's subjective reaction to treatment—that is, changes in breathing effort or pattern.
- Discontinue therapy if patient experiences adverse reactions.

Long Term

- Monitor number and severity of respiratory tract infections, need for antibiotic therapy, emergency visits, and hospitalizations.
- Monitor pulmonary function for improvement or slowing of the rate of deterioration.

General Contraindications

- If the FEV_1 is less than 25% of predicted, it becomes difficult to mobilize and expectorate secretions. Theoretically, with profound airflow compromise, secretion clearance could decrease.
- Use mucoactive therapy with caution in patients with severely compromised vital capacity and expiratory flow, such as in the presence of end-stage pulmonary disease or neuromuscular disorders.

- Gastroesophageal reflux and inability of the patient to protect the airway are risk factors for postural drainage.
- Mucoactive agents should be discontinued if there is evidence of clinical deterioration.
- Patients with acute bronchitis or exacerbation of chronic disease (e.g., CF and COPD) may be less responsive to mucoactive therapy, possibly because of infection and muscular weakness, which can reduce airflow-dependent mechanisms further.

? SELF-ASSESSMENT QUESTIONS

Answers can be found in Appendix A.
1. Identify the mucolytic agents approved for inhalation as an aerosol in the United States—give the generic and brand names.
2. What is the mode of action for dornase alfa?
3. What is the clinical indication for use of dornase alfa?
4. What are contraindications to the use of mucolytic medications?
5. How do macrolide antibiotics affect mucus, and what are their indications for use?
6. How should dornase alfa be administered when high-frequency compression is used?
7. What is a common side effect seen with *N*-acetylcysteine (NAC) by aerosol?
8. What are the indications for the use of acetylcysteine?
9. How and when should bicarbonate aerosol or instillation be used?

📖 CLINICAL SCENARIO

Answers can be found in Appendix A.
A 17-year-old woman with CF was admitted to your hospital with an acute respiratory infection (pulmonary exacerbation). She is pleasant, mature, and well informed concerning her disease. She complains of an increased cough, increased sputum production with some hemoptysis, and weight loss over the past 2 weeks.

History: She was diagnosed with CF at the age of 2 years because of failure to thrive and did well clinically until age 12. She has had a nasal polypectomy and had a G-tube placed for night feeding several years ago, which resulted in a weight gain of 30 lb (13.6 kg). She is chronically infected with resistant *Pseudomonas* and *Staphylococcus,* and she has grown atypical *Mycobacterium* in the past. She has been admitted with exacerbations of CF twice in the past year. She has been taking 300 mg of tobramycin (TSI) bid by aerosol at home regularly this year, with courses of oral ciprofloxacin when symptoms of respiratory infection surfaced.

Physical examination: Vital signs are as follows: temperature (T) 37.5° C, pulse (P) 110 beats/min and regular, respiratory rate (RR) 26 breaths/min, blood pressure

(BP) 110/50 mm Hg. Oxygen saturation by pulse oximetry (SpO$_2$) is 0.92 in ambient air. She has mild dyspnea while walking. Auscultation of the chest revealed crackles in all fields, with more in the right upper lobe. Extremities showed moderate digital clubbing with no cyanosis. She has a cough productive of greenish, thick sputum. No nasal polyps are visible to examination.

Laboratory: Electrolytes were normal, hemoglobin is 14.3 g/dL, hematocrit is 44%, and white blood cell count (WBC) is 13.4 × 10^3 cells/mm^3. Chest radiograph shows diffuse chronic changes with thick interstitial markings consistent with bronchiectasis and a normal cardiac silhouette. There is an infiltrate in the right upper lobe. Her pulmonary function test results show the following:

Observed	% Predicted
Forced vital capacity (FVC)	72
Forced expiratory volume in 1 second (FEV$_1$)	55
Functional residual capacity	121

Hospital course: After her admission, she was treated for the next 21 days with intravenous antibiotics in addition to her usual medications of pancreatic enzymes and vitamin supplements, albuterol by aerosol before chest physical therapy (CPT), nocturnal tube feedings, and oxygen 1 LPM (liter per minute) at night. Her symptoms of dyspnea and her weight improved. She continues to have a productive cough with thick sputum, although the hemoptysis has disappeared. She is clinically stable and is ready to be discharged.

Using the SOAP method, assess this clinical scenario.

REFERENCES

1. Denton R, Forsman W, Hwang SH, et al: Viscoelasticity of mucus: Its role in ciliary transport of pulmonary secretions. *Am Rev Respir Dis* 98(3):380–391, 1968.
2. Sackner MA: Effect of respiratory drugs on mucociliary clearance. *Chest* 73(6 Suppl):958–966, 1978.
3. Puchelle E, de Bentzmann S, Zahm JM: Physical and functional properties of airway secretions in cystic fibrosis—therapeutic approaches. *Respiration* 62(Suppl 1):2–12, 1995.
4. Rogers DF: Mucoactive drugs for asthma and COPD: any place in therapy? *Expert Opin Investig Drugs* 11(1):15–35, 2002.
5. Voynow JA, Rubin BK: Mucins, mucus, and sputum. *Chest* 135(2):505–512, 2009.
6. Reid L, Clamp JR: The biochemical and histochemical nomenclature of mucus. *Br Med Bull* 34(1):5–8, 1978.
7. Basbaum CB: Airway mucin: Chairman's summary. *Am Rev Respir Dis* 144(3 Pt 2):S2–S3, 1991.
8. King M, Rubin BK: Mucus-controlling agents: past and present. *Respir Care Clin N Am* 5(4):575–594, 1999.
9. Nowell JA, Tyler WS: Scanning electron microscopy of the surface morphology of mammalian lungs. *Am Rev Respir Dis* 103(3):313–328, 1971.
10. Luk CK, Dulfano MJ: Effect of pH, viscosity and ionic-strength changes on ciliary beating frequency of human bronchial explants. *Clin Sci (Lond)* 64(4):449–451, 1983.
11. Sleigh MA, Blake JR, Liron N: The propulsion of mucus by cilia. *Am Rev Respir Dis* 137(3):726–741, 1988.
12. Pinnock CB, Graham NM, Mylvaganam A, et al: Relationship between milk intake and mucus production in adult volunteers challenged with rhinovirus-2. *Am Rev Respir Dis* 141(2):352–356, 1990.
13. Basbaum C, Carlson D, Davidson E, et al: NHLBI Workshop summary: Cellular mechanisms of airway secretion. *Am Rev Respir Dis* 137(2):479–485, 1988.
14. Lundgren JD, Shelhamer JH: Pathogenesis of airway mucus hypersecretion. *J Allergy Clin Immunol* 85(2):399–417, 1990.
15. Rose MC, Voynow JA: Respiratory tract mucin genes and mucin glycoproteins in health and disease. *Physiol Rev* 86(1):245–278, 2006.
16. Perez-Vilar J, Boucher RC: Reevaluating gel-forming mucins' roles in cystic fibrosis lung disease. *Free Radic Biol Med* 37(10):1564–1577, 2004.
17. Boat TF, Cheng PW: Biochemistry of airway mucus secretions. *Fed Proc* 39:3067–3074, 1980.
18. Kaliner M, Marom Z, Patow C, et al: Human respiratory mucus. *J Allergy Clin Immunol* 73(3):318–323, 1984.
19. Kaliner M, Shelhamer JH, Borson B, et al: Human respiratory mucus. *Am Rev Respir Dis* 134(3):612–621, 1986.
20. Thornton DJ, Sheehan JK, Lindgren H, et al: Mucus glycoproteins from cystic fibrotic sputum: Macromolecular properties and structural "architecture". *Biochem J* 276(Pt 3):667–675, 1991.
21. Sheehan JK, Richardson PS, Fung DC, et al: Analysis of respiratory mucus glycoproteins in asthma: a detailed study from a patient who died in status asthmaticus. *Am J Respir Cell Mol Biol* 13(6):748–756, 1995.
22. Davies JR, Hovenberg HW, Linden CJ, et al: Mucins in airway secretions from healthy and chronic bronchitic subjects. *Biochem J* 313(Pt 2):431–439, 1996.
23. Button B, Cai LH, Ehre C, et al: A periciliary brush promotes the lung health by separating the mucus layer from airway epithelia. *Science* 337(6097):937–941, 2012.
24. Reid CJ, Gould S, Harris A: Developmental expression of mucin genes in the human respiratory tract. *Am J Respir Cell Mol Biol* 17(5):592–598, 1997.
25. Davies JR, Herrmann A, Russell W, et al: Respiratory tract mucins: structure and expression patterns. *Novartis Found Symp* 248:76–88, 2002.
26. Rose MC, Nickola TJ, Voynow JA: Airway Mucus Obstruction: Mucin Glycoproteins, MUC Gene Regulation and Goblet Cell Hyperplasia. *Am J Respir Cell Mol Biol* 25(5):533–537, 2001.
27. Kirkham S, Sheehan JK, Knight D, et al: Heterogeneity of airways mucus: variations in the amounts and glycoforms of the major oligomeric mucins MUC5AC and MUC5B. *Biochem J* 361(Pt 3):537–546, 2002.
28. Wickstrom C, Davies JR, Eriksen GV, et al: MUC5B is a major gel-forming, oligomeric mucin from human salivary gland, respiratory tract and endocervix: identification of glycoforms and C-terminal cleavage. *Biochem J* 334(Pt 3):685–693, 1998.
29. Thornton DJ, Carlstedt I, Howard M, et al: Respiratory mucins: identification of core proteins and glycoforms. *Biochem J* 316(Pt 3):967–975, 1996.
30. Rose MC, Gendler SJ: Airway mucin genes and gene products. In Rogers DF, Lethem MI, editors: *Airway mucus: basic mechanisms and clinical perspectives*, Basel, Switzerland, 1997, Birkhaeuser Publishing Limited, pp 41–66.
31. Leikauf GD, Borchers MT, Prows DR, et al: Mucin apoprotein expression in COPD. *Chest* 121(5 Suppl):166S–182S, 2002.
32. Williams SJ, Wreschner DH, Tran M, et al: Muc13, a novel human cell surface mucin expressed by epithelial and hemopoietic cells. *J Biol Chem* 276(21):18327–18336, 2001.
33. Pallesen LT, Berglund L, Rasmussen LK, et al: Isolation and characterization of MUC15, a novel cell membrane-associated mucin. *Eur J Biochem* 269(11):2755–2763, 2002.
34. Chen Y, Zhao YH, Kalaslavadi TB, et al: Genome-wide search and identification of a novel gel-forming mucin MUC19/

Muc19 in glandular tissues. *Am J Respir Cell Mol Biol* 30(2):155–165, 2004.

35. Higuchi T, Orita T, Nakanishi S, et al: Molecular cloning, genomic structure, and expression analysis of MUC20, a novel mucin protein, up-regulated in injured kidney. *J Biol Chem* 279(3):1968–1979, 2004.

36. Rogers DF: Airway submucosal gland and goblet cell secretion. In Chung KF, Barnes PJ, editors: *Pharmacology of the respiratory tract*, New York, 1993, Marcel Dekker. Inc.

37. Lopez-Vidriero MT: Airway mucus; production and composition. *Chest* 80(6 Suppl):799–804, 1981.

38. Matthews LW, Spector S, Lemm J, et al: Studies on pulmonary secretions: I. The overall chemical composition of pulmonary secretions from patients with cystic fibrosis, bronchiectasis, and laryngectomy. *Am Rev Respir Dis* 88:199–204, 1963.

39. Dulfano MJ, Adler K, Wooten O: Physical properties of sputum: IV. Effects of 100 per cent humidity and water mist. *Am Rev Respir Dis* 107(1):130–132, 1973.

40. Birrer P: Proteases and antiproteases in cystic fibrosis: pathogenetic considerations and therapeutic strategies. *Respiration* 62(Suppl 1):25–28, 1995.

41. Henke MO, John G, Germann M, et al: MUC5AC and MUC5B mucins increase in cystic fibrosis airway secretions during pulmonary exacerbation. *Am J Respir Crit Care Med* 175(8):816–821, 2007.

42. Henke MO, John G, Rheineck C, et al: Serine proteases degrade airway mucins in cystic fibrosis. *Infect Immun* 79(8):3438–3444, 2011.

43. Clarke LL, Boucher R: Ion and water transport across airway epithelia. In Chung KF, Barnes PJ, editors: *Pharmacology of the respiratory tract: Experimental and clinical research*, New York, 1993, Marcel Dekker. Inc.

44. Boucher RC: Human airway ion transport: Part one. *Am J Respir Crit Care Med* 150(1):271–281, 1994.

45. Boucher RC: Human airway ion transport: Part two. *Am J Respir Crit Care Med* 150(2):581–593, 1994.

46. Knowles MR, Olivier KN, Hohneker KW, et al: Pharmacological treatment of abnormal ion transport in the Airway epithelium in cystic fibrosis. *Chest* 107:71S–76S, 1995.

47. Tomkiewicz RP, Biviji A, King M: Effects of oscillating air flow on the rheological properties and clearability of mucous gel simulants. *Biorheology* 31(5):511–520, 1994.

48. Shah SA, Santago P, Rubin BK: Quantification of biopolymer filament structure. *Ultramicroscopy* 104(3–4):244–254, 2005.

49. Henke MO, Renner A, Huber RM, et al: MUC5AC and MUC5B mucins are decreased in cystic fibrosis airway secretions. *Am J Respir Cell Mol Biol* 31(1):86–89, 2004.

50. Rubin BK, van der Schans CP: *Therapy for mucus clearance disorders*, New York, 2004, Marcel Dekker.

51. Hodgkin JE, Balchum OJ, Kass I, et al: Chronic obstructive airway diseases. Current concepts in diagnosis and comprehensive care. *JAMA* 232(12):1243–1260, 1975.

52. Reid L: Measurement of the bronchial mucous gland layer: a diagnostic yardstick in chronic bronchitis. *Thorax* 15:132–141, 1960.

53. Sturgess J, Reid L: An organ culture study of the effect of drugs on the secretory activity of the human bronchial submucosal gland. *Clin Sci* 43(4):533–543, 1972.

54. Rubin BK, Kishioka C, van der Schans CP, et al: Mucus and mucoactive therapy in chronic bronchitis. *Clin Pulm Med* 5:1–14, 1998.

55. Vestbo J, Prescott E, Lange P: Association of chronic mucus hypersecretion with FEV$_1$ decline and chronic obstructive pulmonary disease morbidity. Copenhagen City Heart Study Group. *Am J Respir Crit Care Med* 153(5):1530–1535, 1996.

56. Turner-Warwick M, Openshaw P: Sputum in asthma. *Postgrad Med J* 63(Suppl 1):79–82, 1987.

57. Rubin BK, Tomkiewicz R, Fahy JV, et al: Histopathology of fatal asthma: drowning in mucus. *Pediatr Pulmonol* (Suppl 23):88–89, 2001.

58. Webber SE, Widdicombe JG: The actions of methacholine, phenylephrine, salbutamol and histamine on mucus secretion from the ferret in-vitro trachea. *Agents Actions* 22(1–2):82–85, 1987.

59. Shimura S, Sasaki T, Sasaki H, et al: Chemical properties of bronchorrhea sputum in bronchial asthma. *Chest* 94(6):1211–1215, 1988.

60. Marom Z, Shelhamer J, Alling D, et al: The effects of corticosteroids on mucous glycoprotein secretion from human airways in vitro. *Am Rev Respir Dis* 129(1):62–65, 1984.

61. Tamaoki J, Chiyotani A, Kobayashi K, et al: Effect of indomethacin on bronchorrhea in patients with chronic bronchitis, diffuse panbronchiolitis, or bronchiectasis. *Am Rev Respir Dis* 145(3):548–552, 1992.

62. Marom ZM, Goswami SK: Respiratory mucus hypersecretion (bronchorrhea): a case discussion—possible mechanisms(s) and treatment. *J Allergy Clin Immunol* 87(6):1050–1055, 1991.

63. Rubin BK, MacLeod PM, Sturgess J, et al: Recurrent respiratory infections in a child with fucosidosis: is the mucus too thin for effective transport? *Pediatr Pulmonol* 10(4):304–309, 1991.

64. Madsen P, Shah SA, Rubin BK: Plastic bronchitis: new insights and a classification scheme. *Paediatr Respir Rev* 6(4):292–300, 2005.

65. Avitabile CM, Goldberg DJ, Dodds K, et al: A Multifaceted Approach to the Management of Plastic Bronchitis After Cavopulmonary Palliation. *Ann Thorac Surg* 98(2):634–640, 2014.

66. Rubin BK, Henke MO: Immunomodulatory activity and effectiveness of macrolides in chronic airway disease. *Chest* 125(2 Suppl):70S–78S, 2004.

67. Horsley A, Rousseau K, Ridley C, et al: Reassessment of the importance of mucins in determining sputum properties in cystic fibrosis. *J Cyst Fibros* 13(3):260–265, 2013.

68. Bush A, Payne D, Pike S, et al: Mucus properties in children with primary ciliary dyskinesia: comparison with cystic fibrosis. *Chest* 129(1):118–123, 2006.

69. Albers GM, Tomkiewicz RP, May MK, et al: Ring distraction technique for measuring surface tension of sputum: relationship to sputum clearability. *J Appl Physiol* 81(6):2690–2695, 1996.

70. King M, Rubin BK: Rheology of airway mucus: Relationship with transport. In Takishima T, Shimura S, editors: *Airway secretion: Physiological bases for the control of mucous hypersecretion*, New York, 1994, Marcel Dekker, Inc., pp 283–314.

71. Rubin BK, King M: Mucus physiology and pathophysiology: Therapeutic aspects. In Derenne JP, Similowski T, Whitelaw WA, editors: *Acute Respiratory Failure in Chronic Obstructive Lung Disease*, New York, 1996, Marcel Dekker, pp 391–411.

72. Rubin BK: Frontiers in mucus clearance. In Goldstein AL, editor: *Frontiers in Biomedicine*, New York, 2000, Kluwer Academic / Plenum Publishers, pp 237–250.

73. Puchelle E, Zahm JM, Duvivier C: Spinability of bronchial mucus. Relationship with viscoelasticity and mucous transport properties. *Biorheology* 20(2):239–249, 1983.

74. Lourenco RV: Bronchial mucous secretions—introduction. *Chest* 63(Suppl):56S, 1973.

75. Dulfano MJ, Adler KB: Physical properties of sputum. VII. Rheologic properties and mucociliary transport. *Am Rev Respir Dis* 112(3):341–347, 1975.

76. Hirsch SR: Airway mucus and the mucociliary system. In Middleton E, Jr, Reed CE, Ellis EF, editors: *Allergy: principles and practice*, vol 2, St. Louis, 1983, Mosby.

77. Kilburn KH: A hypothesis for pulmonary clearance and its implications. *Am Rev Respir Dis* 98(3):449–463, 1968.

78. Marin MG: Pharmacology of airway secretion. *Pharmacol Rev* 38(4):273–289, 1986.

79. King M, Gilboa A, Meyer FA, et al: On the transport of mucus and its rheologic simulants in ciliated systems. *Am Rev Respir Dis* 110(6):740–745, 1974.

80. Shah S, Fung K, Brim S, et al: An in vitro evaluation of the effectiveness of endotracheal suction catheters. *Chest* 128(5):3699–3704, 2005.

81. Rogers DF: Mucus hypersecretion in chronic obstructive pulmonary disease. *Novartis Found Symp* 234:65–77, 2001.

82. Barton AD: Aerosolized detergents and mucolytic agents in the treatment of stable chronic obstructive pulmonary disease. *Am Rev Respir Dis* 110(6 Pt 2):104–110, 1974.

83. Wanner A, Rao A: Clinical indications for and effects of bland, mucolytic, and antimicrobial aerosols. *Am Rev Respir Dis* 122(5 Pt 2):79–87, 1980.

84. Macy AM: Preventing hepatotoxicity in acetaminophen overdose. *Am J Nurs* 79(2):301–303, 1979.

85. Decramer M, Rutten-van Molken M, Dekhuijzen PN, et al: Effects of N-acetylcysteine on outcomes in chronic obstructive pulmonary disease (Bronchitis Randomized on NAC Cost-Utility Study, BRONCUS): a randomised placebo-controlled trial. *Lancet* 365(9470):1552–1560, 2005.

86. McCoy K, Hamilton S, Johnson C: Effects of 12-week administration of dornase alfa in patients with advanced cystic fibrosis lung disease. Pulmozyme Study Group. *Chest* 110(4):889–895, 1996.

87. Wilmott RW, Amin RS, Colin AA, et al: Aerosolized recombinant human DNase in hospitalized cystic fibrosis patients with acute pulmonary exacerbations. *Am J Respir Crit Care Med* 153(6 Pt 1):1914–1917, 1996.

88. O'Donnell AE, Barker AF, Ilowite JS, et al: Treatment of idiopathic bronchiectasis with aerosolized recombinant human DNase I. rhDNase Study Group. *Chest* 113(5):1329–1334, 1998.

89. Henke MO, Saha SA, Rubin BK: The Role of Airway Secretions in COPD—Clinical Applications. *COPD* 3:377–390, 2005.

90. Aitken ML, Burke W, McDonald G, et al: Recombinant human DNase inhalation in normal subjects and patients with cystic fibrosis: A phase 1 study. *JAMA* 267(14):1947–1951, 1992.

91. Shak S, Capon DJ, Hellmiss R, et al: Recombinant human DNase I reduces the viscosity of cystic fibrosis sputum. *Proc Natl Acad Sci U S A* 87(23):9188–9192, 1990.

92. Fiel SB, Fuchs HJ, Johnson C, et al: Comparison of three jet nebulizer aerosol delivery systems used to administer recombinant human DNase I to patients with cystic fibrosis. The Pulmozyme rhDNase Study Group. *Chest* 108(1):153–156, 1995.

93. Ramsey BW, Dorkin HL: Consensus conference: practical applications of Pulmozyme. September 22, 1993. *Pediatr Pulmonol* 17(6):404–408, 1994.

94. Rubin BK, Kater AP, Goldstein AL: Thymosin beta4 sequesters actin in cystic fibrosis sputum and decreases sputum cohesivity in vitro. *Chest* 130(5):1433–1440, 2006.

95. Pollard TD, Blanchoin L, Mullins RD: Molecular mechanisms controlling actin filament dynamics in nonmuscle cells. *Annu Rev Biophys Biomol Struct* 29:545–576, 2000.

96. Vasconcellos CA, Allen PG, Wohl ME, et al: Reduction in viscosity of cystic fibrosis sputum in vitro by gelsolin. *Science* 263(5149):969–971, 1994.

97. Dasgupta B: Rheological properties in cystic fibrosis and airway secretions with combined rhDNase and gelsolin treatment. In Singh M, Savena VP, editors: *Advances in physiological fluid dynamics*, New Delhi, 1996, Narosa, pp 74–78.

98. Pavia D, Agnew JE, Glassman JM, et al: Effects of iodopropylidene glycerol on tracheobronchial clearance in stable, chronic bronchitic patients. *Eur J Respir Dis* 67(3):177–184, 1985.

99. Rubin BK, Ramirez O, Ohar JA: Iodinated glycerol has no effect on pulmonary function, symptom score, or sputum properties in patients with stable chronic bronchitis. *Chest* 109(2):348–352, 1996.

100. Rubin BK: An in vitro comparison of the mucoactive properties of guaifenesin, iodinated glycerol, surfactant, and albuterol. *Chest* 116(1):195–200, 1999.

101. Kagan L, Lavy E, Hoffman A: Effect of mode of administration on guaifenesin pharmacokinetics and expectorant action in the rat model. *Pulm Pharmacol Ther* 22(3):260–265, 2009.

102. Hoffer-Schaefer A, Rozycki HJ, Yopp MA, et al: Guaifenesin has no effect on sputum volume or sputum properties in adolescents and adults with acute respiratory tract infections. *Respir Care* 59(5):631–636, 2014.

103. LaForce C, Gentile DA, Skoner DP: A randomized, double-blind, parallel-group, multicenter, placebo-controlled study of the safety and efficacy of extended-release guaifenesin/pseudoephedrine hydrochloride for symptom relief as an adjunctive therapy to antibiotic treatment of acute respiratory infections. *Postgrad Med* 120(2):53–59, 2008.

104. Bennett S, Hoffman N, Monga M: Ephedrine- and guaifenesin-induced nephrolithiasis. *J Altern Complement Med* 10(6):967–969, 2004.

105. Waldron-Edward D, Skoryna SC: The mucolytic activity of amides. A new approach to mucus dispersion. *Can Med Assoc J* 94(23):1249–1256, 1966.

106. Marriott C, Richards JH: The effects of storage and of potassium iodide, urea, N-acetyl-cysteine and triton X-100 on the viscosity of bronchial mucus. *Br J Dis Chest* 68(0):171–182, 1974.

107. Feng W, Garrett H, Speert DP, et al: Improved clearability of cystic fibrosis sputum with dextran treatment in vitro. *Am J Respir Crit Care Med* 157(3 Pt 1):710–714, 1998.

108. Minasian C, Wallis C, Metcalfe C, et al: Bronchial provocation testing with dry powder mannitol in children with cystic fibrosis. *Pediatr Pulmonol* 43(11):1078–1084, 2008.

109. Ahmed T, Garrigo J, Danta I: Preventing bronchoconstriction in exercise-induced asthma with inhaled heparin. *N Engl J Med* 329(2):90–95, 1993.

110. Stutts MJ, Fitz JG, Paradiso AM, et al: Multiple modes of regulation of airway epithelial chloride secretion by extracellular ATP. *Am J Physiol* 267(5 Pt 1):C1442–C1451, 1994.

111. Newhouse MT: Primary ciliary dyskinesia: what has it taught us about pulmonary disease? *Eur J Respir Dis Suppl* 127:151–156, 1983.

112. Girod S, Galabert C, Lecuire A, et al: Phospholipid composition and surface-active properties of tracheobronchial secretions from patients with cystic fibrosis and chronic obstructive pulmonary diseases. *Pediatr Pulmonol* 13(1):22–27, 1992.

113. Griese M, Essl R, Schmidt R, et al: Sequential analysis of surfactant, lung function and inflammation in cystic fibrosis patients. *Respir Res* 6:133, 2005.

114. Anzueto A, Jubran A, Ohar JA, et al: Effects of aerosolized surfactant in patients with stable chronic bronchitis: a prospective randomized controlled trial. *JAMA* 278(17):1426–1431, 1997.

115. Schurch S, Gehr P, Im HV, et al: Surfactant displaces particles toward the epithelium in airways and alveoli. *Respir Physiol* 80(1):17–32, 1990.

116. Tamaoki J, Chiyotani A, Tagaya E, et al: Effect of long term treatment with oxitropium bromide on airway secretion in chronic bronchitis and diffuse panbronchiolitis. *Thorax* 49(6):545–548, 1994.

117. Kerstjens HAM, Engel M, Dahl R, et al: Tiotropium in asthma poorly controlled with standard combination therapy. *N Engl J Med* 367(13):1198–1207, 2012.

118. Shinkai M, Rubin BK: A global perspective on macrolide use. *Jpn J Antibiot* 58:129, 2005.

119. Shinkai M, Park CS, Rubin BK: Immunomodulatory effects of macrolide antibiotics. *Clin Pulm Med* 12(6):341–348, 2005.

120. Jaffe A, Bush A: Anti-inflammatory effects of macrolides in lung disease. *Pediatr Pulmonol* 31(6):464–473, 2001.

121. Shinkai M, Henke MO, Rubin BK: Macrolide antibiotics as immunomodulatory medications: Proposed mechanisms of action. *Pharmacol Ther* 117(3):393–405, 2008.

122. Kanoh S, Rubin BK: Mechanisms of action and clinical application of macrolides as immunomodulatory medications. *Clin Microbiol Rev* 23(3):590–615, 2010.

123. Kishioka C, Okamoto K, Kim J, et al: Regulation of secretion from mucous and serous cells in the excised ferret trachea. *Respir Physiol* 126(2):163–171, 2001.

124. McElvaney NG, Nakamura H, Birrer P, et al: Modulation of airway inflammation in cystic fibrosis. In vivo suppression of interleukin-8 levels on the respiratory epithelial surface by aerosolization of recombinant secretory leukoprotease inhibitor. *J Clin Invest* 90:1296–1301, 1992.

125. Griffin KL, Fischer BM, Kummarapurugu AB, et al: 2-O, 3-O-desulfated heparin inhibits neutrophil elastase-induced HMGB-1 secretion and airway inflammation. *Am J Respir Cell Mol Biol* 50(4):684–689, 2014.

126. Donaldson SH, Bennett WD, Zeman KL, et al: Mucus clearance and lung function in cystic fibrosis with hypertonic saline. *N Engl J Med* 354(3):241–250, 2006.

127. Robinson M, Hemming AL, Regnis JA, et al: Effect of increasing doses of hypertonic saline on mucociliary clearance in patients with cystic fibrosis. *Thorax* 52(10):900–903, 1997.

128. Eng PA, Morton J, Douglass JA, et al: Short-term efficacy of ultrasonically nebulized hypertonic saline in cystic fibrosis. *Pediatr Pulmonol* 21(2):77–83, 1996.

129. Daviskas E, Anderson SD, Gomes K, et al: Inhaled mannitol for the treatment of mucociliary dysfunction in patients with bronchiectasis: effect on lung function, health status and sputum. *Respirology* 10(1):46–56, 2005.

130. Elkins MR, Robinson M, Rose BR, et al: A controlled trial of long-term inhaled hypertonic saline in patients with cystic fibrosis. *N Engl J Med* 354(3):229–240, 2006.

131. Wark PA, McDonald V, Jones AP: Nebulised hypertonic saline for cystic fibrosis. *Cochrane Database Syst Rev* (3):CD001506, 2005.

132. Wills P, Greenstone M: Inhaled hyperosmolar agents for bronchiectasis. *Cochrane Database Syst Rev* (1):CD002996, 2002.

133. Suri R, Metcalfe C, Lees B, et al: Comparison of hypertonic saline and alternate-day or daily recombinant human deoxyribonuclease in children with cystic fibrosis: a randomised trial. *Lancet* 358(9290):1316–1321, 2001.

134. Valderramas SR, Atallah AN: Effectiveness and safety of hypertonic saline inhalation combined with exercise training in patients with chronic obstructive pulmonary disease: a randomized trial. *Respir Care* 54(3):327–333, 2009.

135. Knowles MR, Hohneker KW, Zhou Z, et al: A controlled study of adenoviral-vector-mediated gene transfer in the nasal epithelium of patients with cystic fibrosis. *N Engl J Med* 333(13):823–831, 1995.

136. Rochat T, Morris MA: Gene therapy for cystic fibrosis by means of aerosol. *J Aerosol Med* 15(2):229–235, 2002.

137. Flotte TR, Laube BL: Gene therapy in cystic fibrosis. *Chest* 120(3 Suppl):124S–131S, 2001.

138. Moss RB, Rodman D, Spencer LT, et al: Repeated adeno-associated virus serotype 2 aerosol-mediated cystic fibrosis transmembrane regulator gene transfer to the lungs of patients with cystic fibrosis: a multicenter, double-blind, placebo-controlled trial. *Chest* 125(2):509–521, 2004.

139. Copreni E, Penzo M, Carrabino S, et al: Lentivirus-mediated gene transfer to the respiratory epithelium: a promising approach to gene therapy of cystic fibrosis. *Gene Ther* 11(Suppl 1):S67–S75, 2004.

140. Eastman SJ, Scheule RK: Cationic lipid: pDNA complexes for the treatment of cystic fibrosis. *Curr Opin Mol Ther* 1(2):186–196, 1999.

141. Montier T, Delepine P, Pichon C, et al: Non-viral vectors in cystic fibrosis gene therapy: progress and challenges. *Trends Biotechnol* 22(11):586–592, 2004.

142. Flume PA, Robinson KA, O'Sullivan BP, et al: Cystic fibrosis pulmonary guidelines: airway clearance therapies. *Respir Care* 54(4):522–537, 2009.

143. Strickland SL, Rubin BK, Drescher GS, et al: AARC clinical practice guideline: effectiveness of nonpharmacologic airway clearance therapies in hospitalized patients. *Respir Care* 58(12):2187–2193, 2013.

144. King M, Kelly S, Cosio M: Alteration of airway reactivity by mucus. *Respir Physiol* 62(1):47–59, 1985.

145. Gross D, Zidulka A, O'Brien C, et al: Peripheral mucociliary clearance with high-frequency chest wall compression. *J Appl Physiol* 58(4):1157–1163, 1985.

146. Warwick WJ: Mechanisms of mucous transport. *Eur J Respir Dis Suppl* 127:162–167, 1983.

147. Camner P: Studies on the removal of inhaled particles from the lungs by voluntary coughing. *Chest* 80(6 Suppl):824–827, 1981.

148. Irwin RS, Madison JM: The diagnosis and treatment of cough. *N Engl J Med* 343(23):1715–1721, 2000.

149. van der Schans CP: Conventional chest physical therapy for obstructive lung disease. *Respir Care* 52(9):1198–1206, 2007.

150. Thomas J, Cook DJ, Brooks D: Chest physical therapy management of patients with cystic fibrosis. A meta-analysis. *Am J Respir Crit Care Med* 151(3 Pt 1):846–850, 1995.

151. Bach JR: Update and perspective on noninvasive respiratory muscle aids. Part 2: The expiratory aids. *Chest* 105(5):1538–1544, 1994.

152. Homnick DN: Mechanical insufflation-exsufflation for airway mucus clearance. *Respir Care* 52(10):1296–1305, 2007.

153. Fink JB: Forced expiratory technique, directed cough, and autogenic drainage. *Respir Care* 52(9):1210–1221, 2007.

154. Hasani A, Pavia D, Agnew JE, et al: Regional lung clearance during cough and forced expiration technique (FET): effects of flow and viscoelasticity. *Thorax* 49(6):557–561, 1994.

155. Hasani A, Pavia D, Agnew JE, et al: Regional mucus transport following unproductive cough and forced expiration technique in patients with airways obstruction. *Chest* 105(5):1420–1425, 1994.

156. Chevaillier J: Autogenic Drainage (AD). In Lawson D, editor: *Cystic Fibrosis: horizons*, vol 235, Chichester, 1984, John Wiley.

157. Shom MH: Autogenic Drainage: a modern approach to physiotherapy in cystic fibrosis. *J R Soc Med* 82(Suppl 16):32–37, 1989.

158. Salh W, Bilton D, Dodd M, et al: Effect of exercise and physiotherapy in aiding sputum expectoration in adults with cystic fibrosis. *Thorax* 44(12):1006–1008, 1989.

159. Zach MS, Purrer B, Oberwaldner B: Effect of swimming on forced expiration and sputum clearance in cystic fibrosis. *Lancet* 2(8257):1201–1203, 1981.

160. Bilton D, Dodd M, Webb AK: Evaluation of exercise as an adjunct to physiotherapy in the treatment of cystic fibrosis in the treatment of cystic fibrosis. *Thorax* 44:859, 1989.

161. Ricksten SE, Bengtsson A, Soderberg C, et al: Effects of periodic positive airway pressure by mask on postoperative pulmonary function. *Chest* 89(6):774–781, 1986.

162. McIlwaine MP, Alarie N, Davidson GF, et al: Long-term multicentre randomised controlled study of high frequency chest wall oscillation versus positive expiratory pressure mask in cystic fibrosis. *Thorax* 68(8):746–751, 2013.

163. Myers TR: Positive expiratory pressure and oscillatory positive expiratory pressure therapies. *Respir Care* 52(10):1308–1326, discussion 1327, 2007.

164. Aquino ES, Shimura F, Santos AS, et al: CPAP has no effect on clearance, sputum properties, or expectorated volume in cystic fibrosis. *Respir Care* 57(11):1914–1919, 2012.

165. Frischknecht-Christensen E, Norregaard O, Dahl R: Treatment of bronchial asthma with terbutaline inhaled by conespacer combined with positive expiratory pressure mask. *Chest* 100(2):317–321, 1991.

166. Andersen JB, Qvist J, Kann T: Recruiting collapsed lung through collateral channels with positive end-expiratory pressure. *Scand J Respir Dis* 60(5):260–266, 1979.

167. Andersen JB, Jespersen W: Demonstration of intersegmental respiratory bronchioles in normal human lungs. *Eur J Respir Dis* 61(6):337–341, 1980.

168. Dasgupta B, Tomkiewicz RP, Boyd WA, et al: Effects of combined treatment with rhDNase and airflow oscillations on spinnability of cystic fibrosis sputum in vitro. *Pediatr Pulmonol* 20(2):78–82, 1995.

169. van Hengstum M, Festen J, Beurskens C, et al: No effect of oral high frequency oscillation combined with forced expiration manoeuvres on tracheobronchial clearance in chronic bronchitis. *Eur Respir J* 3(1):14–18, 1990.

170. Konstan MW, Stern RC, Doershuk CF: Efficacy of the Flutter device for airway mucus clearance in patients with cystic fibrosis. *J Pediatr* 124(5 Pt 1):689–693, 1994.

171. Gondor M, Nixon PA, Mutich R, et al: Comparison of Flutter device and chest physical therapy in the treatment of cystic fibrosis pulmonary exacerbation. *Pediatr Pulmonol* 28(4):255–260, 1999.

172. Mahesh VK, McDougal JA, Haluszka L: Efficacy of the Flutter device for airway mucus clearance in patients with cystic fibrosis. *J Pediatr* 128(1):165–166, 1996.

173. App EM, Kieselmann R, Reinhardt D, et al: Sputum rheology changes in cystic fibrosis lung disease following two different types of physiotherapy: flutter vs autogenic drainage. *Chest* 114(1):171–177, 1998.

174. Pryor JA, Webber BA, Hodson ME, et al: The Flutter VRP1 as an adjunct to chest physiotherapy in cystic fibrosis. *Respir Med* 88(9):677–681, 1994.

175. Homnick DN, Anderson K, Marks JH: Comparison of the flutter device to standard chest physiotherapy in hospitalized patients with cystic fibrosis: a pilot study. *Chest* 114(4):993–997, 1998.

176. Girard JP, Terki N: The Flutter VRP1: a new personal pocket therapeutic device used as an adjunct to drug therapy in the management of bronchial asthma. *J Investig Allergol Clin Immunol* 4(1):23–27, 1994.

177. Alves LA, Pitta F, Brunetto AF: Performance analysis of the Flutter VRP1 under different flows and angles. *Respir Care* 53(3):316–323, 2008.

178. McInturff SL, Shaw LI: Intrapulmonary Percussive Ventilation. *Respir Care* 30:884–885, 1985.

179. Natale JE, Pfeifle J, Homnick DN: Comparison of intrapulmonary percussive ventilation and chest physiotherapy. A pilot study in patients with cystic fibrosis. *Chest* 105(6):1789–1793, 1994.

180. Homnick DN, White F, de Castro C: Comparison of effects of an intrapulmonary percussive ventilator to standard aerosol and chest physiotherapy in treatment of cystic fibrosis. *Pediatr Pulmonol* 20(1):50–55, 1995.

181. Newhouse PA, White F, Marks JH, et al: The intrapulmonary percussive ventilator and Flutter device compared to standard chest physiotherapy in patients with cystic fibrosis. *Clin Pediatr (Phila)* 37(7):427–432, 1998.

182. King M, Phillips DM, Gross D, et al: Enhanced tracheal mucus clearance with high frequency chest wall compression. *Am Rev Respir Dis* 128(3):511–515, 1983.

183. King M, Zidulka A, Phillips DM, et al: Tracheal mucus clearance in high-frequency oscillation: effect of peak flow rate bias. *Eur Respir J* 3(1):6–13, 1990.

184. Arens R, Gozal D, Omlin KJ, et al: Comparison of high frequency chest compression and conventional chest physiotherapy in hospitalized patients with cystic fibrosis. *Am J Respir Crit Care Med* 150(4):1154–1157, 1994.

185. Kluft J, Beker L, Castagnino M, et al: A comparison of bronchial drainage treatments in cystic fibrosis. *Pediatr Pulmonol* 22(4):271–274, 1996.

186. Hansen LG, Warwick WJ: High-frequency chest compression system to aid in clearance of mucus from the lung. *Biomed Instrum Technol* 24(4):289–294, 1990.

187. Chatburn RL: High-frequency assisted airway clearance. *Respir Care* 52(9):1224–1235, 2007.

188. McCool FD, Rosen MJ: Nonpharmacologic airway clearance therapies: ACCP evidence-based clinical practice guidelines. *Chest* 129(1 Suppl):250S–259S, 2006.

CHAPTER **10**

Surfactant Agents

Douglas S. Gardenhire

OBJECTIVES

After reading this chapter, the reader will be able to:

1. Define key terms that pertain to surfactant agents
2. List all available exogenous surfactant agents used in respiratory therapy
3. Describe the mode of action for exogenous surfactant agents
4. Discuss the route of administration for exogenous surfactant agents
5. Recognize hazards and complications of exogenous surfactant therapy
6. Assess the use of surfactant therapy

KEY TERMS AND DEFINITIONS

Laplace's law Physical principle describing and quantifying the relationship between the internal pressure of a drop or bubble, the amount of surface tension, and the radius of the drop or bubble.

Prophylactic treatment Prevention of respiratory distress syndrome (RDS) in infants with very low birth weight and in infants with higher birth weight but with evidence of immature lungs, who are at risk for developing RDS.

Rescue treatment Retroactive, or "rescue," treatment of infants who have developed RDS.

Surface tension Attraction of molecules in a liquid-air interface, such as the liquid lining in lung tissue and the air, pulling the surface molecules inward.

Surfactants Agents that reduce surface tension.

Chapter 10 reviews pharmacologic agents termed **surfactants**, which are intended to alter the surface tension of alveoli and the resulting pressures needed for alveolar inflation. The physical principles of surfactants and surface tension forces are reviewed as a basis for introducing agents that have been used or are currently used in respiratory care. The use of current exogenous surfactant agents in the treatment of respiratory distress syndrome (RDS) of the newborn is presented.

PHYSICAL PRINCIPLES

 KEY POINT

Surfactant agents regulate *surface tension* in films at gas-liquid interfaces. The interrelationship of surface tension, drop or bubble size, and pressure is described by *Laplace's law*.

Exogenous surfactants are administered to replace missing pulmonary surfactant in RDS of the newborn. Surface-active agents act on liquids to affect surface tension. The following terms and concepts form the basis for an understanding of the application of surfactant preparations and their effects in the airway.

Surfactant

A surfactant is a surface-active agent that reduces surface tension. Examples include soap and various forms of detergent. Surfactants, or surface-active agents, have also been termed *detergents* for this reason.

Surface Tension

Surface tension is the force caused by attraction between like molecules that occurs at liquid-gas interfaces and holds the liquid surface intact. The units of measure for surface tension are usually dynes per centimeter (dyn/cm), indicating the force required to cause a 1-cm rupture in the surface film. Because the molecules in a liquid are more attracted to each other than to the surrounding gas, a droplet or spherical shape usually results (Figure 10-1, A).

Laplace's Law

Laplace's law is the physical principle describing and quantifying the relationship between the internal pressure of a drop or bubble, the amount of surface tension, and the radius of the drop or bubble (Figure 10-1, B). For a bubble, which is a liquid film with gas inside and out, Laplace's law is as follows:

$$\text{Pressure} = (4 \times \text{surface tension})/\text{radius}$$

In alveoli, there is only a single air-liquid interface, and Laplace's law is as follows:

$$\text{Pressure} = (2 \times \text{surface tension})/\text{radius}$$

Application to the Lung

Because an alveolus has a liquid lining, surface tension forces apply. The higher the surface tension of the liquid, the greater is the compressing force inside the alveolus, which can cause collapse or difficulty in opening the alveolus. In foamy, bubbly pulmonary edema, the surface tension of the liquid allows the formation of the bubbly froth. In both cases—low compliance and pulmonary edema—lowering the surface tension eases alveolar opening or causes the foam bubbles to collapse and liquefy.

CLINICAL INDICATIONS FOR EXOGENOUS SURFACTANTS

Exogenous surfactants are clinically indicated for the treatment or prevention of RDS in the newborn. There are two such treatments:

- **Prophylactic treatment:** Prevention of RDS in infants with very low birth weight and in infants with higher birth weight but with evidence of immature lungs, who are at risk for developing RDS
- **Rescue treatment:** Retroactive, or "rescue," treatment of infants who have developed RDS

The basic problem in RDS is lack of pulmonary surfactant as a result of lung immaturity. This lack of pulmonary

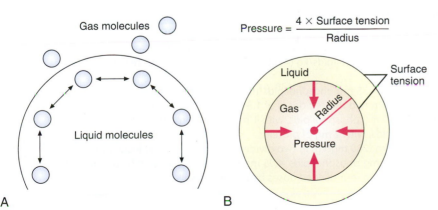

Gas molecules

Liquid molecules

$$\text{Pressure} = \frac{4 \times \text{Surface tension}}{\text{Radius}}$$

Liquid

Gas Radius

Pressure

Surface tension

A B

Figure 10-1 A, The concept of like liquid molecules producing the attractive force resulting in surface tension. **B,** Laplace's law illustrated for a bubble with two air-liquid interfaces. For alveoli (with only one air-liquid interface), the relationship is as follows: Pressure = (2 × surface tension)/radius.

surfactant results in high surface tensions in the liquid-lined, gas-filled alveoli. Increased ventilating pressure is required to expand the alveoli during inspiration, which leads to ventilatory and respiratory failure in an infant without ventilatory support. This concept and the effect of an exogenous surfactant are shown in Figure 10-2. Exogenous surfactants are also being investigated for efficacy in the treatment of acute respiratory distress syndrome (ARDS), acute lung injury (ALI), bronchopulmonary dysplasia (BPD), and meconium aspiration syndrome (MAS).[1] Exog-enous surfactant is not FDA approved for any application in adults or pediatrics.

IDENTIFICATION OF SURFACTANT PREPARATIONS

Table 10-1 lists surfactant formulations that currently have U.S. Food and Drug Administration (FDA) approval for general clinical use in the United States. Detailed differences between these formulations and details of their

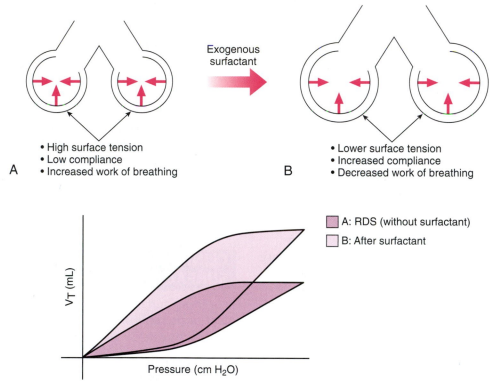

Figure 10-2 *Top:* **A,** Lack of pulmonary surfactant in respiratory distress syndrome *(RDS)* of the newborn results in high surface tension of the alveolar liquid lining and the need for high inspiratory pressures to expand alveoli. **B,** Exogenous surfactants reduce the high surface tension to reduce the pressures needed for alveolar expansion. *Bottom:* Graph illustrating change in the pressure-volume relationship without pulmonary surfactant *(A)* and after exogenous surfactant therapy *(B)*. *V_T,* Tidal volume.

TABLE 10-1	Exogenous Surfactant Preparations Currently Approved for Use in the United States*

DRUG	BRAND NAME	FORMULATION AND INITIAL DOSE
Beractant	Survanta	4- and 8-mL vial, 25 mg phospholipids/mL with 0.5 to 1.75 mg/mL triglycerides, 1.4 to 3.5 mg/mL free fatty acids, and <1 mg/mL protein *Dose:* 100 mg phospholipids/kg (4 mL/kg birth weight) in four divided doses by tracheal instillation
Calfactant	Infasurf	3- and 6-mL vial, 35 mg phospholipids/mL, with 0.65 mg proteins *Dose:* 3 mL/kg in two divided doses of 1.5 mL/kg by tracheal instillation
Poractant alfa	Curosurf	1.5-mL vial, 80 mg phospholipids, with 1 mg of proteins, or 3-mL vial, 160 mg phospholipids, with 2 mg of proteins *Dose:* 2.5 mL/kg (200 mg/kg) in two divided doses by tracheal instillation
Lucinactant	Surfaxin	8.5-mL vial, 30 mg phospholipids, 4.05 mg of palmitic acid, and 0.862 sinapultide *Dose:* 5.8 mL/kg in four divided doses by tracheal instillation

*Individual agents are discussed in a separate section. Detailed information on each agent should be obtained from the manufacturer's drug insert.

dosing and administration are discussed subsequently for each agent in separate sections.

> **KEY POINT**
>
> Four surfactant agents are currently used for treatment of *neonatal RDS*. Beractant (Survanta), calfactant (Infasurf), and poractant alfa (Curosurf) are *modified natural* agents and lucinactant (Surfaxin) is a synthetic agent.

The term *exogenous*, used to describe this class of drugs, refers to the fact that these are surfactant preparations from outside the patient's own body. These preparations may be obtained from other humans, from animals, or by laboratory synthesis. The clinical use of exogenous surfactants has been to replace the missing pulmonary surfactant of the premature or immature lung in RDS of the newborn. These agents have also been investigated for use in ARDS and have been beneficial in improving oxygenation, although results have been inconsistent.[2,3]

Composition of Pulmonary Surfactant

>
>
> **KEY POINT**
>
> Endogenous *pulmonary surfactant* is 90% lipids and 10% protein. The major phospholipid is *dipalmitoylphosphatidylcholine (DPPC)*.

Pulmonary surfactant is a complex mixture of lipids and proteins (Box 10-1). The surfactant mixture is produced by alveolar type II cells. Their primary function, although not their only function, is to regulate the surface tension forces of the liquid alveolar lining. Surfactant regulates surface tension by forming a film at the air-liquid interface. Surfactant reduces surface tension because it is compressed during expiration, reducing the amount of pressure and inspiratory effort required to reexpand the alveoli during a succeeding inspiration. The amount of extracellular (i.e., outside the type II cell) surfactant in animals is 10 to 15 mg/kg of body weight in adults and 5 to 10 times that in mature newborns.[4] Figure 10-3 illustrates the source, basic composition, and regulation of pulmonary surfactant in the alveolus. Each of the major components is described in the following sections.

Lipids

Lipids make up about 85% to 90% of surfactant by weight. The lipid component of surfactant is approximately 90% phospholipids, such as phosphatidylcholine, phosphatidylglycerol, sphingomyelin, and others, and 10% other lipids, most of which is cholesterol.[5] Phospholipids have lipophilic and hydrophilic properties and are able to achieve low surface tensions at air-liquid interfaces. Phosphatidylcholine constitutes about 75% to 80% of the

---

BOX 10-1   Composition of Whole Surfactant From Bronchoalveolar Lavage Fluid (% by Weight)

Lipids (85%-90%)
- Phospholipids (approximately 90%)
- Phosphatidylcholine—half is dipalmitoylphosphatidylcholine (DPPC)
- Phosphatidylglycerol
- Phosphatidylethanolamine
- Phosphatidylserine
- Phosphatidylinositol
- Sphingomyelin
- Neutral lipids (10%)
- Cholesterol and others

Proteins (10%)
- Surfactant protein A (SP-A)
- Surfactant protein B (SP-B)
- Surfactant protein C (SP-C)
- Surfactant protein D (SP-D)

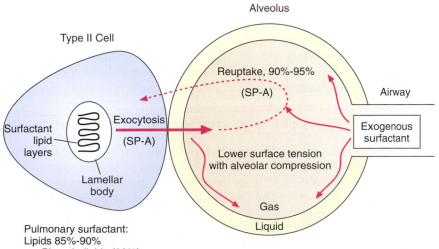

Figure 10-3 Production and reuptake of surfactant by type II cells. Exogenous surfactant is also taken up to become part of the surfactant pool for alveoli.

phospholipids in surfactant, and about half of this is dipalmitoylphosphatidylcholine (DPPC), which is also known as *lecithin*. DPPC is the surfactant component predominantly responsible for the reduction of alveolar surface tension. The hydrophilic choline residue of DPPC is associated with the liquid phase in alveoli, whereas the hydrophobic palmitic acid residue projects into the air phase.[6]

Proteins

> **KEY POINT**
>
> *Surfactant-associated proteins,* such as SP-A, SP-B, and SP-C, regulate the function of endogenous pulmonary surfactant.

The total protein portion of surfactant is about 10% by weight. Approximately 80% of this portion is contaminating serum proteins, and 20% is surfactant-specific proteins (SPs). Four SPs have been identified so far: SP-A, SP-B, SP-C, and SP-D.[4] Proteins of the surfactant mixture are reviewed by Johansson and associates.[7]

All components of surfactant are synthesized by the alveolar type II cell. The type I cell, which is the basic alveolar epithelial cell on 95% of the alveolar surface, has no known role in surfactant synthesis or metabolism. The type II cell also secretes other proteins, such as cytokines, growth factors, and antibacterial proteins, into the alveolar space. The role of the surfactant-associated proteins is well reviewed by Hawgood and Poulain[8] and Possmayer.[9]

Surfactant protein A (SP-A). SP-A is a high-molecular-weight, water-soluble glycoprotein. This protein is specific to surfactant; it has also been denoted as SP-35, apoprotein A, and SAP-35.[4] SP-A seems to regulate secretion and exocytosis of surfactant from the type II cell and the reuptake of surfactant for recycling and reuse.

Surfactant proteins B and C (SP-B and SP-C). SP-B and SP-C are low-molecular-weight, hydrophobic proteins that improve the adsorption and spreading of the phospholipid throughout the air-liquid interface in the alveolus.

Surfactant protein D (SP-D). SP-D is the fourth protein identified in natural endogenous surfactant. Being a large, water-soluble protein, SP-D is similar to SP-A, although differences exist in their molecular configurations.[8] There is no clear role for SP-D in surfactant function at this time, calling into question whether SP-D is correctly designated as a surfactant-associated protein.

Production and Regulation of Surfactant Secretion

> **KEY POINT**
>
> Exogenous surfactant enters the lamellar bodies to replace natural surfactant that is deficient.

The surfactant lipids are synthesized in the alveolar type II cells and stored in vesicles termed *lamellar bodies* (see Figure 10-3). Surfactant in the lamellar bodies is secreted by exocytosis out of the type II cell and into the alveolus. The major stimulus for secretion of lamellar bodies into the alveolar space seems to be inflation of the lung, with a chemically coupled stretch response.[10] SP-A and SP-B facilitate the formation of an intermediate lattice form of surfactant, termed *tubular myelin,* before it reaches the air-liquid interface. SP-C also helps to "break" the lipid layers of surfactant so that adsorption and spreading of the compound as a monolayer proceeds quickly through the air-liquid interface. Surfactant is converted to small vesicles, which can be taken back into the type II cell or taken into alveolar macrophages. The two major alveolar forms of surfactant are large surfactant aggregates (lamellar bodies and tubular myelin–like structures) and small vesicles or aggregates.[11] The secretion of surfactant material from the type II cell is estimated as 10% of the intracellular pool every hour,[12] with an alveolar half-life between 15 and 30 hours.[5] The constant secretion of surfactant is balanced by two clearance mechanisms: endocytosis back into the type II cells and clearance via degradation by alveolar macrophages.[8] In addition, clearance can occur by degradation within the alveoli and by mucociliary removal and transport.[5]

A key feature of surfactant production, which is the basis for the success of replacement therapy with exogenous compounds, is the recycling activity in surfactant production. Most surfactant (90% to 95%) is taken back into the alveolar type II cell, reprocessed, and secreted again. For this reason, exogenously administered surfactant is successful in replacing missing surfactant with one or two doses. The exogenous surfactant is taken into the type II cells and becomes the surfactant pool through the reuptake and recycling mechanism. The reuptake is regulated, at least partly, by SP-A. SPs, or apoproteins, are critical for the surface-active functioning of surfactant and the metabolic regulation of the surfactant pool. This process is well described by Wright and Clements.[6] The normal function of endogenous surfactant also depends on the structural organization of the compound. Smaller surfactant aggregates have less SP-A and are less surface active than larger aggregates.[4]

Pulmonary surfactant has also been found to contribute to host defense by increasing bacterial killing, modifying macrophage function, and downregulating the inflammatory response through decreased mediator release from inflammatory cells.[13] Surfactant also enhances ciliary beat frequency and maintains patency of conducting airways.[11]

Types of Exogenous Surfactant Preparations

Exogenous surfactant preparations can be placed into three categories. These categories and examples of each are listed in Table 10-2 and described in the following sections. A more complete technical description is given by Jobe and Ikegami.[4]

Natural and Modified Natural Surfactant

Natural surfactant is an apt descriptive term for the category of surfactants obtained from animals or humans

TABLE 10-2	Types of Surfactant Preparations and Examples	
CATEGORY	DESCRIPTION	EXAMPLES
Natural	Surfactant from natural sources (human or animal) with addition or removal of substances	Survanta (bovine) Curosurf (porcine) Infasurf (bovine)
Synthetic	Surfactant that is prepared by mixing in vitro–synthesized substances that may or may not be in natural surfactant	Surfaxin
Synthetic natural	Surfactant prepared in vitro by genetic engineering	None at present

by alveolar wash or from amniotic fluid. The large surface-active aggregates of natural surfactant are recovered from the fluid by centrifugation or simple filtration. Because these are natural surfactants, the ingredients necessary for effective function to regulate surface tension are present. Specifically, this includes the surface proteins needed for adsorption and spreading. Depending on the source, natural surfactants can be expensive and time consuming to obtain and prepare. In addition, there is concern over contamination with viral infectious agents or immunologic stimulation and antibody production in response to foreign proteins. Natural surfactant preparations are usually modified by the addition or removal of certain components. Examples of natural surfactants are given in Table 10-2.

The natural surfactant *beractant (Survanta)* is obtained as an extract of minced cow lung, supplemented with other ingredients such as DPPC, palmitic acid, and tripalmitin. The modifications to the natural surfactant material are usually designed to improve functioning in the lung, reduce protein contamination, and provide sterility. Although Survanta contains the hydrophobic proteins SP-B and SP-C, the protein SP-A is missing, and this may shorten the duration of effect.

Another example of a modified natural surfactant is *surfactant TA (Surfacten)*, prepared by Mitsubishi Pharma Corporation in Osaka, Japan, and used by Fujiwara and colleagues in their work.[14] Surfactant TA is a reconstituted chloroform-methanol extract from minced cow lungs, with DPPC and other lipids added. Poractant alfa (Curosurf) is another modified natural surfactant, obtained as a pig lung extract. Calfactant (Infasurf) is a chloroform-methanol extract of fluid lavaged from calf lung; similar to Survanta, it contains the surfactant proteins SP-B and SP-C but not SP-A.[15] Bovactant (Alveofact), not available in the United States, is an organic solvent extract of cow lung lavage containing 99% phospholipids and neutral lipids and 1% SP-B and SP-C.[16]

Synthetic Surfactant

Synthetic surfactants are mixtures of synthetic components. The characteristic feature of artificial surfactants is that none of the ingredients are obtained from natural sources, such as human, cow, or pig lung. Synthetic surfactants do not contain any of the surfactant proteins, including SP-B or SP-C, that are found in the natural preparations. A major advantage of this class of surfactant is its freedom from contaminating infectious agents and additional foreign proteins that may be antigenic to the recipient. A possible disadvantage is the lack of equivalent performance between the organic chemicals substituted for the naturally occurring surfactant proteins, such as SP-A, SP-B, or SP-C.

Colfosceril palmitate (Exosurf), which was the only synthetic surfactant on the market, has been removed.[1] A new synthetic surfactant, lucinactant (Surfaxin), was approved by the FDA in March 2012 for the treatment of RDS. Surfaxin contains similar ingredients compared with Exosurf, such as DPPC and palmitic acid. However, the difference is found in the addition of sinapultide (KL_4 peptide), which is able to mimic SP-B function. Moya and colleagues[17] found that Surfaxin was better at reducing RDS and bronchopulmonary dysplasia than Exosurf. However, there was no difference seen between Surfaxin and Survanta at 24 hours. Surfaxin did demonstrate a larger reduction in RDS-related mortality rates than Exosurf or Survanta. Another study by Sinha and co-workers[18] found no difference between Surfaxin and Curosurf. Surfaxin has been given orphan designation by the FDA for treatment of bronchopulmonary dysplasia. Additionally, lucinactant (Surfaxin) is being studied as a replacement surfactant in an aerosolized form (Aerosurf).

Synthetic Natural Surfactant

An ideal solution to the problems of natural and artificial surfactants would be genetically engineered surfactant produced by recombinant DNA technology. In such a preparation, the phospholipid, lipid, and protein ingredients of the natural surfactant aggregate would be produced by characterizing, via in vitro cloning, the gene or genes responsible for human surfactant. No such products are available for general use at this time, but work progresses on their development. The genes and amino acid sequence for each of the surfactant proteins have been characterized.[19-21] A genetically engineered surfactant that closely resembles the structure and effect of natural human surfactant would be the ideal preparation.

SPECIFIC EXOGENOUS SURFACTANT PREPARATIONS

 KEY POINT

Exogenous surfactants are given either *prophylactically* in RDS or as *rescue* treatment.

Three exogenous surfactant preparations have been approved for general clinical use in the United States at the time of this edition. Each of these preparations is described in greater detail.

Beractant (Survanta)

Beractant (Survanta) is considered a modified natural surfactant. It is a natural bovine lung extract mixed with colfosceril palmitate (lecithin), palmitic acid, and tripalmitin. These three ingredients are used to standardize the composition of the drug preparation and to reproduce the surface tension–lowering properties of natural surfactant. The ingredients are suspended in 0.9% saline. The composition of beractant given in the product literature is described in Table 10-1. The extract from minced bovine lung contains natural phospholipids, neutral lipids, fatty acids, and the low-molecular-weight, hydrophobic surfactant proteins SP-B and SP-C. The hydrophilic, high-molecular-weight protein SP-A is not contained in beractant. SP-A helps regulate surfactant reuptake and secretion by alveolar type II cells. However, the addition of SP-A to beractant by Yamada and colleagues[22] did not improve the biophysical activity (spreading and absorption) or the physiologic activity (lung compliance change) of the mixture.

Beractant is available in a vial containing 4ml or 8 mL of suspension, with a concentration of 25 mg/mL, in a 0.9% sodium chloride solution. The suspension does not require reconstitution. This gives a maximal total dose of 100 mg (4 mL) or 200 mg (8 mL) of phospholipids in a single vial of 8 mL of suspension.

Indications for Use

Specific guidelines for use of beractant are as follows:

- Prophylactic therapy of premature infants less than 1250 g birth weight or with evidence of surfactant deficiency and risk of RDS: The agent should be given within 15 minutes of birth or as soon as possible
- Rescue treatment of infants with evidence of RDS: The agent should be given within 8 hours of age

Dosage

The recommended dose of beractant is 100 mg of phospholipids per kilogram of birth weight. Because there are 25 mg of phospholipids per milliliter in the beractant suspension, this is equivalent to a dose of 4 mL/kg of birth weight. For example, a 2000-g (2-kg) infant would require 8 mL, or the entire vial of suspension.

Repeat doses of beractant are given no sooner than 6 hours later if there is evidence of continuing respiratory distress. The manufacturer's literature recommends that manual hand-bag ventilation *not* be used for the repeat dose in place of mechanical ventilation. Ventilator adjustment may be necessary..

Administration

Beractant suspension is off-white to light brown in color. If settling has occurred in the suspension, the vial can be swirled gently, but it should not be shaken. The suspension is kept refrigerated and must be warmed by allowing it to stand at room temperature for at least 20 minutes. Artificial warming methods should not be used.

The calculated dose is given in four divided aliquots from a syringe and instilled into the trachea through a 5-F catheter placed into the endotracheal tube (ETT). The catheter is removed, and the infant is manually ventilated for at least 30 seconds, or until stable, between doses. The remaining doses are given in similar fashion. During each aliquot, the infant is placed in a different position.

Unopened vials that have been warmed to room temperature may be returned to refrigerated storage within 8 hours. This should be done no more than once. Used vials should be discarded with any residual drug.

Calfactant (Infasurf)

Calfactant (Infasurf) is another modified natural surfactant preparation from calf lung (bovine). It is an organic solvent extract of calf lung surfactant obtained by cell-free bronchoalveolar lavage. The extract contains phospholipids, neutral lipids, and the hydrophobic proteins SP-B and SP-C. The preparation is a suspension, which does not require reconstitution. Its composition is given in Table 10-1. Each milliliter contains 35 mg of total phospholipids, including 26 mg of phosphatidylcholine, of which 16 mg is disaturated phosphatidylcholine; and 0.65 mg of proteins, which includes 0.26 mg of SP-B. The protein SP-A is not contained in the preparation. The formulation is heat sterilized and contains no preservatives.

Indications for Use

Specific guidelines for use of calfactant (Infasurf) are as follows:

- Prevention (prophylaxis) of RDS in premature infants less than 29 weeks gestational age and at high risk for RDS
- Treatment (rescue) of premature infants less than or equal to 72 hours of age who develop RDS and require endotracheal intubation

Dosage

The recommended dose of calfactant is 3 mL/kg of body weight at birth. The dose should be delivered as two divided doses of 1.5 mL/kg. Each 3 or 6 mL of suspension contains enough preparation (105 mg or 210 mg of phospholipids) to treat a 1-kg or 2-kg infant. It is noted in the drug insert that calfactant prophylaxis should be administered as soon as possible, preferably no more than 30 minutes after birth.

Repeat doses, up to a total of three doses, can be given 12 hours apart. Repeat doses as early as 6 hours after the previous dose can be given if the infant is still intubated and requires 30% or greater oxygen for an arterial oxygen pressure (PaO_2) of 80 mm Hg or less (manufacturer's literature).

Administration

Calfactant can be administered to an intubated infant either by side-port delivery or with a catheter. The preparation does not require reconstitution. Calfactant is an off-white suspension that requires gentle swirling or agitation, but not shaking, in the vial to ensure dispersion. Flecks may be visible in the suspension with foaming at the surface.

Side-port adapter. The dose is given in two aliquots of 1.5 mL/kg each. The infant should be positioned with either the right or the left side dependent for each aliquot. The suspension is instilled in small bursts timed to coincide with the inspiratory cycle, over 20 to 30 breaths. It is recommended that the infant be evaluated between repositioning for the second aliquot.

Catheter administration. The dose is divided into four equal aliquots, with the catheter removed between each instillation and mechanical ventilatory support given for 0.5 to 2 minutes. Each aliquot is given with the infant in a different position (prone, supine, right lateral, and left lateral).

Poractant Alfa (Curosurf)

Poractant alfa (Curosurf) is a natural surfactant obtained as an extract of porcine lung. It is a suspension consisting of approximately 99% phospholipids (120 mg of phospholipids in the 1.5-mL vial and 240 mg of phospholipids in the 3-mL vial) and about 1% surfactant-associated proteins, including SP-B.

Indications for Use

Specific guidelines for use of poractant alfa (Curosurf) are as follows:

- For the treatment (rescue) of premature infants with RDS, reducing mortality and pneumothoraces
- Unlabeled uses: Severe MAS in term infants; respiratory failure caused by group B streptococcal infection in neonates

Dosage

The initial dose of poractant alfa is 2.5 mL/kg of birth weight. Subsequent doses of 1.25 mL/kg of birth weight can be given twice at 12-hour intervals if needed. The maximum recommended total dose (initial plus repeat doses) is 5 mL/kg.

Administration

Before use, the vial should be slowly warmed to room temperature. The vial should be turned upside down to disperse the suspension uniformly, without shaking. Poractant alfa does not need to be reconstituted. The dose is administered through a 5-F catheter positioned in the ETT, with the tip in the distal end of the ETT but not extended beyond the end of the ETT.

The dose is given in two aliquots. The infant is positioned with either the right or the left side down for the first aliquot. The catheter is then removed, and the infant is manually ventilated with 100% oxygen for 1 minute. When the infant is stable, the second aliquot is instilled with the alternate side down, after which the catheter is removed. The airway should not be suctioned for 1 hour unless significant airway obstruction is evident.

Lucinactant (Surfaxin)

Lucinactant (Surfaxin) is a synthetic peptide containing surfactant replacement therapy. It is a suspension consisting of 30 mg of phospholipids (22.50 mg of DPPC and 7.50 mg of palmitoyloleoyl-phosphatidylglycerol, sodium salt), 4.05 mg of palmitic acid, and 0.862 mg of sinapultide (KL_4).

Indications for Use

Specific guidelines for use of lucinactant (Surfaxin) are as follows:

- For the prevention of RDS in premature infants at high risk for RDS.

Dosage

The dose of lucinactant is 5.8 mL/kg of birth weight. Subsequent doses may be given up to 4 times in the first 48 hours, not closer than 6 hours apart.

Administration

Before use, the vial should be slowly warmed using a block heater to 44°C (111°F) for 15 minutes. The vial may be kept for 2 hours after removal from the heater and should be vigorously shaken before administering. The dose is administered via syringe through a 5-F catheter positioned in the ETT using a Bodai valve or similar device to allow positive pressure during administration.

The dose is given in four aliquots. The infant is positioned in the right lateral decubitus position with head and thorax inclined upward 30 degrees. After one quarter of the dose is given, ventilate patient until vitals return to normal. Then change to a left lateral decubitus position with head and thorax inclined upward 30 degrees and repeat. Continue changing into the same right and left position until all four aliquots have been delivered, pausing between aliquots to assess the patient. After all aliquots have been given, the head of the patient should be at 10 degrees for at least 1 to 2 hours. The airway should not be suctioned for at least 1 hour unless significant airway obstruction is evident.

MODE OF ACTION

The mode of action of exogenous surfactants is to replace and replenish a deficient endogenous surfactant pool in neonatal RDS. As previously described, endogenous surfactant normally secreted by alveolar type II cells leaves the alveolar space and reenters the type II cells in the form of small vesicles. In the intracellular space, surfactant components are recycled. Exogenously administered surfactant that reaches the alveolar space can be recycled into the type II cells and form a surfactant pool to regulate surface tension.

CLINICAL OUTCOME

There can be a dramatic improvement in oxygenation after surfactant administration, but Davis and associates[23] did not report a corresponding increase in compliance. Although exogenous surfactant should reduce surface tension and increase lung compliance, there is disagreement in the literature over whether the primary clinical effect of exogenous surfactant is one of increasing lung compliance.[24] Fujiwara and colleagues[14] noted that there was clearing of the chest radiograph associated with a good clinical response to surfactant, suggesting that surfactant treatment increased the functional residual capacity (FRC). A study by Goldsmith and associates[25] measured an increase in the FRC within 15 minutes of treatment with natural surfactant, correlating with the time of blood gas improvements. The surfactant stabilizes alveoli on expiration and prevents collapse, increasing residual volume and FRC. An increase in oxygenation would be seen with this effect.[24] An increase in lung volume resulting from improved residual volume and FRC shifts the tidal ventilation to a new pressure-volume curve. At higher lung volumes, chest wall elastic recoil is higher. A shift to the flatter part of the pressure-volume curve could give the same tidal volume for a given pressure change, masking the actual increase in static compliance.[21]

HAZARDS AND COMPLICATIONS OF SURFACTANT THERAPY

KEY POINT

Possible *hazards* to the use of exogenous surfactants include airway occlusion, desaturation, bradycardia, overoxygenation and overventilation, apnea, and pulmonary hemorrhage.

Some complications in exogenous surfactant therapy are due to the dosing procedure, and others can be caused by the therapeutic effect of the drug itself. In the dosing procedure, relatively large volumes of suspension are instilled into neonatal-size airways, and this can block gas exchange, causing desaturation and bradycardia.

The effect of the drug in improving pulmonary compliance can lead to overventilation, excessive volume delivery from pressure-limited ventilation, and overoxygenation with dangerously high PaO_2 levels. As a result, the following complications or hazards can occur with surfactant therapy. In general, complications of prematurity may affect the response to exogenous surfactant.

Airway Occlusion, Desaturation, and Bradycardia

Because the current method of administration is by direct tracheal instillation, a large volume of surfactant suspension may cause an acute obstruction of infant airways, with subsequent hypoxemia and bradycardia.[26] Repetitive small additions of the dose and a transient increase in ventilating pressure may help distribute the surfactant to the periphery.

High Arterial Oxygen Values

A good response to exogenous surfactant results in better (higher) lung compliance, increased FRC, and concomitant improvement in oxygenation. Fractional inspired oxygen (FiO_2) settings must be lowered if PaO_2 improves, to prevent overoxygenation and the possibility of retinopathy of prematurity.

Overventilation and Hypocapnia

As lung compliance improves, peak ventilating pressure, expiratory baseline pressures, and ventilatory rate must be adjusted, or overventilation, leading to *hypocapnia* (low blood carbon dioxide) and pneumothorax, may occur.

Apnea

Apnea has been noted to occur with intratracheal administration of surfactant.

Pulmonary Hemorrhage

Pulmonary hemorrhage seems to be the only consistent pulmonary complication associated with surfactant delivery. Pulmonary hemorrhage seems to be more frequent in infants who are younger, smaller, and with a patent ductus arteriosus (PDA). A causative link has not been found between pulmonary hemorrhage and PDA, and it has not been preventable.

FUTURE DIRECTIONS IN SURFACTANT THERAPY

KEY POINT

Exogenous surfactants are being investigated for clinical use in disease states such as *acute respiratory distress syndrome (ARDS)*, *meconium aspiration syndrome (MAS)*, and *pneumonia*.

In addition to RDS of the newborn, surfactant replacement therapy has been considered in treatment of MAS. In a meta-analysis, Soll and Dargaville[27] reported that surfactant therapy may be beneficial in reducing respiratory illness severity and reducing an infant's need for extracorporeal membrane oxygenation (ECMO).

Surfactant therapy had been studied for various adult respiratory disorders. This topic is comprehensively reviewed by Hamm and colleagues.[5] ARDS in adults is a potential target for surfactant therapy. In RDS of the newborn, the primary abnormality of lung function is related to surfactant deficiency. In ARDS in adults, the surfactant deficiency is secondary to lung injury with complex inflammatory responses.[5] This finding would suggest a difference in clinical response to surfactant therapy between premature infants and adults with ARDS. In addition, dose amount and administration techniques may need to be modified for therapy in adults, who have large lung volumes compared with infants. If lung injury in ARDS is nonuniform in distribution, exogenous surfactant, especially if aerosolized, may distribute unevenly to more compliant lung areas instead of to areas needing surfactant the most.[11]

The availability of newer surfactant preparations, specifically human recombinant surfactants, may offer better results to improve outcomes in adults with ARDS.[21] Finer and colleagues[28] found that lucinactant (Aerosurf) has been successful as an aerosol. The agent has been nebulized using a vibrating mesh for the possible treatment of ARDS in adults and neonates. Other adult respiratory disorders in which either surfactant replacement therapy or abnormal surfactant regulation may occur include pneumonia, lung transplants, sarcoidosis, hypersensitivity pneumonitis, idiopathic pulmonary fibrosis, alveolar proteinosis, obstructive lung disease (e.g., asthma), radiation pneumonitis, and drug-induced pulmonary disease.[29]

RESPIRATORY CARE ASSESSMENT OF SURFACTANT THERAPY

Before Treatment

- Assess the need for surfactant therapy.

During Treatment and Short Term

- Monitor pulse and cardiac rhythm during and after administration.
- Monitor the infant for signs of airway occlusion (desaturation and bradycardia) during and after administration; if obstruction is evident, remove the infant from the ventilator and manually ventilate; in addition, saline lavage and aggressive suctioning to clear the airway may be needed.
- Monitor color and activity level of the infant.
- Monitor chest rise for level of ventilation, or use electronic monitor if available.
- Monitor arterial oxygen saturation and adjust FIO_2 accordingly to prevent hyperoxia or hypoxia.
- Monitor transcutaneous PCO_2 if possible, and be prepared to adjust level of ventilation as needed to prevent hypercarbia or hypocarbia.

Long Term

- Assess lung mechanics (exhaled volumes or peak inspiratory pressures) during mechanical ventilation to determine effectiveness of the exogenous agent in normalizing lung compliance. The instilled drug may cause changes within minutes in some cases.
- Assess the need for repeat dosing.

General Contraindications

- Consider possible hazards if pulse, cardiac rhythm, or arterial/transcutaneous blood gas values deteriorate.

? SELF-ASSESSMENT QUESTIONS

Answers can be found in Appendix A.

1. What is the definition of a *surface-active substance*?
2. In general, what is the clinical indication for use of exogenous surfactants?
3. State the type (category) of exogenous surfactant for each of the following: beractant, calfactant, poractant alfa, and lucinactant.
4. What are the major ingredients of natural pulmonary surfactant?
5. Give the dosage schedule of each of the current exogenous surfactants.
6. What is the difference between "rescue" and "prophylaxis" treatment with surfactants?
7. Identify at least three possible adverse effects with the use of exogenous surfactant treatment.
8. Why does the improvement in lung mechanics last after only one or two administrations of exogenous surfactant?
9. How would you assess the effectiveness of exogenous surfactant treatment in a premature newborn with respiratory distress?

📖 CLINICAL SCENARIO

Answers can be found in Appendix A.

A 16-year-old girl gave birth to a 25-week, 515-g girl by vaginal delivery. The mother had no prenatal care, and she had premature rupture of the membranes 12 days before delivery. Immediately at birth, the newborn was intubated with a 2.5-mm oral ETT. Apgar scores after intubation and application of positive-pressure ventilation with a bag and mask were 7 and 9 at 1 minute and 5 minutes, respectively. After transfer to the neonatal intensive care unit, umbilical venous and arterial catheters were inserted, and the newborn was placed on mechanical ventilation with peak inspiratory pressure (PIP) of 20 cm H_2O, positive end-expiratory pressure (PEEP) of 5 cm H_2O, respiratory rate (RR) of 60 breaths/min, inspiratory time of 0.3 second, and FIO_2 of 1. Physical examination revealed pulse (P) of 140 beats/min,

Continued

blood pressure (BP) of 34/22 mm Hg, temperature (T) of 99.6° F, and SpO$_2$ of 85% to 90%. Laboratory results revealed glucose at 39 mg/dL, white blood cell (WBC) count of 11,900/mm^3, hematocrit of 47%, and platelets at 297,000/mm^3. Chest radiograph showed stage II RDS. *Using the SOAP method, assess this clinical scenario.*

REFERENCES

1. Kattwinkel J: Synthetic surfactants: the search goes on. *Pediatrics* 115:1075, 2005.
2. Davidson WJ, Dorscheid D, Spragg R, et al: Exogenous pulmonary surfactant for the treatment for adult patients with respiratory distress syndrome: results of a meta-analysis. *Crit Care* 10:R41, 2006.
3. Kesecioglu J, Beale R, Stewart TE, et al: Exogenous natural surfactant for treatment of acute lung injury and the acute respiratory distress syndrome. *Am J Respir Crit Care Med* 180:989–994, 2009.
4. Jobe A, Ikegami M: Surfactant for the treatment of respiratory distress syndrome. *Am Rev Respir Dis* 136:1256, 1987.
5. Hamm H, Kroegel C, Hohlfeld J: Surfactant: a review of its functions and relevance in adult respiratory disorders. *Respir Med* 90:251, 1996.
6. Wright JR, Clements JA: Metabolism and turnover of lung surfactant. *Am Rev Respir Dis* 135:427, 1987.
7. Johansson J, Curstedt T, Robertson B: The proteins of the surfactant system. *Eur Respir J* 7:372, 1994.
8. Hawgood S, Poulain FR: Functions of the surfactant proteins: a perspective. *Pediatr Pulmonol* 19:99, 1995.
9. Possmayer F: The role of surfactant-associated proteins. *Am Rev Respir Dis* 142:749, 1990. (editorial).
10. Wirtz HR, Dobbs LG: Calcium mobilization and exocytosis after one mechanical stretch of lung epithelial cells. *Science* 250:1266, 1990.
11. Lewis J, Veldhuizen RAW: Surfactant: current and potential therapeutic application in infants and adults. *J Aerosol Med* 9:143, 1996.
12. Wright JR, Wager RE, Hawgood S, et al: Surfactant apoprotein Mr = 26,000-36,000 enhances uptake of liposomes by type II cells. *J Biol Chem* 262:2888, 1987.
13. Pison U, Max M, Neuendank A, et al: Host defence capacities of pulmonary surfactant: evidence for "non-surfactant" functions of the surfactant system. *Eur J Clin Invest* 24:586, 1994.
14. Fujiwara T, Maeta H, Chida S, et al: Artificial surfactant therapy in hyaline membrane disease. *Lancet* 1:55, 1980.
15. Notter RH, Egan EA, Kwong MS, et al: Lung surfactant replacement in premature lambs with extracted lipids from bovine lung lavage: effects of dose, dispersion techniques, and gestational age. *Pediatr Res* 19:569, 1985.
16. Gortner L, Bartmann P, Pohlandt F, et al: Early treatment of respiratory distress syndrome with bovine surfactant in very preterm infants: a multicenter controlled clinical trial. *Pediatr Pulmonol* 14:4, 1992.
17. Moya FR, Gadzinowski J, Bancalari E, et al, International Surfaxin Collaborative Study Group: A multicenter, randomized, masked, comparison trial of lucinactant, colfosceril palmitate, and beractant for the prevention of respiratory distress syndrome among very preterm infants. *Pediatrics* 115:1018–1029, 2005.
18. Sinha SK, Lacaze-Masmonteil T, Valls i Soler A, et al, Surfaxin Therapy Against Respiratory Distress Syndrome Collaborative Group: A multicenter, randomized, controlled trial of lucinactant versus poractant alfa among very premature infants at high risk for respiratory distress syndrome. *Pediatrics* 115:1030–1038, 2005.
19. Floros J, Phelps DS, Taeusch HW: Biosynthesis and in vitro translation of the major surfactant-associated protein from human lung. *J Biol Chem* 260:495, 1985.
20. Avery ME, Merritt TA: Surfactant-replacement therapy. *N Engl J Med* 324:910, 1991.
21. Rodriguez RJ, Martin RJ: Exogenous surfactant therapy in newborns. *Respir Care Clin N Am* 5:595, 1999.
22. Yamada T, Ikegami M, Tabor BL, et al: Effects of surfactant protein-A on surfactant function in preterm ventilated rabbits. *Am Rev Respir Dis* 142:754, 1990.
23. Davis JM, Veness-Meehan K, Notter RH, et al: Changes in pulmonary mechanics after the administration of surfactant to infants with respiratory distress syndrome. *N Engl J Med* 319:476, 1988.
24. Milner AD: How does exogenous surfactant work? *Arch Dis Child* 68:253, 1993.
25. Goldsmith LS, Greenspan JS, Rubenstein SD, et al: Immediate improvement in lung volume after exogenous surfactant: alveolar recruitment versus increased distention. *J Pediatr* 119:424, 1991.
26. Jobe AH: The role of surfactant therapy in neonatal respiratory distress. *Respir Care* 36:695, 1991.
27. Soll RF, Dargaville P: Surfactant for meconium aspiration syndrome in full term infants. *Cochrane Database Syst Rev* (2):CD002054, 2000.
28. Finer NN, Merritt TA, Bernstein G, et al: A multicenter pilot study of Aerosurf delivered via nasal continuous positive airway pressure (nCPAP) to prevent respiratory distress syndrome in preterm neonates. *Pediatr Res* 59:4840, 2006.
29. Avery ME: Surfactant deficiency in hyaline membrane disease: the story of discovery. *Am J Respir Crit Care Med* 161:1074, 2000.

CHAPTER 11

Corticosteroids in Respiratory Care

Douglas S. Gardenhire

CHAPTER OUTLINE

OBJECTIVES

After reading this chapter, the reader will be able to:

1. Define key terms that pertain to corticosteroids
2. Discuss the indications for inhaled corticosteroid use
3. List all available inhaled corticosteroids used in respiratory therapy
4. Differentiate between specific corticosteroid formulations
5. Describe the route of administration available for corticosteroids
6. Describe the mode of action for corticosteroids
7. Discuss the effect corticosteroids have on the white blood cell count
8. Discuss the effect corticosteroids have on β receptors
9. Differentiate between systemic and local side effects of corticosteroids
10. Discuss the use of corticosteroids in the treatment of asthma and chronic obstructive pulmonary disease
11. Be able to clinically assess corticosteroid use in patient care

KEY TERMS AND DEFINITIONS

Adrenal cortical hormones Chemicals secreted by the adrenal cortex, referred to as *steroids*.

Endogenous Refers to *inside*—produced by the body.

Exogenous Refers to *outside*—manufactured to be placed inside the body (e.g., medication).

Immunoglobulin E (IgE) Gamma globulin that is produced by cells in the respiratory tract.

Prostaglandins One of several hormone-type substances circulating throughout the body.

Steroid diabetes Hyperglycemia (i.e., increased plasma glucose levels) resulting from glucocorticoid therapy; glucocorticoids break down proteins and fats to generate building blocks for gluconeogenesis.

Steroids Also known as *glucocorticoids* or *corticosteroids,* agents that produce an antiinflammatory response in the body.

Chapter 11 discusses the use of corticosteroids in respiratory care and provides a brief review of the physiology of endogenous corticosteroid hormones in the body. A brief description of inflammation, and specifically of airway inflammation in asthma, forms the basis for a discussion of the pharmacology of corticosteroids as antiinflammatory drugs. Aerosolized glucocorticoids and their uses and side effects are described.

CLINICAL INDICATIONS FOR USE OF INHALED CORTICOSTEROIDS

Inhaled corticosteroids are available in formulations for oral inhalation (lung delivery) and intranasal delivery. Specific clinical applications are discussed more fully at the end of this chapter. General clinical indications for the use of inhaled corticosteroids are as follows:

- *Orally inhaled agents:* Maintenance and control therapy of chronic asthma, identified as requiring step 2 care or greater by the National Asthma Education and Prevention Program Expert Panel Report 3[1] *Guidelines for the Diagnosis and Management of Asthma* (available at http://www.nhlbi.nih.gov/guidelines/asthma/asthgdln.htm).
  - *Step 2 asthma* is defined as asthma with symptoms occurring more than 2 days/week but not daily; night awakenings occurring 3 to 4 nights/month, with forced expiratory volume in 1 second (FEV_1) or peak expiratory flow (PEF) 80% of predicted or greater.
  - Inhaled agents can be used with systemic corticosteroids in severe asthma and may allow reduction or elimination of systemic corticosteroids for asthma control.
  - Inhaled corticosteroids are recommended by the American Thoracic Society (ATS)[2] (available at: http://www.thoracic.org/statements/resources/copd/copdexecsum.pdf) and the Global Initiative for Chronic Obstructive Lung Disease (GOLD)[3] (available at: http://www.goldcopd.org/uploads/users/files/GOLD_Report_2014_Jun11.pdf) for chronic obstructive pulmonary disease (COPD).
- *Intranasal aerosol agents:* Management of seasonal and perennial allergic and nonallergic rhinitis.

IDENTIFICATION OF AEROSOLIZED CORTICOSTEROIDS

Increased numbers of aerosolized corticosteroid preparations are becoming available for oral inhalation and intranasal delivery. Table 11-1 lists currently available aerosol formulations of corticosteroids for oral inhalation, Table 11-2 lists combination corticosteroid agents for oral inhalation, and Table 11-3 lists intranasal formulations. The rationale for inhaled aerosol agents is discussed and the properties of corticosteroids required for success as topical agents are described subsequently, along with additional detail on individual agents.

PHYSIOLOGY OF CORTICOSTEROIDS

KEY POINT

The *physiology* of *endogenous corticosteroids* involves a sequence of stimulation of the adrenal cortex through the *hypothalamic-pituitary-adrenal (HPA)* axis, in which increased blood levels of corticosteroid inhibit the HPA and adrenal cortex from further secretion.

Identification and Source

Corticosteroids are a group of chemicals secreted by the adrenal cortex and are referred to as **adrenal cortical hormones**. The adrenal or suprarenal gland is composed of two portions (Figure 11-1). The inner zone is the adrenal medulla and produces epinephrine. The outer zone is the cortex, which is the source of corticosteroids. Three types of corticosteroid hormones are produced by the adrenal cortex: glucocorticoids (e.g., cortisol), mineralocorticoids (e.g., aldosterone), and sex hormones (e.g., androgens and estrogens). The mineralocorticoid aldosterone regulates body water by increasing the amount of sodium reabsorption in the renal tubules. The corticosteroids used in pulmonary disease are all analogs of cortisol or *hydrocortisone,* as it is also termed. Glucocorticoid agents are referred to as *glucocorticosteroids* and by the more general term *corticosteroid,* or simply as **steroids**.

KEY POINT

Corticosteroids secreted by the adrenal cortex include *glucocorticoids* (e.g., cortisol), *mineralocorticoids* (e.g., aldosterone), and *sex hormones* (e.g., androgen and estrogen).

KEY POINT

Glucocorticoids, often referred to simply as *steroids,* exert an *antiinflammatory effect* in the body.

Hypothalamic-Pituitary-Adrenal Axis

The side effects of corticosteroids and the rationale for aerosol or alternate-day therapy can be understood if the production and control of **endogenous** (the body's own) corticosteroids are grasped. The pathway for release and control of corticosteroids is the hypothalamic-pituitary-adrenal (HPA) axis (Figure 11-2). Stimulation of the hypothalamus causes impulses to be sent to the area known as the median eminence, where corticotropin-releasing factor (CRF) is released. CRF circulates through the portal vessel to the anterior pituitary gland, which then releases corticotropin, or adrenocorticotropic hormone (ACTH), into the bloodstream. ACTH in turn stimulates the adrenal cortex to secrete glucocorticoids, such as cortisol. Cortisol

TABLE 11-1   Corticosteroids Available by Aerosol for Oral Inhalation*

DRUG	BRAND NAME	FORMULATION AND DOSAGE
Beclomethasone dipropionate HFA	Qvar	*MDI:* 40 and 80 mcg/puff *Adults ≥12 yr:* 40-80 mcg twice daily[†] or 40-160 mcg twice daily[‡] *Children ≥5 yr:* 40-80 mcg twice daily
Flunisolide hemihydrate HFA	AeroSpan	*MDI:* 80 mcg/puff *Adults ≥12 yr:* 2 puffs bid; adults no more than 4 puffs daily *Children 6-11 yr:* 1 puff daily; no more than 2 puffs daily
Fluticasone propionate	Flovent HFA	*MDI:* 44, 110, and 220 mcg/puff *Adults ≥12 yr:* 88 mcg bid,[†] 88-220 mcg bid,[‡] or 880 mcg bid[§] *Children 4-11 yr:* 88 mcg bid[¶]
	Flovent Diskus	*DPI:* 50, 100, and 250 mcg *Adults:* 100 mcg bid,[†] 100-250 mcg bid,[‡] 1000 mcg bid[§] *Children 4-11 yr:* 50-100 mcg twice daily
Fluticasone furoate	Arnuity Ellipta	*DPI:* 100 and 200 mcg *Adults and children ≥12 yr:* 100 or 200 mcg once daily
Budesonide	Pulmicort Flexhaler	*DPI:* 90 mcg/actuation and 180 mcg/actuation *Adults:* 180-360 mcg bid,[†‡] 360-720 mcg bid§ *Children ≥6 yr:* 180-360 mcg bid
	Pulmicort Respules	*SVN:* 0.25 mg/2 mL, 0.5 mg/2 mL, 1 mg/2 mL *Children 1-8 yr:* 0.5 mg total dose given once or twice daily in divided doses;[†‡] 1 mg given as 0.5 mg bid or once daily[§]
Mometasone furoate	Asmanex Twisthaler	*DPI:* 110 and 220 mcg/actuation *Adults and children ≥12 yr:* 220-880 mcg daily *Children 4-11 yr:* 110 mcg daily
	Asmanex HFA	*MDI:* 100 and 200 mcg/actuation *Adults and children ≥ 12 yr:* 100-200 mcg bid
Ciclesonide	Alvesco	*MDI:* 80 and 160 mcg/puff *Adults ≥12 yr:* 80-160 mcg twice daily,[†] or 80-320 mcg twice daily[‡]

DPI, Dry powder inhaler; *HFA,* hydrofluoroalkane; *MDI,* metered dose inhaler; *SVN,* small volume nebulizer.
*Individual agents are discussed in text. Detailed information about each agent should be obtained from the manufacturer's drug insert.
[†]Recommended starting dose if taking only bronchodilators.
[‡]Recommended starting dose if previously taking inhaled corticosteroids.
[§]Recommended starting dose if previously taking oral corticosteroids.
[¶]This dose should be used regardless of previous therapy.

TABLE 11-2   Combination Corticosteroid Agents Available for Oral Inhalation*

Fluticasone propionate/ salmeterol	Advair Diskus	*DPI:* 100 mcg fluticasone/50 mcg salmeterol, 250 mcg fluticasone/50 mcg salmeterol, or 500 mcg fluticasone/50 mcg salmeterol *Adults and children ≥12 yr:* 100 mcg fluticasone/50 mcg salmeterol, 1 inhalation twice daily, about 12 hr apart (starting dose if not currently taking inhaled corticosteroids) Maximal recommended dose is 500 mcg fluticasone/50 mcg salmeterol twice daily *Children ≥4 yr:* 100 mcg fluticasone/50 mcg salmeterol, 1 inhalation twice daily, about 12 hr apart (for patients who are symptomatic while taking inhaled corticosteroid)
	Advair HFA	*MDI:* 45 mcg fluticasone/21 mcg salmeterol, 115 mcg fluticasone/21 mcg salmeterol, or 230 mcg fluticasone/21 mcg salmeterol *Adults and children ≥12 yr:* 2 inhalations twice daily, about 12 hr apart
Budesonide/formoterol fumarate HFA	Symbicort	*MDI:* 80 mcg budesonide/4.5 mcg formoterol and 160 mcg budesonide/4.5 mcg formoterol *Adults and children ≥12 yr:* 160 mcg budesonide/9 mcg formoterol bid, 320 mcg budesonide/9 mcg formoterol bid; daily maximum: 640 mcg budesonide/18 mcg formoterol
Mometasone furoate/ formoterol fumarate HFA	Dulera	*MDI:* 100 mcg mometasone/5 mcg formoterol and 200 mcg mometasone/5 mcg formoterol *Adults and children ≥12 yr:* If previously on medium dose of corticosteroids, ≤400 mcg mometasone/20 mcg formoterol daily; if previously on high dose of corticosteroid, ≤800 mcg mometasone/20 mcg formoterol daily
Fluticasone furoate/vilanterol	Breo Ellipta	*DPI:* 100 mcg fluticasone/25 mcg vilanterol *Adults:* 100 mcg fluticasone/25 mcg vilanterol daily and 200 mcg fluticasone/25 mcg vilanterol

DPI, Dry powder inhaler; *HFA,* hydrofluoroalkane; *MDI,* metered dose inhaler.
*Individual agents are discussed in text. Detailed information about each agent should be obtained from the manufacturer's drug insert.

TABLE 11-3	Aerosol Corticosteroid Preparations Available for Intranasal Delivery*	
DRUG	**BRAND NAME**	**FORMULATION AND DOSAGE**
Beclomethasone	Beconase AQ	*Spray:* 42 mcg/actuation *Adults ≥12 yr:* 1 or 2 sprays in each nostril twice daily *Children 6-11 yr:* 1 spray in each nostril twice daily, may increase to 2 sprays
	Qnasl	*Spray:* 80 mcg/actuation *Adults ≥12 yr:* 2 sprays in each nostril once daily
Triamcinolone acetonide	Nasacort Allergy 24 Hour†	*Spray:* 55 mcg/actuation *Adults and children ≥12 yr:* 2 sprays in each nostril once daily (starting dose). May reduce once symptoms improve. *Children 6-11 yr:* 1 spray in each nostril once daily (starting dose). May increase if symptoms do not improve. *Children 2-6 yr:* 1 spray in each nostril once daily
Flunisolide		*Spray:* 25 mcg/actuation and 29 mcg/actuation *Adults and children ≥14 yr:* 2 actuations in each nostril bid *Children 6-14 yr:* 1 actuation in each nostril tid or 2 actuations in each nostril bid
Budesonide	Rhinocort Aqua	*Spray:* 32 mcg/actuation *Adults and children ≥6 yr:* 1 spray in each nostril daily (starting dose). Adults up to 4 sprays in each nostril daily. Children ≥6 yr: Up to 2 sprays in each nostril daily.
Fluticasone	Flonase Allergy Relief†	*Spray:* 50 mcg/actuation *Adults:* 2 sprays in each nostril once daily (starting dose) *Children ≥4 yr:* 1 spray in each nostril once daily (starting dose)
Mometasone furoate	Nasonex	*Spray:* 50 mcg/actuation *Adults and children ≥12 yr:* 2 sprays in each nostril once daily. Adults ≥18 may use 2 sprays in each nostril bid. *Children 2-11 yr:* 1 spray in each nostril once daily
Fluticasone furoate	Veramyst	*Spray:* 27.5 mcg/actuation *Adults and children ≥12 yr:* 2 sprays in each nostril once daily *Children 2-11 yr:* 1 spray in each nostril once daily
Ciclesonide	Omnaris	*Spray:* 50 mcg/actuation *Adults and children ≥6 yr:* 2 sprays in each nostril once daily
	Zetonna	*Spray:* 37 mcg/actuation *Adults and children ≥12 yr:* 1 spray in each nostril once daily

*Detailed information about each agent should be obtained from the manufacturer's drug insert.
†Only available over-the-counter.

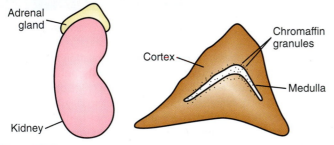

Figure 11-1 Location and cross section of adrenal, or suprarenal, gland. The outer portion, or cortex, of the adrenal gland is the source of corticosteroid hormones.

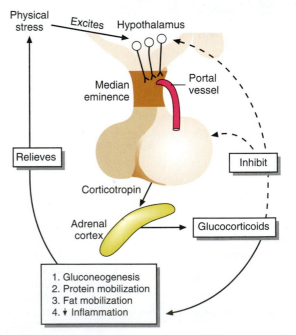

Figure 11-2 Hypothalamic-pituitary-adrenal (HPA) axis regulation of corticosteroid secretion (see text for complete description of function).

and glucocorticoids in general regulate the metabolism of carbohydrates, fats, and proteins, generally to increase levels of glucose for body energy. This is the reason cortisol and its analogs are called *glucocorticoids*. They can also cause lipolysis, redistribution of fat stores, and breakdown of tissue protein stores. These actions are the basis for many of the side effects seen with glucocorticoid drugs. The breakdown of proteins for use of the amino acids (gluconeogenesis) is responsible for muscle wasting, and the effects on glucose metabolism can increase plasma glucose levels. The latter is sometimes referred to as **steroid diabetes**.[4]

Hypothalamic-Pituitary-Adrenal Suppression With Steroid Use

KEY POINT

Exogenous corticosteroid agents can *suppress the HPA axis* and the adrenal gland.

One of the most significant side effects of treatment with glucocorticoid drugs (**exogenous** corticosteroids) is adrenal suppression or, more generally, HPA suppression. When the body produces endogenous glucocorticoids, there is a normal feedback mechanism within the HPA axis to limit production. As glucocorticoid levels increase, release of CRF and ACTH is inhibited, and further adrenal production of glucocorticoids is stopped. This feedback inhibition of the hypothalamus and the pituitary is shown in Figure 11-2 and is analogous to the servo mechanism by which a thermostat regulates furnace production of heat by monitoring temperature levels.

The body cannot distinguish between its own endogenous glucocorticoids and exogenous glucocorticoid drugs. Administration of glucocorticoid drugs increases the body's level of these hormones, and this inhibits the hypothalamus and pituitary glands, which decreases adrenal production. This inhibition is referred to as *HPA suppression* or, specifically, *adrenal suppression*. It is seen with systemic administration of corticosteroids, begins after 1 day of treatment, and is significant after 1 week of oral therapy at usual doses. A primary reason for using aerosolized glucocorticoids is to minimize adrenal, or HPA, suppression by minimizing the dosage and localizing the site of treatment.

If a patient has received oral corticosteroids and adrenal suppression has occurred, weaning from the exogenous corticosteroids through use of tapered dose therapy allows time for recovery of the body's own adrenal secretion. It should be noted that aerosolized corticosteroids do not deposit sufficient amounts of drug to replace the missing output of a suppressed adrenal gland. Therefore a patient with adrenal suppression cannot be abruptly withdrawn from oral corticosteroids and placed on an aerosol dosage. The aerosol should be started while the oral agent is tapered off slowly at the same time.

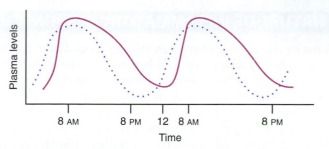

Figure 11-3 Diurnal variations in adrenocorticotropic hormone *(dotted line)* and cortisol *(solid line)* (see text for detailed description).

Diurnal Steroid Cycle

KEY POINT

Levels of endogenous corticosteroids follow a daily, or *diurnal*, rhythm.

The production of the body's own glucocorticoids follows a rhythmic cycle, termed a *diurnal* or *circadian rhythm*. This daily rise and fall of glucocorticoid levels in the body is shown in Figure 11-3. On a daily schedule of daytime work and nighttime sleep, cortisol levels are highest in the morning around 8 AM. These high plasma levels inhibit further production and release of glucocorticoids and ACTH by the HPA axis because of the feedback mechanism previously described. During the day, plasma levels of ACTH (see Figure 11-3, *dotted line*) and cortisol (see Figure 11-3, *solid line*) gradually decrease. As the glucocorticoid level decreases, the anterior pituitary is reactivated to begin releasing ACTH, which stimulates production of cortisol by the adrenal cortex. This lag between increased ACTH and cortisol levels is illustrated in Figure 11-3. One of the reasons for jet lag and the delay in adjusting to night shift from day shift is that this diurnal and regular rhythm of corticosteroid levels becomes out of synchronization with the time zone and the work time. Although a worker needs to sleep at 8 AM after working all night, the body is wide awake, with energy stores being released.

Alternate-Day Steroid Therapy

Alternate-day therapy mimics the natural diurnal rhythm by giving a steroid drug early in the morning, when normal tissue levels are high. Suppression of the HPA system occurs at the same time it normally would with the body's own steroid, and on the alternate day the regular diurnal secretion in the HPA system can resume. Tissue side effects are minimized because the drug is administered at the time when tissues are normally exposed to elevated corticosteroid levels by the body's rhythm. Use of an intermediate-acting corticosteroid drug, with a duration of 12 to 36 hours, allows drug therapy to be restricted to alternate days.

NATURE OF INFLAMMATORY RESPONSE

A major therapeutic effect seen with analogs of the natural (endogenous) adrenal cortical hormone hydrocortisone is an antiinflammatory action. Glucocorticoid analogs of endogenous hydrocortisone are used for this effect in treating asthma, which is an inflammatory process in the lungs. To understand the antiinflammatory activity of the glucocorticoid drugs used in asthma, the nature of inflammation in general and of airway inflammation in particular are reviewed briefly.

KEY POINT

Inflammation produces general symptoms of redness, swelling, heat, and pain.

A general definition of *inflammation* is the response of vascularized tissue to injury. An excellent and still applicable description of inflammation was given in the first century AD by Celsus: *"rubor et tumor cum calore et dolore,"* which is translated as "redness and swelling with heat and pain." This is the most general description of an inflammatory reaction to injury, such as a cut, wound infection, splinter, burn, scrape, or bee sting.

An update of Celsus' description occurred in the 1920s with Lewis' characterization known as the *triple response:*

1. *Redness:* Local dilation of blood vessels, occurring in seconds
2. *Flare:* Reddish color several centimeters from the site, occurring 15 to 30 seconds after injury
3. *Wheal:* Local swelling, occurring in minutes

The process of inflammation producing the visible results described by Celsus, Lewis, and others is caused by the following four major categories of activity:

1. *Increased vascular permeability:* An exudate is formed in the surrounding tissues.
2. *Leukocytic infiltration:* White blood cells emigrate through capillary walls (diapedesis) in response to attractant chemicals (chemotaxis).
3. *Phagocytosis:* White blood cells and macrophages (in the lungs) ingest and process foreign material, such as bacteria.
4. *Mediator cascade:* Histamine and chemoattractant factors are released at the site of injury, and various inflammatory mediators, such as complement and arachidonic acid products, are generated.

Inflammation in the Airway

KEY POINT

In the airway, inflammation is mediated by various cells, such as *eosinophils, basophils, macrophages, mast cells, T lymphocytes,* and *epithelial* or *endothelial cells* in response to the release of *mediators of inflammation.* This process is

KEY POINT—cont'd

complex and involves several mediators, including the *arachidonic acid cascade* (**prostaglandins** and leukotrienes); *histamine;* and various *cytokines,* such as interleukins. These mediators further amplify the inflammatory response by attracting the cells mentioned previously to the airway and inducing the release of *adhesion* factors (e.g., intercellular adhesion molecule [ICAM]) to bind inflammatory cells to the airway surface.

Inflammation can occur in the lungs in response to various causes, including direct trauma (gunshot wound, stabbing), indirect trauma (blunt chest injury), inhalation of noxious or toxic substances (chlorine gas, smoke), respiratory infections and systemic infections producing septicemia and septic shock with acute respiratory distress syndrome (ARDS), and allergenic or nonallergenic stimulation in asthma. The two most common inflammatory diseases of the airway seen in respiratory care are chronic bronchitis, usually caused by tobacco smoking, and asthma, which can be caused by a range of triggers and involves a complex pathophysiology.

Because glucocorticoids are a mainstay for treating asthma, the multiple pathways and mediators for the genesis of airway inflammation seen in asthma are briefly described. Asthma is currently understood as a disease in which there is chronic inflammation of the airway wall, causing airflow limitation and a hyperresponsiveness to various stimuli[4,5] (Box 11-1). The airway inflammation is mediated by inflammatory cells, such as mast cells, eosinophils, T lymphocytes, and macrophages. The mast cell and the eosinophil are considered to be the major effector cells of the inflammatory response, regardless of whether the asthma is allergic or nonallergic.[6] T lymphocytes may be pivotal in coordinating the inflammatory response by releasing numerous proinflammatory cytokines (proteins that regulate immune and inflammatory responses), which act on basophils, epithelial cells, and endothelial cells in the airway to further the inflammatory process. The potent mediators released during an asthmatic reaction cause airway smooth muscle contraction (bronchospasm),

---

BOX 11-1 Operational Definition of Asthma

Asthma is a chronic inflammatory disorder of the airways in which many cells and cellular elements play a role, in particular, mast cells, eosinophils, T lymphocytes, macrophages, neutrophils, and epithelial cells. In susceptible individuals, this inflammation causes recurrent episodes of wheezing, breathlessness, chest tightness, and coughing, particularly at night or in the early morning. These episodes are usually associated with widespread but variable airflow obstruction that is often reversible either spontaneously or with treatment. The inflammation also causes an associated increase in the existing bronchial hyperresponsiveness to various stimuli.

National Asthma Education and Prevention Program, National Heart, Lung, and Blood Institute, National Institutes of Health: *Expert Panel Report 3: guidelines for the diagnosis and management of asthma,* NIH Publication No. 08-4051, Bethesda, Md, 2007, National Institutes of Health.

increased microvascular leakage and airway wall swelling, mucus secretion, and remodeling of the airway wall over the longer term. In an acute state, people with asthma exhibit wheezing, breathlessness, chest tightness, and cough, especially at night or early morning. The acute symptoms produced by the airway inflammation are at least partly reversible either spontaneously or with pharmacologic treatment. Treatment with antiinflammatory agents such as glucocorticoids is important to reduce the basal level of airway inflammation, airway hyperresponsiveness, and the predisposition to acute episodes of obstruction.

Asthmatic reactions are biphasic, including an early phase and a late phase. Figure 11-4 shows a conceptual representation of the overall process. After an insult to the asthmatic airway by an allergen, cold air, viral infection, or noxious gas, there is evidence that the early asthmatic response is caused by **immunoglobulin E (IgE)**–dependent activation of airway mast cells, which can release inflammatory mediators such as histamine, prostaglandin D_2 (PGD_2), and leukotriene C_4.[5] The immediate response of the airway to chemicals such as histamine is bronchospasm. This response peaks at about 15 minutes and then declines over the next hour; this produces the early phase decrease in expiratory flow rates illustrated in Figure 11-4.

Although the early bronchoconstriction of smooth muscle may self-limit or respond to β agonists, the progression of cellular events can continue. Mast cell mediators and the release of cytokines recruit other inflammatory cells (eosinophils, basophils, monocytes/macrophages, and lymphocytes) by activating epithelial cells and endothelial cells to release adhesion molecules (e.g., intercellular adhesion molecule [ICAM]) and other cytokines to cause the late-phase reaction. During the late-phase response, mast cells and recruited eosinophils, lymphocytes, or macrophages that have infiltrated the airway release a range of inflammatory mediators. Neutrophils are not generally associated with asthma and allergic reactions in the absence of infection. The late asthmatic response occurs 6 to 8 hours after a challenge, and it may last for 24 hours. The late-phase reaction is thought to be reflective of the chronic inflammation characterizing asthma between acute episodes.[6]

Phospholipids in the cell membrane of mast cells and other cells are converted by phospholipase A_2 (PLA_2) to arachidonic acid and then to various bronchoactive and vasoactive substances by the two metabolic paths shown in Figure 11-4: the cyclooxygenase and lipoxygenase pathways. The term *eicosanoid* is used to refer to the products of the two pathways. The migration of eosinophils and lymphocytes and further development of inflammation-producing chemicals such as the arachidonic acid metabolites and cytokines all contribute to build an inflammatory response in the lung.[7] In addition to smooth muscle spasm, mucus secretion occurs, along with mucosal swelling resulting from increased vascular permeability. Shedding of airway

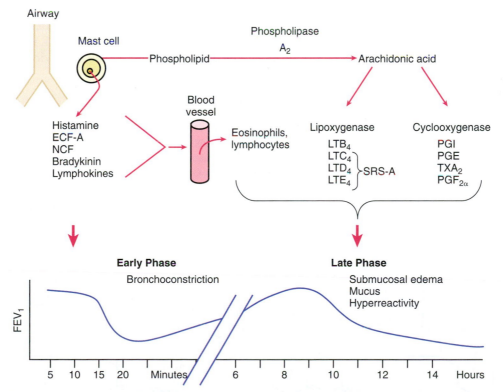

Figure 11-4 Conceptual illustration of inflammatory asthmatic response in the airway, producing a biphasic deterioration in expiratory flow rates described as an early-phase and late-phase response to triggering stimuli. *ECF-A*, Eosinophilic chemotactic factor; *FEV$_1$*, forced expiratory volume in 1 second; *LTB$_4$*, leukotriene B$_4$; *LTC$_4$*, leukotriene C$_4$; *LTD$_4$*, leukotriene D$_4$; *LTE$_4$*, leukotriene E$_4$; *NCF*, neutrophil chemotactic factor; *PGE*, prostaglandin E; *PGF$_2$α*, prostaglandin F$_2$α; *PGI*, prostaglandin I; *SRS-A*, slow-reacting substance of anaphylaxis; *TXA$_2$*, thromboxane A$_2$.

cells (*desquamation*) and goblet cell hyperplasia are seen. The result is mucous plugging of the airway, complicated by the cellular debris in the bronchial lumen. The pathology of bronchial asthma has been described as "chronic desquamating eosinophilic bronchitis."[8] These airway changes lead to further bronchial hyperreactivity seen in asthma. There is evidence of airway remodeling, with increased tenascin (an extracellular matrix protein for cell development), collagens, and fibronectin, all of which can cause thickening of the basement membrane in the airway wall. This airway remodeling deregulates communication between cells, promoting epithelial damage and enhancing the inflammatory response.[9]

AEROSOLIZED CORTICOSTEROIDS

Several corticosteroid preparations are available, such as hydrocortisone, cortisone, prednisone, prednisolone, and methylprednisolone, all of which have antiinflammatory activity. However, these agents produce undesirable systemic side effects when used to treat asthma, COPD, and inflammation of the lung. As with all inhaled agents, topical application of corticosteroids is intended to provide direct application of the drug to the lung or nasal passages and reduce systemic side effects.

Aerosolized Corticosteroid Agents

Several aerosol steroid agents, all of which are glucocorticoids, are available for inhalational use in the United States at the time of this edition. These are identified in Table 11-1, which summarizes steroids used for oral inhalation, corticosteroids in combination with other agents are found in

Table 11-2 and Table 11-3, lists agents for intranasal delivery, giving strengths and recommended doses. Originally, in the United States, all of the orally inhaled corticosteroids were available as metered dose inhaler (MDI) formulations. However, dry powder inhalers (DPIs)—Diskus (fluticasone), Arnuity Ellipta (fluticasone), Pulmicort Flexhaler (budesonide), and Asmanex Twisthaler (mometasone furoate)—have also been introduced, along with the only approved small volume nebulizer (SVN) formulation (budesonide [Pulmicort Respules]). At the time of this edition, all of the MDI formulations are available with hydrofluoroalkane (HFA) propellant (beclomethasone, flunisolide, fluticasone, and ciclesonide).

These agents possess a high topical-to-systemic potency ratio, which makes them suitable for control of asthma or COPD with minimal systemic side effects. The chemical structures of the aerosol agents available for oral and nasal inhalation are shown in Figure 11-5. Each of the aerosol agents is briefly described next.

Beclomethasone Dipropionate (Qvar)

Beclomethasone dipropionate (Qvar) has been known by several names, including Vanceril and Beclovent; however, with the transition from chlorofluorocarbon (CFC)-propelled MDI formulations, beclomethasone dipropionate has been reformulated with an HFA propellant in a 40- and 80-mcg MDI strength as Qvar (see Table 11-1). Along with the change in propellant, many components of the MDI system were reengineered, significantly increasing the efficiency of this drug delivery system. Lung deposition with Qvar has been measured at 50% to 60% of the emitted dose (see discussion of MDIs in Chapter 3). The usual starting dose of Qvar is 40 to 80 mcg twice daily (see Table 11-1).

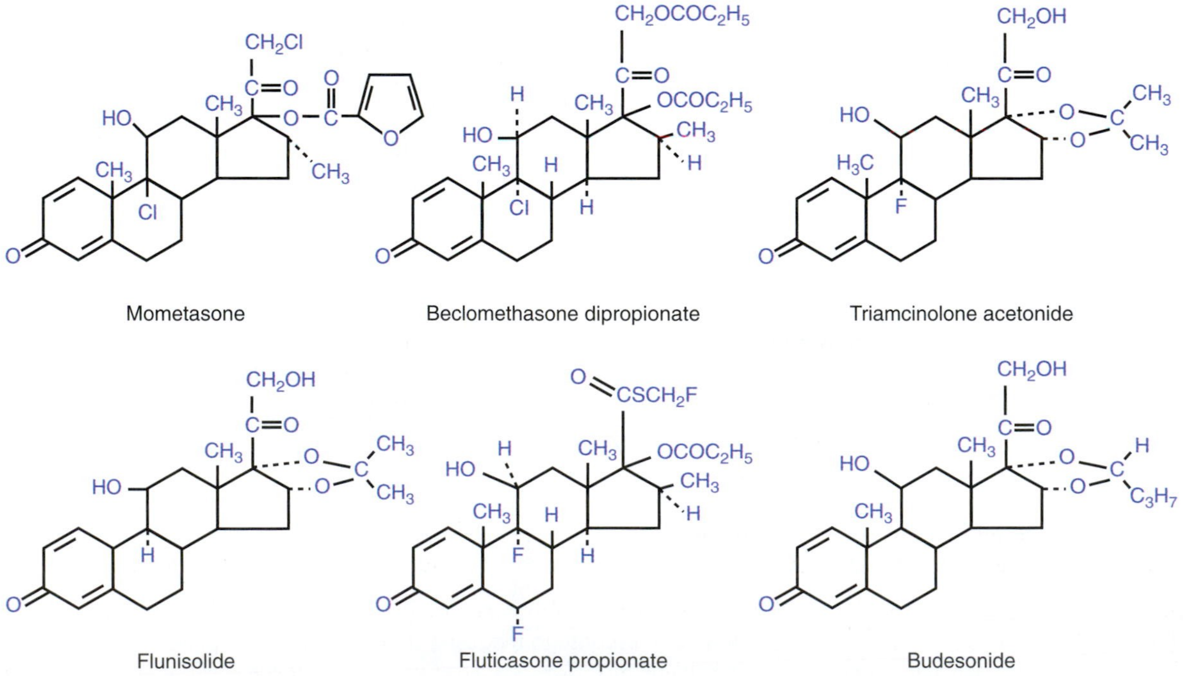

Figure 11-5 Structures of aerosolized corticosteroids, showing the common steroid nucleus, and modifications to enhance topical antiinflammatory action.

An aerosol dose of 400 mcg is approximately equivalent to 5 to 10 mg of oral prednisone. When inhaled by aerosol, the swallowed drug is slowly absorbed from the gastrointestinal tract, and most of what is absorbed is quickly (half-life in the liver is 10 minutes) broken down in its first passage through the liver, preventing high plasma levels.

Absorption of the drug across the pulmonary epithelium is good, but rapid inactivation prevents systemic accumulation. After inhalation of a 2-mg dose, plasma levels of beclomethasone dipropionate are very low, but the active metabolite, beclomethasone monopropionate (often designated 17-BMP), reaches significant plasma levels of 1.8 to 2.5 ng/mL.[10]

Flunisolide (AeroSpan)

Flunisolide (AeroSpan) is another topically active aerosol preparation, similar in potency to triamcinolone and said to have a longer duration of action. Because of the phase-out of CFC propellant and the increased deposition seen with other HFA MDIs, flunisolide is currently available as an HFA MDI (AeroSpan). AeroBid (Flunisolide) was discontinued as of June 30, 2011. AeroSpan is prescribed twice daily at 80 mcg/puff, but may be used up to four times daily. AeroSpan is available in 60 or 120 actuation canisters. AeroSpan is manufactured with a spacer attached to the actuation device.[11]

Flunisolide shows a peak plasma level after inhalation at between 2 and 60 minutes, indicating good absorption from the lungs, as with beclomethasone. The half-life in plasma with inhalation is approximately 1.8 hours and similar to that with oral or intravenous dosing, indicating a rapid first-pass metabolism.[12]

Fluticasone Propionate (Flovent HFA, Flovent Diskus)

Fluticasone propionate (Flovent HFA, Flovent Diskus) is a synthetic, trifluorinated glucocorticoid with high topical antiinflammatory potency and is available in MDI and DPI forms. The MDI is available in three different strengths: 44 mcg, 110 mcg, and 220 mcg. The DPI is also available in three different strengths: 50 mcg, 100 mcg, and 250 mcg. The drug is a further analog of previous agents with high topical potency, synthesized in an attempt to avoid systemic side effects. Fluticasone is derived from the 17β-carbothioate series of androstane analogs, a group that has very weak HPA inhibitory activity but high antiinflammatory effect.[13] Using fluocinolone acetonide as a reference standard, fluticasone propionate was found to have an antiinflammatory potency of 91 in mice,[14] with an HPA-inhibitory activity of only 1, giving a therapeutic index (antiinflammatory potency/HPA potency) of 91. By comparison, beclomethasone dipropionate has an antiinflammatory potency of 21, with an HPA-inhibitory potency of 49 in mice.[15] If given by subcutaneous injection to mice, fluticasone propionate exhibits HPA inhibition; however, the oral route gives only weak HPA suppression; this is useful with inhaled aerosols because a portion of the aerosol may be swallowed and contribute to systemic activity of a drug. An explanation for the weak HPA suppression when given orally may be its high first-pass effect, resulting in less than 1% of active drug dose in the circulation because fluticasone is rapidly metabolized in the liver into the inactive product 17β-carboxylic acid.[14]

Fluticasone Furoate (Arnuity Ellipta)

Fluticasone furoate (Arnuity Ellipta) is available as a DPI delivering 100 mcg/inhalation and 200 mcg/inhalation for once-daily maintenance treatment of asthma in patients aged 12 years and older. Fluticasone furoate differs from fluticasone propionate in that they are different salts or esters from different acids. The difference appears to be that the furoate salt has better affinity for the glucocorticoid receptor, thus providing a longer duration of action. Because of this affinity, fluticasone furoate lends itself to once daily dosing.

Budesonide (Pulmicort, Pulmicort Respules)

Budesonide (Pulmicort, Pulmicort Respules) is available as a DPI (Pulmicort) or as an inhalation solution (Pulmicort Respules). The DPI delivers two strengths—90 mcg/metered dose and 180 mcg/metered dose—and Pulmicort Respules is available in doses of 0.25 mg, 0.5 mg, and 1 mg. The benefit of using Respules is that it can be mixed with other agents, such as bronchodilators (e.g., albuterol, levalbuterol, and ipratropium). Numerous studies have shown that mixing the agents had no effect on the drugs mixed.[15]

Budesonide is a topically active inhaled corticosteroid with a potency greater than beclomethasone dipropionate, triamcinolone, or flunisolide, but it is less potent than fluticasone, as estimated by skin vasoconstriction assay. With oral administration, only 10% of budesonide enters the systemic circulation because of high (approximately 89%) first-pass metabolism in the liver. After inhalation with a spacer device, peak plasma concentrations occur between 15 and 45 minutes. The plasma half-life is 2 hours. There appears to be minimal metabolism in the lung, with approximately 70% of the inhaled dose reaching the circulation.[16] Budesonide was found to exhibit about half the adrenal suppression of fluticasone, on a microgram equivalent basis in asthmatic patients.[17]

Mometasone Furoate (Asmanex Twisthaler, Asmanex HFA)

Mometasone furoate is available as a MDI and DPI. McCormack and Plosker[18] reviewed its use in asthma. Asmanex can be given once or twice daily. Single-day dosing may be beneficial to increase consistency in usage of an inhaled corticosteroid. Karpel and others[19] found that pulmonary function results increased in patients receiving once-daily Asmanex compared with a placebo in patients previously using twice-daily doses of inhaled corticosteroids. Asmanex is approved for patients as young as 4 years of age.

Ciclesonide (Alvesco)

Ciclesonide (Alvesco) is a prodrug; once it enters the body, it is enzymatically converted to des-ciclesonide. Ciclesonide has been shown to decrease the development of Candida albicans infection in the mouth. Although it is listed to be dispensed twice daily, the literature describes once-daily dosing to be as effective as twice-daily dosing with other inhaled corticosteroids. Des-ciclesonide has a 120 times greater affinity for the glucocorticoid receptor. Ciclesonide is approved by the U.S. Food and Drug Administration (FDA) only for individuals older than 12 years; however, several pediatric studies exist, which may offer potential to prescribe off-label.

Fluticasone Propionate/Salmeterol (Advair)

Fluticasone propionate/salmeterol (Advair) is a combination product of the corticosteroid fluticasone with the long-acting β_2-agonist bronchodilator salmeterol. Advair is available as a DPI and HFA MDI in three different strengths (fluticasone/salmeterol): DPI, 100 mcg/50 mcg, 250 mcg/50 mcg, and 500 mcg/50 mcg; HFA MDI, 45 mcg/21 mcg, 115 mcg/21 mcg, and 230 mcg/21 mcg. The combination of inhaled steroid and long-acting $\beta2$ agonist in a convenient dose package is useful in patients with asthma requiring step 3 care or higher who need both types of drug. In a large multicenter clinical study by Shapiro and colleagues, 20 patients with asthma who were taking medium doses of inhaled corticosteroids were treated with 250 mcg of fluticasone in combination with 50 mcg of salmeterol from the DPI Diskus device for 12 weeks. Patients in the treatment group had significantly better FEV_1 profiles over 12 hours, a significantly greater probability of remaining in the study and not withdrawing because of worsening symptoms, a significantly increased morning PEF, reduced asthma symptom scores, reduced rescue albuterol use, and significantly fewer nights with no awakenings compared with patients taking salmeterol or fluticasone alone or a placebo.

Mometasone Furoate/Formoterol (Dulera)

Mometasone furoate/formoterol (Dulera) is a combination product of the corticosteroid mometasone with the long-acting β_2-agonist bronchodilator formoterol (see Chapter 6 for a discussion of formoterol). Dulera is available as an MDI in two strengths (mometasone/formoterol): 100 mcg/5 mcg and 200 mcg/5 mcg. In two randomized, double-blind, placebo-controlled studies involving more than 1500 patients, Dulera was able to increase lung function as a combination drug better than formoterol alone or a placebo. Fewer patients reported a deterioration on Dulera than formoterol alone (manufacturer's literature).

Budesonide/Formoterol (Symbicort)

Budesonide/formoterol (Symbicort) is a combination product of the corticosteroid budesonide with the long-acting β_2-agonist bronchodilator formoterol (see Chapter 6 for a discussion of formoterol). Symbicort is available as an MDI in two strengths (budesonide/formoterol): 80 mcg/4.5 mcg and 160 mcg/4.5 mcg. In two large, double-blind, placebo-controlled studies involving more than 100 patients, Symbicort was able to increase lung function as a combination drug better than either drug separately or a placebo, and it was found that the combination therapy was able to increase lung function 15 minutes after administration (manufacturer's literature).

Although combination products have the disadvantage of not allowing changes in dose for each drug separately and have been discouraged, there is evidence of a beneficial, complementary interaction between glucocorticoids and β-adrenergic agonists. The addition of long-acting bronchodilators to inhaled corticosteroids has no negative effect and shows improvements in lung function and symptom control, as shown in the clinical trial by Shapiro and associates,[20] by Chung[21] for Advair, and by Jenkins and colleagues[22] for Symbicort.

The interaction results from the following known or investigational actions of steroids and β agonists:

- Steroids increase β_2-adrenergic receptor transcription (upregulation of β receptors).[21,23]
- Inhaled corticosteroid therapy can provide partial protection against the development of tolerance to β_2-adrenergic agonists.[21]
- Salmeterol has been shown to promote binding of the glucocorticoid receptor to the response element of the cell's nuclear DNA, *without the glucocorticoid present*, in vascular cells, initiating the antiinflammatory effect at least partially.[23]

If management of asthma requires a long-acting β agonist and an inhaled corticosteroid, the combination products fluticasone propionate/salmeterol and budesonide/formoterol offer the advantage of more convenient, single-formulation dosing.

Fluticasone Furoate/Vilanterol (Breo Ellipta)

Breo Ellipta is a combination product of the corticosteroid fluticasone furoate with the long-acting β_2-agonist bronchodilator vilanterol (see Chapter 6 for a discussion of vilanterol). Breo Ellipta is a DPI containing two double-foil blister strips of powder formulation for oral inhalation. One strip contains 100 or 200 mcg of fluticasone furoate per blister and the other contains 25 mcg of vilanterol per blister. The combination product is approved for once-daily treatment of COPD and patients with asthma who are 18 years old or older.

Intranasal Corticosteroids

All of the steroids available as orally inhaled agents are also available in an intranasal formulation. Exact indications for the intranasal preparations vary by specific agent, but intranasal steroids generally are used to treat allergic or inflammatory nasal conditions and seasonal or perennial allergic or nonallergic rhinitis and to prevent recurrence of nasal polyps. Available preparations are listed in Table 11-3, with strengths and recommended doses. Other agents that are used to treat seasonal allergic rhinitis include H_1-receptor antagonists (e.g., loratadine), cromolyn sodium (see Chapter 12), topical vasoconstrictors such as oxymetazoline or ephedrine, and anticholinergics such as ipratropium bromide.

KEY POINT

Aerosolized glucocorticoids all are topically active drugs and include beclomethasone dipropionate, triamcinolone acetonide, flunisolide, budesonide, fluticasone propionate, fluticasone furoate, and mometasone furoate. Aerosol agents are available for *oral inhalation* in the control of *asthma* and *COPD* and *intranasal* administration for *rhinitis*.

PHARMACOLOGY OF CORTICOSTEROIDS

KEY POINT

Glucocorticoids are lipid soluble and act on intracellular receptors to produce antiinflammatory effects.

The inflammatory process can be reduced or blocked by the antiinflammatory effects of glucocorticoids. The beneficial effect of glucocorticoids in asthma and other inflammatory diseases is due to their ability to inhibit the activity of inflammatory cells and mediators of inflammation.

Mode of Action

KEY POINT

The *mode of action* of glucocorticoids is through the *upregulation* of antiinflammatory proteins (e.g., β receptors and lipocortin) and the *downregulation* of proinflammatory proteins (e.g., cytokines and substance P).

Glucocorticoids are highly lipophilic and enter airway cells to bind to intracellular receptors.[24] This mechanism of drug signaling action was described briefly in Chapter 2 in the discussion of the pharmacodynamics of lipid-soluble drugs that interact with intracellular receptors. Originally, investigators thought that corticosteroids or, more simply, steroids exerted antiinflammatory activity by stabilizing lysosomes within neutrophils; this prevented degranulation and an inflammatory response. In the mid-1960s, steroid receptors were discovered, and it was realized that steroids modify the inflammatory response by inducing gene expression within the cell. By the 1980s, it was shown that glucocorticoids induce gene expression for the antiinflammatory protein lipocortin, which inhibits the enzyme PLA_2, preventing the arachidonic acid cascade, which leads to prostaglandin synthesis and lipoxygenase products. However, now it is understood that PLA_2 inhibition is only one of multiple mechanisms by which steroids attenuate the inflammatory response.[6,25-27]

Steroids suppress a local or systemic inflammatory response by at least three general actions; these actions are illustrated in Figure 11-6. Generally, steroids diffuse into

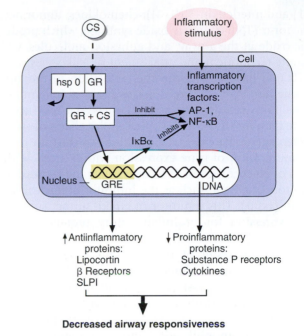

Decreased airway responsiveness

Figure 11-6 Proposed mechanism of action by which glucocorticoids exert an antiinflammatory effect. *AP-1*, Activator protein-1; *CS*, corticosteroid; *DNA*, deoxyribonucleic acid; *GR*, glucocorticoid receptor; *GRE*, glucocorticoid response element; *hsp90*, heat shock protein 90; *IκBα*, inhibitor of nuclear factor-κBα; *NF-κB*, nuclear factor-κB; *SLPI*, secretory leukocyte protease inhibitor.

the cell and bind to a glucocorticoid receptor. Before binding by a steroid, the glucocorticoid receptor is in an inactive state and is bound to a protein complex termed *heat shock protein 90 (hsp90)*, which prevents the unoccupied receptor from translocating to the nucleus of the cell. When the steroid binds to the receptor, hsp90 dissociates, and the steroid-receptor complex translocates to the cell nucleus. One general action (not always the first temporally) of a glucocorticoid is to upregulate the transcription of antiinflammatory genes for substances such as lipocortin, as previously described.[25-27] In the nucleus, the steroid produces this part of its effect on the cell by binding to portions of the nuclear DNA termed *glucocorticoid response elements*. Binding of the drug-receptor complex to glucocorticoid response elements upregulates, or induces, transcription of antiinflammatory substances such as lipocortin, neutral endopeptidase, secretory leukocyte protease inhibitor (SLPI), or inhibitors of plasminogen activator.[6] These are all antiinflammatory substances. A second general action of glucocorticoids is the suppression of factors such as activator protein-1 (AP-1) and nuclear factor-κB (NF-κB), which cause transcription of genes involved in inflammation. This suppression may be by means of a direct interaction with these transcription factors, by which the transcription factor is inactivated before it induces gene expression in the nucleus.[25] Direct inactivation of AP-1 and NF-κB leads to downregulation of gene expression for proinflammatory mediators, such as cytokines. NF-κB regulates genes that have increased expression in asthma, including genes for cytokines such as interleukins (e.g., interleukin-1

[IL-1] and interleukin-3 [IL-3]); chemokines; tumor necrosis factor-α (TNF-α); nitric oxide synthase, which produces nitric oxide in the airway; and adhesion molecules, which promote recruitment and attachment of leukocytes (eosinophils and basophils) from the circulation to the airway endothelium.[14,25,26] A direct inactivation of inflammatory transcription factors such as AP-1 or NF-κB may account for the rapidity with which some cellular effects of steroids are seen and that are not well explained by the time needed for modification of gene expression within a cell. A third action of glucocorticoids is to upregulate the expression of inhibitors of NF-κB, such as the inhibitor of nuclear factor protein (IκBα). This inhibitor of NF-κB further suppresses gene expression for proinflammatory proteins, such as cytokines.[26-28]

The general result of these actions is to *induce* gene expression for antiinflammatory proteins and receptors and to *suppress* gene expression for proinflammatory proteins. Overall, glucocorticoids inhibit the cytokine production responsible for recruitment and migration of inflammatory cells such as eosinophils and lymphocytes into the airway. Examples of cytokines that are suppressed through gene suppression activity of steroids are listed in Box 11-2.

Glucocorticoids inhibit many of the cells involved in airway inflammation, including macrophages, T lymphocytes, eosinophils, and mast cells, in the bronchial airway epithelium and submucosa, and reverse the shedding of epithelial cells and goblet cell hyperplasia seen in asthma.[25,29] By decreasing cytokine-mediated survival of eosinophils, apoptosis of eosinophils occurs, reducing the number of eosinophils in the circulation and in the airway of subjects with asthma. Glucocorticoids also reduce the number of mast cells within the airways; mast cells are sources of histamine and other mediators of inflammation and inhibit plasma exudation and mucus secretion in inflamed airways.[24,29-30]

Effect on White Blood Cell Count

Leukocytes, such as monocytes, macrophages, neutrophils, and basophils, are also essential to the inflammatory response and are attracted to an area of injury by the chemotactic factors identified among the mediators of inflammation. Neutrophils usually adhere ("marginate") to the capillary endothelium of storage sites in the lung. Glucocorticoids cause depletion of these stores and reduce their accumulation at inflammatory sites and in exudates. This is termed *demargination* and can increase the number of neutrophils in circulation when the cells leave their storage sites. An overall increase in the white blood cell count can be seen in patients receiving glucocorticoids. Glucocorticoids affect other leukocytes by inhibiting the number of monocytes, basophils, and eosinophils; this can also be seen in the differential count of these cells. A person with allergic asthma who would otherwise have a higher than normal eosinophil count would show a low count after initiation of drug therapy. Finally, glucocorticoids constrict the microvasculature to reduce leakage of the previously cited cells and fluids into inflammatory sites.

Effect on β Receptors

β-Adrenergic agents are among the most potent inhibitors of mast cell release; yet an individual with asthma in an acute episode may be unresponsive to these drugs. A beneficial effect of glucocorticoids is their ability to restore responsiveness to β-adrenergic stimulation.[23,30] This effect can be seen within 1 to 4 hours after intravenous administration of glucocorticoids and is the rationale for administering a bolus of steroid in status asthmaticus as part of acute treatment. Although steroid action is slow, the sooner steroids are given, the sooner the asthmatic patient begins to respond to β-adrenergic drugs, and supported ventilation may be avoided. Glucocorticoids enhance β-receptor stimulation by increasing the number and availability of β receptors on the cell surfaces and by increasing affinity of the receptors for β agonists. There is also evidence that glucocorticoids prolong endogenous circulatory catecholamine action by inhibiting the uptake-2 mechanism. The mechanisms for a positive interaction between β_2 agonists and corticosteroids

---

BOX 11-2   Cytokines* Involved in Airway Inflammation That Are Suppressed by Glucocorticoids

Tumor necrosis factor-α (TNF-α), interleukin-1 (IL-1)	Released from macrophages, monocytes, and other cells to activate endothelial cells to recruit neutrophils, eosinophils, and basophils from circulation
Interleukin-4 (IL-4), interleukin-13 (IL-13)	Released from lymphocytes and basophils and associated with allergic diseases; cause endothelium to bind basophils, eosinophils, monocytes, and lymphocytes
Interleukin-3 (IL-3), interleukin-5 (IL-5), granulocyte-macrophage colony-stimulating factor (GM-CSF), interferon-γ (IFN-γ)	Cause eosinophil priming, resulting in prolonged eosinophil survival and potentiated degranulation to release inflammatory substances
Chemokines	Family of small cytokines (molecules with masses of 8-10 kDa) having many chemotactic properties to attract cells to a site. *Example:* Regulated on activation, normal T-cell expressed and secreted (RANTES), one of the most potent chemokines, which induces eosinophil and lymphocyte migration and attraction

*Cytokines are proteins secreted by various cells, such as lymphocytes, that regulate local and systemic inflammatory responses.

are described in the discussion on aerosolized corticosteroid agents at the end of the section.

HAZARDS AND SIDE EFFECTS OF STEROIDS

Systemic Administration of Steroids

KEY POINT

Hazards associated with *systemically* administered steroids include HPA suppression, immunosuppression, fluid retention, muscle wasting, and others.

The complicating side effects of systemic steroid treatment are well known and provide the motivation to switch to aerosolized, inhaled steroids when possible. These complications arise from the physiologic effects of steroids on the body. These physiologic effects are often exaggerated with systemic drug therapy because potency and plasma levels are higher than with the body's own steroids. Complications of systemic therapy are reviewed by Truhan and Ahmed.[31] These complications are summarized in Box 11-3 and are briefly described here:

- Suppression of the HPA axis may occur, causing inhibition of ACTH release and cortisol secretion from the adrenal gland. The length of time to recover from this suppression varies with patient, dose, and duration of treatment.
- With sufficient dose and duration, immunosuppression can be caused; this can lead to increased susceptibility to infection by bacterial, viral, or fungal agents.
- Psychiatric reactions can occur, including insomnia, mood changes, and bipolar or schizophrenic psychoses.
- Cataract formation has been noted, and, rarely, intraocular pressure may increase.
- Myopathy of striated skeletal muscle can occur.
- Steroid-induced osteoporosis is debated, but is thought to be a limitation of extended steroid therapy. Aseptic necrosis of the bone is also caused by steroid therapy.

- Peptic ulcer is thought to be a complication, but evidence for this is debated. Patients may often be receiving other ulcerogenic medications such as aspirin or nonsteroidal antiinflammatory drugs (NSAIDs).
- Fluid retention can occur as a result of the sodium-sparing effects of glucocorticoids, giving a puffy appearance.
- Hypertension may accompany the fluid retention or be aggravated by it.
- Corticosteroids given systemically can increase the white blood cell count, with an increase in neutrophils and a decrease in lymphocytes and eosinophils.
- Dermatologic changes can occur, including a redistribution of subcutaneous fat causing the cushingoid appearance of central obesity, humpback, and moon face.
- Growth of children can be slowed by prolonged systemic therapy because corticosteroids retard bone growth and epiphyseal maturation.
- Corticosteroids lead to gluconeogenesis and antagonize glucose uptake, causing hyperglycemia. This can lead to reversible steroid-induced diabetes.

Systemic Side Effects With Aerosol Administration

KEY POINT

HPA suppression is minimal or absent with inhaled agents, although high doses can cause adrenal suppression in a dose-dependent fashion.

The rationale for the introduction of inhaled aerosol steroids was to eliminate or reduce the side effects seen with systemic therapy. Although aerosol steroids are administered in low doses because of their high topical activity, local side effects may occur, and certain systemic side effects, listed in Box 11-4, are also a concern. Some side effects may occur with transfer from oral therapy to the inhaled route. Three systemic effects of concern with inhaled steroids are

---

BOX 11-3 Side Effects Seen With Systemic Administration of Corticosteroids

- Hypothalamic-pituitary-adrenal (HPA) suppression
- Immunosuppression
- Psychiatric reactions
- Cataract formation
- Myopathy of skeletal muscle
- Osteoporosis
- Peptic ulcers
- Fluid retention
- Hypertension
- Increased white blood cell count
- Dermatologic changes
- Growth restriction
- Increased glucose levels

BOX 11-4 Potential Hazards and Side Effects With Inhaled Aerosol Corticosteroids

Systemic
- Adrenal insufficiency*
- Extrapulmonary allergy*
- Acute asthma*
- HPA suppression (minimal, dose-dependent)
- Growth restriction (dose-dependent)

Local (Topical)
- Oropharyngeal fungal infections
- Dysphonia
- Cough, bronchoconstriction
- Incorrect use of MDI (inadequate dose)

HPA, Hypothalamic-pituitary-adrenal; *MDI*, metered dose inhaler.
*After transfer from systemic corticosteroid therapy.

HPA suppression, loss of bone density, and growth restriction in children. Possible systemic side effects with inhaled steroids are the following:

- Adrenal insufficiency may occur after transfer from systemic to inhaled aerosol steroids. Weaning from systemic steroids to allow recovery of adrenal cortex and HPA function and careful monitoring of pulmonary function can help control this problem.
- There may be a recurrence of allergic inflammation in other organs, such as nasal polyps or atopic dermatitis, after cessation of systemic steroids.
- Acute severe episodes of asthma may occur after withdrawal from oral steroids and transfer to inhaled forms. Aerosolized steroids may be inadequate to control asthma, especially during periods of stress, and short courses of oral drug may be necessary ("burst" therapy).
- Suppression of HPA function is nonexistent or low at small doses of inhaled aerosol steroids and increases with higher doses. Clinically significant suppression is rare at inhaled doses less than 800 mcg/day in adults and less than 400 mcg/day in children.[32] Goldberg and associates[33] investigated MDI beclomethasone administration in children with and without a reservoir. They found that 7 of 15 subjects using the MDI alone (average dose 474 ± 220 mcg/day) showed adrenal suppression as measured by 24-hour urinary free cortisol excretion. Only 2 of 24 subjects using an MDI-reservoir system (average dose 563 ± 249 mcg/day) showed such suppression. These results indicated that inhalation of low to moderate doses can cause some adrenal suppression and that use of a reservoir can reduce this, probably by reducing the amount of drug swallowed. Although higher inhaled doses of steroid have a greater risk of adrenal suppression, the dose at which the risk for toxicity outweighs the beneficial effect of an inhaled steroid is unknown.[32]
- Questions have been raised about the effect of inhaled steroids on growth when used in prepubertal children. A study by Wolthers and Pedersen[34] found a reduction in rate of lower leg growth with inhaled budesonide compared with a placebo. Growth restriction was seen in some studies with beclomethasone dipropionate, but other studies have found no effect on growth with the same drug by inhalation. Results may be confounded by the moderate growth restriction and delay in puberty seen as a result of asthma.[3] The authors cite a meta-analysis that found no association between growth impairment and inhaled beclomethasone dipropionate, even at higher doses.[35] Sharek and Bergman[36] found in a meta-analysis that the use of beclomethasone and fluticasone resulted in a decrease in growth. The benefits of inhaled corticosteroids in the treatment of asthma outweigh the possible consequence of growth reduction, however.
- No data have shown clearly the effect of inhaled glucocorticoids in asthma on bone density and osteoporosis. However, Israel and others[37] discovered that the higher the dose of inhaled corticosteroid, the greater the effect on bone density seen in premenopausal, asthmatic women.

It is logical that the risks of steroid-induced adverse effects are lower with the relatively low doses of inhaled steroids compared with systemic administration. However, the threshold doses by inhalation causing adrenal suppression or other effects are unknown. These effects generally are rare with doses of 800 mcg/day or less in adults and 400 mcg/day or less in children. Absorption of inhaled steroid leads to systemic bioavailability from both the swallowed portion and the inhaled portion reaching the lung. Table 11-4 summarizes data on the bioavailability of four agents. When administered orally, bioavailability ranges from less than 1% to more than 20% of the total dose; this is due to the high first-pass metabolism of the swallowed drug. In contrast, all of the inhaled dose reaching the lung is absorbed and enters the systemic circulation, where it is ultimately metabolized in the liver or extrapulmonary tissues.[11] The efficiency of the delivery device in depositing drug in the lungs determines the amount of drug entering the systemic circulation from the airway. Thorsson and colleagues[38] reported that an MDI of budesonide delivered 18% of the dose to the lungs, whereas a DPI preparation (Turbuhaler) delivered nearly twice as much (32%). Leach and colleagues[39] found that HFA formulations gave more than CFC formulations, with 53% of HFA beclomethasone deposited in the lung.

The higher deposition is related to the particle size distribution of the device. HFA inhalers give a much better particle size distribution than CFC devices. Unless lower doses are used with HFA devices and DPIs, greater systemic drug levels result compared with those produced with an equal dose from MDIs. Total bioavailability—and the amount of drug that can cause systemic side effects such as HPA suppression—is a function of the swallowed amount, with its bioavailability, and the inhaled amount, all of which is absorbed into the circulation. Many HFA corticosteroid doses are lower than CFC corticosteroid doses. Use of a reservoir device and mouth rinsing can minimize the oropharyngeal loss and amount of swallowed drug contributing to systemic bioavailability and potential side effects. It is necessary to adjust doses on the basis of

TABLE 11-4	Bioavailability of Oral and Inhaled Corticosteroid Agents	
	ORAL (%)*	INHALED (%)†
Beclomethasone dipropionate	<20	≈20
Triamcinolone acetonide	22.5	21.5
Budesonide	1.0	25.0
Fluticasone propionate	<1	20.0

Modified from Johnson M: Pharmacodynamics and pharmacokinetics of inhaled glucocorticoids, *J Allergy Clin Immunol* 97(suppl):169, 1996.
*Figures represent percentages of a 100% oral dose.
†Figures represent the 20% of an inhaled dose that reaches the lungs and indicate complete absorption of that fraction.

the efficiency of the delivery system and the amount reaching the airway.

Topical (Local) Side Effects With Aerosol Administration

KEY POINT

Inhaled agents may cause local *oral candidiasis, hoarseness, cough,* and *bronchoconstriction* in some cases.

Two of the most common side effects caused by topical application of inhaled steroids in the respiratory tract are oropharyngeal candidiasis (oral thrush) and dysphonia. Several other complications and precautions with the inhaled route are summarized subsequently.

Oropharyngeal Fungal Infections

Infections with *C. albicans* or *Aspergillus niger* may occur in the mouth, pharynx, or larynx with aerosolized steroid treatment. Some form of this may be seen in one third of patients taking the aerosol formulations; however, these infections respond to topical antifungal agents and seem to diminish with continued aerosol steroid use.[8] Occurrence and severity are dose-related and are more likely in patients who are also taking oral steroids. The use of a spacer device and gargling after treatment can reduce oropharyngeal deposition of the steroid and the incidence or severity of oropharyngeal fungal infections.

Dysphonia

Hoarseness and changes in voice quality also may occur with inhaled steroids in one third of patients. This dysphonia can be minimized by use of a spacer and by gargling. The effect is caused primarily by adductor vocal cord paresis, which is thought to be a local steroid-induced myopathy.[40]

Other Complications or Precautions

- *Cough and bronchoconstriction:* Occasionally, cough or bronchoconstriction may occur after inhalation of an aerosol steroid.[8]
- *Incorrect use:* Incorrect use of the MDI delivery vehicle represents a possible risk factor because inadequate amounts of the topical inhaled steroid are delivered.

With inhaled steroids, the following can minimize the risk of local and systemic adverse effects:

- Use of minimal doses (400 mcg/day in children and 800 mcg/day in adults), or the lowest effective dose
- Use of a reservoir device
- Mouth rinsing after treatments

KEY POINT

Side effects with inhaled steroids can be *minimized* by use of a reservoir device, rinsing of the mouth after treatments, and use of minimal doses.

CLINICAL APPLICATION OF AEROSOL STEROIDS

Corticosteroids are used for a wide variety of conditions with the therapeutic goal of reducing inflammation. These applications include clinical conditions such as contact dermatitis, rheumatoid arthritis, and systemic lupus erythematosus, as well as asthma and COPD, and include topical cream application and oral, parenteral, and inhaled formulations.

Use in Asthma

KEY POINT

Inhaled steroids are used in asthma as a *first-line therapy* for mild to moderate asthma.

The 2014 Global Initiative for Asthma (GINA)[4] and the 2007 National Asthma Education and Prevention Program Expert Panel Report 3 (NAEPP EPR-3), *Guidelines for the Diagnosis and Management of Asthma,*[1] identify corticosteroids as long-term control agents rather than quick-relief agents. Corticosteroids traditionally have been used in asthma by the oral route for maintenance therapy of severe asthma, by the oral or intravenous route for treatment of status asthmaticus, and by inhalation for maintenance of asthma control. However, increased emphasis on asthma as a disease of inflammation leading to bronchial hyperresponsiveness has shifted the use of inhaled aerosol steroids from second- or third-line therapy to first-line, primary therapy. The use of corticosteroids can control asthma and improve asthma symptoms by reducing exacerbations and improving lung function.[1]

The principles of corticosteroid use in asthma, based on the previously mentioned guidelines, are summarized as follows:

- Bronchial hyperresponsiveness is characteristic of asthma and is related to the degree of airway inflammation.
- The basic pathology of asthma, previously emphasized as bronchospasm, is now understood to be a chronic inflammatory disorder of the airways resulting from a complex interaction among inflammatory cells, mediators, and airway tissue.[1] The phrase "chronic desquamating eosinophilic bronchitis" has been used to describe asthma.[8]
- Inhaled corticosteroids are considered to be the most effective long-term therapy for mild, moderate, or severe persistent asthma, and they are well tolerated and safe at recommended dosages.[1,4] Several points are related to the use of inhaled steroids:
  - Barnes[41] suggested starting inhaled corticosteroids at a high-enough dose to be effective and then reducing the dose. Alternatively, a short course of systemic corticosteroids can be used to gain control of symptoms followed by a step-down in therapy.[1] Loss of patient confidence and compliance with prescribed use of

inhaled corticosteroids may be avoided in this way, especially because steroids do not give an immediate effect as a bronchodilator does. Any reduction in pharmacologic management should be monitored by symptoms, concomitant need for β_2 agonists, and peak flow rates.

- An increase in dose of inhaled corticosteroids, such as doubling of the current dose, if PEF rates decline 25% to 30% may avoid the need for oral steroids. However, controlled studies are needed to confirm the effectiveness of such practices.[41]
- If asthma is not controlled by inhaled corticosteroids and other types of drug therapy, a short burst of oral steroids may be required to regain control of the asthma and to help clear the airways.[1,9]

Early Use of Corticosteroids in Asthma

There is evidence that the addition of an inhaled corticosteroid to first-line β-agonist maintenance treatment of asthma reduces morbidity and airway hyperresponsiveness.[1,42] Haahtela and associates[43] showed that subjects with mild asthma maintained on inhaled budesonide (1200 mcg/day for 2 years and then 400 mcg/day) had decreased bronchial response to histamine challenge compared with subjects taking inhaled terbutaline (375 mcg twice daily) over a 2-year period. Perhaps the most significant finding was that the later addition of inhaled budesonide after use of a β_2 agonist was unable to give as high a level of bronchoprotection as achieved by subjects who had started with and continued taking the inhaled steroid. This finding suggests that irreversible changes had occurred during the 2 years of β_2-agonist therapy and supports earlier use of inhaled steroids.

Pauwels and colleagues[44] found that early treatment in mild persistent asthma with low-dose corticosteroids decreased exacerbations, increased symptom-free days, improved FEV_1, and decreased the need for systemic corticosteroids. In a meta-analysis, Masoli and colleagues[45] reported that inhaled corticosteroids are best in treating asthma when kept to a therapeutic range of 400 mcg/day. Although inhaled corticosteroids are first-line antiinflammatory agents and acceptable for primary therapy of moderate asthma in children, the antiasthmatic prophylactic agents cromolyn sodium, nedocromil sodium, and leukotriene modifiers may be used as an initial choice for long-term control therapy of mild persistent asthma (step 2 therapy) in children because these medications have excellent safety profiles.[1]

Inhaled Corticosteroids for Acute Severe Asthma

Inhaled corticosteroids have not been considered useful for treatment of acute, severe asthma episodes, and drug labeling contraindicates this use because there is no bronchodilator effect. In addition, the dose of inhaled steroids is low compared with oral administration. A study by Rodrigo and Rodrigo[46] examined the addition of high, cumulative doses of inhaled flunisolide added to albuterol in emergency department treatment of acute adult asthma. Both drugs

were given by MDI with a spacer. Flunisolide was given as four puffs (250 mcg/actuation) every 10 minutes. Their protocol allowed 3 hours of this treatment, with a cumulative dose of 6 mg of flunisolide each hour, and equally aggressive albuterol dosing. The use of flunisolide resulted in better lung function at 90 minutes and afterward compared with the use of albuterol alone. Although preliminary, these results suggest that the contraindication to the use of inhaled corticosteroids for treating acute severe asthma may need to be reconsidered.

Clinical Use of Inhaled Corticosteroids

Other considerations in the clinical application of inhaled corticosteroids are as follows:

- High-dose inhaled steroids can be tried in cases of severe, persistent asthma to replace or reduce oral corticosteroid dependence. High doses of inhaled steroids are two to four times the usual recommended dose. Oral steroid therapy can be reduced slowly while monitoring the patient's pulmonary function.[1] (Note that relative inhaled doses considered low, medium, and high are given in the NAEPP guidelines.)
- Although more control may be achieved with high doses of inhaled steroids, side effects, including systemic effects, are also likely to increase with inhaled doses greater than 1 mg/day. However, if oral steroids can be replaced or even reduced, this can be an overall improvement in the risk-to-benefit ratio.
- MDI-formulated corticosteroids should be administered for oral inhalation using a reservoir device (preferably a holding chamber rather than a spacer), and all formulations should include mouth rinsing to reduce the risk of oropharyngeal candidiasis or other fungal infections and to reduce systemic absorption from swallowed drug.
- Use of a long-acting β_2 agonist such as salmeterol in subjects with inadequate symptom control, who are already receiving low to moderate doses of inhaled corticosteroids, may prevent the need to increase the inhaled corticosteroid dose.[1]
- The use of long-term β-agonist therapy with a corticosteroid can improve lung function.[1]
- Compliance with prescribed steroid therapy by inhalation seems to be poor and can be a complicating factor in the management of asthma and COPD. The ability to reduce agents or move to once-a-day dosing may be helpful.

Use in Chronic Obstructive Pulmonary Disease

KEY POINT

Glucocorticoids may be useful in chronic obstructive pulmonary disease (COPD) and are often administered systemically for acute exacerbations. Inhaled glucocorticoids are prescribed for long-term results.

The use of steroids in COPD is recognized as having potential action in relieving symptoms and exacerbations, but steroid use has little to no effect on FEV_1. The use of corticosteroids is described in the 2004 ATS guidelines[2] and in the 2009 GOLD guidelines.[3] A review and update on COPD have been provided by Fabbri and colleagues.[47]

COPD is characterized by a different pattern of inflammatory cells than is seen in asthma.[48,49] Eosinophils predominate in asthma, whereas neutrophils predominate in COPD. Oral and inhaled corticosteroids do not influence the inflammatory changes driven by neutrophils.[26,48,49]

Available studies show that corticosteroid use in COPD reduces exacerbations, symptoms, and mortality[50] but has little effect on pulmonary function results.[51-54] Other studies have found that inhaled corticosteroids may slow the decline of FEV_1.[53,55]

In acute exacerbations of COPD, oral or parenteral steroids are often given. Short-term corticosteroid therapy has shown benefits in hospitalized patients.[3,4] Maltais and associates[56] found that 2 mg of liquid nebulized budesonide improved FEV_1 compared with a placebo and had similar results to 30 mg of oral prednisolone. Use of inhaled corticosteroids is much safer than oral steroid use. Patients with stable COPD should not be given systemic corticosteroids.[2]

RESPIRATORY CARE ASSESSMENT OF INHALED CORTICOSTEROID THERAPY

Before Treatment

- Instruct patient in correct use of the aerosol delivery system (MDI, holding chamber, SVN, or DPI), and then verify.
- Assess breathing rate and pattern.
- Assess breath sounds by auscultation before and after treatment.
- Assess pulse before and after treatment.
- Assess patient's subjective reaction to treatment for any change in breathing effort or pattern.

During Treatment and Short Term

- Verify that patient understands that a corticosteroid is a controller agent and is aware of its difference from a rescue bronchodilator (relieving agent); assess patient's understanding of the need for consistent use of an inhaled corticosteroid (compliance with therapy).
- In asthma, instruct patient in use of a peak flow meter to monitor baseline PEF and changes. Verify that there is a specific action plan, based on symptoms and peak flow meter results. Patient should be clear on when to contact a physician with deterioration in PEF or exacerbation of symptoms.

Long Term

- Assess severity of symptoms (coughing, wheezing, nocturnal awakenings); symptoms during exertion; use of rescue bronchodilator; number of exacerbations; missed work or school days; and pulmonary function. Modify level of therapy with reference to NAEPP or GINA guidelines for asthma and ATS or GOLD guidelines for COPD.
- Assess for presence of side effects with inhaled steroid therapy (oral thrush, hoarseness or voice changes, cough or wheezing with MDI use); have patient use a reservoir (preferably a holding chamber) with MDI use and verify correct use.

General Contraindications

- In general, corticosteroids are safe. However, using the lowest effective dose is best practice.
- Patients should rinse mouth after inhalation of a corticosteroid.

? SELF-ASSESSMENT QUESTIONS

Answers can be found in Appendix A.

1. Identify all corticosteroids using generic names approved for clinical use by oral inhalation in the United States.
2. What is the major therapeutic effect of corticosteroids?
3. Name two common respiratory diseases in which inhaled corticosteroids are prescribed.
4. What is the rationale for administering corticosteroids by the inhalation route, rather than by the oral route, in asthma?
5. Contrast the effects of β agonists with the effects of corticosteroids on the early phase and late phase of asthma.
6. What is the effect of orally administered corticosteroids on growth, bone density, and adrenal function?
7. What is the purpose of alternate-day steroid therapy?
8. Can you transfer an asthmatic patient from oral steroid use to inhaled steroid use? Explain the precautions or reasons, as appropriate.
9. State two common side effects with inhaled steroids.
10. Identify two methods of minimizing the side effects identified in question 9.
11. Have inhaled corticosteroids traditionally been used with an asthmatic during an acute episode?

📖 CLINICAL SCENARIO

Answers can be found in Appendix A.

A 55-year-old white woman presents to the emergency department with a chief complaint of cough, wheezing, shortness of breath, and chest pain. She is well nourished and educated. She is a known asthmatic, with one hospitalization in the previous year for asthma exacerbation. She reported experiencing rhinorrhea, sore

Continued

throat, sinus congestion, and subsequent increase in dyspnea and wheeze 2 days earlier.

Physical examination on admission to the emergency department revealed wheezing on auscultation, use of accessory muscles, no cyanosis or diaphoresis, and mild respiratory distress. Vital signs were as follows: temperature (T) of 98.4° F, pulse (P) of 96 beats/min, regular, respiratory rate (RR) of 22 breaths/min, and blood pressure (BP) of 92/68 mm Hg.

A chest radiograph showed hyperinflation but no infiltrates or other abnormalities. An electrocardiogram revealed sinus tachycardia. Arterial blood gas determination on room air indicated the following: pH of 7.44, arterial carbon dioxide pressure ($PaCO_2$) of 38 mm Hg, arterial oxygen pressure (PaO_2) of 54 mm Hg, base excess (BE) at 2.2, bicarbonate (HCO_3^-) of 25.9 mEq/L, and arterial oxygen saturation (SaO_2) of 89.4%. Hemoglobin was at 13.3 g/dL, and the white blood cell count (WBC) was $8.8 \times 10^3/mm^3$. Administration of MDI albuterol by reservoir showed little improvement in her peak flow rates.

Using the SOAP method, assess this clinical scenario.

REFERENCES

1. National Asthma Education and Prevention Program, National Heart, Lung, and Blood Institute, National Institutes of Health: *Expert Panel Report 3: guidelines for the diagnosis and management of asthma*, NIH Publication No. 08-4051, Bethesda, MD, 2007, National Institutes of Health. Available at: <http://www.nhlbi.nih.gov/guidelines/asthma/asthgdln.htm>.

2. Celli BR, MacNee W, ATS/ERS Task Force: Standards for the diagnosis and treatment of patients with COPD: a summary of the ATS/ERS position paper. *Eur Respir J* 23:932, 2004. Available at: <http://www.thoracic.org/statements/resources/copd/copdexecsum.pdf>.

3. Global Initiative for Chronic Obstructive Lung Disease: *Global strategy for the diagnosis, management, and prevention of COPD*, National Heart, Lung, and Blood Institute (Bethesda, MD) and World Health Organization (Geneva, Switzerland), 2014. Available at: <http://www.goldcopd.org/uploads/users/files/GOLD_Report_2014_Jun11.pdf>.

4. Global Initiative for Asthma (GINA), National Heart, Lung, and Blood Institute, National Institutes of Health: *Global strategy for asthma management and prevention*, NIH Publication No. 02-1561, Bethesda, MD, 2014, National Institutes of Health. Available at: <http://www.ginasthma.org/local/uploads/files/GINA_Report_2014_Jun11.pdf>.

5. Holgate ST: The immunopharmacology of mild asthma. *J Allergy Clin Immunol* 98:S7, 1996.

6. Schwiebert LM, Beck LA, Stellato C, et al: Glucocorticosteroid inhibition of cytokine production: relevance to antiallergic actions. *J Allergy Clin Immunol* 97:143, 1996.

7. Kay AB: Mediators and inflammatory cells in allergic disease. *Ann Allergy* 59:35, 1987.

8. Reed CE: Aerosol glucocorticoid treatment of asthma: adults. *Am Rev Respir Dis* 141(Suppl):S82, 1990.

9. Laitinen LA, Laitinen A: Remodeling of asthmatic airways by glucocorticosteroids. *J Allergy Clin Immunol* 97:153, 1996.

10. Johnson M: Pharmacodynamics and pharmacokinetics of inhaled glucocorticoids. *J Allergy Clin Immunol* 97:169, 1996.

11. Berger WE, Tashkin P: Flunisolide hydrofluoroalkane with integrated spacer for treating asthma: An updated review. *Allergy Asthma Proc* 36:2, 2015.

12. Chaplin MD, Rooks W, II, Swenson EW, et al: Flunisolide metabolism and dynamics of a metabolite. *Clin Pharmacol Ther* 27:402, 1980.

13. Holliday SM, Faulds D, Sorkin EM: Inhaled fluticasone propionate: a review of its pharmacodynamic and pharmacokinetic properties, and therapeutic use in asthma. *Drugs* 47:318, 1994.

14. Phillipps GH: Structure-activity relationships of topically active steroids: the selection of fluticasone propionate. *Respir Med* 84(Suppl A):19, 1990.

15. McKenzie JE, Cruz-Rivera M: Compatibility of budesonide inhalation suspension with four nebulizing solutions. *Ann Pharmacother* 38:967, 2004.

16. Barnes PJ, Pedersen S: Efficacy and safety of inhaled corticosteroids in asthma: report of a workshop held in Eze, France, October 1992. *Am Rev Respir Dis* 148(Suppl):S1, 1993.

17. Clark DJ, Grove A, Cargill RI, et al: Comparative adrenal suppression with inhaled budesonide and fluticasone propionate in adult asthmatic patients. *Thorax* 51:262, 1996.

18. McCormack PL, Plosker GL: Inhaled mometasone furoate: a review of its use in persistent asthma in adults and adolescents. *Drugs* 66:1151, 2006.

19. Karpel JP, Busse WW, Noonan MJ, et al: Effects of mometasone furoate given once daily in the evening on lung function and symptom control in persistent asthma. *Ann Pharmacother* 39:1977, 2005.

20. Shapiro G, Lumry W, Wolfe J, et al: Combined salmeterol 50 μg and fluticasone propionate 250 μg in the Diskus device for the treatment of asthma. *Am J Respir Crit Care Med* 161:527, 2000.

21. Chung KF: The complementary role of glucocorticosteroids and long-acting β-adrenergic agonists. *Allergy* 53:7, 1998.

22. Jenkins C, Kolarikova R, Kuna P, et al: Efficacy and safety of high-dose budesonide/formoterol (Symbicort) compared with budesonide administered either concomitantly with formoterol or alone in patients with persistent symptomatic asthma. *Respirology* 11:276, 2006.

23. Anderson GP: Interactions between corticosteroids and β-adrenergic agonists in asthma disease induction, progression, and exacerbation. *Am J Respir Crit Care Med* 161:S188, 2000.

24. Barnes PJ: Inhaled glucocorticoids for asthma. *N Engl J Med* 332:868, 1995.

25. Barnes PJ: Molecular mechanisms of steroid action in asthma. *J Allergy Clin Immunol* 97(Suppl):159, 1996.

26. Barnes PJ, Pedersen S, Busse WW: Efficacy and safety of inhaled corticosteroids: new developments. *Am J Respir Crit Care Med* 157:S1, 1998.

27. Barnes NC, Qiu YS, Pavord ID, et al: SCO30005 Study Group: antiinflammatory effects of salmeterol/fluticasone propionate in chronic obstructive lung disease. *Am J Respir Crit Care Med* 173:736, 2006.

28. Baraniuk JN: Molecular actions of glucocorticoids: an introduction. *J Allergy Clin Immunol* 97:141, 1996.

29. Allen DB, Bielory L, Derendorf H, et al: Inhaled corticosteroids, past lessons and future issues. *J Allergy Clin Immunol* 112(Suppl 3):s1, 2003.

30. Svedmyr N: Action of corticosteroids on β-adrenergic receptors, clinical aspects. *Am Rev Respir Dis* 141(Suppl):S31, 1990.

31. Truhan AP, Ahmed AR: Corticosteroids: a review with emphasis on complications of prolonged systemic therapy. *Ann Allergy* 62:375, 1989.

32. Kamada AK, Szefler SJ, Martin RJ, et al: Issues in the use of inhaled glucocorticoids. *Am J Respir Crit Care Med* 153:1739, 1996.

33. Goldberg S, Algur N, Levi M, et al: Adrenal suppression among asthmatic children receiving chronic therapy with inhaled corticosteroid with and without spacer device. *Ann Allergy Asthma Immunol* 76:234, 1996.

34. Wolthers OD, Pedersen S: Controlled study of linear growth in asthmatic children during treatment with inhaled glucocorticoids. *Pediatrics* 89:839, 1992.

35. Allen DB, Mullen M, Mullen B: A meta-analysis of the effect of oral and inhaled corticosteroids on growth. *J Allergy Clin Immunol* 93:967, 1994.

36. Sharek PJ, Bergman DA: The effect of inhaled steroids on the linear growth of children with asthma: a meta-analysis. *Pediatrics* 106:e8, 2000.

37. Israel E, Banerjee TR, Fitzmaurice GM, et al: Effects of inhaled glucocorticoids on bone density in premenopausal women. *N Engl J Med* 345:941, 2001.

38. Thorsson L, Edsbacker S, Conradson T-B: Lung deposition of budesonide from Turbuhaler is twice that from a pressurized metered-dose inhaler P-MDI. *Eur Respir J* 7:1839, 1994.

39. Leach CL, Davidson PJ, Hasselquist BE, et al: Lung deposition of hydrofluoroalkane-134a beclomethasone is greater than that of chlorofluorocarbon fluticasone and chlorofluorocarbon beclomethasone. *Chest* 122:510, 2002.

40. Williams AJ, Baghat MS, Stableforth DE, et al: Dysphonia caused by inhaled steroids: recognition of a characteristic laryngeal abnormality. *Thorax* 38:813, 1983.

41. Barnes PJ: Inhaled glucocorticoids: new developments relevant to updating of the Asthma Management Guidelines. *Respir Med* 90:379, 1996.

42. Kerstjens HA, Brand PL, Hughes MD, et al: A comparison of bronchodilator therapy with or without inhaled corticosteroid therapy for obstructive airways disease. *N Engl J Med* 327:1413, 1992.

43. Haahtela T, Jarvinen M, Kava T, et al: Effects of reducing or discontinuing inhaled budesonide in patients with mild asthma. *N Engl J Med* 331:700, 1994.

44. Pauwels RA, Pedersen S, Busse WW, et al: Early intervention with budesonide in mild persistent asthma: a randomized, double-blind trial. *Lancet* 361:1071–1076, 2003.

45. Masoli M, Holt S, Weatherall M, et al: Dose-response relationship of inhaled budesonide in adult asthma: a meta-analysis. *Eur Respir J* 23:552–558, 2004.

46. Rodrigo G, Rodrigo C: Inhaled flunisolide for acute severe asthma. *Am J Respir Crit Care Med* 157:698, 1998.

47. Fabbri LM, Luppi F, Beghe B, et al: Update in chronic obstructive pulmonary disease 2005. *Am J Respir Crit Care Med* 173:1056, 2006.

48. Barnes PJ: Mechanisms in COPD: differences from asthma. *Chest* 117:10S, 2000.

49. Jeffery PK: Remodeling in asthma and chronic obstructive lung disease. *Am J Respir Crit Care Med* 164:s28, 2001.

50. Sin DD, Man SFP: Inhaled corticosteroids and survival in chronic obstructive pulmonary disease: does the dose matter? *Eur Respir J* 21:260, 2003.

51. Hattotuwa KL, Gizycki MJ, Ansari TW, et al: The effects of inhaled fluticasone on airway inflammation in chronic obstructive pulmonary disease, a double-blind, placebo-controlled biopsy study. *Am J Respir Crit Care Med* 165:1592, 2002.

52. Alsaeedi A, Sin DD, McAlister FA: The effects of inhaled corticosteroids in chronic obstructive pulmonary disease: a systematic review of randomized, placebo-controlled trials. *Am J Med* 113:59, 2002.

53. Highland KB, Strange C, Heffner JE: Long term effects of inhaled corticosteroids on FEV_1 in patients with chronic obstructive disease: a meta-analysis. *Ann Intern Med* 138:969, 2003.

54. Calverley PA: Effect of corticosteroids on exacerbations of asthma and chronic obstructive pulmonary disease. *Proc Am Thorac Soc* 1:161, 2004.

55. Sutherland ER, Allmers H, Ayas NT, et al: Inhaled corticosteroids reduce the progression of airflow limitation in chronic obstructive pulmonary disease: a meta-analysis. *Thorax* 58:937, 2003.

56. Maltais F, Ostinelli J, Bourbeau J, et al: Comparison of nebulized budesonide and oral prednisolone with placebo in the treatment of acute exacerbations of chronic obstructive pulmonary disease: a randomized controlled trial. *Am J Respir Crit Care Med* 165:298–703, 2002.

CHAPTER 12

Nonsteroidal Antiasthma Agents

Douglas S. Gardenhire

OBJECTIVES

After reading this chapter, the reader will be able to:

1. Discuss the indications for nonsteroidal antiasthma agents.
2. List available nonsteroidal antiasthma agents used in respiratory therapy.
3. Differentiate between the specific nonsteroidal antiasthma agents.
4. Describe routes of administration available for various nonsteroidal antiasthma agents.
5. Describe the mechanism of action for various nonsteroidal antiasthma agents.
6. Discuss the use of nonsteroidal antiasthma agents in the treatment of asthma.

KEY TERMS AND DEFINITIONS

Antileukotrienes Agents that block the inflammatory response in asthma.
Immunoglobulin E (IgE) Gamma globulin that is produced by cells in the respiratory tract.
Leukotrienes Chemical mediators that cause inflammation.

Mast cells Connective tissue cells that contain heparin and histamine.
Mast cell stabilizers Also known as *cromolyn-like agents*, agents used prophylactically to treat the inflammatory response in asthma.

In Chapter 11, to present the antiinflammatory actions of glucocorticoids, the concept of airway inflammation was introduced, and some of the numerous cells and chemicals involved in an inflammatory response were described. Chapter 12 presents drug groups that also have an antiinflammatory effect through mechanisms different from those of the corticosteroids. Three subgroups of agents are included in the nonsteroidal antiasthma group: cromolyn-like drugs (**mast cell stabilizers**), **antileukotrienes**, and monoclonal antibodies. A brief summary of the immune mechanisms involved in allergic responses is given as an introduction to the specific mechanisms of action for the drug groups discussed in this chapter.

CLINICAL INDICATIONS FOR NONSTEROIDAL ANTIASTHMA AGENTS

The general indication for clinical use of nonsteroidal antiasthma agents described in this chapter is *prophylactic* management (control) of mild persistent asthma (asthma requiring step 2 care, according to the classification presented in the 2007 National Asthma Education and Prevention Program [NAEPP] guidelines[1]).

The following are qualifications to the general indication for use of these agents:

- Cromolyn and antileukotrienes are alternatives to low-dose inhaled corticosteroids in asthma requiring step 2 care.[1]
- Cromolyn is often used with infants and young children as an alternative to inhaled corticosteroids in asthma requiring step 2 care because of the safety profiles of inhaled corticosteroids.[1]
- Antileukotrienes can be beneficial when used in combination with inhaled corticosteroids to reduce the dose of the steroid.

All of the nonsteroidal antiasthma drugs described in this chapter are controllers, not relievers, and are used in asthma requiring antiinflammatory drug therapy. Box 12-1 summarizes reliever and controller agents used in drug therapy for asthma, listing cromolyn sodium, antileukotrienes, and monoclonal antibodies as controllers. Use of rescue β_2-agonist agents more than twice a week (i.e., asthma requiring step 2 care) is an indicator of the need to initiate controller drug therapy.

IDENTIFICATION OF NONSTEROIDAL ANTIASTHMA AGENTS

Individual agents in the cromolyn-like agent group, antileukotriene group, and monoclonal antibody group are presented in Table 12-1 with generic and brand names, formulations and strengths, and usual recommended dosages.

BOX 12-1 Drug Groups Used in Pharmacologic Management of Asthma (Categorized as Controllers or Relievers)

Controllers	Relievers
Inhaled corticosteroids	Short-acting inhaled β_2 agonists
Oral corticosteroids	
Cromolyn sodium	Systemic corticosteroids (oral burst therapy, intravenous)
Long-acting inhaled β_2 agonists	
Long-acting oral β_2 agonists	
Leukotriene modifiers	Inhaled anticholinergic bronchodilators
Sustained-release theophylline	
Monoclonal antibodies (omalizumab)	

MECHANISMS OF INFLAMMATION IN ASTHMA

KEY POINT

Asthma is an inflammatory disorder of the airways in which *allergic stimuli* often trigger *immunoglobulin E (IgE)—mediated mast cell* release of mediators of inflammation. Airway reactivity also can be triggered by *nonspecific stimuli,* such as cold air or dust.

Asthma is a chronic inflammatory disorder of the airways.[1] Asthma has been divided into extrinsic and intrinsic forms on the basis of the triggers for asthma. *Extrinsic* asthma is dependent on allergy, or *atopy,* whereas *intrinsic* asthma shows no evidence of sensitization to common inhaled allergens.[2] The allergic form of asthma, which is **immunoglobulin E (IgE)**–mediated, is associated with younger subjects, and the intrinsic, or nonallergic, form is associated with later onset in adults in whom childhood asthma may not have been present. Corren[3] described asthma as an "evolving paradigm" disease in childhood, when viruses are an important trigger, whereas in school and teen years, allergens stimulate an immune response. As asthma progresses and in adults, the disease becomes intrinsic and may be driven by T cells (lymphocytes) that release various cytokines, as described in Chapter 11. Asthma is chronic and persistent, with continuous inflammation and episodes of acute obstruction.

In both forms of asthma, allergic and nonallergic mediators and enzymes are released to act on target tissues in the airway, and cells involved in inflammation are recruited and activated in the airway. Airway inflammation is manifested in the responses of bronchoconstriction, airway swelling, mucus secretion and obstruction, and subsequent airway wall remodeling that furthers the responsiveness of the airway.[4]

KEY POINT

The *clinical result* of asthma is chronic persistent airway inflammation and occasional acute episodes of wheezing and airway obstruction caused by *bronchoconstriction, mucosal swelling*, and *mucus secretion.*

Immunologic (Allergic) Response

Most instances of asthma are primarily an allergic response, which involves **mast cells** and IgE.[1] The immunologic response is outlined in Box 12-2. An understanding of the immune response is fundamental to discussing asthma and the mediator antagonists presented in this chapter because allergy is essentially a mistaken immune response.

Generation of an immune response and specifically an allergic asthmatic response is considered to be *initiated* by the interaction of T lymphocytes with an antigen presented by other cells, such as macrophages or B lymphocytes.[4] Activation of T lymphocytes results in production of IgE by

TABLE 12-1   Nonsteroidal Antiasthma Medications: Generic and Brand Names, Formulations, and Usual Recommended Dosages*

GENERIC DRUG	BRAND NAME	FORMULATION AND DOSAGE
Cromolyn-Like Agents (Mast Cell Stabilizers)		
Cromolyn sodium	Generic only	*Small volume nebulizer (SVN):* 20 mg/ampule or 20 mg/2 mL (1%)
		Adults and children ≥ 2 yr: 20 mg inhaled 4 times daily
		Spray: 5.2 mg per actuation. Available over the counter (OTC)
		Adults and children ≥ 2 yr: 1 spray in each nostril, 3-6 times daily, every 4-6 hr
		Oral concentrate: 100 mg/5 mL
		Adults and children ≥ 13 yr: 2 ampules 4 times daily, 30 min before meals and at bedtime
		Children 2-12 yr: 1 ampule 4 times daily, 30 min before meals and at bedtime
Antileukotrienes		
Zafirlukast	Generic; Accolate	*Tablets:* 10 and 20 mg
		Adults and children ≥ 12 yr: 20 mg twice daily, without food
		Children 5-11 yr: 10 mg twice daily
Montelukast	Generic; Singulair	*Tablets:* 10 mg and 4- and 5-mg cherry-flavored chewable; 4-mg packet of granules
		Adults and children ≥ 15 yr: One 10-mg tablet daily
		Children 6-14 yr: One 5-mg chewable tablet daily
		Children 2-5 yr: One 4-mg chewable tablet or one 4-mg packet of granules daily
		Children 6-23 mo: One 4-mg packet of granules daily
Zileuton	Zyflo; Zyflo CR	*Tablets:* 600 mg
		Adults and children ≥ 12 yr: One 600-mg tablet 4 times per day; CR, two tablets twice daily, within 1 hr of morning and evening meals
Monoclonal Antibody		
Omalizumab	Xolair	*Adults and children ≥ 12 yr:* Subcutaneous injection every 4 wk; dose depends on weight and serum IgE level

*Detailed prescribing information should be obtained from manufacturer's package insert.
IgE, Immunoglobulin E.

BOX 12-2   Overview of Immune Mechanisms Involved in Allergy and Inflammation

Cell-Mediated

T lymphocytes (from bone marrow stem cells, processed in the thymus) mediate the immune response by several mechanisms, including cytotoxicity and secretion of cytokines. Members of the family of T lymphocytes are the basis of cellular immunity:

- *Helper/T4 (CD4+) cells,* which are subdivided into the following:
  - *Type 1 (Th1) cells:* Regulate classic delayed-type hypersensitivity reactions and other actions related to macrophage activation and T cell–mediated immunity by the production of interferon-γ and interleukin-2 (IL-2)
  - *Type 2 (Th2) cells:* Translate mRNAs for interleukin-4 (IL-4) and interleukin-5 (IL-5) and are involved in atopic allergy. IL-4 is essential for production of immunoglobulin E (IgE) by B cells; IL-5 and granulocyte-macrophage colony-stimulating factor (GM-CSF) and interleukin-3 (IL-3) promote eosinophil maturation, activation, and survival
- *Suppressor/T8 (CD8+) cells:* Inhibit immune response to an antigen after the immune response has begun
- *Cytotoxic T cells:* Bind to viral antigen on the surface of infected cells to destroy the cells

- *Natural killer cells:* Lymphocytes related to cytotoxic T cells; their targets are thought to be tumor cells or cells infected with organisms other than viruses

Antibody-Mediated

Antibodies are serum globulins (proteins) modified specifically to combine and react with an antigen (substance capable of provoking antibodies or cellular immunity).

- *B lymphocytes:* Antibody-producing plasma cells; memory cells for later antibody production
- *Classes of antibody:* Classes of immunoglobulins are as follows:
  - *Immunoglobulin G (IgG)*
  - *Immunoglobulin A (IgA)*
  - *Immunoglobulin M (IgM)*
  - *Immunoglobulin D (IgD)*
  - *Immunoglobulin E (IgE):* Cytophilic antibody (binds to effector cells such as mast cells); termed *reaginic antibody;* involved in allergic responses and atopy

---

B lymphocytes. Antigen-specific IgE binds to effector cells such as mast cells and is termed a *cytophilic* antibody because of this. When activated by subsequent exposure to an antigen or allergen, mast cells release physiologically active mediators of inflammation, such as prostaglandins, **leukotrienes**, proteases, histamine, platelet-activating factor (PAF), and certain cytokines.[4] The cytokines released, which include tumor necrosis factor–alpha (TNF-α) and interleukin-4 (IL-4), can upregulate endothelial adhesion molecules.[3]

This cascade of mediators causes an inflammatory response manifested by vascular leakage, bronchoconstriction, mucus secretion, and mucosal swelling, all of which obstruct airflow in the bronchioles. T lymphocytes also release cytokines (e.g., interleukins), causing accumulation and activation of eosinophils, which also release chemicals to damage the airway. The process of initiating the inflammatory response and continuing it through amplification, as discussed next, is illustrated in Figure 12-1.

After being initiated by exposure to antigen, the inflammatory response in the airway is *amplified* by chemoattraction of more lymphocytes, eosinophils, basophils, and neutrophils and by an increase in mast cells. Adhesion molecules increase after stimulation of lymphocytes and mast cells by antigen or allergen. These molecules, found in epithelial cells (intercellular adhesion molecule-1 [ICAM-1]) and vascular endothelial cells (vascular cell adhesion molecule-1 [VCAM-1]) in the airway, are responsible for eosinophil, neutrophil, and lymphocyte recruitment from the microvascular circulation into the airways. The adhesion molecules enable leukocytes to marginate, cross the blood vessel wall, and migrate to the airway mucosa, continuing and further amplifying the inflammation that has begun.[5] The increase and activation of eosinophils are associated with increased inflammation and severity in asthma.[3]

Nonspecific stimuli, such as fog, sulfur dioxide, dust, and cold air, can stimulate sensory receptors and cause reflex bronchoconstriction[4] (see Chapter 7). Patients with asthma are more sensitive to such stimuli, which reflects altered neural control or chronic inflammation sensitizing the airway, or both. Nerve fibers of the noncholinergic, nonadrenergic excitatory system, containing potent peptide mediators, contribute to local effects on smooth muscle and mucous glands and reflexively stimulate cholinergic activity. Some of these peptides include substance P (SP), neurokinin A (NKA), and neurokinin B (NKB); they are released from sensory C-fiber nerve endings. These neuropeptides can also contribute to inflammation and the features of asthma previously described, such as mucus hypersecretion, smooth muscle contraction, plasma leakage, inflammatory cell activation, and adhesion. Neutral endopeptidase (NEP) is an enzyme that inactivates neuropeptides to limit their activity; NEP is found on the surface of cells that contain receptors for neuropeptides (smooth muscle, airway epithelium, and vascular endothelium). An increased release of excitatory neuropeptides may be involved in asthma.[4]

Nitric oxide is formed in airway tissue through the action of the enzyme nitric oxide synthase (NOS). There is evidence that in asthma NOS is upregulated in airway epithelium.[4] Nitric oxide, a potent vasodilator and bronchodilator, may be the neurotransmitter for the nonadrenergic, noncholinergic inhibitory nervous system (see Chapter 5). Nitric oxide, which can damage cells, possibly is induced by proinflammatory cytokines in asthma and contributes to the observed epithelial damage[5,6] seen in Figure 12-1.

A better understanding of the inflammatory process just described has spurred the development of drugs targeted at

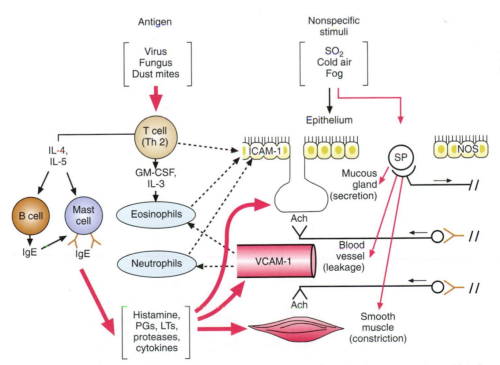

Figure 12-1 Illustration of complex interaction of cells and mediators that are thought to initiate and amplify inflammation of the airway in asthma, resulting in acute episodes of bronchoconstriction and persistent airway damage. *Ach,* Acetylcholine; *GM-CSF,* granulocyte-macrophage colony-stimulating factor; *ICAM-1,* intercellular adhesion molecule-1; *IgE,* immunoglobulin E; *IL-3, IL-4, IL-5,* interleukin-3, interleukin-4, interleukin-5; *LTs,* leukotrienes; *NOS,* nitric oxide synthase; *PGs,* prostaglandins; *SO₂,* sulfur dioxide; *SP,* substance P; *Th2,* helper T cell type 2; *VCAM-1,* vascular cell adhesion molecule-1.

interrupting the inflammatory processes and blocking the asthmatic response. These drugs include cromolyn sodium, mast cell stabilizer; montelukast, zafirlukast, and zileuton, which are antileukotrienes; and omalizumab, a monoclonal antibody.

> **KEY POINT**
>
> Allergic inflammation of the airway is the product of an *immune* response, and the *T lymphocyte* plays a central role in attracting *mast cells* and *eosinophils*, which in turn release mediators that attract other cells and damage epithelial cells.

CROMOLYN-LIKE (MAST CELL–STABILIZING) AGENTS

Cromolyn sodium, also termed *disodium cromoglycate,* is used as an inhaled prophylactic aerosol drug to prevent the inflammatory response in asthma. These drugs differ in structure and activity from the drug groups considered in previous chapters. Their chemical structures are illustrated in Figure 12-2. The basic catecholamine xanthine and steroid structures are given for comparison. Cromolyn is not related to the β agonists, xanthines, theophylline, or antiinflammatory glucocorticoids. Cromolyn has no intrinsic bronchodilating capability.

Cromolyn Sodium (Disodium Cromoglycate)

Cromolyn sodium is used as a prophylactic agent in the treatment of asthma. Although it may not be used as often in clinical practice today as it was previously, this agent is an alternative in mild persistent asthma.[1] The antiinflammatory, mast cell–stabilizing effect of cromolyn has led to uses other than asthma prophylaxis, including the following:

- Allergic rhinitis (nasal solution)
- Mastocytosis—to improve diarrhea, abdominal pain, headaches, nausea, and itching (oral)

Administration and dosage for these alternative applications are presented briefly in the next section, along with inhaled formulations for asthma and allergic rhinitis.

Dosage and Administration

Table 12-1 lists the inhaled, oral, and nasal formulations of cromolyn sodium and recommended doses.

Solution for nebulization. The ampoule or vial contains 20 mg in 2 mL of aqueous solution (a 1% strength). This solution can be nebulized in any small reservoir device powered by compressed air to produce suitably small particles of 3 to 5 μm in size. Additional diluent may be needed for most nebulizers to function well. Slow tidal breathing reduces the need for inspiratory maneuvers as seen with the

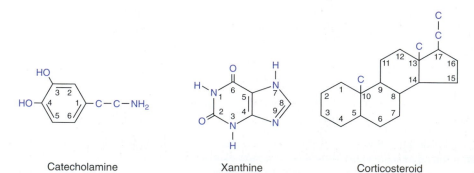

Figure 12-2 Chemical structures of cromolyn sodium (disodium cromoglycate) compared with basic catecholamine, xanthine, and corticosteroid structures.

metered dose inhaler (MDI), although longer administration times and lack of portability become a disadvantage.

Metered dose inhaler. The chlorofluorocarbon (CFC) version of cromolyn sodium was removed from the market as of December 31, 2010.

Nasal solution (NasalCrom). Cromolyn is available as 5.2 mg per actuation for treatment of seasonal and perennial allergic rhinitis. As with the inhaled solution, protection requires prior administration, although the drug does not need to be taken outside of seasonal exposure to allergens. The solution is delivered by means of a metered pump spray device that is available over the counter (OTC).

Mechanism of Action

Cromolyn sodium is considered an antiasthmatic agent, an antiallergic agent, and a mast cell stabilizer. Pretreatment with inhaled cromolyn sodium results in inhibition of mast cell degranulation, blocking release of the chemical

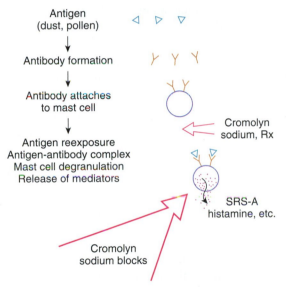

Figure 12-3 Mechanism of action of cromolyn sodium in preventing mast cell degranulation. *SRS-A,* Slow-reacting substance of anaphylaxis, consisting of leukotrienes C_4, D_4, and E_4.

mediators of inflammation (Figure 12-3). By its action, cromolyn is effective in blocking the late phase reaction in asthma. (The late phase reaction in asthma is discussed in the review of corticosteroids in Chapter 11.)

Cromolyn prevents the extrusion of granules containing the mediators of inflammation to the cell exterior. For this reason, cromolyn is often classified as a mast cell stabilizer. The exact mechanism by which this inhibition is accomplished is not completely understood, but the following details of cromolyn activity and mast cell function are known:

- The mechanism of action of cromolyn sodium is *prophylactic;* pretreatment is necessary for inhibition of mast cell degranulation.
- Cromolyn sodium may inhibit mediator release by preventing calcium influx necessary for microfilament contraction and extrusion of mast cell granules.
- Cromolyn sodium does not have an antagonist effect on any of the chemical mediators themselves.
- Cromolyn sodium does not operate through the cyclic adenosine 3′,5′-monophosphate (cAMP) system and does not affect α or β receptors.
- Antibody formation, attachment of antibodies (IgE) to the mast cell, and antigen-antibody union are *not* prevented by cromolyn; cromolyn does prevent release of mediators.
- Cromolyn sodium can prevent or attenuate the late phase response in an asthmatic episode, which can otherwise cause more severe airway obstruction 6 to 8 hours after initial bronchoconstriction.

The protective effect of cromolyn in inhibiting mast cell degranulation has been captured by scanning electron microscopy and is shown in the sequence in Figure 12-4. Initial understanding of the activity of cromolyn focused on allergy-triggered mast cell release of mediators, and the drug came to be considered useful primarily in allergic asthma. There is evidence that the activity of cromolyn is not limited to preventing allergen-stimulated asthma. Cromolyn inhibits mast cell mediator release caused by

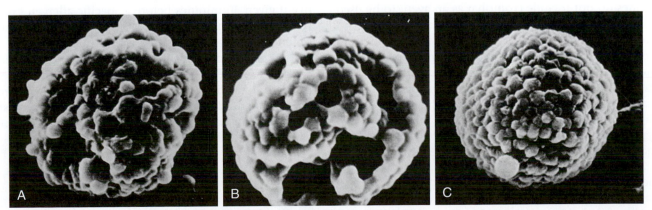

Figure 12-4 Degranulation of a mast cell. **A,** Mast cell undergoing gross degranulation shows free granules. **B,** The pores occupy a large area of the cytoplasm. **C,** Sensitized mast cell fails to degranulate after challenge when pretreated with cromolyn sodium. (Courtesy Rhone-Poulenc Rorer Pharmaceuticals, Inc, Collegeville, Pa.)

nonallergic stimuli and may reduce reflex-induced asthma. The latter requires about twice the usual dose of cromolyn. Understanding of the broader protection given by cromolyn has supported its successful use in allergic and nonallergic asthma and specifically in exercise-induced asthma.

Pharmacokinetics

As with other inhaled aerosols, cromolyn sodium is distributed to the airway and to the stomach via a swallowed portion. Distribution to the stomach (swallowed portion) can be modified by use of reservoir devices with the MDI formulation. The dose reaching the airway is absorbed from the lung and quickly excreted unchanged in the bile and urine. The lung portion does not seem to be metabolized in the airway. The swallowed portion is largely unabsorbed from the gastrointestinal tract and excreted in the feces.

Cromolyn sodium is a safe drug. It has an effectiveness similar to theophylline in controlling asthma, with a better therapeutic margin than theophylline.[1] Nasal congestion may be seen after beginning cromolyn sodium use. Dermatitis, myositis (muscle tissue inflammation), and gastroenteritis occurred in a very few patients.

Use of the *nebulizer solution* has been associated with cough, nasal congestion, wheezing, sneezing, nasal itching, epistaxis, or nose burning. Use of the *nasal solution* has most commonly been associated with sneezing, nasal stinging or burning, and a bad taste. Side effects with the *oral capsules* for mastocytosis are difficult to differentiate from effects of the disease itself. Adverse events with this use of cromolyn sodium were transient and included headache and diarrhea.

Clinical Efficacy of Cromolyn Sodium

The NAEPP guidelines provide a number of studies describing cromolyn sodium's effectiveness.[1] However, the guidelines do point out that other studies have not found it to be effective in the treatment of asthma. van der Wouden and colleagues[7] have reviewed 23 studies and found that most of the studies done had small samples that provided negative results; however, clinically relevant effects of sodium cromoglycate could not be excluded. What may be more telling is that the Global Initiative for Asthma (GINA) guidelines do not include cromolyn as an agent to be used in the treatment of asthma.[4]

Use for cough associated with angiotensin-converting enzyme inhibitor. Hargreaves and Benson[19] reported that cromolyn sodium, administered as two actuations four times daily of the 5-mg MDI formulation, provided protection against the cough often seen as a side effect with use of angiotensin-converting enzyme (ACE) inhibitors.[8] Cromolyn sodium significantly improved cough scores (frequency and severity) in 9 of the 10 patients in the study after 2 weeks. Cough was not completely suppressed in any of the 10 patients.

Anti–sickle cell effects. Both the intranasal solution and the 20-mg inhaled powder capsule of cromolyn given as a single dose were observed to cause a striking decrease in sickle cell percentage in nine African children with severe sickle cell disease. Improvement was seen 24 hours after administration of the single dose. The reduction in sickling is hypothesized to be due to the blocking of calcium-activated potassium channels, which play a major part in water loss and erythrocyte dehydration.[9]

Clinical Application of Cromolyn Sodium

Three points should be emphasized concerning the clinical application of cromolyn sodium with asthma and hyperreactive airway states:

1. The drug is prophylactic only and should not be used during acute bronchospasm. This is based on its mechanism of action because the drug must already be present to prevent mast cell degranulation. *It has no bronchodilating action* and may cause further bronchial irritation as an aerosol.
2. Abrupt withdrawal of oral corticosteroids and substitution of cromolyn sodium in patients with asthma can result in inadequate adrenal function. Cromolyn has no effect on the adrenal system, and tapered withdrawal of corticosteroids is necessary while beginning cromolyn use with patients.
3. It may take 2 to 4 weeks for improvement in the patient's symptoms that enable a decrease in concomitant therapy, such as bronchodilator or steroid use.

Guidelines for the management of asthma indicate that cromolyn sodium is used in subjects requiring regular use of β agonists for control of symptoms. It is considered an alternative to the use of inhaled corticosteroids, especially in children.[1]

Dosage regulation. The protective effect of cromolyn in allergic, nonallergic, or reflex-induced asthma is dose-dependent. The usual dosage of 20 mg four times daily (80 mg/day) with the nebulized solution in some cases can be reduced to a maintenance dosage of 40 to 60 mg/day after the patient is stabilized for 1 or 2 months. Likewise, if stimuli for asthma increase in severity (e.g., heavy exercise in cold weather [skiing] as opposed to walking in warm weather), higher dosages or addition of a β agonist may be required. For seasonal allergy, cromolyn should be started at least 1 week before allergen exposure. The drug is protective if given 30 minutes before a specific allergen exposure (e.g., cat fur), and a single dose 15 minutes before exercise on an occasional, rather than a continuous, basis is effective. As stated previously, the degree of exercise and the conditions must be considered in estimating the protection required. Long-term continuous maintenance with cromolyn may be needed for patients with reflex-induced asthma or for patients with late-phase reactions or severe bronchial reactivity and lability.[10]

KEY POINT

Cromolyn is an *alternative* treatment for asthma in children. However, low-dose inhaled corticosteroids are *preferred.*

Nedocromil Sodium (Tilade)

The CFC version of nedocromil sodium was removed from the market as of June 14, 2010.

ANTILEUKOTRIENE AGENTS

The name *leukotriene* is based on the fact that these molecules were originally isolated from leukocytes, and the carbon backbone has three double bonds in series, termed a *triene*. Chemical structures of the three antileukotriene drugs currently available in the United States are shown in Figure 12-5. Three antileukotriene agents (zafirlukast, montelukast, and pranlukast) attach to and block the receptor for leukotrienes; however, only zafirlukast and montelukast are approved for use in the United States. A fourth agent (zileuton) inhibits the synthesis of leukotrienes.

Leukotrienes and Inflammation

The leukotrienes are members of a group of biologically active fatty acids, including prostaglandins, thromboxanes, and lipoxins, that are known as eicosanoids. These molecules are lipid mediators of inflammation that are synthesized from the fatty acid precursor arachidonic acid (5,8,11,14-eicosatetraenoic acid). Arachidonic acid (AA) is found in cell nuclear membrane phospholipids. The leukotrienes mediate directly or indirectly at least some of the inflammatory process seen in asthma. They are potent bronchoconstrictors and stimulate other cells to cause airway edema, mucus secretion, ciliary beat inhibition, and recruitment of other inflammatory cells into the airway.[11]

Cell Sources of Leukotrienes

The leukotrienes and other lipid mediators are not preformed and stored in cells but rather are synthesized after a mechanical, chemical, or physical stimulus that activates phospholipase A_2 (PLA_2), an enzyme. These stimuli include antigen challenge of sensitized tissues and exposure to PAF or other cytokines. Certain cells, including eosinophils, mast cells, monocytes, macrophages, basophils, neutrophils, and B lymphocytes,[12] have the necessary enzymes to synthesize leukotrienes and other mediators. Eosinophils, mast cells, and macrophages are present and recruited to the lung in asthma.[13]

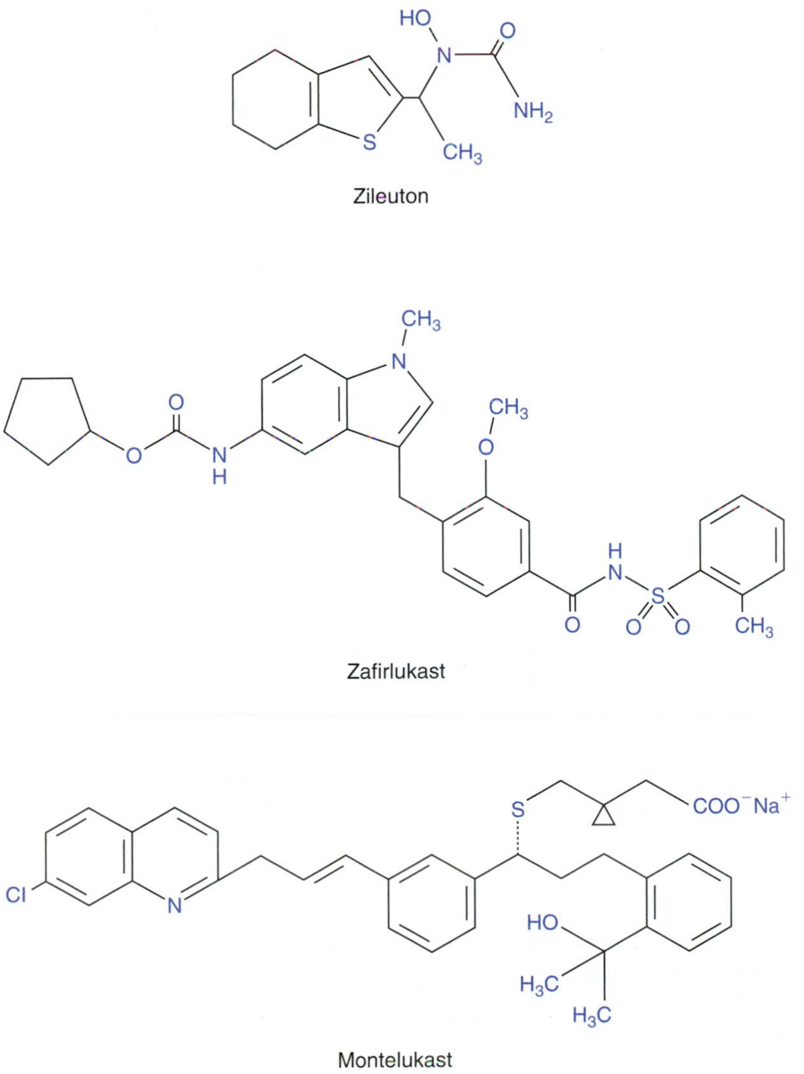

Zileuton

Zafirlukast

Figure 12-5 Chemical structures of the three antileukotriene agents: zileuton, zafirlukast, and montelukast.

Montelukast

Biochemical Pathways

A simplified diagrammatic view of the AA cascade, which results in the various lipid mediators, is given in Figure 12-6. Essentially, free AA is converted to various lipid mediators by two routes: the cyclooxygenase (COX) and 5-lipoxygenase (5-LO) pathways. The COX pathway results in the prostaglandins and thromboxane, and the 5-LO pathway results in the leukotrienes. Aspirin and other nonsteroidal antiinflammatory drugs (NSAIDs), such as ibuprofen, inhibit the COX enzyme, blocking prostaglandin and thromboxane production. There are two forms of the COX enzyme: COX-1 and COX-2. Many NSAIDs are mainly COX-1–selective, such as aspirin, ketoprofen, and indomethacin; some are slightly COX-1–selective, such as ibuprofen and naproxen. Other agents, such as celecoxib and rofecoxib, used to treat arthritis, have primarily selective inhibition of COX-2. The 5-LO pathway results in the synthesis of leukotrienes; this pathway is the target for drugs in the antileukotriene group.

Leukotriene Production

The lipoxygenase pathway resulting in leukotriene production is illustrated in Figure 12-7. After stimulation of an appropriate cell, the enzyme PLA_2, which is located in the cell cytoplasm, moves to the cell nuclear membrane. In the nuclear membrane, PLA_2 hydrolyzes phospholipids to liberate free AA. AA binds to 5-LO–activating protein (FLAP) (AA-FLAP). Another enzyme, 5-LO, moves from both the nucleus and the cell cytoplasm to the nuclear membrane and interacts with the AA-FLAP complex to oxygenate the

AA. This results in 5-hydroperoxyeicosatetraenoic acid (5-HPETE), which is converted to the unstable intermediate leukotriene A_4 (LTA_4). LTA_4 is the source of all the other leukotrienes. LTA_4 is converted either into leukotriene B_4 (LTB_4) or the cysteinyl leukotriene C_4 (LTC_4). LTB_4 and LTC_4 are exported from the cell to the extracellular space; LTC_4 is converted to leukotrienes D_4 and E_4 (LTD_4 and LTE_4). These three leukotrienes are termed *cysteinyl leukotrienes (CysLTs)* because they each have the amino acid cysteine in their chemical structure. The three CysLTs—LTC_4, LTD_4, and LTE_4—have been identified as the components of the previously termed slow-reacting substance of anaphylaxis (SRS-A).

Cysteinyl Leukotriene Receptors and Effects of Leukotrienes

Leukotrienes bind to leukotriene receptors to exert their inflammatory effects. Several different receptor types have been identified to date. LTB_4 binds to a seven transmembrane–spanning receptor, termed the *B leukotriene (BLT) receptor*. The BLT receptor is involved in cellular recruitment (chemotaxis), probably of neutrophils, and may be involved in acute respiratory distress syndrome (ARDS).

CysLTs attach to two subtypes of receptors: *$CysLT_1$* and *$CysLT_2$ receptors*. The proasthmatic actions of CysLTs are

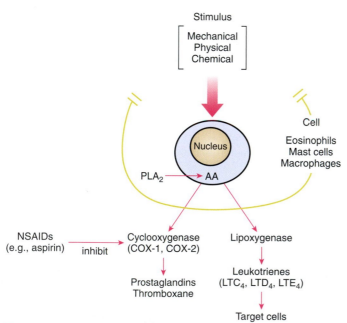

Figure 12-6 Simplified diagrammatic overview of stimuli and cell types involved in the arachidonic acid cascade, resulting in cyclooxygenase products, such as prostaglandins, and lipoxygenase products (the leukotrienes). *AA,* Arachidonic acid; *COX-1, COX-2,* isoenzyme forms of cyclooxygenase; *LTC_4, LTD_4, LTE_4,* leukotrienes C_4, D_4, E_4; *NSAIDs,* nonsteroidal antiinflammatory drugs; *PLA_2,* phospholipase A_2.

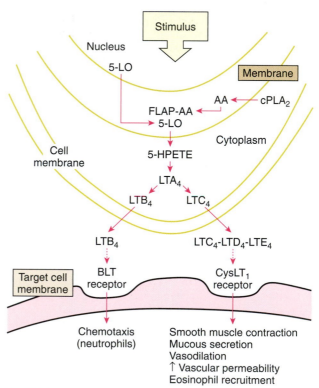

Figure 12-7 Detailed model of synthesis of leukotrienes through the 5-lipoxygenase *(5-LO)* pathway and their effects on target cells. See text for a detailed description. *AA,* Arachidonic acid; *BLT receptor,* B leukotriene (LTB_4) receptor; *$cPLA_2$,* cytosolic phospholipase A_2; *$CysLT_1$ receptor,* cysteinyl leukotriene receptor subtype 1; *FLAP,* 5-lipoxygenase-activating protein; *5-HPETE,* 5-hydroperoxyeicosatetraenoic acid; *LTA_4, LTB_4, LTC_4, LTD_4, LTE_4,* leukotrienes A_4, B_4, C_4, D_4, E_4.

mediated by the CysLT$_1$ receptor, which is located on smooth muscle cells in the airway and other cell types. The human CysLT$_1$ receptor has been cloned and characterized.[14] Stimulation of the CysLT$_1$ receptor causes bronchoconstriction, and CysLTs are more potent airway constrictors than histamine.[15] In addition to direct bronchoconstriction, there is an increase in bronchial hyperresponsiveness to other irritants, such as histamine. Other effects include mucus secretion in the airway, increased vascular permeability causing airway wall edema, and plasma exudation into the airway lumen. The resulting protein and cellular debris in the airway, together with the mucus secretion, increases secretion viscosity and may lead to airway occlusion such as that seen in asthma. CysLTs may also have an eosinophilic chemoattractant effect. Drugs that block the binding of leukotrienes to CysLT$_1$ receptors are named with the generic suffix -lukast (e.g., zafirlukast, montelukast, and pranlukast). The CysLT$_2$ receptor subtype mediates constriction of pulmonary vascular smooth muscle.[15]

CysLTs are produced largely by eosinophils, mast cells, and macrophages, all of which are cell types seen in the airways of people with asthma. Elevated levels of CysLTs may be markers of asthma. Leukocytes of people with asthma release more CysLTs than the leukocytes of people who do not have asthma. Plasma levels of LTE$_4$ correlate with asthma severity and are elevated in the urine of patients during an asthma attack, during exercise-induced asthma, and in the presence of nocturnal asthma symptoms.[13] Urinary LTE$_4$ is also elevated after challenge with an allergen in atopic asthma or with aspirin in aspirin-sensitive people with asthma.[11]

Zileuton (Zyflo)

Zileuton, available as Zyflo or Zyflo CR, is an orally active inhibitor of 5-LO. Its structure is shown in Figure 12-5. This drug is indicated for prophylaxis and long-term treatment of asthma and is approved for use in adults and children 12 years of age or older. It is considered a controller agent rather than a reliever and has no indication for use in an acute asthma episode.

Dosage and Administration

Dosage of Zileuton can found in Table 12-2. Zileuton is taken at meals and at bedtime. Hepatic transaminase enzymes should be measured and evaluated before initiation of treatment, once a month for the first 3 months, and every 2 to 3 months thereafter for the first year, with periodic monitoring for longer term therapy. If clinical signs of liver injury (right upper quadrant pain, nausea, fatigue, lethargy, pruritus, jaundice, or flulike symptoms) develop, the drug should be discontinued.

Mechanism of Action

Taken orally, zileuton inhibits the 5-LO enzyme, which would otherwise catalyze the formation of leukotrienes from AA. Specifically, 5-LO in the presence of FLAP catalyzes the conversion of AA to the intermediate 5-HPETE, which is converted to LTA$_4$ and ultimately the other leukotrienes. By interrupting the synthesis of these biologically active leukotrienes, their contribution to the inflammatory responses in asthma is effectively blocked. Both the (R)-enantiomers and the (S)-enantiomers are active as 5-LO inhibitors. The mechanism of action of zileuton is illustrated along with that of the other antileukotrienes in Figure 12-8.

Pharmacokinetics

Zileuton is rapidly absorbed when taken orally, with an apparent volume of distribution of 1.2 L/kg. The drug is about 93% bound to plasma proteins, including albumin. The drug has a half-life of 2.5 hours, is metabolized to glucuronide conjugates and an N-dehydroxylated metabolite in the liver by cytochrome P450 enzymes, and is eliminated in the urine and feces.

TABLE 12-2	Summary of Comparative Features of the Three Currently Available Antileukotriene Agents		
	ZILEUTON (ZYFLO)	**ZAFIRLUKAST (ACCOLATE)**	**MONTELUKAST (SINGULAIR)**
Action	5-LO inhibitor	CysLT$_1$ receptor block	CysLT$_1$ receptor block
Age range	≥12 yr	≥5 yr	≥6 mo
Dosage	600-mg tablet qid or bid if extended release	10-mg or 20-mg tablet bid	*Adult:* 10-mg tablet every evening *Children 6-14 yr:* 5-mg tablet every evening *Children 2-5 yr:* 4-mg tablet every evening
Administration	Can be taken with food	1 hr before or 2 hr after meal	Taken with or without food
Drug interactions	Yes; theophylline, warfarin, propranolol	Yes; warfarin, theophylline, aspirin	No
Common side effects	Headache, dyspepsia, unspecified pain, liver enzyme elevations	Headache, infection, nausea, possible liver enzyme changes	Headache, influenza, abdominal pain
Contraindications	Active liver disease or elevated liver enzymes; hypersensitivity to components	Hypersensitivity to components	Hypersensitivity to components

CysLT$_1$, Cysteinyl leukotriene receptor subtype 1; *5-LO,* lipoxygenase.

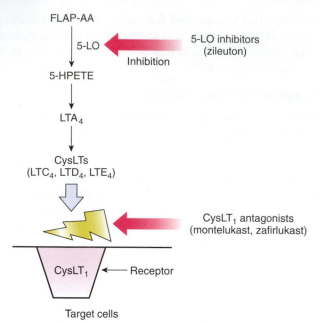

Figure 12-8 Illustration of the mechanism and site of action of the antileukotriene agents zileuton, zafirlukast, and montelukast. Zileuton inhibits the 5-lipoxygenase *(5-LO)* enzyme to prevent leukotriene production, and zafirlukast and montelukast antagonize the action of the cysteinyl leukotrienes *(CysLTs)* at the leukotriene receptor, *CysLT₁*. *FLAP-AA*, 5-Lipoxygenase-activating protein complexed with arachidonic acid; *5-HPETE*, 5-hydroperoxyeicosatetraenoic acid; *LTA₄, LTC₄, LTD₄, LTE₄,* leukotrienes A_4, C_4, D_4, E_4.

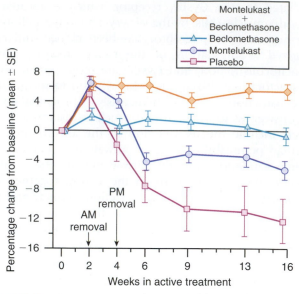

Figure 12-9 Mean (±SE) percent change from baseline in four treatment groups receiving combined inhaled beclomethasone and oral montelukast, beclomethasone alone, montelukast alone, or a placebo. The AM and PM beclomethasone inhalers were replaced with a placebo in the montelukast and placebo groups during the run-in period. (From Laviolette M, Malmstrom K, Lu S, et al: *Am J Respir Crit Care Med* 160:1862, 1999.)

Hazards and Side Effects

Side effects with oral zileuton that are greater than side effects with a placebo include headache, general pain, abdominal pain, loss of strength, and dyspepsia. Elevations of one or more liver function test values have occurred with zileuton, and it is recommended that hepatic transaminases be monitored before and during treatment. Liver enzyme levels may decrease or return to normal either during therapy or after discontinuation. Serum alanine transaminase (ALT), also known as serum glutamate pyruvate transaminase (SGPT), is a good indicator of liver injury. Zileuton is contraindicated in subjects with acute liver disease or transaminase elevations greater than three times the upper limit of normal.

Zileuton interacts with two important drugs in respiratory care: theophylline and warfarin. Zileuton can increase serum theophylline concentrations and can increase prothrombin time when given concomitantly with warfarin. Dosage adjustments of theophylline and oral warfarin may be needed.

Zafirlukast (Accolate)

Zafirlukast (Accolate) is a synthetic asthma prophylactic agent (its structure is illustrated in Figure 12-5). It is indicated for prophylaxis and long-term treatment of asthma and has been approved for use in children 5 years of age or older. This drug inhibits asthma reactions induced by exercise, cold air, allergen, and aspirin.

Dosage and Administration

Dosage of zafirlukast can be found in Table 12-2. Zafirlukast's bioavailability can be reduced with the consumption of food, therefore it should be taken at least 1 hour before or 2 hours after eating.

Mechanism of Action

Zafirlukast and montelukast are both leukotriene receptor antagonists and block the inflammatory effects of leukotrienes (Figure 12-9). Specifically, zafirlukast binds to the CysLT₁ receptors, with no agonist effect. This activity causes competitive inhibition of LTC₄, LTD₄, and LTE₄ and subsequent blockade of the inflammatory effects described previously in the section on leukotrienes and inflammation.

Pharmacokinetics

Zafirlukast is rapidly absorbed when taken orally. Peak plasma levels are reached 3 hours after dosing, with an elimination half-life of approximately 10 hours. Zafirlukast is metabolized in the liver, with 10% excreted in the urine and the remainder excreted in the feces. Administration of zafirlukast with food reduces mean bioavailability by about 40%.

Hazards and Side Effects

The most common side effects reported in healthy volunteers and patients were headache, infection, nausea, diarrhea, and generalized and abdominal pain. Infections were predominantly respiratory. Because zafirlukast is metabolized by liver enzymes, hepatic impairment (e.g., in cirrhosis) increases drug plasma levels. Although not noted in

6-month trials of zafirlukast, postmarketing surveillance indicated that doses greater than the 40-mg daily dose can cause elevations in serum aminotransferase concentrations.[15] A case of hepatitis and hyperbilirubinemia with no other attributable cause has been reported in a patient receiving 40 mg a day for 100 days, indicating the possibility of liver enzyme dysfunction with the drug (this case was reported in the manufacturer's drug literature).

Montelukast (Singulair)

Montelukast (Singulair) is an orally active leukotriene receptor antagonist (its structure is illustrated in Figure 12-5). It is indicated for prophylaxis and long-term treatment of asthma (a controller) and has no bronchodilating effect for use in acute asthma treatment. Montelukast is also approved for allergic rhinitis. Montelukast is the only one of the three currently available antileukotriene agents that is approved for use in infants 6 months of age. Montelukast has been shown to have clinical efficacy in treating mild to moderate asthma and exercise-induced bronchoconstriction. Compared with a placebo, montelukast significantly improved asthma control in children 12 to 23 months old, children 2 to 14 years old, adolescents older than 15 years of age, and adults.[16-20] To date, no safety issues have appeared with pediatric use. The manufacturer states that the drug has not been proven safe and effective in infants younger than 6 months of age. However, Knorr and associates[21] found that the 4-mg dose of granules was just as safe and effective in infants 3 to 6 months old as in children 6 to 24 months old.

Dosage and Administration

Dosage of Montelukast can be found in Table 12-2.

Montelukast can be taken with or without meals. Bioavailability when taken orally is not altered by a standard meal.

The oral granules can be directly poured into the mouth of the child or can be mixed with liquid or soft food. Infant formula, breast milk, applesauce, ice cream, and soft foods such as carrots and rice were used in studies. The manufacturer suggests only these foods should be used.

Mechanism of Action

Similar to zafirlukast, montelukast is a competitive antagonist for the CysLTs LTC_4, LTD_4, and LTE_4. It binds with high affinity and selectivity to the $CysLT_1$ receptor subtype (see Figure 12-8). Blockade of the $CysLT_1$ receptor prevents leukotriene stimulation of the receptor on target cells such as airway smooth muscle and secretory glands. Montelukast has been shown to inhibit both early and late phase bronchoconstriction caused by antigen challenge.

Pharmacokinetics

Montelukast is rapidly absorbed after oral administration. With a 10-mg dose, peak plasma concentration occurred in 3 to 4 hours, with a mean oral bioavailability of 64%. This bioavailability was not influenced by a standard meal in the morning. Concentration levels were slightly higher with the

5-mg chewable tablet taken while fasting in adults. For the 4-mg chewable tablet, the peak plasma concentration was reached in 2 hours. The drug is metabolized extensively in the liver and excreted via the bile, with little urinary excretion. Mean plasma half-life in adults ranged from 2.7 to 5.5 hours. Mild to moderate hepatic insufficiency increases plasma levels, but no dosage adjustment is required. Severe hepatic impairment was not evaluated.

Hazards and Side Effects

The safety profile of montelukast was similar to a placebo in drug testing. Adverse events that occurred in 2% or more of cases included diarrhea, laryngitis, pharyngitis, nausea, otitis, sinusitis, and viral infection. Hypersensitivity reactions were reported. Liver enzymes were not altered compared with a placebo. Phenobarbital decreases the plasma level of montelukast, but the manufacturer suggests no dosage adjustment. If potent cytochrome P450 enzyme inducers such as phenobarbital or rifampin are used, appropriate clinical monitoring is suggested.

Role of Antileukotriene Drugs in Asthma Management

Antileukotriene agents are recommended in the NAEPP guidelines for the treatment of mild to moderate asthma.[1] Table 12-2 summarizes comparative features of the three currently available antileukotriene agents. Drazen and colleagues[15] published an excellent review of asthma management with these agents.

KEY POINT

Drugs that act to *inhibit the mediators* of inflammation include *cromolyn sodium, zafirlukast, montelukast,* and *zileuton*. These agents are *prophylactic* and intended for the management of chronic asthma rather than for relief of acute airway obstruction. They do not provide bronchodilation in an acute asthma episode. *Cromolyn* is available as a nebulizer solution and a metered nasal spray and acts as a mast cell stabilizer. The agents discussed are indicated in the management of *mild to moderate asthma*, when more than occasional β-agonist use is needed.

Zafirlukast and *montelukast* are available as oral agents and act by competitive antagonism of cysteinyl leukotriene receptor subtype 1 ($CysLT_1$) to prevent bronchoconstriction, vascular permeability, and mucus secretion. *Zileuton* is another oral agent and acts by inhibiting the 5-lipoxygenase (5-LO) enzyme to prevent generation of leukotrienes.

Protection Against Specific Asthma Triggers

Antileukotrienes are particularly useful in controlling asthma resulting from certain triggers, including exercise-induced asthma, aspirin-induced asthma, and, to a lesser extent, allergen-induced asthma.[15,22]

- *Exercise-induced asthma:* In exercise-induced asthma, cooling and drying of the airway promotes the generation of leukotrienes, resulting in bronchoconstriction.

Although protection varies from complete to very little, the antileukotrienes develop no tolerance and may benefit patients who want to exercise or whose jobs require exercise under cold and dry conditions, without the use of short-acting rescue β agonists.

- *Aspirin-induced asthma:* In 3% to 8% of asthma cases, aspirin or NSAIDs can cause bronchoconstriction as a result of an increase in LTC_4 synthase activity. On the basis of such pathophysiology, which involves leukotriene production, leukotriene modifiers are the treatment of choice of patients with aspirin-induced asthma.
- *Allergen-induced asthma:* Antileukotrienes also block the early asthma response to allergen challenge and attenuate airway obstruction in the late-phase response. They are not completely effective in abolishing the late response that is also due to histamine release.

Chronic Persistent Asthma

The evidence to date supports the use of antileukotriene agents in the management of mild, moderate, or severe chronic asthma.[15,23,24] In mild to moderate asthma, antileukotrienes improve lung function, reduce the need for rescue β-agonist use, and decrease asthma symptoms, including nocturnal symptoms. In moderate to severe asthma, the additive effect between antileukotrienes and inhaled corticosteroids is the basis for asthma control with lower steroid doses or without an increase in steroid dosing (inhaled or oral). The advantages and disadvantages of antileukotriene drug therapy in asthma are summarized in Box 12-3.

Antileukotriene drug therapy is effective in approximately 50% of patients (although this proportion is greater for aspirin-sensitive individuals), but there is no method to predict which patients will be responders.[25,26] Considerable intersubject variability in response has been seen. In a study of exercise challenge, 20 mg of zafirlukast gave complete

protection in three subjects, partial protection in four subjects, and no protection in one subject.[27]

Antileukotrienes in Relation to Corticosteroids

Asthma guidelines agree that corticosteroids are the most effective antiinflammatory drugs for use in asthma, and they have broader antiinflammatory activity than the more limited effect of antileukotrienes. Leukotriene modifiers affect only one biochemical pathway—the lipoxygenase path and resulting leukotriene effects. Two aspects of antileukotriene therapy should be considered in relation to the use of corticosteroids in asthma:

1. Choosing between an inhaled steroid and an antileukotriene in mild persistent asthma is based on offsetting advantages: the superior efficacy of inhaled steroids with possibly poor compliance versus the anticipated superior compliance of the orally administered antileukotrienes with their more limited antiinflammatory action.[15]
2. There is an additive effect between antileukotriene and inhaled corticosteroid therapy in mild to moderate asthma. A study by Laviolette and colleagues[28] showed a greater response to inhaled beclomethasone alone compared with oral montelukast alone; however, the combination of the two treatments resulted in the greatest improvement in lung function, as seen in Figure 12-9. In another study, use of montelukast by adults with asthma taking inhaled steroids long-term resulted in a 47% reduction in steroid dose compared with a 30% reduction in the placebo group.[29]

Churg-Strauss Syndrome

Churg-Strauss syndrome has been reported in a few patients treated with zafirlukast[30] or montelukast (postmarketing letter).[31] Churg-Strauss syndrome is a vasculitis of unknown etiology, usually occurring in adults 20 to 40 years old, marked by peripheral eosinophilia, eosinophilic infiltration of tissues, and necrotizing vasculitis that can result in major organ damage and death if left untreated. The syndrome is rare, with a prevalence of about 1 case per 15,000 to 20,000 patient-years of treatment. Patients to date who developed this syndrome have had difficult-to-control asthma and have been taking oral or high doses of inhaled corticosteroids.

It is unclear whether development of Churg-Strauss syndrome is an effect of antileukotriene treatment, or whether the syndrome is unmasked by a reduction in corticosteroid therapy allowed by the antileukotriene therapy.[15] A review by Wechsler and associates[31] of eight patients concluded that the occurrence of Churg-Strauss syndrome in asthmatic patients receiving antileukotriene treatment seemed to be due to unmasking of an underlying vasculitic syndrome diagnosed as moderate to severe asthma and treated with corticosteroids. Nevertheless, experience in humans with antileukotriene drugs, specifically $CysLT_1$ receptor antagonists, is still new, and not all of the processes associated with 5-LO products are completely understood. For example, $CysLT_2$, which is *not* blocked by the $CysLT_1$

BOX 12-3   Advantages and Disadvantages of Antileukotriene Drug Therapy in Managing Asthma

Advantages
- Oral administration, possible once-daily dosing
- Safe, with few side effects to date
- Effective in aspirin sensitivity and often in exercise-induced asthma
- Systemic distribution reaches entire lung through the circulation
- Additive effect with inhaled steroids
- May reduce steroid dose or prevent an increase in steroid dose
- Formulation approved for pediatric dosing (montelukast)

Disadvantages
- Antiinflammatory action limited to one mediator pathway
- Unknown long-term toxicity
- Variable response; effective in about 50%-70% of patients
- No predictor of patients who will respond
- Systemic drug exposure, not limited to lung
- Generally not useful as monotherapy

antagonists such as zafirlukast or montelukast, has been identified on human pulmonary vasculature.[13] The effect of introducing a potential imbalance with $CysLT_1$ antileukotriene therapy is not well understood. Although antileukotriene drugs seem to be safe and effective, additional clinical experience is needed.

Summary of Clinical Use of Antileukotriene Therapy

The following points summarize the current understanding of the role of antileukotriene drug therapy in asthma:

- Antileukotriene agents are prophylactic, controller drugs used in persistent asthma, including mild, moderate, and severe states; they are not indicated for acute relief or rescue therapy.
- Antileukotrienes can be tried as an alternative to inhaled corticosteroids or cromolyn-like agents in mild persistent asthma requiring more than as-needed β_2 agonists.
- Antileukotrienes may not be optimal as monotherapy in persistent asthma.
- Antileukotrienes may allow reduction of high-dose inhaled corticosteroids or prevent an increase in the dose of inhaled corticosteroids, and they reduce or prevent the need for oral corticosteroids.
- Evidence to date shows these agents are safe and often effective choices in managing a wide range of asthma severity.

Monoclonal Antibodies

KEY POINT

Omalizumab (Xolair), a monoclonal antibody, is used to treat moderate to severe asthma.

Omalizumab (Xolair) is a subcutaneously injected monoclonal antibody. This drug is indicated for the treatment of moderate to severe asthma in adults and adolescents 12 years of age and older who have a positive skin test or in vitro reactivity to a perennial aeroallergen. It may be beneficial in treating seasonal allergic rhinitis.[32]

Dosage and Administration

Omalizumab is available as a powder that must be reconstituted; after reconstitution, it has a concentration of 150 mg/1.2 mL. Dosing is every 2 or 4 weeks and depends on the weight and serum IgE level of the patient. Refer to the manufacturer's package insert for specific dosing instructions.

Mechanism of Action

Omalizumab is a recombinant DNA-derived humanized IgG1(κ) murine monoclonal antibody that selectively binds to human IgE. The drug blocks the binding of IgE to the IgE receptor on the surface of mast cells and basophils (Figure 12-10). This blocking allows the reduction of mediators that can be released in an allergic response.

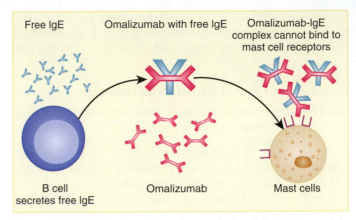

Figure 12-10 Model of omalizumab complexing to free immunoglobulin E *(IgE)* to stop attachment to a mast cell, stopping mast cell degranulation. (Modified from Rosenwasser LJ, Nash DB: *Pharm Therap* 28:400-441, 2003.)

Pharmacokinetics

After parenteral administration, omalizumab is absorbed with an average bioavailability of 62%. Omalizumab is absorbed slowly, reaching peak concentrations after an average of 7 to 8 days. If doses greater than 0.5 mg/kg are given, a linear correlation exists, meaning the more given, the greater the drug availability. Omalizumab is eliminated primarily via the liver. The half-life of the drug averages 26 days and may be weight-related: increasing weight increases clearance.[33]

Hazards and Side Effects

The most severe reactions occurring in clinical trials with omalizumab were anaphylaxis and malignancies; however, these were rare. Other, more commonly observed reactions included injection site reactions, viral infection, upper respiratory tract infection, and pharyngitis.

Omalizumab is not for acute asthmatic conditions. Patients taking inhaled or systemic corticosteroids and considering omalizumab should note that this drug is not a replacement for regular corticosteroid use.

Role of Omalizumab in Asthma Management

The literature at the time of this edition supports the use of omalizumab in uncontrolled moderate to severe asthma. Busse and colleagues[34] found that omalizumab reduced asthma exacerbations and decreased corticosteroid and rescue medication use. Soler and colleagues[35] found similar results in that asthma exacerbations per patient were reduced, and use of corticosteroids had decreased. Of patients taking omalizumab, 79% were able to decrease their steroid dose by 50% or more compared with only 55% in the placebo group. In an extension phase of a clinical trial for omalizumab, Buhl and associates[36] found that patients receiving omalizumab had fewer exacerbations and that their corticosteroid use had decreased by approximately 180 mcg/day. Lanier and colleagues[37] discovered that patients being treated with omalizumab reduced their corticosteroid use by 108 mcg/day compared with patients receiving a placebo. It was noted that many patients in the placebo group were given more long-term β agonists and leukotriene inhibitors compared with the omalizumab group.

Summary of Clinical Use of Omalizumab

The following points summarize the current understanding of the role of omalizumab in asthma:

- Omalizumab is a prophylactic agent used in uncontrolled moderate to severe persistent asthma; it is not indicated for acute relief or rescue therapy.
- Omalizumab is not a replacement for inhaled corticosteroids.
- Omalizumab is not optimal as monotherapy in persistent asthma.
- Omalizumab may allow reduction of high-dose inhaled corticosteroids or prevent an increase in the dose of inhaled corticosteroids.
- Omalizumab may allow reduction of asthmatic rescue agents.

RESPIRATORY CARE ASSESSMENT OF NONSTEROIDAL ANTIASTHMA AGENTS

Before Treatment

- Evaluate patient for optimal aerosol delivery formulation for inhaled medications, if more than one delivery system is available (e.g., small volume nebulizer [SVN] or MDI). Note age, ability to understand instructions, and need for reservoir with MDI.

During Treatment and Short Term

- Initially for aerosol medications: Instruct patient in use of aerosol delivery system selected (MDI, reservoir, SVN) and then verify correct use.
- Assess breathing rate and pattern.
- Assess breath sounds by auscultation before and after treatment.
- Assess pulse before and after treatment.
- Assess patient's subjective reaction to treatment for any change in breathing effort or pattern.
- Verify that patient understands that nonsteroidal antiasthma agents are controller drugs and understands their difference from a rescue bronchodilator (relieving agent); assess patient's understanding of the need for consistent use of these agents (compliance with therapy).
- Instruct patient in use of a peak flow meter to monitor baseline peak expiratory flow (PEF) and changes. Verify that there is a specific action plan based on symptoms and peak flow results. The patient should be clear on when to contact a physician with deterioration in PEF or exacerbation of symptoms.

Long Term

- Assess severity of symptoms (coughing, wheezing, nocturnal awakenings, and symptoms during exertion); use

of rescue medication; number of exacerbations and missed work or school days; and pulmonary function. Modify level of asthma therapy (up or down, as described in NAEPP Expert Panel Report 3 [EPR-3] guidelines for step therapy).

- Assess for presence of side effects with nonsteroidal antiasthma agents (refer to particular agent and its side effects, as listed previously).

General Contraindications

- In general, antiasthmatic agents are safe. However, each type of agent may affect each patient differently.
- Patients should understand that these agents are long-acting agents; if a crisis occurs, they should use short-acting medication.

❓ SELF-ASSESSMENT QUESTIONS

Answers can be found in Appendix A.

1. Identify four nonsteroidal antiasthma drugs used in the management of chronic asthma; give generic and brand names.
2. Which immunoglobulin is implicated in allergy and is termed *cytophilic*?
3. Which type of asthma involves allergic reaction to an antigenic stimulus?
4. Which type of helper T cell, Th1 or Th2, is involved primarily in the atopic allergic response?
5. A resident wishes to order nebulized cromolyn sodium for a young asthmatic patient in the emergency department who is wheezing and in moderate distress. Would you agree?
6. Which of the following could be recommended as possible choices for the asthmatic patient in question 5: inhaled albuterol, inhaled salmeterol, inhaled ipratropium bromide, theophylline (either orally or intravenously)?
7. An patient with asthma has been taking 40 mg of oral prednisone for 1 week after an acute asthma attack and an emergency department visit. His physician now wants to switch him to inhaled cromolyn and discontinue the oral prednisone. What is the risk in doing this, and what would you recommend?
8. How does the mechanism of action of zafirlukast and montelukast differ from that of zileuton?
9. What is the recommended dosage and route of administration for zafirlukast, montelukast, and zileuton?
10. Which of the three antileukotriene agents in question 9 offers the most convenient dosing and the fewest drug interactions?
11. When would you recommend using omalizumab?
12. A 17-year-old patient with asthma has been treated for symptoms for the last 12 months. His

SELF-ASSESSMENT QUESTIONS—cont'd

symptoms have not improved despite the use of the highest dosage of an inhaled corticosteroid agent and regular use of salmeterol; in addition, trials on montelukast, cromolyn sodium, and oral theophylline have been unsuccessful. What would you recommend for this patient?

CLINICAL SCENARIO

Answers can be found in Appendix A.

A 45-year-old white woman is seen in the emergency department with a complaint of chest tightness, shortness of breath, and wheezing for the past 1.5 days. She also complains of a cough, with only occasional thin, whitish sputum during that period. She denies any fever or chills. She was diagnosed with adult-onset asthma 3 years ago and is sensitive to aspirin. She has no history of tobacco use. She had a nasal polypectomy 2 years ago. She has been taking over-the-counter (OTC) racemic epinephrine for the past 4 months as needed because her albuterol prescription ran out. She was taking oral theophylline 300 mg twice daily from about 4 months ago. She is alert but mildly anxious.

Her vital signs are as follows: temperature (T) of 97° F, pulse (P) of 112 beats/min, regular blood pressure (BP) of 135/90 mm Hg, and respiratory rate (RR) of 22 breaths/min with no laboring. Expiration is slightly prolonged, but there is no use of accessory muscles. No cyanosis is evident. Auscultation reveals diffuse wheezes, greater on expiration than inspiration, and rhonchi bilaterally. Routine blood work later showed the following: hemoglobin at 13.5 g/dL and white blood cell count (WBC) at $6.1 \times 10^3/mm^3$ with 13% eosinophils. Electrolytes were also normal except for a plasma glucose level of 281 mg/dL. A chest radiograph showed some hyperinflation bilaterally, with no infiltrates, no pneumothorax, and normal heart size. Results of an arterial blood gas measurement on room air were: pH of 7.38, arterial carbon dioxide pressure ($PaCO_2$) of 42 mm Hg, arterial oxygen pressure (PaO_2) of 72 mm Hg, base excess +0.3 mEq/L, and arterial oxygen saturation (SaO_2) of 96%.

On questioning, the patient states that she has been using her OTC racemic epinephrine almost every 2 hours over the past 24 hours, with little improvement. She states that she has been experiencing many headaches, upset stomach, some lack of appetite, and insomnia often during the week. It has been 2 to 3 hours since she last used her OTC racemic epinephrine.

Using the SOAP method, assess this clinical scenario.

REFERENCES

1. National Asthma Education and Prevention Program, National Heart, Lung, and Blood Institute, National Institutes of Health: *Expert Panel Report 3: guidelines for the diagnosis and management of asthma*, NIH Publication No. 08-4051, Bethesda, MD, 2007, National Institutes of Health. Retrieved from: <http://www.nhlbi.nih.gov/guidelines/asthma/asthgdln.htm>.
2. Platts-Mills TA, Woodfolk JA, Chapman MD, et al: Changing concepts of allergic disease: the attempt to keep up with real changes in lifestyles. *J Allergy Clin Immunol* 98:S297, 1996.
3. Corren J: Asthma phenotypes and endotypes: an evolving paradigm for classification. *Discov Med* 5(83):243–249, 2013.
4. Global Initiative for Asthma (GINA): Global Strategy for Asthma Management and Prevention 2014. Retrieved from: <http://www.ginasthma.org>.
5. Flak TA, Goldman WE: Autotoxicity of nitric oxide in airway disease. *Am J Respir Crit Care Med* 154:S202, 1996.
6. Liggett SB, Levi R, Metzger H: G-protein coupled receptors, nitric oxide, and the IgE receptor in asthma. *Am J Respir Crit Care Med* 152:394, 1995.
7. van der Wouden JC, Uijen JH, Bernsen RM, et al: Inhaled sodium cromoglycate for asthma in children. *Cochrane Database Syst Rev* (4):CD002173, 2008.
8. Hargreaves MR, Benson MK: Inhaled sodium cromoglycate in angiotensin-converting-enzyme inhibitor cough. *Lancet* 345:13, 1995.
9. Toppet M, Fall AB, Ferster A, et al: Antisickling activity of sodium cromoglycate in sickle-cell disease. *Lancet* 356:309, 2000.
10. Bernstein IL: Cromolyn sodium in the treatment of asthma: coming of age in the United States. *J Allergy Clin Immunol* 76:381, 1985.
11. Busse W: The role and contribution of leukotrienes in asthma. *Ann Allergy Asthma Immunol* 81:17, 1998.
12. Busse W: Leukotrienes and inflammation. *Am J Respir Crit Care Med* 157(Suppl):S210, 1998.
13. Bisgaard H: Role of leukotrienes in asthma pathophysiology. *Pediatr Pulmonol* 30:166, 2000.
14. Lynch KR, O'Neill GP, Liu Q, et al: Characterization of the human cysteinyl leukotriene CysLT$_1$ receptor. *Nature* 399:789, 1999.
15. Drazen JM, Israel E, O'Byrne PM: Treatment of asthma with drugs modifying the leukotriene pathway. *N Engl J Med* 340:197, 1999.
16. Knorr B, Matz J, Bernstein JA, et al: Montelukast for chronic asthma in 6- to 14-year-old children: a randomized, double-blind trial. *JAMA* 279:1181, 1998.
17. Reiss TF, Chervinsky P, Dockhorn RJ, et al: Montelukast, a once-daily leukotriene receptor antagonist, in the treatment of chronic asthma: a multicenter, randomized, double-blind trial. *Arch Intern Med* 158:1213, 1998.
18. Leff JA, Busse WW, Pearlman D, et al: Montelukast, a leukotriene-receptor antagonist, for the treatment of mild asthma and exercise-induced bronchoconstriction. *N Engl J Med* 339:147, 1998.
19. Bisgaard H, Zielen S, Garcia-Garcia ML, et al: Montelukast reduces asthma exacerbations in 2 to 5 year old children with intermittent asthma. *Am J Respir Crit Care Med* 171:315, 2004.
20. Knorr B, Franchi LM, Bisgaard H, et al: Montelukast, a leukotriene receptor antagonist, for the treatment of persistent asthma in children aged 2 to 5 years. *Pediatrics* 108:E48, 2001.
21. Knorr B, Maganti L, Ramakrishnan R, et al: Pharmacokinetics and safety of montelukast in children aged 3 to 6 months. *J Clin Pharmacol* 46:620, 2006.
22. Dahlen SE, Malmstrom K, Nizankowska E, et al: Improvement of aspirin intolerant asthma by montelukast, a leukotriene antagonist: a randomized, double blind, placebo-controlled trial. *Am J Respir Crit Care Med* 165:9, 2002.
23. Becker A: Leukotriene receptor antagonists: efficacy and safety in children with asthma. *Pediatr Pulmonol* 30:183, 2000.
24. Kemp J: Role of leukotriene receptor antagonists in pediatric asthma. *Pediatr Pulmonol* 30:177, 2000.

25. Ind PW: Anti-leukotriene intervention: is there adequate information for clinical use in asthma? *Respir Med* 90:575, 1996.

26. Smith LJ: Newer asthma therapies. *Ann Intern Med* 130:531, 1999.

27. Finnerty JP, Wood-Baker R, Thomson H, et al: Role of leukotrienes in exercise-induced asthma. *Am Rev Respir Dis* 145:746, 1992.

28. Laviolette M, Malmstrom K, Lu S, et al: Montelukast added to inhaled beclomethasone in treatment of asthma. *Am J Respir Crit Care Med* 160:1999, 1862.

29. Lofdahl CG, Reiss TF, Leff JA, et al: Randomised, placebo controlled trial of effect of a leukotriene receptor antagonist, montelukast, on tapering inhaled corticosteroids in asthmatic patients. *BMJ* 319:87, 1999.

30. Wechsler ME, Garpestad E, Flier SR, et al: Pulmonary infiltrates, eosinophilia, and cardiomyopathy following corticosteroid withdrawal in patients with asthma receiving zafirlukast. *JAMA* 279:455, 1998.

31. Wechsler ME, Finn D, Gunawardena D, et al: Churg-Strauss syndrome in patients receiving montelukast as treatment for asthma. *Chest* 117:708, 2000.

32. Kaliner MA: Omalizumab and the treatment of allergic rhinitis. *Curr Allergy Asthma Rep* 4:237, 2004. (abstract).

33. Davis LA: Omalizumab: a novel therapy for allergic asthma. *Ann Pharmacother* 38:1236, 2004.

34. Busse W, Corren J, Lanier BQ, et al: Omalizumab, anti-IgE recombinant humanized monoclonal antibody, for the treatment of severe allergic asthma. *J Allergy Clin Immunol* 108:184, 2001.

35. Soler M, Matz J, Townley R, et al: The anti-IgE antibody omalizumab reduces exacerbations and steroid requirement in allergic asthmatics. *Eur Respir J* 18:254, 2001.

36. Buhl R, Soler M, Matz J, et al: Omalizumab provides long-term control in patients with moderate-to-severe allergic asthma. *Eur Respir J* 20:73, 2002.

37. Lanier BQ, Corren J, Lumry W, et al: Omalizumab is effective in the long-term control of severe allergic asthma. *Ann Allergy Asthma Immunol* 91:154, 2003.

CHAPTER 13

Aerosolized Antiinfective Agents

Douglas S. Gardenhire

CHAPTER OUTLINE

OBJECTIVES

After reading this chapter, the reader will be able to:

1. Define terms that pertain to aerosolized antiinfective agents
2. Discuss the indications for inhaled antiinfective agents
3. List all available inhaled antiinfective agents used in respiratory therapy
4. Differentiate between specific antiinfective agent formulations
5. Discuss the route of administration available for the various antiinfective agents
6. Describe the mechanism of action for the various antiinfective agents
7. Recognize side effects for the various antiinfective agents
8. Discuss the use of each antiinfective agent in the treatment of lung disease

KEY TERMS AND DEFINITIONS

Cystic fibrosis (CF) Inherited disease of the exocrine glands affecting the pancreas, respiratory system, and apocrine glands. Symptoms usually begin in infancy and are characterized by increased electrolytes in the sweat, chronic respiratory infection, pancreatic insufficiency, and reduced fertility (females) and sterility (males).

Pneumocystis pneumonia (PCP) Interstitial plasma cell pneumonia caused by the organism *Pneumocystis carinii* (now known as *Pneumocystis jiroveci*). This pneumonia is common among patients with lowered immune system response.

Respiratory syncytial virus (RSV) Virus that causes formation of syncytial masses in infected cell structures.

Virostatic Stopping a virus from replicating.

Virucidal Killing a virus.

Virus Obligate intracellular parasite, containing either DNA or RNA, that reproduces by synthesis of subunits within the host cell and causes disease as a consequence of this replication.

Chapter 13 discusses antiinfective agents currently approved for administration as inhaled aerosols: pentamidine isethionate (NebuPent), ribavirin (Virazole), tobramycin (TOBI), aztreonam (Cayston), and zanamivir (Relenza). Pentamidine is used to prevent and treat *Pneumocystis* pneumonia (PCP) in patients with acquired immunodeficiency syndrome (AIDS), and ribavirin is used to treat respiratory syncytial virus (RSV). A single or monoclonal antibody preparation, palivizumab (Synagis) offers prophylaxis and treatment for RSV infection. Inhaled tobramycin and aztreonam are available for the management of *Pseudomonas aeruginosa* infections in patients with cystic fibrosis (CF). Zanamivir is an inhaled antiviral agent used to treat influenza.

CLINICAL INDICATIONS FOR AEROSOLIZED ANTIINFECTIVE AGENTS

Clinical indications for each of the aerosolized antiinfective agents available at the time of this edition are given. Each agent is discussed separately in detail.

Indication for Aerosolized Pentamidine

Pentamidine by inhalation is indicated for the *prevention* of PCP in high-risk human immunodeficiency virus (HIV)–infected patients who have a history of one or more episodes of PCP or a peripheral CD4+ (T4 helper cell) lymphocyte count of 200/mm^3 or less.

Indication for Aerosolized Ribavirin

Aerosolized ribavirin is indicated for the *treatment* of hospitalized infants with severe lower respiratory tract infection caused by RSV.

Indication for Aerosolized Tobramycin

Aerosolized tobramycin is indicated for the *management* (control) of chronic *P. aeruginosa* infection in CF.

Indication for Aerosolized Aztreonam

Aerosolized aztreonam is indicated to improve pulmonary symptoms in CF patients with *P. aeruginosa* infection.

Indication for Inhaled Zanamivir

Inhaled zanamivir is indicated for the *treatment* of uncomplicated acute illness caused by the influenza virus in adults and children age 7 years and older who have been symptomatic for no more than 2 days. It may also be used prophylactically in children 5 years and older against the influenza virus.

IDENTIFICATION OF AEROSOLIZED ANTIINFECTIVE AGENTS

The antiinfective agents available for inhalation are listed in Table 13-1 with details of formulation, usual recommended dosage, and clinical use. Each of these agents is discussed in more detail.

Aerosolized Pentamidine (NebuPent)

Pentamidine isethionate (NebuPent) is an antiprotozoal agent that is active against *Pneumocystis carinii* (now known as *Pneumocystis jiroveci*), the causative organism for *Pneumocystis jiroveci* pneumonia (PJP). The chemical structure of pentamidine is shown in Figure 13-1. Pentamidine can be

TABLE 13-1	Currently Available Inhaled Antiinfective Agents With Formulations, Usual Recommended Dosage, and Clinical Use*		
DRUG	**BRAND NAME**	**FORMULATION AND DOSAGE**	**CLINICAL USE**
Pentamidine isethionate	NebuPent	300 mg of powder in 6 mL of sterile water; 300 mg once every 4 wk	PCP prophylaxis
Ribavirin	Virazole	6 mg of powder in 300 mL of sterile water (20-mg/mL solution); given 12-18 hr/day for 3-7 days by SPAG-2 nebulizer	RSV
Tobramycin	TOBI; Bethkis	TOBI: 300 mg/5 mL ampule Bethkis: 300 mg/4 mL ampule *Adults and children ≥6 yr:* 300 mg bid, 28 days on/28 days off drug	*Pseudomonas aeruginosa* in CF
Aztreonam	Cayston	75 mg/1 mL *Adults and children ≥7 yr:* 75 mg tid, 28 days on/28 days off drug	*Pseudomonas aeruginosa* in CF
Zanamivir	Relenza	*DPI:* 5 mg/inhalation *Adults and children ≥5 yr:* 2 inhalations (one 5-mg blister per inhalation) bid <12 hr apart for 5 days	Influenza

CF, Cystic fibrosis; *DPI,* dry powder inhaler; *PCP, Pneumocystis* pneumonia; *RSV,* respiratory syncytial virus; *SPAG,* small particle aerosol generator.
*Details on use and administration should be obtained from manufacturer's drug insert material before use.

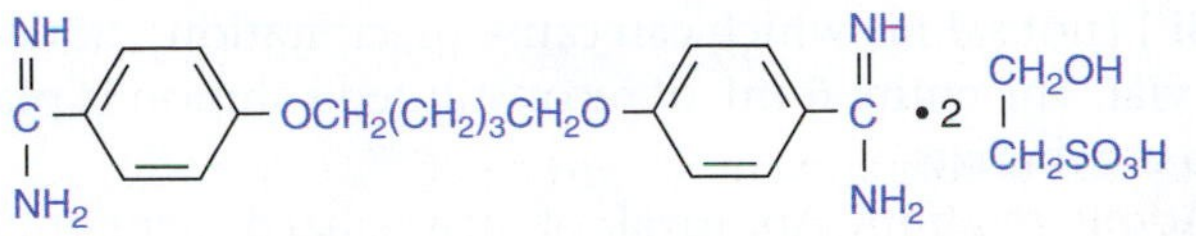

Figure 13-1 Chemical structure of pentamidine isethionate (Nebu-Pent).

given either parenterally or as an inhaled aerosol, but it is not absorbed with oral administration. When given parenterally, either intravenously or intramuscularly, the drug distributes quickly to the major organs (liver, kidneys, lung, and pancreas).

Introduction of Aerosolized Pentamidine

KEY POINT

Aerosolized pentamidine isethionate is approved for use as second-line prophylactic therapy in patients with acquired immunodeficiency syndrome (AIDS) to prevent *Pneumocystis* pneumonia (PCP). Clinical experience with the aerosolized drug has resulted in significant side effects and less efficacy than with the oral agent trimethoprim-sulfamethoxazole (TMP-SMX). TMP-SMX is indicated for prophylaxis of PCP unless side effects are not tolerated, in which case the aerosol drug should be considered.

KEY POINT

The mechanism of action of pentamidine is not fully understood but seems to interfere with nuclear metabolism and inhibits DNA, RNA, phospholipids, and protein synthesis.

KEY POINT

Side effects with aerosolized pentamidine include local airway effects, such as cough, bronchospasm, and dyspnea, and bad taste and systemic effects.

KEY POINT

Aerosolized pentamidine should be administered with a nebulizer capable of producing small particle sizes (mass median diameter [MMD] 1 to 2 μm), with a scavenging system to protect the environment. Precautions against the spread of tuberculosis (TB) with HIV patients should be taken, such as containment booths or isolation rooms.

Both systemic administration and aerosol administration of pentamidine have been used for the treatment of **Pneumocystis pneumonia (PCP)**, which occurs as a common opportunistic respiratory infection in patients with AIDS. In addition to the prophylactic use of aerosolized pentamidine, the aerosol form has been used for the treatment of acute episodes. The first report by Montgomery and associates[1] was for therapy of acute episodes of PCP.

Rationale for Aerosol Administration

The rationale for aerosol administration of pentamidine to treat or prevent PCP is based on the same rationale for other inhaled aerosol drugs used to treat the pulmonary system: local targeted lung delivery, with fewer or less severe side effects compared with systemic administration. Aerosolized pentamidine produces significantly higher lung concentrations than intravenous administration.[2] The San Francisco prophylaxis trial showed that 300 mg of aerosolized pentamidine every 4 weeks was effective in preventing PCP in patients with HIV infection.[3] Subsequent clinical experience with aerosolized pentamidine did not show improved clinical efficacy compared with oral drugs such as TMP-SMX(Septra and Bactrim), and toxic side effects still occurred.

Description of *Pneumocystis* Pneumonia

The organism *P. carinii* (now termed *P. jiroveci*) was first noted in the lungs of guinea pigs by Chagas in 1909 and Carini in 1910. It was named as a new organism by Delanöe and Delanöe in 1912 as *Pneumocystis carinii* to describe the cystic form in the lungs and its earlier discoverer. Mammals are commonly infected with the organism at an early age, probably through an airborne vector. Disease occurs when there is suppression of the immune system. When not contained by a competent immune system, *P. jiroveci* causes PCP. Before the AIDS pandemic, PCP was reported in malnourished infants in the 1940s and 1950s and in the 1970s in premature infants able to survive.[4] PCP produces a foamy intraalveolar exudate that contains cysts of *P. jiroveci*. The life cycle of *P. jiroveci* and the resulting pneumonia are illustrated in Figure 13-2. Both pentamidine and TMP-SMX are effective against PCP and are usually given parenterally to treat an acute episode.

Conflicting names for *P. carinii* may be found in scientific reading. Stringer and associates[5] described the name change to *Pneumocystis jiroveci* in honor of Otto Jírovec, a Czech parasitologist. However, in a letter to the editor, Hughes[6] pointed out that the name change is not valid or final because it has not been registered in the International Code of Botanical Nomenclature. Hughes[6] also pointed out that the name change would cause confusion with discussion of *P. carinii* because many clinicians still use this terminology. In a letter, Gigliotti[7] continued the stance taken by Hughes that no clear evidence exists that an official name change has occurred.

What is known is that *P. carinii* or *P. jiroveci* is a fungus. The acronym *PCP* for *Pneumocystis* pneumonia remains the same[5]; however, most utilize *Pneumocystis jiroveci* pneumonia (PJP), which will be used in this text.

Dosage and Administration

Details of dose and administration of NebuPent, the aerosolized brand name of pentamidine, can be found in the manufacturer's literature. The following summary is not intended to replace the more detailed instructions that accompany the drug.

Dosage. The approved dose of aerosolized pentamidine (NebuPent) for prophylaxis of PCP in AIDS patients is 300 mg given by inhalation once every 4 weeks. This dose may be altered by physicians in treating individual patients.

NebuPent is supplied as a dry powder with 300 mg in a single vial. This powder must be reconstituted with 6 mL of sterile water for injection, United States Pharmacopeia (USP) (not saline, which can cause precipitation), added to the vial. The entire 6 mL of reconstituted solution is placed into a nebulizer.

Administration. Approval of aerosolized pentamidine by the U.S. Food and Drug Administration (FDA) was for administration with the Respirgard II nebulizer (Vital Signs, Inc., Totowa, N.J.). This is a small volume nebulizer (SVN) system, powered by compressed gas, fitted with a series of one-way valves and an expiratory filter (Figure 13-3). This nebulizer system has been described by Montgomery and associates.[2] The Respirgard II nebulizer should be powered with a flow rate of 5 to 7 L/min from a 50-pounds per square inch (psi) source or, alternatively, by controlling the flow with a 22- to 25-psi pressure source connected to the small-bore tubing of the nebulizer. Pressures below 20 psi are insufficient to produce the desired particle size necessary for peripheral delivery of the drug. These requirements with Respirgard II are found in the manufacturer's literature and discussed further by Corkery and colleagues.[8] It may also be noted that pentamidine may also be administered in a room or tent that acts as a "vacuum" to draw any particles that have escaped to a filter. Capturing of these particles results in less exposure to the respiratory therapist.

Nebulizer performance. Although nebulized pentamidine was approved for general clinical use with the Respirgard II nebulizer system, other nebulizers have been used to administer the drug. At present, the manufacturer recommends use with a Respirgard II nebulizer system.

The general requirement for effective nebulization of pentamidine is a particle size or distribution of sizes with a mass median diameter (MMD) of 1 to 2 μm. This particle size is needed for the following two reasons[5]:

1. To achieve peripheral intraalveolar deposition targeted at the location of the microorganism
2. To reduce or prevent airway irritation seen with larger particle sizes, which deposit more in larger airways

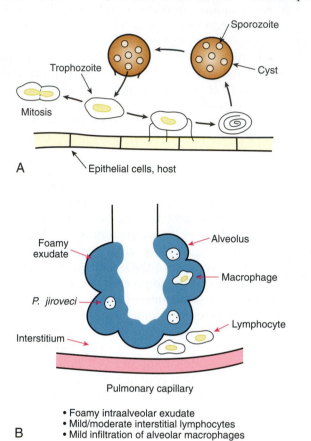

Figure 13-2 Pathogenesis of *Pneumocystis jiroveci*, the organism that causes *Pneumocystis* pneumonia (PCP). **A,** Life cycle of *P. jiroveci*. **B,** PCP pathology.

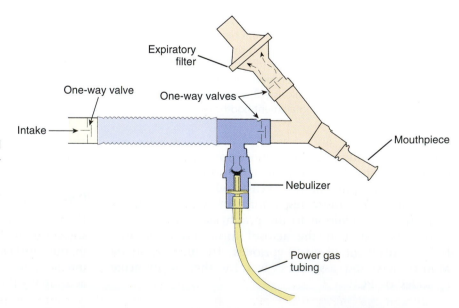

Figure 13-3 Diagrammatic illustration of Respirgard II nebulizer system, showing one-way valves and expiratory filter to scavenge exhaust aerosol.

Studies by Vinciguerra and Smaldone[9] and by Smaldone and associates[10] have examined nebulizer performance and compared treatment time and patient tolerance of aerosolized pentamidine with Respirgard II versus other nebulizers. Treatment times and efficiency in drug availability were greater with the AeroTech II (CIS-US, Bedford, Mass.) than the approved Respirgard II.

Mechanism of Action

The exact mechanism of action of pentamidine is unknown. The toxic effect of the drug on *P. jiroveci* may be due to multiple actions. Pentamidine blocks RNA and DNA synthesis, inhibits oxidative phosphorylation, and interferes with folate transformation.[4,11,12]

When given by inhaled aerosol, pentamidine reaches significantly higher concentrations in the lung than when given intravenously.[2] The inhaled drug first binds to lung tissue. Although plasma levels are much less than with parenteral administration, the drug is slowly absorbed into the circulation and distributed to body tissues, as with parenteral administration. As a result, prolonged aerosol administration can result in systemic accumulation. Approximately 75% of the drug is excreted in urine and 25% in feces over the months after administration.

Side Effects

The side effects seen with systemic therapy of PCP using either pentamidine or TMP-SMX provided part of the rationale for aerosol administration of pentamidine. Although both of these drugs are effective in most patients with PCP when given systemically, more than 50% of patients experience adverse side effects.

Side effects with parenteral pentamidine. Side effects with parenteral administration of pentamidine have been summarized in several reviews, with numerous references.[8,11] *Parenteral* use of pentamidine has resulted in the following:

- Pain, swelling, and abscess formation at the site of injection with intramuscular administration
- Thrombophlebitis and urticarial eruptions with intravenous administration
- Hypoglycemia (up to 62% of patients), with a cumulative cytotoxic effect on pancreatic beta cells
- Impaired renal function and azotemia
- Hypotension
- Leukopenia
- Hepatic dysfunction

Side effects with aerosol administration. Side effects with aerosol administration can be differentiated into local airway effects and systemic effects. *Local airway effects* with aerosol administration have included the following:

- Cough and bronchial irritation in 36% of patients in one study[3]
- Shortness of breath
- Bad taste (bitter or burning) from the aerosol impacting in the oropharynx
- Bronchospasm and wheezing in 11% of patients[3]
- Spontaneous pneumothoraces[13]

In addition, the following *systemic reactions* have occurred with aerosolized pentamidine:

- Conjunctivitis
- Rash
- Neutropenia
- Pancreatitis[14]
- Renal insufficiency
- Dysglycemia (hypoglycemia and diabetes)
- Digital necrosis in both feet[15]
- Appearance of extrapulmonary *P. jiroveci* infection

Because of the pharmacokinetics of pentamidine, long-term treatment with the aerosol can lead to tissue accumulation in the body, causing some of the same side effects as with parenteral administration. Suppression of *P. jiroveci* with local targeting of the lung has resulted in the appearance of infection elsewhere in the body.

Preventing airway effects. Use of a β-adrenergic bronchodilator before inhaling aerosolized pentamidine can reduce or prevent local airway reaction, including reduction of coughing or wheezing. Ipratropium has also been shown by Quieffin and colleagues[16] to prevent bronchoconstriction. The airway reaction may be caused by the sulfite moiety in isethionate (see Figure 13-1), which is known to cause airway irritation, or by the drug itself.[17,18] This effect can be reduced by use of a nebulizing system producing very small particle sizes, which lessen airway deposition and increase alveolar targeting.[8]

Environmental Contamination by Nebulized Pentamidine

The following concerns exist regarding environmental contamination from nebulized pentamidine:

- Exposure to the drug itself from the exhaust aerosol
- Risk of infection with tuberculosis (TB), a disease associated with AIDS, from patients being treated with aerosolized pentamidine

Pentamidine is not known to be teratogenic, based on its use in pregnant women with African sleeping sickness (trypanosomiasis), although detailed clinical data were not kept. The drug is not mutagenic, and its carcinogenic potential is considered minimal.[11] Studies have shown that low levels of pentamidine can be detected in health care workers exposed to the drug during treatments.[19,20] The investigators concluded that exposure probably occurred during treatment interruptions, usually caused by coughing episodes. Health care workers have also complained of conjunctivitis and bronchospasm when aerosolizing the drug.[11] On the basis of these reports and the long tissue half-life of pentamidine, contact with the drug should be kept to a minimum or prevented if possible.

The risk of contracting TB when treating AIDS patients with nebulized pentamidine is based on the association of TB and AIDS, the airborne mode of transmission of TB, and the fact that pentamidine aerosol can cause coughing and expulsion of droplet nuclei containing TB bacilli during aerosol treatments.

Environmental precautions. The following precautionary measures are suggested when administering aerosolized pentamidine to reduce the risk of drug exposure and TB infection[21-24]:

- Use a nebulizer system with one-way valves and an expiratory filter.
- Stop nebulization if the patient takes the mouthpiece out of the mouth (a thumb control on the power gas tubing gives more control).
- Use nebulizers producing an MMD of 1 to 2 μm to increase alveolar targeting and lessen large airway deposition and cough production.
- Always use a suitable expiratory filter and one-way valves with the nebulizer. Instruct patients to turn off the nebulizer when talking or when taking it out of the mouth.
- Screen patients for cough history and pretreat with a β agonist, with sufficient lead time for effect in reducing the bronchial reactivity.
- Administer aerosol in a negative-pressure room, with six air changes per hour, or consider using an isolation booth/hood assembly with an exhaust fan and air directed through a high-efficiency filter.
- Health care workers should use barrier protection (gloves, mask, and eyewear).
- Screen patients with HIV infection for TB, and treat where evidence of infection exists.
- Do not allow treatment patients to mix with others until coughing subsides.
- Health care workers should periodically screen themselves for TB.
- Pregnant women and nursing mothers should avoid exposure to the drug, and all practitioners should limit exposure to the extent possible.

Although measures exist to radically limit environmental contamination with aerosolized pentamidine, many of these are expensive, such as negative-pressure rooms and improved ventilation exchange in older buildings. Other measures are difficult, such as the wearing of effective high-efficiency masks in a busy clinical setting for a prolonged period. The use of room disinfection with ultraviolet light has been reviewed[25] but is debated.[22]

Aerosol Therapy for Prophylaxis of *Pneumocystis* Pneumonia: Clinical Application

Comparisons of the efficacy of aerosolized pentamidine with oral TMP-SMX, together with reports of serious adverse effects with aerosolized pentamidine, led to a reevaluation of aerosol therapy with pentamidine for prophylaxis of PCP. General recommendations for prophylaxis of PCP have been published by the U.S. Centers for Disease Control and Prevention (CDC) in *MMWR Recommendations and Reports* for HIV-positive children[26] and guidelines for adults.[27] In the 2013 CDC recommendations, oral TMP-SMX is preferred for prophylaxis of PCP as long as adverse side effects from TMP-SMX were absent or acceptable.[27] Aerosolized pentamidine is recommended as an alternative therapy for prophylaxis of PCP if TMP-SMX cannot be tolerated.

Ribavirin (Virazole)

KEY POINT

Ribavirin is an aerosolized antiviral drug used with respiratory syncytial viral (RSV) infections in children and infants at risk for severe or complicated disease.

KEY POINT

Ribavirin acts as a nucleoside analog to terminate viral DNA replication. The aerosol is administered with a small particle aerosol generator, model 2 (SPAG-2) unit.

KEY POINT

Side effects with ribavirin include pulmonary deterioration and equipment malfunction (ventilator occlusion and endotracheal tube occlusion). Environmental containment systems are available to protect caregivers.

Ribavirin (Virazole) is classified as an antiviral drug; it is active against RSV, influenza viruses, and the herpes simplex virus. Chemically, it is a nucleoside analog and resembles guanosine and inosine.[28] Ribavirin is **virostatic**, not **virucidal**, and inhibits DNA and RNA (retrovirus) viruses.

Ribavirin has been used throughout the world for various viral infections, including RSV and influenza types A and B. Clinical trials of aerosolized ribavirin for severe RSV infection conducted by Hall and associates[29] have shown significant improvement with ribavirin treatment compared with a placebo; however, Guerguerian and colleagues[30] have noted its ineffectiveness.

Clinical Use

Infection with RSV in children results in either bronchiolitis or pneumonia. Guidelines concerning the use of ribavirin were published by the Committee on Infectious Diseases of the American Academy of Pediatrics in 2009. Generally, the drug is not recommended for routine RSV infection, but it may be considered for life-threatening infections.[31] The Agency for Healthcare Research and Quality (AHRQ) has designated ribavirin as "possibly ineffective."[32]

Ribavirin treatment by aerosol is expensive and risks environmental exposure to the drug by personnel. Studies have given conflicting results on whether the use of ribavirin significantly reduces outcomes such as ventilator days, oxygen needs, intensive care unit days, hospital days, or mortality.[33,34]

Nature of Viral Infection

A summary of viruses and viral infection is presented to establish key principles and concepts needed for understanding the difficulties in treating viral diseases and the mechanism of action of ribavirin. A **virus** can be defined as an obligate intracellular parasite, containing either DNA or RNA, that reproduces by synthesis of subunits within the host cell and causes disease as a consequence of this replication.

Figure 13-4 illustrates the simple structure of a virus. These are primitive members of the animal kingdom, submicronic in size, that consist of a strand of DNA or RNA that is surrounded by a protein coat. A virus may or may not be surrounded by an envelope, whose glycoprotein spikes are partially obtained from the host cell.

The concept and sequence of a viral infection are shown in Figure 13-5. A virus enters the body through various routes (oral, inhaled, mucous membranes) and invades a host cell. This is a multistep process consisting of phases in which the virus adsorbs to the cell; penetrates the cell; uncoats itself; goes through a process of recoding cell DNA (transcription, translation, synthesis); assembles itself; and sheds from the cell. The host cell usually dies in the process. Clinically, signs of a viral infection do not occur until after

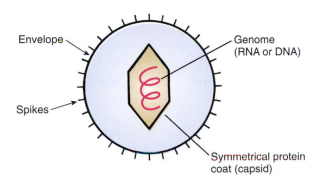

Virion: extracellular virus particle

Figure 13-4 Structure of a virus, showing nuclear material (DNA or RNA), protein coat, and envelope.

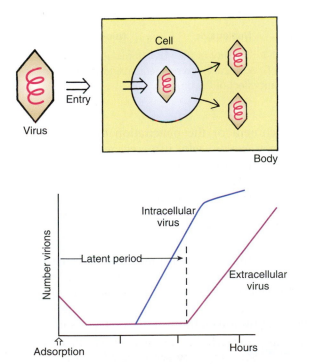

Figure 13-5 Sequence of viral infection, illustrating intracellular replication before dissemination in the body.

the initial latent period, when the virus leaves the cell (see Figure 13-5). At this point, infection is well established. The diagnosis of viral illness is usually based on clinical signs, including the symptoms, age of the patient, and time of year. Definitive diagnosis requires isolating the virus or showing an antibody titer increase. Diseases produced by viruses include chickenpox, smallpox, fever blisters (herpes simplex virus), genital herpes, poliomyelitis, the common cold, AIDS, influenza, mumps, and measles.

Because of the nature of viral infection, as just outlined, antiviral drug treatment, whether for the common cold or for HIV infection, is difficult. In particular, there are three complications in treating viral disease with drugs, as follows:

1. Attacking the intracellular virus may harm the host cell.
2. Viral replication is maximal before the appearance of symptoms.
3. Viruses have the property of antigenic mutability; that is, they change their appearance to the immune system.

Respiratory syncytial virus infection. **Respiratory syncytial virus (RSV)** can cause bronchiolitis and pneumonia. Almost all children are exposed to RSV by their second year of life, and in most the infection is mild and self-limiting. Outbreaks of RSV pneumonia are seasonal and peak during winter months (November to March), with some variation according to geographic region.

The name of the virus reflects its effects on cells, which is to cause the formation of large, multinucleated cells, or a *syncytium*. The virus spreads easily by personal contact or hand contamination from surfaces. No effective vaccine exists to prevent RSV respiratory disease. Prepared antibody to RSV is available and is discussed subsequently (RSV immune globulin intravenous).

Dosage and Administration

Following is a summary of ribavirin dosage and administration. It is not intended to replace detailed instructions contained in the manufacturer's literature, which should be reviewed before administering this drug. This includes the operating manual for the small particle aerosol generator, model 2 (SPAG-2) nebulizing system.

Dosage. Ribavirin is given as a 20-mg/mL solution, which is administered by nebulizer (SPAG-2) for 12 to 18 hours per day, for a minimum of 3 days and not more than 7 days. The drug is supplied as 6 g of powder in a 100-mL vial. The powder is reconstituted in the vial with sterile water for injection or inhalation, transferred to the large volume (500-mL) reservoir of the nebulizer, and diluted further to a total volume of 300 mL with sterile water. This gives a concentration of 6 g/300 mL, or 20 mg/mL, a 2% strength solution.

Administration. Clinical trials of ribavirin aerosol were carried out with a large volume nebulizing system, the SPAG-2. The drug was approved for general use with this aerosol generator. A diagram of the SPAG-2 unit is shown in Figure 13-6. It is a large volume, pneumatically powered nebulizer operating on a jet shearing principle, with baffling of aerosol particles and a drying chamber to reduce

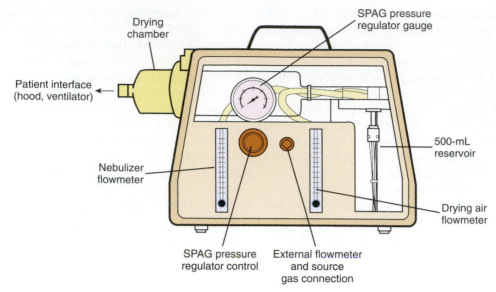

Figure 13-6 Diagrammatic illustration of small particle aerosol generator (SPAG-2) unit used for nebulizing ribavirin.

particle size further to a level of approximately 1.3 μm MMD. Solutions in the SPAG-2 reservoir should be replaced after 24 hours. Residual solution in the reservoir should be discarded before adding newly reconstituted solution. The drug solution should always be visually inspected for particulate matter or discoloration before use.

The nebulizer is connected to a hood as the patient interface. The manufacturer specifically warns against administration of the drug to infants requiring mechanical ventilation because of the risk of drug precipitation occluding expiratory valves and sensors or the endotracheal tube. The sickest infants with RSV are likely to need ventilatory support; however, there are reports of drug use with mechanical ventilation. Demers and colleagues[35] provided detailed information concerning precautions with ventilator use during administration of the drug. A clinical study of aerosol administration with mechanical ventilation of infants with severe RSV infection was reported by Smith and associates[33]; these authors showed that treatment reduced duration of ventilation, oxygen support, and hospital stay. Although labor-intensive, mechanical ventilatory administration of ribavirin actually simplifies environmental control.

Mechanism of Action

The mechanism of action by which ribavirin exerts its virostatic effect is not completely understood. Viral inhibition is probably based on its structural resemblance to the nucleosides used to construct the DNA chain.[28] Figure 13-7 shows the structures of the natural nucleoside guanosine with ribavirin, which is a synthetic nucleoside analog. During the formation and assembly of new viral protein within the cell, ribavirin is most likely taken up instead of the natural nucleoside to form the DNA chain; this prevents construction of viable viral particles and subsequent shedding of virus into the bloodstream. Figure 13-8 is a conceptual illustration of the process. Ribavirin does not prevent

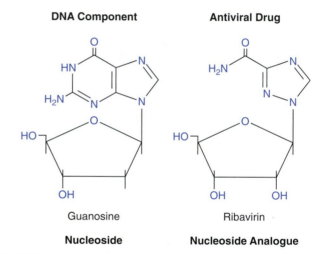

Figure 13-7 Similarity of the ribavirin molecule to the (deoxyribonucleic acid) DNA precursor component, guanosine, may be the basis for the virostatic effect of the drug.

the attachment or the penetration of RSV into the cell, which may explain why it merely reduces the severity of illness rather than preventing or abolishing it altogether.[28]

When given by inhaled aerosol, ribavirin levels are much greater in respiratory secretions than in the bloodstream. Waskin[11] provided a referenced summary of ribavirin kinetics. With 8 to 20 hours of aerosol treatment, peak plasma levels are 1 to 3 mcg/mL, and respiratory secretion levels are greater than 1000 mcg/mL. The minimal inhibitory concentration (MIC) for RSV is 4 to 16 mcg/mL. The half-life of ribavirin is about 9 hours in plasma and about 1 to 2 hours in respiratory secretions, which is the rationale for almost-continuous administration by aerosol.

Side Effects

Side effects seen with aerosolized ribavirin are listed in the product literature and have been reviewed by Waskin.[11] The

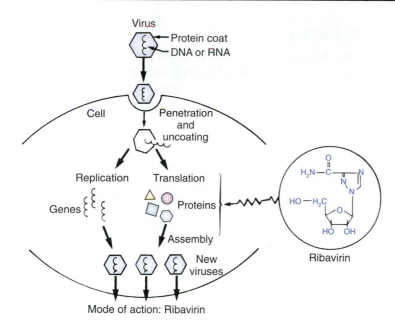

Figure 13-8 Illustration of mechanism of action of ribavirin in blocking viral replication.

following list summarizes adverse effects reported, including those seen with adults receiving the drug:

- *Pulmonary:* Deterioration of pulmonary function and worsening of asthma or chronic obstructive pulmonary disease (COPD) occur; pneumothorax, apnea, and bacterial pneumonia have been described.
- *Cardiovascular:* Cardiovascular instability, including hypotension, cardiac arrest, and digitalis toxicity, has been noted.
- *Hematologic:* Effects on blood cells have been reported with oral or parenteral administration but not with aerosol use. Reticulocytosis (excess of young erythrocytes in the circulation) has been reported with aerosol use.
- *Dermatologic/topical:* Rash, eyelid erythema, and conjunctivitis have been noted.
- *Equipment-related:* Equipment-related adverse effects with ribavirin treatment include occlusion and impairment of expiratory valves and sensors with ventilator use and endotracheal tube blockage from drug precipitate.

Although all of the previously listed effects have been reported, common effects clinically are pulmonary function deterioration, equipment malfunction from drug precipitate, and skin irritation from excess drug precipitation.

Environmental Contamination With Aerosolized Ribavirin

There is concern among health care workers over exposure to ribavirin. The drug has potential for mutagenic and carcinogenic effects based on in vitro and animal studies.[11] The effect on fertility is uncertain, but the drug has caused testicular lesions in rats. The effect on pregnancy is of particular concern because the drug is teratogenic or embryocidal in animal species. Acute effects from aerosolized ribavirin reported by health care workers have included precipitation on contact lenses and conjunctivitis, headache (51%), rhinitis, nausea, rash, dizziness, pharyngitis,

and lacrimation (10% to 20%). Several cases of bronchospasm or chest pain have been reported by individuals with reactive airways disease. The symptoms noted have resolved within hours after discontinuing exposure to the drug.[36]

Minimal levels of ribavirin exposure are difficult to specify because of the lack of dose-response data for humans.[37] Corkery and others[38] stated that the California Department of Health Services recommended an acceptable occupational airborne concentration for 8 hours of limited exposure to be $\frac{1}{1000}$ of the lowest no-observed-effect level, which would be 2.5 mcg/m^3.

Although there are no reports to date of serious effects from drug exposure by aerosol, precautions to limit or avoid exposure to the drug are well indicated, as advocated by Kacmarek.[39] Pregnant females, or those wishing to become pregnant, should avoid exposure to the drug if possible. In addition, environmental containment is superior to personnel barrier protection alone. Standard surgical masks do not prevent inhalation of 1- to 2-µm particles. Dermal absorption of ribavirin seems to be negligible.[40] It may be helpful to use a containment system when the drug is aerosolized to an oxygen hood; several systems have been proposed in the literature.[41-43] All have common features of enclosure around the hood, with vacuum extraction and filtering of gas from the enclosure. Details needed for use can be found in the references given. It is recommended that the drug be administered in well-ventilated areas—that is, six or more air changes per hour.

Palivizumab (Synagis)

Palivizumab (Synagis) represents the new drug class of therapeutic monoclonal antibodies.[44] The drug was approved for the prevention and treatment of RSV in premature infants and infants with bronchopulmonary dysplasia (BPD).

Clinical Use

Palivizumab is indicated for the prevention of serious lower respiratory tract disease caused by RSV in children and infants at high risk. Safety and efficacy were established for infants with BPD, infants born prematurely (less than 35 weeks), and children with congenital heart disease.[45]

Dosage and Administration

The powder for injection is lyophilized or freeze-dried and is available at 50 mg/mL or 100 mg/mL. A premixed injection of 100 mg/mL is also available. The recommended dose is 15 mg/kg given intramuscularly once a month before the start of and throughout the RSV season.

Mechanism of Action

Palivizumab is a humanized monoclonal antibody produced by recombinant DNA techniques, directed against the F protein of RSV. As an antibody against RSV, palivizumab provides neutralizing and fusion-inhibiting activity, preventing viral replication.

Adverse Reactions

The most serious adverse reaction is anaphylaxis; however, this occurs in less than 1 per 100,000 cases. Other reactions that occurred in treatment and placebo groups included fever, upper respiratory infection, otitis media, rhinitis, rash, pain, hernia, and coughing and wheezing.[36]

Clinical Efficacy

In a large multicenter trial of infants at high risk of RSV infection, palivizumab given intravenously at 15 mg/kg reduced the rate of hospitalization resulting from RSV infection to 4.8% compared with 10.6% in placebo recipients.[46] Adverse events were similar in placebo and treatment groups.

Feltes and colleagues[47] found that palivizumab is safe and effective for RSV-positive children with congenital heart disease. In this study, 53% of the children had reduced hospital stays, and 73% had fewer days of supplemental oxygen use.

Aerosolized Tobramycin (TOBI; Bethkis)

KEY POINT

Nebulized tobramycin is used to manage chronic *Pseudomonas aeruginosa* infection in patients with **cystic fibrosis (CF)** as an alternative to intravenous therapy. The nebulized form is attractive because of poor oral bioavailability for respiratory tract infections.

KEY POINT

Side effects with tobramycin include tinnitus and voice changes. Inhaled tobramycin should be used with caution in the presence of renal impairment, auditory or vestibular problems, or neuromuscular dysfunction.

Clinical Use

One disease state in which aerosolized antibiotics have been used more consistently for pulmonary infections is CF. Patients with CF are chronically infected with gram-negative organisms, such as *P. aeruginosa*, and the gram-positive bacterium *Staphylococcus aureus*, as well as other microorganisms. In particular, chronic *Pseudomonas* infection leads to recurring acute respiratory infections. With the exception of the quinolone derivatives such as ciprofloxacin, antibiotics that are effective against *Pseudomonas* do not give sufficient lung levels to inhibit bacteria when taken orally. Antibiotics with poor oral bioavailability for lung tissue include aminoglycosides, penicillin derivatives, and cephalosporins. Consequently, either the intravenous or the inhaled aerosol route must be used.

Baran and colleagues[48] administered 40 mg of gentamicin by aerosol to eight children with CF and found high levels of drug (more than 20 mcg/mL) in the bronchial secretions of seven of the children. Blood levels with the inhaled drug were low, supporting the case for minimal systemic toxicity by aerosol. Similar results with nebulized tobramycin (300 mg) were reported by Le Conte and associates.[49] By contrast, intramuscular injection of 1.5 mg/kg gave low levels of less than 2 mcg/mL in bronchial secretions and, in some cases, undetectable levels.[48]

Aerosol administration is attractive because of reduced cost potential and ease of use at home compared with intravenous therapy. Furthermore, fluoroquinolones such as ciprofloxacin and norfloxacin, which are active when taken orally, are not as suitable for prolonged maintenance or preventive therapy as the agents given by inhalation because of the risk of drug-resistant strains of bacteria.[50] A report of the clinical trial establishing the safety and efficacy of inhaled tobramycin in managing *P. aeruginosa* in patients with CF was published by Ramsey and colleagues.[51] Inhaled tobramycin is used to manage chronic infection with *P. aeruginosa* in CF, as follows:

- Treat or prevent early colonization with *P. aeruginosa*
- Maintain present lung function or reduce the rate of deterioration

Efficacy with *Burkholderia cepacia* has not been shown using the inhaled route of administration.

Dosage and Administration

Inhaled tobramycin is recommended for children 6 years of age or older. The usual dosage is 300 mg twice daily approximately 12 hours apart and not less than 6 hours apart for 28 days consecutively, with the next 28 days off the drug. This cycle is repeated on a maintenance basis. Inhaled tobramycin has been studied with specific nebulizers. Any nebulizer other than one recommended by the manufacturer should be tested to ensure adequate drug output and particle size.

Patients should be instructed not to mix dornase alfa or any other drug with tobramycin in the nebulizer because of incompatibility with other drugs. Tobramycin should be inhaled after other therapies usually administered in CF, such as chest physiotherapy measures and other inhaled medications including bronchodilators or dornase alfa to allow for the greatest deposition of drug at the alveolar level.

The drug should be stored at refrigerated temperatures of 2° to 8° C (36° to 46° F). After removal from refrigeration or if refrigeration is unavailable, the pouches in which the drug is provided can be stored at room temperatures less than 25° C (77° F) for up to 28 days. Drug ampoules should not be exposed to intense light. The solution may darken with aging if not refrigerated, although this does not change the drug activity if the manufacturer's guidelines are followed.

Mechanism of Action

Tobramycin is a member of the aminoglycoside family of antibiotics. These antibiotics are effective in treating gram-negative infections and have a bactericidal effect, blocking protein synthesis in the bacteria and causing cellular death. Serum tobramycin levels are approximately 1 mcg/mL 1 hour after inhalation in patients with normal renal function.

Side Effects

Side effects for parenteral and inhaled administration of tobramycin are listed in Box 13-1. Adverse effects with *nebulized* delivery are based on the clinical trial of Ramsey and colleagues[51] and on 2 years of experience after the approval of inhaled tobramycin.

Side effects with parenteral administration. Adverse effects that can occur with *parenteral* administration of aminoglycosides are reviewed briefly because the presence of impaired renal function or other conditions may increase the risk of these effects with inhaled administration.

Ototoxicity. Ototoxicity is associated with parenteral use of aminoglycosides. Ototoxicity is manifested as auditory (cochlear) damage with small loss of hearing at the higher frequencies or vestibular dysfunction with vertigo, nausea, or nystagmus (involuntary movement of eyeball).

Nephrotoxicity. Nephrotoxicity is also possible with aminoglycosides, which are excreted as unchanged drug by

glomerular filtration. Although toxicity risk increases with dose, it may occur even with conventional doses in patients with prerenal azotemia or impaired renal function. Because excretion is by the renal system, impaired renal function can also increase risk of the other side effects noted.

Neuromuscular blockade. Neuromuscular blockade is another side effect resulting from the potential curare-like effect of aminoglycosides on the neuromuscular junction. Neuromuscular blockade can aggravate muscle weakness, cause further worsening of neuromuscular disorders, or prolong and intensify neuromuscular blockade by curare-like paralyzing agents (see Chapter 18). *Hypomagnesemia* can occur in patients who have a poor diet or whose diet is restricted.

Cross-allergenicity. Cross-allergenicity exists among the aminoglycosides, and hypersensitivity to one agent in this group constitutes a contraindication to the use of other agents. The side effects cited are more likely with overdosage, poor renal function, and dehydration (resulting from higher renal concentrations with possible nephrotoxicity).

Fetal harm. Fetal harm can occur with aminoglycosides, and these drugs can cross the placenta. Irreversible bilateral congenital deafness has been reported in children of mothers who received streptomycin, another aminoglycoside.[36]

Side effects with nebulized tobramycin. The only adverse effects reported after the 6-month clinical trial of Ramsey and colleagues[51] were *tinnitus* and *voice alteration*. There was no hearing loss associated with nebulized use of tobramycin or changes in serum creatinine indicative of renal toxicity. There was a modest decrease in susceptibility of *P. aeruginosa* to tobramycin in the treatment group but not the placebo group in the study by Ramsey and colleagues.[51] However, this was not associated with a lack of clinical response to inhaled therapy with tobramycin. Use of an alternating schedule of administration may reduce the risk of drug resistance. Ramsey and associates[51,52] noted that their rationale for intermittent administration of tobramycin was the observation that "drug holidays" allow susceptible pathogens to repopulate the airway in patients with CF. Because tobramycin is delivered by inhalation, the airway concentration can be 100 times as high as systemic levels. Thresholds of pathogen susceptibility with parenteral administration do not apply well to direct inhalation doses.

Precautions in Use of Nebulized Tobramycin

- Inhaled tobramycin should be administered with caution to patients with preexisting renal, auditory, vestibular, or neuromuscular dysfunction.
- Admixture incompatibility exists between β-lactam antibiotics (penicillins and cephalosporins) and aminoglycosides when mixed directly together; tobramycin solution should not be mixed with antibiotics in this group, and mixing with other drugs generally is discouraged.
- Factors that could increase the risk of hearing damage with prolonged tobramycin use are renal impairment;

BOX 13-1 Side Effects With Aminoglycosides and Tobramycin

Parenteral Administration
- Ototoxicity (auditory and vestibular)
- Nephrotoxicity
- Neuromuscular blockade
- Hypomagnesemia
- Cross-allergenicity
- Fetal harm (deafness)

Inhaled Nebulized Tobramycin
- Voice alteration
- Tinnitus
- Nonsignificant increase in bacterial resistance

concomitant dosage of parenteral aminoglycosides; dehydration; and concomitant use of ethacrynic acid, furosemide, or other ototoxic drugs.

- Nebulization of antibiotics during hospitalization should be performed under conditions of containment, as previously described for pentamidine and ribavirin, to prevent environmental saturation and development of resistant organisms in the hospital.
- Aminoglycosides can cause fetal harm if administered to pregnant women; exposure to ambient aerosol drug should be avoided by women who are pregnant or trying to become pregnant.
- *Local airway irritation* resulting in cough and bronchospasm with decreased ventilatory flow rates is a possibility with inhaled antibiotics and seems to be related to the osmolality of the solution.[53-56] Peak flow rates and chest auscultation should be used before and after treatments to evaluate airway changes. Pretreatment with a β agonist may be needed.
- *Allergies* in the patient, staff, or family should be considered, if exposure to the aerosolized drug is not controlled. The use of a nebulizing system with scavenging filter, one-way valves, and thumb control could reduce ambient contamination with the drug, as previously described.

Clinical Efficacy

Clinical efficacy of inhaled tobramycin by nebulization was shown in the randomized controlled study by Ramsey and colleagues.[51] In that study, which compared inhaled tobramycin with placebo in 521 patients with CF, 6 months of alternating inhaled tobramycin together with standard therapy for CF resulted in the following:

- Improved pulmonary function (Figure 13-9)
- Decreased density of *P. aeruginosa* in expectorated sputum

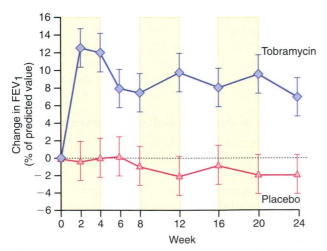

Figure 13-9 Mean change in forced expiratory volume in 1 second (FEV$_1$) from baseline for patients receiving inhaled tobramycin versus placebo. Bars represent 95% confidence intervals. (Modified from Ramsey BW, Pepe MS, Quan JM, et al: *N Engl J Med* 340:23, 1999.)

- Reduced need for intravenous antipseudomonal antibiotics and hospitalizations
- No development of significant bacterial resistance

Other studies, such as that by Gibson and colleagues,[57] have produced similar results indicating that inhaled tobramycin is safe and effective in treating *P. aeruginosa* in patients with CF.

Because inhaled tobramycin is effective in patients with CF, is it effective in other patients with *P. aeruginosa* infection? LoBue[58] reported that studies to date have been small or that the drug has not been used long-term. Inhaled tobramycin cannot be recommended for treatment other than for CF patients with *P. aeruginosa* infection.

Aerosolized Aztreonam (Cayston)

 KEY POINT

Aerosolized aztreonam is used to improve *Pseudomonas aeruginosa* infection in patients with CF. Patients should be pretreated with a bronchodilator before administering aerosolized aztreonam.

Clinical Use

Aztreonam was approved in December 1986 by the FDA as a monobactam, a synthetic bactericidal antibiotic; it is given as an intravenous solution. Inhaled aztreonam (Cayston) was approved in February 2010 to improve pulmonary symptoms in CF patients colonized with *P. aeruginosa*. Cayston is not indicated for patients younger than 7 years of age, or those with *B. cepacia*. It has been studied only in patients with a forced expiratory volume in 1 second (FEV$_1$) greater than 25% or less than 75% of predicted.

Dosage and Administration

Cayston is supplied in a form that must be reconstituted. In a 28-day kit, each 2-mL single-use glass vial contains 75 mg of lyophilized aztreonam and must be mixed with the provided 1 mL of sterile diluent (0.17% sodium chloride). The reconstituted agent is delivered by itself using the Altera Nebulizer System (PARI Respiratory Equipment, Midlothian, Virginia).

Each patient should be pretreated with a bronchodilator before each dosing. Cayston is given three times a day for 28 days on and 28 days off. The kit should be refrigerated; however, when the kit is ready to use, it can be stored at room temperature for 28 days.

Any prescribed mucolytic should also be given before Cayston. In addition, any bronchial hygiene should be done before administration of Cayston. Cayston has the potential for use as part of an alternating cycle of therapy with other inhaled therapy, such as inhaled tobramycin.

Mechanism of Action

Aztreonam displays in vitro activity against gram-negative aerobic bacteria. It binds to penicillin-binding proteins of pathogens such as *P. aeruginosa*, inhibiting bacterial cell wall synthesis and ultimately causing death of the cell.

Precautions in Use of Nebulized Aztreonam

As mentioned earlier, Cayston can cause bronchospasm and decrease a patient's FEV_1. All patients should be screened for baseline pulmonary function results and be treated with a bronchodilator before administering Cayston.

It has been reported that patients have experienced severe allergic reactions with injectable aztreonam. Careful observation is warranted when first using Cayston because it could cause an allergic reaction. If any signs occur during the delivery of Cayston, the treatment should be stopped immediately and the health care team should be informed.

The use of antibiotics in the absence of infection may lead to the development of drug-resistant bacteria. Cayston should not be used in CF patients not infected with *P. aeruginosa*.

General Considerations in Aerosolizing Antibiotics

Several points should be noted when nebulizing antibiotic drugs, especially if an injectable formulation is used, although this is *not* recommended for routine clinical use.

- Antibiotic solutions, such as gentamicin, are more viscous than bronchodilator solutions, and this may affect nebulizer performance. Compressors must be suitably powerful; high-flow compressors are suggested.[59] Flow rates of 10 to 12 L/min have also been suggested by Newman and associates[60] for suitably small particle sizes with antibiotic solutions.
- Environmental contamination in health care agencies and practitioner exposure to the aerosolized drug can be reduced by using expiratory filters with one-way valves and a thumb control, as with aerosolized pentamidine.
- Hata and Fick[61] noted physical incompatibility between some antibiotics. Aminoglycosides, such as gentamicin, are chemically inactivated by carbenicillin and piperacillin when mixed together. These drugs should be given in separate nebulizer treatments, which has the disadvantage of requiring twice the patient treatment time. Any antibiotic combination and other drug combinations

should at least be inspected for visible changes such as discoloration or precipitation and should not be used if such changes are observed. Ideally, drug mixtures for nebulization should be tested for chemical compatibility in addition to a visual inspection.

Inhaled Zanamivir (Relenza)

KEY POINT

Zanamivir is available for administration with a dry powder inhaler (DPI) to treat acute symptoms of influenza.

KEY POINT

The mechanism of action of zanamivir is to inhibit viral neuraminidase (NA), causing viral aggregation to the cell and each other.

KEY POINT

Side effects include possible bronchospasm of lung deterioration, especially in preexisting airways disease and undertreatment or inappropriate treatment of nonviral bacterial respiratory infections.

Clinical Use

Zanamivir (Relenza) is an antiviral agent approved for use in the treatment of uncomplicated influenza illness in adults and children older than 7 years of age during the early onset (within the first 2 days) of infection. Children as young as 5 years of age may use the medication prophylactically. The agent has an off-label use for treatment and prophylaxis of H1N1 influenza A ("swine flu"). An oral antiinfluenza agent, oseltamivir phosphate (Tamiflu) is also available as 30-mg, 45-mg, and 75-mg capsules and 12 mg/mL oral liquid. It is indicated in the treatment and prophylaxis of influenza in patients 1 year of age and older. Tamiflu has an off-label use in H1N1 influenza A. In addition, two older drugs, amantadine and rimantadine, have been used for prophylaxis and treatment of acute symptoms of influenza. Table 13-2 summarizes information about these four

TABLE 13-2	Antiviral Agents Used to Treat or Prevent Influenza					
DRUG	BRAND NAME	FDA APPROVAL	ACTIVITY	CLINICAL USE	ROUTE OF ADMINISTRATION	ADULT DOSAGE
Amantadine	Symmetrel	1966	Influenza A	Prophylaxis, acute treatment	Oral: tablet, syrup	200 mg/day
Rimantadine	Flumadine	1993	Influenza A	Prophylaxis, acute treatment	Oral: tablet, syrup	100 mg bid
Oseltamivir	Tamiflu	1999	Influenza A and B; H1N1 ("swine flu")	Prophylaxis, acute treatment	Oral: capsule, liquid suspension	12 mg,* 75 mg bid, for 5 days
Zanamivir	Relenza	1999	Influenza A and B; H1N1 ("swine flu")	Prophylaxis, acute treatment	DPI: Diskhaler	10 mg (2 inhalations) bid, for 5 days

DPI, Dry powder inhaler; *FDA*, U.S. Food and Drug Administration.
*Depends on weight of child; see manufacturer's dosing schedule.

agents, only one of which (zanamivir) is available by inhalation. Prophylactic vaccination against influenza, especially in high-risk patients with cardiovascular or respiratory disease, remains the unqualified recommendation, despite the availability of drugs to treat acute infection.

Dosage and Administration

Zanamivir is available in a dry powder inhaler (DPI), the Diskhaler device, for oral inhalation. Each blister contains 5 mg of drug, providing a dose of 5 mg per inhalation. There are four blisters in a Rotadisk, and the drug package contains five Rotadisks with one Diskhaler device. The dose for adults and children 5 years of age or older is two inhalations (two blisters, for a total of 10 mg) taken twice a day approximately 12 hours apart for 5 days. The complete drug package has the equivalent of 5 days of treatment because each Rotadisk contains 1 day's dosage. Patients should finish the entire 5-day course of drug.

Mechanism of Action

The general mechanism of viral infection was described previously with ribavirin (see discussion of the nature of viral infection). Zanamivir represents a new class of antiviral agents, termed *neuraminidase inhibitors,* which act by binding to the viral enzyme neuraminidase (NA) and blocking the action of the enzyme. The influenza virus has an envelope and a protein coat surrounding the viral RNA and targets the respiratory tract. Briefly, as illustrated in Figure 13-10, the virus envelope for both *influenza A* and *influenza B* has two surface glycoproteins, *hemagglutinin (HA)* and *NA.*

HA binds to a sugary molecule, *sialic acid (SA),* on the surface of a cell to be infected. This binding leads to fusion of virus and cell membranes and allows adsorption and penetration of the virus into the cell. However, when the newly minted viral particles bud from the cell and are ready to be released, the viral envelope acquires SA from the cell, along with its own HA and NA receptors. Without NA, the viral HA would combine with the SA again, "sticking" the viral particles to each other and to the cell surface, preventing further infection. NA cleaves part of the SA to prevent HA and SA combination and prevents viral aggregation (clumping). NA is essential for virus release from infected cells, prevents virus aggregation, and may decrease virus inactivation by respiratory mucus. Zanamivir is able to bind to NA and block the enzyme action. By inhibiting NA, zanamivir inhibits viral particle separation and cellular release needed for systemic infection to proceed.[62]

Zanamivir is given by inhalation because the binding ability of the drug also prevents good absorption when given orally. Inhalation also delivers the drug to the affected organ directly. Approximately 4% to 17% of an inhaled dose is absorbed systemically. Zanamivir has limited plasma protein binding (less than 10%) and is excreted unchanged in the renal system. It is apparently not metabolized to other products in vivo. Its serum half-life is 2.5 to 5.1 hours. Any unabsorbed drug is excreted in the feces.

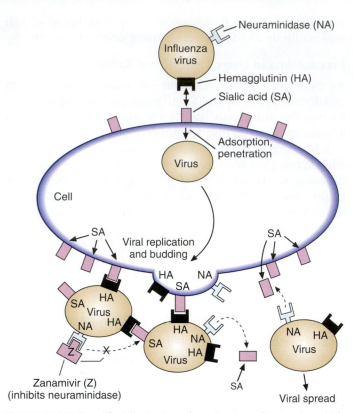

Figure 13-10 Simplified illustration of mechanism of action by which inhaled zanamivir (Z) provides its antiviral effect in influenza viral infection. As a sialic acid (SA) analog, zanamivir binds to the enzyme neuraminidase (NA) and inhibits its usual inactivation of SA. As a result, the viral hemagglutinin (HA) receptor continues to combine with both cell and viral SA, causing viral aggregation and preventing viral release and spread.

Adverse Effects

The side effects discussed in the following sections have been noted during clinical trials and after release of zanamivir.

Bronchospasm and deterioration of lung function. Patients with underlying respiratory disease such as asthma or COPD may experience bronchospasm after inhaling zanamivir. Respiratory difficulty and wheezing have been reported in a patient with COPD[63] and an asthma patient inhaling zanamivir.[64] Apparently neither of these patients had influenza at the time of treatment. A clinical trial of zanamivir by Cass and colleagues[65] in 11 patients with mild to moderate asthma with no influenza showed no symptoms of bronchospasm or airway responsiveness. However, such data do not establish the safety of zanamivir in asthmatics with influenza infection, which can cause mucosal damage and airway reactivity from the viral inflammation.[66-67] In ongoing treatment studies of patients with COPD or asthma who had influenza-like illness, more patients receiving zanamivir compared with patients receiving a placebo had a greater than 20% decline in FEV_1 or peak expiratory flow rate.[62] Zanamivir should be discontinued if bronchospasm or a decline in lung function occurs in any patient, and the managing physician should be consulted. The manufacturer recommends that any patient with underlying airways disease not take zanamivir.[36]

Undertreatment of bacterial infection. Bacterial respiratory infections can manifest with influenza-like symptoms, and viral respiratory infections can progress to serious bacterial secondary infections.[67] Treatment with an antiviral agent such as zanamivir is ineffective against bacterial infection and could possibly allow progression of the infection to serious illness such as pneumonia. Two deaths from bacterial infection in subjects taking zanamivir have been reported,[68] although the reasons have not been determined.[69] In a patient with COPD exacerbation who is treated inappropriately, risk of serious complications and the need for hospitalization can result.[67]

Allergic reactions. As with any drug, patients should be monitored for allergic or allergic-like reactions with zanamivir.

Other adverse effects. Adverse reactions occurring in a small percentage of patients included gastrointestinal (diarrhea, nausea, vomiting) and respiratory (bronchitis; cough; sinusitis; ear, nose, and throat infections) effects, dizziness, and headaches. These reactions did not differ substantially from reactions with placebos and may have been caused by the same lactose vehicle used in the active drug and the placebo.

Overdosage. There have been no reports of overdosage from use of zanamivir.

Clinical Efficacy and Safety

Clinical efficacy of zanamivir has been established in trials showing that inhaled zanamivir can significantly shorten the duration of influenza symptoms.[66,69,70] With uncomplicated influenza-like illness, treatment with 10 mg of zanamivir twice daily resulted in approximately 1 day of shortening of the median time to improvement in symptoms compared with a placebo.[66] The time to improvement in major symptoms was defined as no fever and no or mild headache, myalgia, cough, and sore throat. Among patients who were febrile and began treatment 30 hours or less after onset of symptoms, treatment with zanamivir resulted in a shortening of 3 days in the median time to alleviation of symptoms.[66] There are no data on efficacy when zanamivir is started after more than 2 days of symptoms of influenza.

There was no consistent difference in treatment effect between patients with influenza A versus influenza B. However, the clinical trials of zanamivir enrolled predominantly patients with influenza A (89% influenza A versus 11% influenza B in one clinical trial). Patients with lower temperature and less severe symptoms in general derived less benefit from treatment with zanamivir.

Clinical trials of zanamivir were performed mainly with previously healthy subjects.[66,69,70] The manufacturer's literature states that safety and efficacy of zanamivir for treating influenza have not been shown in patients with COPD. Zanamivir may carry risk for patients with COPD or asthma, as indicated in the discussion of side effects. Revised labeling for zanamivir adds a warning that zanamivir is *not generally recommended for patients with underlying airways disease because of the risk of serious adverse effects.*[66]

Zanamivir is not approved for prophylaxis to prevent influenza, and it does not reduce the risk of transmission of the virus to others. However, some data suggest a prophylactic benefit with zanamivir in influenza A and influenza B in university and nursing home communities.[71] Results of a controlled study of inhaled zanamivir for treatment and prevention of influenza in families in which one member developed influenza-like illness showed that zanamivir did reduce the rate of developing influenza in other family members. The proportion of families in which an initially healthy member developed influenza was 4% with zanamivir compared with 19% with a placebo.[72] In the trial, treatment of the index cases with zanamivir in families reduced the median duration of symptoms from 7.5 to 5.0 days, a significant reduction. Oseltamivir (Tamiflu) was approved for prevention of influenza A and influenza B in children 1 year of age or older who are in close contact with influenza. Adverse reactions were similar in both groups.[36]

The safety and efficacy of zanamivir have been tested in children. In a study by Hedrick and others,[73] zanamivir was tested on children 5 to 12 years old. In the study of 471 children, 224 were given zanamivir, and the remaining children, the control group, were given a placebo. The children taking zanamivir had reduced influenza symptoms 1.25 days before children in the placebo group. The zanamivir group returned to normal activities in less time and took fewer relief medications than the placebo group.

A final issue with the use of zanamivir or other antiinfluenza agents as acute treatment is the lack of a clinically easy and inexpensive diagnostic tool to confirm the presence of influenza infection. Zanamivir is not beneficial in patients with infections other than influenza. In the clinical trial by Hayden and colleagues,[66] 262 of 417 patients (63%) with influenza-like illness had confirmed influenza virus infection. As a result, symptoms alone can result in inappropriate use of antiinfluenza drugs, with attendant risks as outlined in the discussion of adverse effects. Inappropriate use contributes to increased cost.

The cost versus efficacy of zanamivir has been debated. There is modest reduction in symptoms for the cost of the drug; there is no readily available test to confirm the presence of influenza viral infection for use of the drug, resulting in possibly inappropriate use; and the drug carries increased risk for the patients who might benefit most—patients with reactive airways disease.

RESPIRATORY CARE ASSESSMENT OF AEROSOLIZED ANTIINFECTIVE AGENTS

Before Treatment

The following assessment applies to all of the aerosolized antiinfective agents discussed.

- Assess for the presence of disease indicating appropriate use of the agent:
  - *Pentamidine:* Risk of PCP
  - *Ribavirin:* Presence of severe RSV infection in infants or children at risk

- *Tobramycin:* Chronic *P. aeruginosa* infection compromising lung function in CF patients
- *Aztreonam:* Chronic *P. aeruginosa* infection compromising lung function in CF patients
- *Zanamivir:* Symptoms of acute influenza infection within first 2 days of onset

- Assess the correct configuration and function of aerosol equipment for ribavirin; instruct and verify correct use of aerosol delivery device for other agents.
- On initial aerosol treatment, assess respiratory rate and pattern, pulse, and breath sounds; evaluate for the presence of airway irritation resulting in wheezing and bronchospasm.

During Treatment and Short Term

Pentamidine

- Monitor for coughing and bronchospasm, and if these are present, provide a short-acting β agonist or an anticholinergic bronchodilator such as ipratropium with inhaled pentamidine.
- Monitor for occurrence rate of PCP and rate of hospitalizations long term.
- Monitor for presence of side effects (shortness of breath, possible pneumothorax, conjunctivitis, rash, neutropenia, dysglycemia) or appearance of extrapulmonary *P. jiroveci* infection.

Ribavirin

- Monitor signs of RSV infection severity for improvement, including vital signs, respiratory pattern and work of breathing (clinically), level of fraction of inspired oxygen (FIO_2) needed, level of ventilatory support, arterial blood gases, body temperature, and other indicators of pulmonary gas exchange.
- Monitor patient for evidence of side effects such as deterioration in lung function, bronchospasm, occlusion of endotracheal tube if present, cardiovascular instability, skin irritation from the aerosol drug, and equipment malfunction caused by drug residue.

Tobramycin

- Verify that patient understands that nebulized tobramycin should be given after other inhaled medications for CF.
- Check whether patient has renal, auditory, vestibular, or neuromuscular problems or is taking other aminoglycosides or ototoxic drugs. Consider whether tobramycin should be given to the patient, based on severity of preexisting or concomitant risk factors.
- Monitor lung function to note improvement in FEV_1.
- Assess rate of hospitalization before and after institution of inhaled tobramycin.
- Assess need for intravenous antipseudomonal therapy.
- Assess improvement in weight.
- Monitor for occurrence of side effects such as tinnitus or voice alteration; have patient rinse mouth after aerosol treatments.

- Evaluate for changes in hearing function or renal function during use of inhaled tobramycin.

Aztreonam

- Verify that patient understands that nebulized aztreonam should be given after other inhaled medications for CF.
- Monitor lung function to note improvement in FEV_1.
- Assess rate of hospitalization before and after institution of inhaled aztreonam.
- Monitor for occurrence of side effects, such as an allergic reaction; have patient rinse mouth after aerosol treatments.

Zanamivir

- Assess improvement in influenza symptoms: fever reduction, less myalgia and headache, reduced coughing and sore throat, and less systemic fatigue.
- Monitor for airway irritation and symptoms of bronchospasm, especially during initial use of the dry powder aerosol. Provide a short-acting β agonist if needed or if patient is at risk for airway reactivity (COPD, asthma).

Long Term

- Monitor pulmonary function studies of lung volumes, capacities, and flows.
- Instruct CF patients in the use and interpretation of disposable peak flow meters to assess the severity of CF episodes and to ensure there is an action plan for treatment modification.
- Instruct and verify correct use of the aerosol delivery device (SVN, MDI, reservoir, DPI).
- Instruct patients in the use, assembly, and especially cleaning of aerosol inhalation devices.

General Contraindications

Pentamidine

- Bronchospasm and cough are common; pretreat with a bronchodilator.
- Use with a nebulizer system with a one-way valve and expiratory filter system to decrease caregiver exposure.

Ribavirin

- Caregivers who are pregnant or wish to become pregnant should avoid exposure; the effect on fertility is uncertain.

Tobramycin

- Drug resistance is the greatest risk with the use of this agent; using an alternating schedule should help.

Aztreonam

- Drug resistance is the greatest risk with the use of this agent; using an alternating schedule should help.
- Aztreonam should not be used in CF patients not infected with *P. aeruginosa*.

Zanamivir

- Patients with preexisting and uncontrolled airways disease should not use this agent; bronchospasm and lung deterioration may occur.

SELF-ASSESSMENT QUESTIONS

Answers can be found in Appendix A.

1. Identify the disease states for which each of these drugs is used when inhaled as an aerosol: pentamidine, ribavirin, tobramycin, aztreonam, and zanamivir.
2. Briefly explain the rationale for aerosolizing an antibiotic such as tobramycin or aztreonam in cystic fibrosis.
3. What is the brand name of aerosolized pentamidine?
4. What is the dose and frequency for aerosolized pentamidine?
5. What device is approved for aerosolization of pentamidine?
6. Identify the common airway effects with aerosolized pentamidine, and suggest a method for preventing or lessening these effects.
7. What is a major risk to the caregiver when aerosolizing pentamidine to a patient with AIDS?
8. What is the current Centers for Disease Control and Prevention (CDC) recommended prophylactic treatment for PCP in AIDS patients?
9. What is the brand name and dose for aerosol ribavirin?
10. What is the mechanism of action of ribavirin?
11. Name two serious hazards when ribavirin is given to a patient undergoing mechanical ventilation.
12. In general, how can you prevent environmental contamination when delivering ribavirin to an oxygen hood?
13. What is the recommended dosage for inhaled tobramycin?
14. Identify common side effects that have been observed with aerosolized tobramycin.
15. Name two potential hazards to family members with aerosolized tobramycin at home.
16. What is the recommended dosage for inhaled aztreonam?
17. What should be done before a patient is prescribed inhaled aztreonam?
18. Give the brand name and dosage for zanamivir.
19. In one sentence, describe the mechanism of action of zanamivir.
20. Identify common hazards in the use of inhaled zanamivir.
21. What factors cause debate over the use of zanamivir in treating influenza?

CLINICAL SCENARIO

Answers can be found in Appendix A.

Brody Hendrix is a 29-year-old man with cystic fibrosis (CF). The history of his disease and its previous treatment are well known to his pulmonary physician. He has been admitted to the hospital with complaints of increasing cough, shortness of breath, and sputum production. He reports that his sputum is greenish. His recent history reveals that his last admission for exacerbation of CF was approximately 6 months ago. He has used albuterol by metered dose inhaler (MDI), with two puffs qid, and recently began to use salmeterol, two puffs bid. He maintains himself on a regular regimen of CF medications, including iron and vitamin supplements and pancrelipase (Pancrease). Approximately 3 weeks ago, he complained of increasing pulmonary secretions and noted a mild elevation of his temperature (99.1° F). At that time, his physician prescribed ciprofloxacin, 500 mg orally bid, and he completed a course of 14 days, ending 5 days ago.

He is alert, oriented, and in no acute distress at this time. His skin is warm and dry. Vital signs are as follows: blood pressure (BP) of 106/66 mm Hg, pulse (P) of 88 beats/min, regular respiratory rate (RR) of 20 breaths/min, and temperature (T) of 98.9° F. His respiratory pattern is normal, and there is no use of accessory muscles. Auscultation reveals scattered rales and wheezes bilaterally, both anteriorly and posteriorly. His cough is nonproductive during the examination.

A chest radiograph shows hyperexpanded lung fields, with linear fibrotic changes bilaterally over the lung fields. Cardiac silhouette shows mild right atrial hypertrophy. No consolidation or pleural effusion is seen. Complete blood count (CBC) results are as follows: hemoglobin of 13.2 g/dL, hematocrit at 38.6%, and white blood cell count (WBC) of $13.5 \times 10^3/mm^3$. Remaining blood values are normal. Pulse oximetry measures 89% saturation on room air. Pulmonary function testing, performed approximately 2 months ago and available in his chart, shows the following:

	Observed	Predicted	Percent Predicted
Total lung capacity (TLC), L	7.66	6.67	115
Forced vital capacity (FVC), L	3.52	5.23	67
Forced expiratory volume in 1 second (FEV$_1$), L	1.41	3.51	40

Continued

CLINICAL SCENARIO—cont'd

	Observed	Predicted	Percent Predicted
Mean forced expiratory flow during middle half of FVC (FEF$_{25-75}$), L/sec	0.49	2.93	17
Expiratory reserve volume (ERV), L	0.94	1.69	56
Residual volume (RV), L	4.0	1.54	260

A sputum culture is taken and sent to the laboratory. Mr. Hendrix is admitted for acute exacerbation of his pulmonary symptoms.

Using the SOAP method, assess this clinical scenario.

REFERENCES

1. Montgomery AB, Debs RJ, Luce JM, et al: Aerosolized pentamidine as sole therapy for *Pneumocystis carinii* pneumonia in patients with acquired immunodeficiency syndrome. *Lancet* 2:480, 1987.
2. Montgomery AB, Debs RJ, Luce JM, et al: Selective delivery of pentamidine to the lung by aerosol. *Am Rev Respir Dis* 137:477, 1988.
3. Leoung GS, Feigal DW, Jr, Montgomery AB, et al: Aerosolized pentamidine for prophylaxis against *Pneumocystis carinii* pneumonia. *N Engl J Med* 323:769, 1990.
4. Levine SJ, White DA: *Pneumocystis carinii*. *Clin Chest Med* 9:395, 1988.
5. Stringer JR, Beard CB, Miller RF, et al: A new name (*Pneumocystis jiroveci*) for pneumocystis from humans. *Emerg Infect Dis* 8:891, 2002.
6. Hughes WT: *Pneumocystis carinii* vs. *Pneumocystis jiroveci:* another misnomer (response to Stringer et al.). *Emerg Infect Dis* 9:276, 2003.
7. Gigliotti F: *Pneumocystis carinii:* has the name really changed? *Clin Infect Dis* 41:1752, 2005.
8. Corkery KJ, Luce JM, Montgomery AB: Aerosolized pentamidine for treatment and prophylaxis of *Pneumocystis carinii* pneumonia: an update. *Respir Care* 33:676, 1988.
9. Vinciguerra C, Smaldone G: Treatment time and patient tolerance for pentamidine delivery by Respirgard II and AeroTech II. *Respir Care* 35:1037, 1990.
10. Smaldone GC, Perry RJ, Deutsch DG: Characteristics of nebulizers used in the treatment of AIDS-related *Pneumocystis carinii* pneumonia. *J Aerosol Med* 1:113, 1988.
11. Waskin H: Toxicology of antimicrobial aerosols: a review of aerosolized ribavirin and pentamidine. *Respir Care* 36:1026, 1991.
12. Mathewson HS: *Pneumocystis carinii* pneumonia: chemotherapy and prophylaxis. *Respir Care* 34:360, 1989.
13. Martinez CM, Romanelli A, Mullen MP, et al: Spontaneous pneumothoraces in AIDS patients receiving aerosolized pentamidine. *Chest* 94:1317–1318, 1988. (letter).
14. Hart CC: Aerosolized pentamidine and pancreatitis. *Ann Intern Med* 111:691, 1989. (letter).
15. Davey RT, Jr, Margolis D, Kleiner D, et al: Digital necrosis and disseminated *Pneumocystis carinii* infection after aerosolized pentamidine prophylaxis. *Ann Intern Med* 111:681, 1989.
16. Quieffin J, Hunter J, Schechter MT, et al: Aerosol pentamidine-induced bronchoconstriction: predictive factors and preventive therapy. *Chest* 100:624, 1991.
17. Fine JM, Gordon T, Sheppard D: The roles of pH and ionic species in sulfur dioxide and sulfite-induced bronchoconstriction. *Am Rev Respir Dis* 136:1122, 1987.
18. Corkery KJ, Montgomery AB, Montanti R, et al: Airway effects of aerosolized pentamidine isethionate. *Am Rev Respir Dis* 141:A152, 1990. (abstract).
19. Smaldone GC, Vinciguerra C, Marchese J: Detection of inhaled pentamidine in health care workers. *N Engl J Med* 325:891, 1991.
20. O'Riordan TG, Smaldone GC: Exposure of health care workers to aerosolized pentamidine. *Chest* 101:494, 1992.
21. Fallat RJ, Kandal K: Aerosol exhaust: escape of aerosolized medication into the patient and caregiver's environment. *Respir Care* 36:1008, 1991.
22. Chaisson RE, McAvinue S: Control of tuberculosis during aerosol therapy administration. *Respir Care* 36:1017, 1991.
23. Centers for Disease Control: Guidelines for preventing the transmission of tuberculosis in health-care settings, with special focus on HIV-related issues. *MMWR Recomm Rep* 39(RR–17):1, 1990.
24. American Respiratory Care Foundation: *Pentamidine aerosols and care giver safety*, Dallas, TX, 1992, American Association for Respiratory Care.
25. Riley RL, Nardell EA: Clearing the air: the theory and application of ultraviolet air disinfection. *Am Rev Respir Dis* 139:1286, 1989.
26. Mofenson LM, Brady MT, Danner SP, et al; Centers for Disease Control and Prevention; National Institutes of Health; HIV Medicine Association of the Infectious Diseases Society of America; Pediatric Infectious Diseases Society; American Academy of Pediatrics: Guidelines for the Prevention and Treatment of Opportunistic Infections among HIV-exposed and HIV-infected children: recommendations from CDC, the National Institutes of Health, the HIV Medicine Association of the Infectious Diseases Society of America, the Pediatric Infectious Diseases Society, and the American Academy of Pediatrics. *MMWR Recomm Rep* 58(RR–11):1–166, 2009.
27. Panel on Opportunistic Infections in HIV-Infected Adults and Adolescents. Guidelines for the prevention and treatment of opportunistic infections in HIV-infected adults and adolescents: recommendations from the Centers for Disease Control and Prevention, the National Institutes of Health, and the HIV Medicine Association of the Infectious Diseases Society of America. Available at: <http://aidsinfo.nih.gov/contentfiles/lvguidelines/adult_oi.pdf>.
28. Reines ED, Gross PA: Antiviral agents. *Med Clin North Am* 72:691, 1988.
29. Hall CB, McBride JT, Walsh EE, et al: Aerosolized ribavirin treatment of infants with respiratory syncytial viral infection: a randomized double-blind study. *N Engl J Med* 308:1443, 1983.
30. Guerguerian AM, Gauthier M, Lebel MH, et al: Ribavirin in Ventilated Respiratory Syncytial Virus Bronchiolitis. *Am J Respir Crit Care Med* 160(3):829–834, 1999.
31. American Academy of Pediatrics Committee on Infectious Diseases: Respiratory syncytial virus. In Pickering LK, editor: *Red Book: 2009 report of the Committee on Infectious Diseases*, ed 28, Elk Grove Village, Ill, 2009, American Academy of Pediatrics.
32. Agency for Healthcare Research and Quality: *Management of bronchiolitis in infants and children evidence report/technology assessment: number 69*, AHRQ Publication No. 03-E014, Rockville, MD, 2003, Agency for Healthcare Research and Quality. Available at: <http://www.ahrq.gov/clinic/epcsums/broncsum.htm>.

33. Smith DW, Frankel LR, Mathers LH, et al: A controlled trial of aerosolized ribavirin in infants receiving mechanical ventilation for severe respiratory syncytial virus infection. *N Engl J Med* 325:24, 1991.

34. Meert KL, Sarnaik AP, Gelmini MJ, et al: Aerosolized ribavirin in mechanically ventilated children with respiratory syncytial virus lower respiratory tract disease: a prospective, double-blind, randomized trial. *Crit Care Med* 22:566, 1994.

35. Demers RR, Parker J, Frankel LR, et al: Administration of ribavirin to neonatal and pediatric patients during mechanical ventilation. *Respir Care* 31:1188, 1986.

36. *Drug facts and comparisons*, St Louis, MO, 2014, Facts & Comparisons, Wolters Kluwer Health.

37. Centers for Disease Control: Assessing exposures of health-care personnel to aerosols of ribavirin: California. *MMWR Morb Mortal Wkly Rep* 37:560, 1988.

38. Corkery K, Eckman D, Charney W: Environmental exposure of aerosolized ribavirin. *Respir Care* 34:1027, 1989. (abstract).

39. Kacmarek RM: Ribavirin and pentamidine aerosols: caregiver beware! *Respir Care* 35:1034, 1990. (editorial).

40. American Academy of Pediatrics Committee on Infectious Diseases: Use of ribavirin in the treatment of respiratory syncytial virus infection. *Pediatrics* 92:501, 1993.

41. Cefaratt JL, Steinberg EA: An alternative method for delivery of ribavirin to nonventilated pediatric patients. *Respir Care* 37:877, 1992.

42. Kacmarek RM, Kratohvil J: Evaluation of a double-enclosure double-vacuum unit scavenging system for ribavirin administration. *Respir Care* 37:37, 1992.

43. Charney W, Corkery KJ, Kraemer R, et al: Engineering and administrative controls to contain aerosolized ribavirin: results of simulation and application to one patient. *Respir Care* 35:1042, 1990.

44. Breedveld FC: Therapeutic monoclonal antibodies. *Lancet* 355:735, 2000.

45. American Academy of Pediatrics Committee on Infectious Diseases and Committee on Fetus and Newborn: Revised indications for the use of palivizumab and respiratory syncytial virus immune globulin intravenous for the prevention of respiratory syncytial virus infections. *Pediatrics* 112:1442, 2003.

46. Palivizumab, a humanized respiratory syncytial virus monoclonal antibody, reduces hospitalization from respiratory syncytial virus infection in high-risk infants. The Impact-RSV Study Group. *Pediatrics* 102:531, 1998.

47. Feltes TF, Cabalka AK, Meissner HC, et al; Cardiac Synagis Study Group: Palivizumab prophylaxis reduces hospitalizations due to respiratory syncytial virus in young children with hemodynamically significant congenital heart disease. *J Pediatr* 143:532, 2003.

48. Baran D, Dachy A, Klastersky J: Concentration of gentamicin in bronchial secretions of children with cystic fibrosis or tracheostomy. *Int J Clin Pharmacol Biopharm* 12:336, 1975.

49. Le Conte P, Potel G, Peltier P, et al: Lung distribution and pharmacokinetics of aerosolized tobramycin. *Am Rev Respir Dis* 147:1279, 1993.

50. Neu HC: Quinolones: a new class of antimicrobial agents with wide potential uses. *Med Clin North Am* 72:623, 1988.

51. Ramsey BW, Pepe MS, Quan JM, et al: Intermittent administration of inhaled tobramycin in patients with cystic fibrosis. *N Engl J Med* 340:23, 1999.

52. Smith AL, Ramsey B: Aerosol administration of antibiotics. *Respiration* 62(Suppl 1):19, 1995.

53. Littlewood JM, Smye SW, Cunliffe H: Aerosol antibiotic treatment in cystic fibrosis. *Arch Dis Child* 68:788, 1993.

54. Dickie KJ, de Groot WJ: Ventilatory effects of aerosolized kanamycin and polymyxin. *Chest* 63:694, 1973.

55. Dally MB, Kurrle S, Breslin ABX: Ventilatory effects of aerosol gentamicin. *Thorax* 33:54, 1978.

56. Wilson FE: Acute respiratory failure secondary to polymyxin-B inhalation. *Chest* 79:237, 1981.

57. Gibson RL, Emerson J, McNamara S, et al: Significant microbiological effect of inhaled tobramycin in young children with cystic fibrosis. *Am J Respir Crit Care Med* 167:841, 2003.

58. LoBue PA: Inhaled tobramycin not just for cystic fibrosis anymore? *Chest* 127:1098, 2005.

59. Standaert TA, Vandevanter D, Ramsey BW, et al: The choice of compressor effects the aerosol parameters and the delivery of tobramycin from a single model nebulizer. *J Aerosol Med* 13:147, 2000.

60. Newman SP, Pellow PGD, Clarke SW: Choice of nebulisers and compressors for delivery of carbenicillin aerosol. *Eur J Respir Dis* 69:160, 1986.

61. Hata JS, Fick RB, Jr: Pseudomonas aeruginosa and the airways disease of cystic fibrosis. *Clin Chest Med* 9:679, 1988.

62. Gubareva LV, Kaiser L, Hayden FG: Influenza virus neuraminidase inhibitors. *Lancet* 355:827, 2000.

63. Williamson JC, Pegram PS: Respiratory distress associated with zanamivir. *N Engl J Med* 342:661, 2000.

64. Winquist AG, Fukuda K, Bridges CB, et al; Centers for Disease Control and Prevention: Neuraminidase inhibitors for treatment of influenza A and B infections. *MMWR Recomm Rep* 48(RR–14):1, 1999. Available at: <http://www.cdc.gov/mmwr/preview/mmwrhtml/rr4814a1.htm>.

65. Cass LM, Gunawardena KA, Macmahon MM, et al: Pulmonary function and airway responsiveness in mild to moderate asthmatics given repeated inhaled doses of zanamivir. *Respir Med* 94:166, 2000.

66. Hayden FG, Osterhaus AD, Treanor JJ, et al: Efficacy and safety of the neuraminidase inhibitor zanamivir in the treatment of influenzavirus infections. *N Engl J Med* 337:874, 1997.

67. U.S. Food and Drug Administration: Revised labeling for zanamivir. *JAMA* 284:1234, 2000.

68. Yamey G: Drug company issues warning about flu drug. *BMJ* 320:334, 2000.

69. O'Riordan TG: Inhaled antimicrobial therapy: from cystic fibrosis to the flu. *Respir Care* 45:836, 2000.

70. Randomised trial of efficacy and safety of inhaled zanamivir in treatment of influenza A and B virus infections. The MIST (Management of Influenza in the Southern Hemisphere Trialists) Study Group. *Lancet* 352:1877, 1998.

71. Dunn CJ, Goa KL: Zanamivir: a review of its use in influenza. *Drugs* 58:761, 1999.

72. Hayden FG, Gubareva LV, Monto AS, et al; Zanamivir Family Study Group: Inhaled zanamivir for the prevention of influenza in families. *N Engl J Med* 343:1282, 2000.

73. Hedrick JA, Barzilai A, Behre U, et al: Zanamivir for treatment of symptomatic influenza A and B infection in children five to twelve years of age: a randomized controlled trial. *Pediatr Infect Dis J* 19:410, 2000.

CHAPTER **14**

Antimicrobial Agents

Christopher A. Schriever, Susan L. Pendland

CHAPTER OUTLINE

OBJECTIVES

After reading this chapter, the reader will be able to:

1. Define terms that pertain to antimicrobial agents
2. Define antibiotic
3. Describe the process involved in bacterial susceptibility testing
4. Discuss possible outcomes of antimicrobial combinations
5. List the various classes of the penicillins
6. List the various classes of the cephalosporins
7. Recognize similarities between members of the macrolides, azalides, and ketolides
8. Recognize similarities between members of the fluoroquinolones
9. List four mechanisms of action of antibacterials
10. List five commonly used antimycobacterials
11. Describe the commonly used azole antifungals and how they differ in spectrum of activity
12. Discuss similarities between members of the echinocandins
13. Describe the mechanism of action of the antiretrovirals

KEY TERMS AND DEFINITIONS

Antagonism Antibiotic combination in which the activity of one antibiotic interferes with the activity of the other (block receptor site, enzymatic inactivation), resulting in less activity with the combination than with the individual drugs.

Antibiotics Substance derived or produced from a microorganism that inhibits or kills other microorganisms.

Antimicrobials Natural and synthetic compounds that either inhibit or kill microorganisms.

Synergy The combined effect of two antimicrobials is greater than their added effect (i.e., increased permeability by one agent allows the second agent access to the bacterial target).

Antimicrobials are among the most widely used therapeutic agents in the world. A variety of antimicrobial agents have been developed from naturally occurring compounds or created synthetically. The development of new classes of antimicrobials (i.e., those with a novel mechanism of action) has declined in recent years, with most new agents coming from chemical modification of older agents. This presents a challenge to clinicians as microbes are developing resistance to many commonly used antimicrobial agents.

Techniques to identify organisms[1] and to determine their susceptibility[2,3] have evolved over the years and are vital for selection of effective antimicrobial therapy. In addition, other factors, such as the host, antimicrobial pharmacodynamics, antimicrobial combinations, and methods of monitoring therapy, are important parameters that need consideration before selecting an antimicrobial agent.[4-6] This chapter focuses on these basic principles of antimicrobial therapy, provides a synopsis of mechanism of action and adverse effects, and emphasizes the clinical use of the various antimicrobial classes for the treatment of respiratory infections.

PRINCIPLES OF ANTIMICROBIAL THERAPY

Several factors require careful consideration before choosing a particular antimicrobial agent.[4-6] Identification of the organism or organisms responsible for the infection is the first step toward treatment. Before initiating antimicrobial therapy, diagnostic specimens should be properly collected and promptly submitted to the microbiology laboratory.[1,4,6] Results from these tests may not be available for 24 to 72 hours, so initial therapy is guided by the clinical presentation of the patient.[4-6] Empiric therapy is often based on evidence-based practice guidelines. The Infectious Diseases Society of America (IDSA) and the American Thoracic Society (ATS) have published guidelines for the management of community-acquired (CAP), hospital-acquired (HAP), ventilator-associated (VAP), and health-care associated pneumonia (HCAP).[7,8] Once an organism is isolated, antimicrobial susceptibility is determined according to standardized methods that can be replicated between laboratories, such as those established by the Clinical and Laboratory Standards Institute (CLSI). The susceptibility pattern of the organism narrows the choice of potential agents. The choice of a specific agent is also influenced by host factors (drug allergies, organ function, infection site) and drug factors (available dosage forms, cost).

Identification of Pathogen

The first step toward identification of potential pathogens is the collection of specimens for culture. Specimens commonly collected include blood, urine, sputum, cerebrospinal fluid, pleural fluid, synovial fluid, peritoneal fluid, and stool.[6] Several methods are employed to identify the pathogens rapidly using various chemical stains, immunologic assays, and microscopic examination.[1] The simplest and most common preparation is the Gram stain. This stain designates bacteria into two major classes: gram positive (which stain purple) or gram negative (which stain red). Bacteria stain differently depending on the structural components of their cell walls. These structural components also affect their susceptibility to antimicrobials. The Gram stain also distinguishes bacteria from one another by their morphology. Spheric bacteria, such as *Staphylococcus* and *Streptococcus* species, are cocci, and rod-shaped bacteria, such as *Escherichia coli* and *Pseudomonas aeruginosa*, are bacilli. Other bacteria, such as *Mycobacterium tuberculosis*, require the use of an acid-fast stain to penetrate their wax-like cell walls. Mycobacteria generally require 10 to 14 days for growth, but may take as long as 6 weeks, which makes the acid-fast stain vital for the rapid diagnosis of tuberculosis.[6] Certain fungi can be quickly identified using India ink (for *Cryptococcus neoformans*) and potassium hydroxide (KOH) preparations. Urinary antigen tests are routinely performed for rapid identification of *Streptococcus pneumoniae* and *Legionella pneumophila*. Rapid antigen tests for influenza allow detection, as well as to distinguish between influenza A and B.[1,7,9]

In many clinical cases, the exact identity of the infecting organism is unknown. As a result, patients are treated empirically with an antimicrobial agent active against the organism or organisms that are most likely causing the infection.[6] For example, 40% or more of patients with CAP fail to expectorate sputum, which prevents identification of a specific pathogen.[7] Collective data from numerous studies have shown that the most common pathogens responsible for CAP include *S. pneumoniae*; *Haemophilus influenzae*; and atypical (intracellular) organisms such as *Mycoplasma pneumoniae*, *Chlamydrophila* (formerly *Chlamydia*) *pneumoniae*, and *L. pneumophila*. As a result, empiric therapy for CAP involves antimicrobials active against this spectrum of organisms.[7,9,10] Conversely, identification of an organism from culture material does not necessarily indicate an infection.[6] For example, hospitalized patients often have growth of gram-negative bacilli in sputum samples. However, these organisms may only represent colonization and not HAP (also known as *nosocomial* pneumonia). In addition, specimens obtained after initiation of antimicrobial therapy may not be reliable, as *S. pneumoniae* and other pathogens may be masked by overgrowth of normal microbial flora.[1,7,8]

Common pathogens and treatment of specific respiratory infections are listed in Table 14-1.

Susceptibility Testing and Resistance

KEY POINT

The susceptibility of an organism to an antimicrobial is quantified as the *minimal inhibitory concentration (MIC)* and the *minimal bactericidal concentration (MBC)*.[2-4] The science of understanding the optimal effect of an antimicrobial as a function of its concentration to the MIC against the microorganism is known as *pharmacodynamics*.[4-6]

Once an organism is isolated, susceptibility test results can usually be obtained within 24 hours. Several methods are commonly used to determine the susceptibility of isolated pathogens.[2-3] The Kirby-Bauer disk diffusion test involves the use of antibiotic-impregnated disks that are placed on an agar plate heavily inoculated (10^5 colony-forming units [cfu]/mL) with the isolated bacteria. If the organism is susceptible to the antibiotic, a clear zone of inhibition (no growth of the organism) develops around the disk. Published breakpoints for the diameter of the clear zones are used to determine whether the organism is susceptible or resistant to the antimicrobial agent. However, they do not provide specific data on the concentration needed to kill or inhibit growth of the organism. Another disk diffusion test is the elliptical test, or E-test. The E-test strip is placed on an agar plate heavily inoculated with the isolated organism. The strip creates an antimicrobial gradient, which results in a clear elliptical zone of inhibition. This method allows the determination of the *minimal inhibitory concentration (MIC)*. MIC is defined as the least concentration of antimicrobial that prevents visible growth.[2-4] The Kirby-Bauer and E-test methods are illustrated in Figure 14-1.

Other methods include inoculation of the organism into serial dilutions of an antimicrobial in agar or, more commonly, in broth culture media (Figure 14-2). Automated systems such as Vitek (bioMérieux, Durham, North Carolina), MicroScan (Siemens Medical Solutions, Malvern, Pennsylvania), and BD Phoenix (Becton Dickinson, Franklin Lakes, New Jersey) take advantage of broth microdilution methods to provide efficient and rapid susceptibility results. When susceptibility testing is performed in broth media, a small sample can be removed from the test tubes or microwells with no growth and used to inoculate agar plates. The lowest concentration of antimicrobial agent that prevents growth of the organism on the agar plate after 24 hours of incubation is termed the *minimal bactericidal concentration (MBC)*.[3] Most laboratories do not routinely perform MBC testing, but these tests can be performed in specialized laboratories. They are often employed in research studies of new or investigational antimicrobial agents to determine whether these drugs are bacteriostatic or bactericidal. Drugs that inhibit the growth of bacteria but do not kill them are termed *bacteriostatic*. A *bactericidal* drug is one that kills the bacteria.[3,5] Examples of bacteriostatic and bactericidal drugs are listed in Box 14-1.

Susceptibility testing is a crucial part of antimicrobial therapy because the empiric regimen may fail when used to treat infections with resistant organisms.[2] Microorganisms have genetic variability that affects their susceptibility to antimicrobials. Selective pressure from extensive clinical and agricultural use of antibiotics is thought to play an important role in the emergence of resistant bacteria.[6] Mechanisms of bacterial resistance include the production of enzymes that degrade or modify antibiotics; the alteration of bacterial cell walls or membranes, resulting in decreased permeability; upregulation of antimicrobial efflux pumps; and alteration of the target site of antimicrobial action.[6] Table 14-2 lists important emerging resistant bacteria.

Host Factors

KEY POINT

The outcome of antimicrobial therapy depends on *host factors, susceptibility* or *resistance* to the antimicrobial, and *pharmacodynamics*.

Host factors play a significant role in the selection of optimal antimicrobial therapies. Consideration must be given to such factors as history of allergy or intolerance, age, organ dysfunction, pregnancy and lactation, and site of infection. Other important factors include immune status, travel history, recent exposure (approximately 3 months) to antimicrobials, as well as concomitant drugs and disease states. In addition, drug factors, such as available dosage forms, ease of administration, pharmacokinetic and pharmacodynamic properties, tissue penetration, drug toxicities, and cost, influence the choice of a specific agent.[4-6]

The safety and efficacy of an antimicrobial agent varies, based on the population of patients being treated.[4,6] For example, bone marrow transplant recipients with an active infection may not improve despite use of the ideal antimicrobial agent because of their impaired immune function. Similarly, other immunocompromised hosts, such as patients with acquired immunodeficiency syndrome (AIDS), recipients of cancer chemotherapy or steroids, solid organ transplant recipients, and diabetics, are also at risk of failing to improve on a regimen of antimicrobial therapy.[6] Patients with infections involving foreign bodies or necrotic tissue often require surgical removal of the foreign device or necrotic tissue despite appropriate antimicrobial therapy. Other factors such as the altered pharmacokinetics of an antimicrobial can affect response to therapy. For example, the absorption of certain antimicrobials, such as itraconazole (an antifungal agent), is increased in the presence of gastric acid; others, such as

TABLE 14-1	Common Pathogens and Treatment of Respiratory Infections in Adults*	

RESPIRATORY INFECTION	COMMON PATHOGENS	POTENTIAL ANTIBIOTIC REGIMENS
Rhinosinusitis[11,12]		
Acute (community acquired)	*Streptococcus pneumoniae, Haemophilus influenzae, Moraxella catarrhalis,* viruses (rhinovirus, adenovirus, coronavirus)	Amoxicillin-clavulanate is drug of choice; doxycycline or a respiratory fluoroquinolone (levofloxacin or moxifloxacin) for penicillin-allergic patients
Acute (hospital acquired)	*Pseudomonas aeruginosa, Staphylococcus aureus,* Enterobacteriaceae	Antipseudomonal β-lactam (ceftazidime, cefepime, or aztreonam) or an antipseudomonal carbapenem (imipenem, meropenem, or doripenem) and vancomycin
Chronic	Predominantly anaerobes (*Prevotella* spp., *Porphromonas* spp., *Peptostreptococcus* spp., *Fusobacterium* spp.), *S. aureus, P. aeruginosa*	Antibiotics are usually not indicated; amoxicillin-clavulanate and azithromycin often used
Bronchitis[13-14]		
Acute	Predominantly respiratory viruses (influenza A and B, parainfluenza, RSV), *Mycoplasma pneumoniae, Chlamydrophila pneumoniae, Bordetella pertussis*	Antibiotics are usually not indicated; however, doxycycline or azithromycin may be considered
Exacerbation of chronic bronchitis	*S. pneumoniae, H. influenzae, M. catarrhalis*	Value of antibiotics is controversial; doxycycline or azithromycin may be considered
Pneumonia[7-10,15-19]		
Outpatient	*S. pneumoniae, M. pneumonia, H. influenzae, C. pneumonia,* and respiratory viruses	Azithromycin, doxycycline, respiratory fluoroquinolone, or β-lactam (amoxicillin-clavulante, cefuroxime) plus, azithromycin
Inpatient (non-ICU)	As indicated for Outpatient, plus *Legionella pneumophilia*	Respiratory fluoroquinolone or β-lactam (cefotaxime, ceftriaxone, ampicillin-sulbactam) plus azithromycin
Inpatient (ICU)	*S. pneumoniae, S. aureus, L. pneumophilia, H. influenzae,* Enterobacteriaceae	β-Lactam (cefotaxime, ceftriaxone, ampicillin-sulbactam) plus azithromycin or respiratory fluoroquinolone
	If risk for *P. aeruginosa*	Antipneumococcal, antipseudomonal β-lactam (piperacillin-tazobactam, cefepime, ceftazidime, or antipseudomonal carbapenem) plus ciprofloxacin, levofloxacin, or aminoglycoside
	If risk for *S. aureus*	Add vancomycin or linezolid
Hospital acquired and health-care associated (nonneutropenic patient)	*S. pneumoniae, S. aureus* including MRSA, *P. aeruginosa,* Enterobacteriaceae	Cefepime, ceftazidime, piperacillin-tazobactam, aztreonam, or antipseudomonal carbapenem ± aminoglycoside, ciprofloxacin, or levofloxacin ± vancomycin or linezolid
Hospital acquired (neutropenic patient)	As listed for nonneutropenic patients, and fungi such as *Candida* spp., *Aspergillus* spp., and if HIV positive, *Pneumocystis jiroveci* (formerly *P. carinii* [PCP])	As listed for nonneutropenic ± amphotericin B (commonly lipid formulations), azoles (fluconazole or voriconazole), or echinocandins (caspofungin, micafungin, anidulafungin) ± TMP-SMX
Aspiration suspected	Anaerobes (*Bacteroides* spp., *Fusobacterium* spp., *Peptostreptococcus* spp.) and aerobes (*S. aureus, S. pneumoniae, H. influenzae,* Enterobacteriaceae)	β-Lactam/ β-lactamase inhibitor (Amoxicillin-clavulanate, ampicillin-sulbactam, piperacillin-tazobactam), or clindamycin, carbapenem, or moxifloxacin.
Patient with cystic fibrosis	*P. aeruginosa, S. aureus, Burkholderia cepacia* complex, *Achromobacter xylosoxidans, Stenotrophomonas maltophilia*	Aminoglycoside or ciprofloxacin plus piperacillin-tazobactam or ceftazidime, cefepime or antipseudomonal carbopenem ± TMP-SMX (*B. cepacia* complex, *S. maltophilia*) ± vancomycin
Empyema[5,20]	*Streptococcus milleri* group, *Bacteroides fragilis* group, *Prevotella* spp., *Fusobacterium* spp., *Peptostreptococcus* spp., *S. pneumoniae, S. aureus,* Enterobacteriaceae	β-Lactam/ β-Lactamase inhibitor, carbapenem, or third-generation cephalosporin (ceftriaxone) plus clindamycin or metronidazole ± vancomycin

HIV, Human immunodeficiency virus; *TMP-SMX*, trimethoprim-sulfamethoxazole; *MRSA*, methicillin-resistant *S. aureus*; *RSV*, respiratory syncytial virus.
*The potential treatments listed here are not listed in order of superiority. Choice of antimicrobials depends on the individual susceptibility pattern of the suspected organisms within the specific institution or community and host factors.
See Table 14-7 for antimycobacterial regimens.

benzylpenicillin (penicillin G), are degraded in the presence of acid. The pH of the stomach varies with age; older patients tend to have achlorhydria, and young children tend to have a higher gastric pH. As a result, these two populations may have enhanced absorption of penicillin and decreased absorption of itraconazole relative to the rest of the population.

The function of the liver and the kidney also changes with age. These two organs play a major role in the metabolism and elimination of drugs from the body. Premature and newborn infants have diminished renal function at birth. Drugs such as β-lactams and aminoglycosides that are eliminated unchanged in the urine require less frequent application because of their reduced clearance. Similarly, renal function declines with age, necessitating dosage reductions in elderly patients to prevent potential toxicities from antimicrobial accumulation.[4-6]

Prevention of toxicity to the fetus or infant while treating a pregnant or nursing mother is also a crucial consideration.[4,6] Generally, most β-lactams and macrolides are believed to be safe in pregnancy. The teratogenic potential of most other antimicrobials is unknown. However, the tetracyclines have been shown to affect fetal dentition and to affect pregnant women adversely.[4] Antimicrobials are often eliminated in breast milk and so have the potential to affect nursing infants adversely. For example, premature infants are often jaundiced at birth because they are unable to conjugate and eliminate bilirubin efficiently. Even a

---

BOX 14-1   Examples of Bactericidal/Fungicidal and Bacteriostatic/Fungistatic Antimicrobials

"Cidal"	"Static"
• Aminoglycosides	• Azoles
• Carbapenems	• Chloramphenicol
• Cephalosporins	• Clindamycin
• Colistin	• Linezolid*
• Daptomycin	• Macrolides, azalides, ketolides
• Isoniazid	• Nitrofurantoin
• Metronidazole	• Quinupristin/dalfopristin*
• Penicillins	• Tetracyclines
• Polyenes	• Tigecycline
• Fluoroquinolones	• Trimethoprim-sulfamethoxazole
• Rifampin, rifabutin	
• Vancomycin*	

*Agents that are bactericidal against *Staphylococcus aureus* but bacteriostatic against *Enterococcus* species.

TABLE 14-2   Emerging Resistant Bacterial Pathogens

CLASS OF BACTERIA	NAME
Gram positive	MRSA
	VISA
	VRSA
	Penicillin-resistant *Streptococcus pneumoniae*
	VRE
Gram negative	MDR nonenteric bacilli (*Pseudomonas aeruginosa, Stenotrophomonas maltophilia, Acinetobacter* spp.)
	Third-generation cephalosporin-resistant *Enterobacter* and *Citrobacter* spp.
	ESBL-producing *Escherichia coli* and *Klebsiella* spp.
	Ampicillin-resistant *Haemophilus* spp.
	Carbapenemase-producing Enterobacteriaceae and *Acinetobacter* spp.

ESBL, Extended-spectrum β-lactamase; *MDR,* multidrug-resistant; *MRSA,* methicillin-resistant *Staphylococcus aureus; VISA,* vancomycin-intermediate *S. aureus; VRE,* vancomycin-resistant *Enterococcus; VRSA,* vancomycin-resistant *S. aureus.*

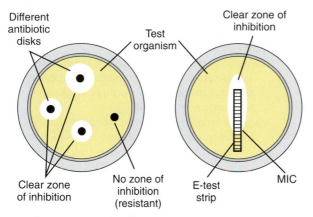

Figure 14-1 Disk diffusion test and E-test methods.

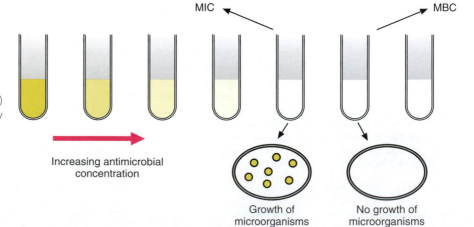

Figure 14-2 Minimal inhibitory concentration (MIC) and minimal bactericidal concentration (MBC) by broth macrodilution.

small dose of sulfonamides ingested through breast milk from a treated mother can displace the albumin-bound bilirubin and predispose the infant to kernicterus. Kernicterus is marked by a pattern of cerebral palsy with uncoordinated movements, deafness, disturbed vision, and speech difficulties resulting from deposition of bilirubin in the developing brain.

Antimicrobials concentrate in varying degrees within organ systems and can influence the outcome of therapy.[4,6] Clindamycin achieves excellent bone concentrations and is very useful for treatment of osteomyelitis resulting from susceptible organisms. Similarly, drugs such as the aminoglycosides, most fluoroquinolones, and penicillins achieve very high concentrations in the urine and are useful for the treatment of urinary tract infections (UTIs). Conversely, certain drugs, although active against the organism in vitro, cannot achieve adequate concentrations at the site of infection. For example, aminoglycosides cannot penetrate the blood-brain barrier to treat meningitis adequately in adults. The blood-brain barrier represents tight junctions between the epithelial cells of the capillary wall that prevent drugs from entering the central nervous system.[6]

Some antimicrobials are not clinically effective at certain infection sites. Daptomycin, which has excellent in vitro activity against methicillin-resistant *Staphylococcus aureus* (MRSA), is not effective for treatment of pneumonia because it is inactivated by lung surfactant.[4] Aminoglycosides are less effective in low-oxygen, low-pH environments such as abscesses. Drainage remains the most effective treatment for abscesses.[4]

Pharmacodynamics

Pharmacodynamics refers to the science of understanding the optimal effect of a drug as a function of its concentration and the in vitro activity (MIC) against an organism. The pharmacodynamic properties of an antimicrobial are measured in vitro by using time-kill studies. Time-kill tests are not performed in most microbiology laboratories, but instead in research facilities studying the optimal dosages of antimicrobial agents. These studies measure the rate and extent of microorganism killing over time when exposed to varying concentrations of antimicrobials.[3] If the microbial kill rate increases proportionally with drug concentration, the antimicrobial is said to have a *concentration-dependent* effect. If the microbial kill rate is influenced by the time of drug concentration above the MIC, the antimicrobial is defined as *time-dependent* (or *concentration-independent*).[5,6] Another pharmacodynamic phenomenon exhibited by antimicrobials is known as the *postantibiotic effect (PAE)*. The PAE refers to the sustained suppression of bacterial growth even after the concentration of the antibiotic declines below detectable levels. The length of the PAE varies by the type of organism and the drug. Generally, time-dependent drugs, such as β-lactams and vancomycin, have short PAEs, whereas concentration-dependent drugs, such as aminoglycosides, metronidazole, and fluoroquinolones, have longer PAEs. Agents with a short PAE should be

given frequently, and longer intervals should be used for antimicrobials having a long PAE. These pharmacodynamic properties have been shown in vitro and in numerous animal studies.[6] Clinical trials validating these principles are ongoing, and practical guidelines to incorporate pharmacodynamics in clinical practice have been published, resulting in increased use of extended infusions for piperacillin-tazobactam and carbapenems.

Antimicrobial Combinations

Empiric regimens must often cover a broad spectrum of organisms, which occasionally requires the use of two or more classes of antimicrobials. Ideally, the regimen should be narrowed after the specific organism has been isolated and susceptibilities are determined. Certain infections are polymicrobial, and in certain settings the use of antimicrobial combinations is justified. When antimicrobials are used in combination, it is important to know whether these agents act synergistically or are antagonistic.[5,6] **Synergy** is shown in vitro when the combined effect of two antimicrobials is greater than their added effects. Synergistic combinations have played a vital role in the treatment of resistant *Pseudomonas* infections in patients with cystic fibrosis (CF). These patients have recurrent bouts of pseudomonal pneumonia and are often colonized with resistant species. Certain synergistic combinations of β-lactams and aminoglycosides have been shown to curb the development of resistance and to improve outcomes.[5,6] **Antagonism** occurs when the effect of the combined drugs is lower than the sum of their independent activities when measured separately.[4] Antagonism may result in an unfavorable response, and such drug combinations should be avoided. A classic example of antagonism was the use of tetracycline (static) and penicillin (cidal) in children with pneumococcal meningitis. The mortality associated with the use of combination therapy was three times higher than the use of penicillin alone. However, not all combinations of static and cidal antimicrobials are detrimental. Ceftriaxone (cidal) plus a static agent such as a macrolide, azalide, or tetracycline are considered drugs of choice for CAP.[7]

Monitoring Response to Therapy

KEY POINT

Treatment failure may manifest as continued fever spikes, elevated white blood cell count (WBC), repeated positive cultures, and nonresolution of symptoms.

Certain laboratory parameters can be monitored to assess the efficacy of an antimicrobial regimen, but ultimately the clinical assessment of the patient is the best measure of response to therapy. Treatment failure may manifest as continued fever spikes, elevated white blood cell count (WBC), repeated positive cultures, or nonresolution of symptoms (shortness of breath, cough, sputum production).[6] The reasons for failure can be multifactorial and require consideration of all the aforementioned factors. In addition, noncompliance with the treatment regimen can play a significant role in outpatient treatment failures.

The use of antimicrobials can be associated with significant toxicities. The agent amphotericin B, which is used to treat fungal infections such as pulmonary aspergillosis, can cause significant renal dysfunction. Aminoglycosides can also cause renal dysfunction. Serum concentrations of aminoglycosides are routinely monitored to ensure therapeutic, but nontoxic levels.[6] Similarly, other agents can have adverse effects on the liver, gastrointestinal tract, neuromuscular system, hematologic system, heart, and lungs. The incidence of these adverse events varies among agents and is often reversible. Careful monitoring of patients receiving antimicrobials can prevent serious and potentially life-threatening adverse events.

ANTIBIOTICS

Numerous **antibiotics**, substances derived or produced from a microorganism that inhibit or kill other microorganisms, are available to treat infectious diseases. A synopsis of the mechanism of action, clinical uses, and adverse reactions of each class is described in the following sections.

Penicillins

KEY POINT

The β-lactams are a large class of antibiotics that includes penicillins, cephalosporins, carbapenems, and monobactams (aztreonam).

The discovery of penicillin in 1928 by Fleming ultimately led to the creation of a broad class of antibiotics commonly referred to as β-lactams. β-Lactam antibiotics include the penicillins, cephalosporins, monobactams, and carbapenems.[21,22] The main constituent of these antibiotics is the β-lactam ring structure. Chemical manipulation of β-lactam side chains led to the development of new agents with enhanced spectra of antimicrobial activity compared with penicillin. Specific side-chain modifications of penicillin have resulted in a broad class that includes the natural penicillins, aminopenicillins, penicillinase-resistant penicillins, carboxypenicillins, and ureidopenicillins (Table 14-3). Penicillins have also been combined with β-lactamase inhibitors to overcome a common mechanism of bacterial resistance.

TABLE 14-3   Classification and Clinical Uses of Penicillins[21-23]

β-LACTAM CLASS (GENERIC NAME)	BRAND NAME	ROUTE	COMMON USES (MICROORGANISM)
Natural Penicillins			
Penicillin G (potassium)	Pfizerpen	IM, IV	*Streptococcus pyogenes, Neisseria meningitidis, Bacillus*
Penicillin G (procaine)	Wycillin	IM	*anthracis* (anthrax), *Clostridium perfringens* (gangrene),
Penicillin G (benzathine)	Bicillin L-A	IM	*Pasteurella multocida, Treponema pallidum* (syphilis)
Penicillin V (potassium)	Pen-Vee K	PO	
Penicillinase-Resistant Penicillins			
Oxacillin	Prostaphlin	PO, IM, IV	MSSA, MSSE
Nafcillin	Unipen	IV	
Dicloxacillin	Dynapen	PO	
Aminopenicillins			
Ampicillin	Omnipen	PO, IM, IV	*Listeria monocytogenes, Proteus mirabilis, Eikenella corrodens, Borrelia burgdorferi, Haemophilus influenzae, Escherichia coli*
Amoxicillin	Amoxil, Wymox	PO	
Carboxypenicillins			
Ticarcillin	Ticar	IV, IM	
Ureidopenicillins			
Piperacillin	Pipracil	IM, IV	*Pseudomonas aeruginosa*, Enterobacteriaceae, *Stenotrophomonas* spp.
Penicillin plus β-Lactamase Inhibitors			
Amoxicillin–clavulanic acid	Augmentin, Unasyn	PO, IM, IV	Increased activity against β-lactamase–producing strains
Ampicillin-sulbactam			*S. aureus, H. influenzae, Moraxella catarrhalis, Proteus* spp., *Bacteroides* spp.
Ticarcillin–clavulanic acid	Timentin	IV	*P. aeruginosa*, Enterobacteriaceae
Piperacillin-tazobactam	Zosyn	IV	

IM, Intramuscular; *IV,* intravenous; *MSSA,* methicillin-sensitive *Staphylococcus aureus; MSSE,* methicillin-sensitive *Staphylococcus epidermidis; MRSA,* methicillin-resistant *Staphylococcus aureus; PO,* oral.

The penicillins generally are widely distributed throughout the body and are associated with relatively low levels of toxicity. Most penicillins are acid-labile (destroyed in the stomach) and therefore are poorly absorbed after oral administration. Most agents in this class are not metabolized but are excreted unchanged in the urine. Therefore most penicillins require reductions in dosage for patients with renal dysfunction.[21,22]

Mode of Action

Penicillins exert their pharmacologic activity by inhibiting cell wall synthesis. Penicillins bind to enzymes (penicillin-binding proteins) located within the cell wall and prevent cross-linking of the peptidoglycan structure necessary for cell wall development. In addition, penicillins activate an endogenous autolytic system within bacteria, which subsequently leads to cell lysis and death. Penicillins are bactericidal, exhibit time-dependent killing, and can act synergistically with aminoglycosides against some bacteria (i.e., *P. aeruginosa* and enterococci).[21,22]

Clinical Uses

Natural penicillins. Penicillin G is the parent compound of this class. Natural penicillins are effective primarily against gram-positive bacteria and anaerobes. Penicillin G is the drug of choice for the treatment of primary and secondary syphilis (*Treponema pallidum*) and pharyngitis caused by group A streptococci (*Streptococcus pyogenes*). Because of the increasing frequency of resistance in *S. aureus, S. pneumoniae,* and *Neisseria gonorrhoeae,* penicillin G should no longer be considered for infections caused by these organisms.[21,22]

Penicillinase-resistant penicillins. In an attempt to overcome the emergence of penicillinase-producing (β-lactamase–producing) staphylococci, semisynthetic penicillinase-resistant antibiotics were developed. These agents are commonly referred to as *antistaphylococcal* agents because of their excellent activity against *S. aureus.* Methicillin was the first agent in this class of antibiotics, followed by oxacillin, nafcillin, cloxacillin, and dicloxacillin. Chemical modification of penicillin by the addition of an acyl side chain prevents hydrolysis of the agents in the presence of penicillinase. This class has activity against gram-positive cocci (staphylococci and streptococci) and is routinely used in skin and soft tissue infections. These agents are ineffective in the treatment of infections caused by gram-negative organisms or anaerobes. Until the 1980s, these antibiotics were the mainstay of treatment against staphylococci. However, the emergence of methicillin-resistant staphylococci has greatly reduced the clinical effectiveness of these agents.[21,22]

Aminopenicillins. Aminopenicillins were the first penicillin class developed that were considered clinically active against some gram-negative bacteria (*E. coli, H. influenzae*). Ampicillin and amoxicillin are the primary antibiotics in this class. In contrast to penicillin, ampicillin and amoxicillin are stable in gastric acid and therefore are suitable for oral administration. Both ampicillin and amoxicillin are frequently used in infections with susceptible organisms of the respiratory (*S. pneumoniae, H. influenzae*) and urinary (*E. coli*) tracts.[21,22]

Carboxypenicillins. With the emergence of more resistant gram-negative bacilli, penicillins with increased gram-negative activity were needed. Carbenicillin was the first penicillin to have activity against *P. aeruginosa.* It was also active against most members of the family Enterobacteriaceae, including *E. coli, Enterobacter, Proteus, Morganella,* and *Serratia.* Subsequent modification of carbenicillin resulted in ticarcillin, which has even greater in vitro activity against *P. aeruginosa* and members of Enterobacteriaceae (including *Klebsiella*). Neither of these agents is considered to have appreciable activity against gram-positive organisms (staphylococci or streptococci). These agents are administered primarily in the intravenous form because high serum concentrations cannot be achieved with the oral formulations.[21,22]

Ureidopenicillins. Although carbenicillin and ticarcillin provided increased gram-negative coverage, antimicrobial agents with enhanced antipseudomonal activity were still needed. The ureidopenicillins were developed to fill this need. Piperacillin is a penicillin antibiotic with enhanced gram-negative activity (especially against *P. aeruginosa*) and with fewer adverse reactions than carboxypenicillins. Ureidopenicillins also exhibit activity against streptococci and enterococci and many anaerobes. Piperacillin is the primary agent of this class and has been efficacious in the treatment of pneumonia, bacteremia, UTIs, osteomyelitis, and soft tissue infections.[21,22]

β-Lactam and β-lactamase inhibitor combinations. Certain bacteria have the ability to produce enzymes (β-lactamases) that destroy the activity of penicillins by disrupting the β-lactam structure. β-Lactamase inhibitors were developed to overcome this form of resistance. Combination β-lactams and β-lactamase inhibitors have a large spectrum of activity, making them particularly useful in polymicrobial infections. At present, three β-lactamase inhibitors are approved for combination with penicillins: clavulanic acid, sulbactam, and tazobactam. β-Lactamase inhibitors enhance the activity of β-lactams against β-lactamase–producing strains of *S. aureus, Moraxella catarrhalis, E. coli, H. influenzae, Klebsiella* species, and *Bacteroides* species.[23]

Adverse Reactions and Precautions

The most common adverse reaction to penicillins is hypersensitivity. Approximately 3% to 10% of the population are allergic to penicillin. Reactions vary in severity from a mild rash to life-threatening anaphylaxis. Patients allergic to a penicillin could be potentially allergic to all classes of β-lactams (cephalosporins, carbapenems). In addition to allergic reactions, hematologic reactions such as thrombocytopenia and increased bleeding times have been reported. Gastrointestinal disturbances (nausea, vomiting, and diarrhea) are more common with oral dosage forms of penicillins, especially ampicillin. Interstitial nephritis has occurred most commonly with methicillin (not commercially available) but may occur with other penicillins as well. Central nervous system toxicities (e.g., seizures) have been reported with penicillins. Patients with an underlying seizure disorder and patients with renal insufficiency are at greatest risk for developing this complication.

Cephalosporins

 KEY POINT

Cephalosporins have been loosely grouped into "generations" based on their spectrum of activities. At present there are five generations (classes) of cephalosporins.

The cephalosporins include a large group of antimicrobials that are structurally related to the penicillins. Discovered in the 1940s as a microbial byproduct of the fungus *Cephalosporium acremonium*, this class is now widely used in clinical practice. Similar to the penicillins, this class exhibits bactericidal activity, is distributed throughout the body, and produces relatively few adverse effects. Cephalosporins are used for various clinical indications and are available in oral and intravenous formulations[24] (Table 14-4). Agents

from this class have been loosely grouped into "generations" based on their spectrum of activities. At present there are five generations (classes) of cephalosporins.

Mechanism of Action

Cephalosporins inhibit bacterial cell wall synthesis in a manner similar to penicillins. Cephalosporins bind to the penicillin-binding proteins within the cell wall and inhibit the cross-linking of peptidoglycan. This inhibition compromises the structural integrity of the bacterial cell wall, resulting in cell lysis (bactericidal).

Clinical Uses

As a class, cephalosporins are active against a wide variety of organisms. Because of their broad spectrum of activity and low level of toxicity, these agents are commonly used for a wide variety of infections. The spectrum of activity differs for each cephalosporin generation. All cephalosporins are ineffective against enterococci.[24]

First-generation cephalosporins. The first-generation cephalosporin agents are very active against a wide variety of gram-positive organisms, including methicillin-sensitive *S. aureus* (MSSA) and streptococci. They have moderate

TABLE 14-4   Classification and Clinical Uses of Cephalosporins[24-28]

CEPHALOSPORIN (GENERIC NAME)	BRAND NAME	ROUTE	COMMON USES (MICROORGANISM)
First Generation			
Cefadroxil	Duricef	PO	MSSA, streptococci
Cephalexin	Keflex, Biocef	PO	
Cefazolin	Ancef, Kefzol	IM, IV	
Second Generation			
Cefaclor	Ceclor	PO	MSSA, MSSE, *Streptococcus pneumoniae*, *Klebsiella* spp.,
Cefprozil	Cefzil	PO	*Escherichia coli*, *Proteus* spp., *Haemophilus influenzae*
Cefuroxime axetil	Ceftin	PO	
Cefuroxime	Zinacef, Kefurox	IM, IV	
Cefotetan	Cefotan	IM, IV	As above plus *Bacteroides fragilis*
Cefoxitin	Mefoxin	IM, IV	
Third Generation			
Cefixime	Suprax,	PO	Better activity than second-generation cephalosporins against
Cefpodoxime proxetil	Vantin	PO	*Klebsiella, E. coli, Proteus* spp., *H. influenzae, Enterobacter* spp.
Ceftibuten	Cedax	PO	
Cefdinir	Omnicef	PO	
Cefotaxime	Claforan	IM, IV	
Ceftriaxone	Rocephin	IM, IV	
Ceftizoxime	Cefizox	IM, IV	
Ceftazidime	Fortaz, Tazidime	IM, IV	As above plus *Pseudomonas aeruginosa*
Cefoperazone	Cefobid	IM, IV	
Fourth Generation			
Cefepime	Maxipime	IM, IV	MSSA, *S. pneumoniae, Klebsiella, E. coli, Proteus* spp., *H. influenzae,* *P. aeruginosa, Enterobacter* spp.
Fifth Generation			
Ceftaroline	Teflaro	IM, IV	MRSA, *S. pneumoniae, Klebsiella, E. coli, Proteus* spp., *H. influenzae,* *Enterobacter* spp.

IM, Intramuscular; *IV,* intravenous; *MSSA,* methicillin-sensitive *Staphylococcus aureus; MSSE,* methicillin-sensitive *Staphylococcus epidermidis; MRSA,* methicillin-resistant *Staphylococcus aureus; PO,* oral.

activity against community-acquired, gram-negative organisms such as *E. coli, Klebsiella pneumoniae, H. influenzae, M. catarrhalis,* and some *Proteus* species. They are also considered effective against many oral anaerobes (e.g., *Peptostreptococcus*). Commonly used agents within this class are cephalexin, cefazolin, and cefadroxil. These agents are not active against *Bacteroides fragilis, P. aeruginosa,* and most members of Enterobacteriaceae. Generally, first-generation cephalosporins are appropriate for treatment of infections of skin and soft tissue, uncomplicated community-acquired UTIs, streptococcal pharyngitis, and surgical prophylaxis.[24]

Second-generation cephalosporins. Second-generation cephalosporins comprise two groups: true cephalosporins and synthetic cephamycins. Cefuroxime and cefaclor are among the more widely used true cephalosporins. In contrast to first-generation cephalosporins, these agents display enhanced gram-negative activity and maintain comparable gram-positive activity. This group provides improved activity against *H. influenzae, M. catarrhalis, Neisseria meningitidis, N. gonorrhoeae,* and some members of Enterobacteriaceae. These agents are considered effective in treating CAP, otitis media, pharyngitis, skin and soft tissue infections, and uncomplicated UTIs.[24]

Cephamycins, consisting of cefotetan and cefoxitin, have enhanced activity against gram-negative members of Enterobacteriaceae and anaerobic activity against many *Bacteroides* species. They are not considered effective against gram-positive organisms such as staphylococci and streptococci. Cephamycins are also useful in the treatment of intraabdominal, pelvic, and gynecologic infections; decubitus ulcers; diabetic foot syndrome; and mixed aerobic-anaerobic soft tissue infections.[24]

Third-generation cephalosporins. Commonly used third-generation cephalosporins are cefixime, cefpodoxime, ceftibuten, cefoperazone, cefotaxime, ceftazidime, ceftriaxone, and ceftizoxime. These agents are active against most gram-negative organisms. However, only ceftazidime and to a lesser extent cefoperazone have activity against *P. aeruginosa.* Third-generation cephalosporins show excellent activity against *S. pneumoniae, S. pyogenes, H. influenzae, N. meningitidis, N. gonorrhoeae,* and *M. catarrhalis.* Although activity varies with individual agents, this group is not considered to have significant activity against anaerobes. Ceftriaxone, cefotaxime, and to a lesser extent ceftizoxime achieve clinically significant concentrations within the meninges, making them ideal agents for the treatment of meningitis. In addition, ceftriaxone has replaced penicillin as the agent of choice in treating all forms of gonococcal (*N. gonorrhoeae*) infection because of the increased prevalence of β-lactamase–producing strains. Third-generation cephalosporins are commonly used to treat nosocomial pneumonia, bacteremia, UTIs, osteomyelitis, and soft tissue infections.[24]

Fourth-generation cephalosporins. Fourth-generation cephalosporins have extended gram-positive and gram-negative coverage. Cefepime is presently the only agent available in the United States. It is parentally administered and active against most gram-negative aerobic organisms, including *P. aeruginosa.* In addition, it has excellent activity against MSSA, *Neisseria* species, *H. influenzae, S. pneumoniae,* and *S. pyogenes.* Cefepime has been used primarily for the treatment of patients with uncomplicated and complicated UTIs, patients with skin and soft tissue infections, and for empiric treatment of patients with neutropenic fever, nosocomial pneumonia, and other serious bacterial infections.[24,25]

Fifth-generation cephalosporins. Ceftaroline is the first and only member of the latest class of cephalosporins. Similar to the fourth-generation cephalosporins, it has broad gram-negative and gram-positive activity. Unlike cefepime, ceftaroline has activity against MRSA, but is inactive against *P. aeruginosa.* It is approved for use in CAP, as well as skin and skin structure infections. It appears to have a role in treating various types of polymicrobial infections, especially those with MRSA.[25,26]

Adverse Reactions and Precautions

Similar to penicillins, the cephalosporins as a group are well tolerated. Hypersensitivity reactions occur in 1% to 3% of patients, with cross-reactivity of cephalosporins in patients with penicillin allergy ranging from 5% to 15%. Generally, patients with a penicillin allergy (limited to a rash) may be challenged with a cephalosporin. Cephalosporin use is contraindicated, however, in patients with a history of anaphylaxis to β-lactams. Desensitization should be performed if no therapeutic alternative exists for the use of a cephalosporin.[27] Oral cephalosporins have been associated with minor gastrointestinal complaints such as nausea, vomiting, and diarrhea. Hypoprothrombinemia has been reported, especially with agents (cefotetan and cefoperazone) with a methylthiotetrazole (MTT) side chain. The MTT side chain may also induce a disulfiram-like reaction in patients who concurrently ingest alcohol (disulfiram inhibits the metabolism of alcohol). The symptoms of this uncomfortable reaction include flushing, nausea, thirst, palpitations, chest pain, vertigo, and death in some cases. Most cephalosporins are eliminated through the kidneys and require dosage adjustment in the presence of renal insufficiency.[28]

Carbapenems

The *carbapenems* are the newest class of β-lactam antibiotics. At present four carbapenems—imipenem-cilastatin, meropenem, doripenem, and ertapenem—are available for use in the United States. Cilastatin is used to inhibit the metabolism of imipenem within the kidney to prolong the half-life of this agent. Carbapenems are broad-spectrum antibiotics, displaying activity against a wide variety of gram-positive, gram-negative, and anaerobic bacteria.[29,30]

Mechanism of Action

The mechanism of action of carbapenems is similar to other β-lactam antibiotics. These agents demonstrate bactericidal activity.

Clinical Uses

Imipenem, meropenem, and doripenem all are active against *P. aeruginosa*, multidrug-resistant (MDR) gram-negative bacilli, and most anaerobes. Ertapenem differs from other carbapenems in that it possesses no activity against *P. aeruginosa*. All four carbapenems have activity against gram-positive organisms such as MSSA and the *Streptococcus* species, including pneumococci *(S. pneumoniae)*. Imipenem, meropenem, and doripenem have been used clinically for empiric treatment of bacteremia and sepsis, CAP and nosocomial pneumonia, skin and skin structure infections, complicated UTIs, intraabdominal infections, obstetric and gynecologic infections, osteomyelitis, and infections in patients with cancer and neutropenia. Because ertapenem is ineffective against *P. aeruginosa*, it should not be used in the treatment of nosocomial pneumonia, neutropenic fever, or any other infection in which *P. aeruginosa* is a likely pathogen. Because of their excellent in vitro activity and broad spectrum of coverage, these agents are often reserved to treat infections that are caused by bacteria resistant to most other agents.[29,30]

Adverse Reactions and Precautions

Carbapenems are generally well tolerated, with a low incidence of adverse reactions. Because carbapenems are structurally related to other β-lactam antibiotics, cross-reactivity may occur when they are used in patients with allergies to β-lactams. The occurrence of seizures has been reported with carbapenems, more frequently with imipenem than with meropenem, doripenem, or ertapenem. Seizures are most commonly seen in patients with decreased renal function and patients with an underlying seizure disorder. Dosage adjustment is necessary in the presence of renal insufficiency to prevent accumulation of the drug and to reduce the potential for seizures.[29,30]

Monobactams (Aztreonam)

Aztreonam is a synthetic monocyclic β-lactam antibiotic. It is the only commercially available agent belonging to the class of antibiotics known as the *monobactams*.[30]

Mechanism of Action

The mechanism of action of aztreonam is similar to other β-lactam antibiotics, and it also exhibits bactericidal activity.

Clinical Uses

Aztreonam is active only against gram-negative aerobic bacilli (most Enterobacteriaceae and *P. aeruginosa*). It is ineffective against gram-positive and anaerobic bacteria. The strict gram-negative spectrum of aztreonam limits its use as a single agent. It has been used for the treatment of serious UTIs and bacteremia. Aztreonam has more extensive use in combination therapy for treatment of patients with intraabdominal infections, spontaneous bacterial peritonitis, gram-negative osteomyelitis, HAP, and neutropenic fever.[30]

Adverse Reactions and Precautions

Aztreonam is well tolerated and is thought to have little to no cross-reactivity to β-lactams. Rare cases of rashes and anaphylactic reactions have been reported when aztreonam was used in patients with a β-lactam allergy.[30]

Aminoglycosides

Streptomycin was discovered in 1943 and was the first antimicrobial agent available to treat tuberculosis. Numerous other *aminoglycosides* have been developed since and include gentamicin, tobramycin, netilmicin, and amikacin. These agents are used for gram-negative infections, including infections caused by *P. aeruginosa*. These antimicrobials have poor gastrointestinal absorption and require parenteral administration.[31]

Table 14-5 lists aminoglycosides and their clinical uses.

Mechanism of Action

Aminoglycosides bind irreversibly to the 30S bacterial ribosome and inhibit the translation of ribonucleic acid (RNA) into proteins. Aminoglycosides also competitively displace cations that link lipopolysaccharides in the outer cell wall of gram-negative bacteria. This destabilization of the cell

TABLE 14-5	Clinical Uses of Aminoglycosides*[31-34]	
GENERIC NAME (TRADE NAME)	**BRAND NAME**	**MOST COMMON CLINICAL USES**
Streptomycin		Brucellosis, tuberculosis, endocarditis caused by gentamicin-resistant enterococci
Gentamicin	Garamycin	Nosocomial Enterobacteriaceae and *Pseudomonas aeruginosa* infections, tularemia, brucellosis; endocarditis caused by susceptible enterococci or viridans streptococci, *Staphylococcus aureus*, *Corynebacterium* spp., penicillin-susceptible *Streptococcus*
Tobramycin	Nebcin	
Amikacin	Amikin	Similar to gentamicin and tobramycin but useful against *Acinetobacter* spp., *Nocardia* spp., *Mycobacterium avium-intracellulare*, *Mycobacterium chelonae*, *Mycobacterium fortuitum*

*The aminoglycosides (most commonly gentamicin and tobramycin) are used to treat infections caused by gram-negative bacteria.

wall results in increased cell permeability and lysis. Aminoglycosides are bactericidal agents and exhibit concentration-dependent killing. They are often synergistic when used in combination with β-lactam antibiotics.[31-34]

Clinical Uses

Gentamicin, tobramycin, and amikacin all have been used for nosocomial gram-negative infections, such as VAPs. However, aminoglycosides do not achieve high concentrations in bronchial secretions when administered systemically; this is thought to be particularly problematic for patients infected with resistant gram-negative organisms. As a result, aminoglycosides (particularly tobramycin and now amikacin) have been administered by inhalation to control *P. aeruginosa* infections in patients with CF (see Chapter 13). Amikacin is currently more expensive and is generally reserved for organisms resistant to other aminoglycosides. Aminoglycosides are used synergistically with β-lactams when treating endocarditis caused by the *Streptococcus* species and *Enterococcus* species. Aminoglycosides are also used extensively to treat intraabdominal infections. Streptomycin is used in combination with other antitubercular antimicrobials, especially for MDR tuberculosis.[31-34]

Adverse Reactions and Precautions

> **KEY POINT**
>
> Primary toxicities associated with the use of *aminoglycosides* are nephrotoxicity and ototoxicity.

The primary toxicities associated with the use of aminoglycosides are nephrotoxicity and ototoxicity. Nephrotoxicity usually develops after at least 5 to 7 days of therapy and occurs more commonly in patients with hypotension, liver disease, advanced age, and coadministration of other nephrotoxic agents. Ototoxicity (both cochlear toxicity and vestibular toxicity) may be irreversible because significant damage must occur before it can be detected. The most common symptoms associated with the development of cochlear toxicity include tinnitus (ringing in the ears); vestibular toxicity manifests as dizziness and nausea. Another serious but rare toxicity is neuromuscular blockade associated with peritoneal irrigation and rapid high-dose aminoglycoside use. Underlying conditions such as myasthenia gravis or concomitant use of neuromuscular blockers may potentiate this side effect, requiring supportive measures such as intubation and possible ventilation support.[31-34]

Tetracyclines

> **KEY POINT**
>
> *Tetracyclines* are broad-spectrum antibiotics with activity against gram-positive and gram-negative microorganisms and many rickettsiae, chlamydiae, mycoplasmas, spirochetes, protozoa, and mycobacteria.

Tetracyclines are broad-spectrum antibiotics with activity against gram-positive and gram-negative microorganisms and many rickettsiae, chlamydiae, mycoplasmas, spirochetes, protozoa, and mycobacteria. The most commonly used agent in this class is doxycycline because it can be administered twice daily and is relatively inexpensive. Other available tetracyclines include minocycline and tetracycline. The agents are available in oral and parenteral formulations.[35]

Mechanism of Action

Tetracyclines bind reversibly on the 30S ribosome and inhibit the attachment of transfer RNA to an acceptor site on the messenger RNA–ribosome complex. This inhibition blocks protein synthesis and results in a bacteriostatic effect.

Clinical Uses

Clinical conditions in which tetracyclines are used include respiratory tract infections and other systemic infections. Acute exacerbation of chronic bronchitis (AECB) and CAP caused by typical (*S. pneumoniae, H. influenzae*) and atypical (*C. pneumoniae, M. pneumoniae, L. pneumophila*) bacteria can be treated with a tetracycline. Tetracyclines are also useful for the treatment of *Chlamydia trachomatis* (sexually transmitted disease), Rocky Mountain spotted fever, Q fever, typhus, brucellosis, Lyme disease, ehrlichiosis, relapsing fever, and cholera. Tetracyclines tend to concentrate in the skin and are useful for the treatment of acne. Tetracyclines have also been used as sclerosing agents for the treatment of malignant and refractory pleural effusions.[35]

Adverse Reactions and Precautions

Gastrointestinal symptoms such as nausea, vomiting, and diarrhea are the most common side effects associated with tetracyclines. Tetracyclines bind to growing bone and can temporarily inhibit their growth. Because of the latter side effect, use of tetracyclines is contraindicated in women during pregnancy and when breastfeeding and in children younger than 8 years of age. Tetracyclines bind to divalent and trivalent cations (calcium, magnesium, aluminum, and iron), which decreases their gastrointestinal absorption when given with antacids, iron supplements, and dairy products. Avoiding the coadministration of tetracyclines with these agents by 1 to 2 hours can prevent this interaction.[35]

Tigecycline

Tigecycline, a glycylcycline antibiotic, is similar in structure to tetracycline antibiotics. Because of substitution of a central four-ring carbocyclic nucleus, tigecycline has a greater spectrum of activity than tetracyclines. Tigecycline is active against most gram-positive bacteria, including *S. pneumoniae*, enterococci (including vancomycin-resistant strains), coagulase-negative staphylococci, MSSA, and MRSA. Tigecycline also has activity against most gram-negative bacteria, including *H. influenzae, M. catarrhalis*, most members of the Enterobacteriaceae family (including extended-spectrum β-lactamase [ESBL]–producing organisms), and *Acinetobacter* species. It is also active against many anaerobic bacteria. However, tigecycline is not active against *P. aeruginosa* and *Proteus* species.[36,37]

Mechanism of Action

Tigecycline displays a similar mechanism to tetracycline antibiotics by inhibiting bacterial protein synthesis at the 30S ribosome. Because of the large, bulky constituent at ring position 9, tigecycline maintains antimicrobial activity against organisms that carry resistance to tetracycline antibiotics. Tigecycline is generally considered to be bacteriostatic against most organisms except *S. pneumoniae*, to which it is bactericidal.[36-37]

Clinical Uses

Tigecycline is currently approved for the treatment of complicated skin and skin structure infections, complicated intraabdominal infections, and bacterial CAP. Of note, the FDA recommends using alternatives to tigecycline in severe infections after decreased cure rates and increased mortality in a study involving VAP patients receiving tigecycline compared with imipenem.[37] Tigecycline is available only as an intravenous formulation.

Adverse Reactions and Precautions

During clinical trials, the most common side effects observed with the use of tigecycline were gastrointestinal and included nausea, vomiting, diarrhea, and abdominal pain. Other frequently reported adverse effects were headache, thrombocytopenia, and elevations of liver enzymes. Because tigecycline is a structural derivative of minocycline, it is appropriate to monitor for side effects associated with other tetracycline antibiotics, such as phototoxicity and dental disorders. Tigecycline should not be used in individuals with hypersensitivity reactions to tetracycline antibiotics.[36,37]

Macrolides, Azalides, and Ketolides

> **KEY POINT**
>
> *Macrolides, azalides, and ketolides* exhibit activity against gram-positive bacteria (streptococci and MSSA), gram-negative bacteria (*H. influenzae* and *M. catarrhalis*), and atypical bacteria (mycoplasmas, rickettsiae, *Legionella*, and *Chlamydia*).

Erythromycin was the first agent of this class to be used for infections with atypical organisms and for infections in patients intolerant to penicillin G. Early work with erythromycin involved production of various salt derivatives to improve its gastrointestinal tolerability and absorption. Clarithromycin, azithromycin (an azalide), and telithromycin (a ketolide) were introduced in subsequent years. These agents exhibit activity against gram-positive bacteria (streptococci, MSSA), gram-negative bacteria (*H. influenzae*, *M. catarrhalis*), and atypical bacteria (mycoplasmas, rickettsiae,

Legionella, and *Chlamydia*). Clarithromycin and azithromycin are also active against *Mycobacterium avium* and other mycobacterial species.[36]

Mechanism of Action

Macrolides, azalides, and ketolides inhibit protein synthesis by reversibly binding to the 50S ribosomal subunit and induce the dissociation of transfer RNA from the ribosome during the elongation phase. As a result, bacterial growth is inhibited (bacteriostatic).

Clinical Uses

These agents are used for the treatment of pneumonia caused by the atypical pathogens *C. pneumoniae*, *M. pneumoniae*, and *L. pneumophila*. Macrolides and azalides are considered a safer alternative to tetracyclines for the treatment of chlamydial (*C. trachomatis*) pelvic infections in pregnant women. Clarithromycin is the preferred agent in combination with ethambutol or rifabutin for the treatment of *M. avium* complex (MAC) in patients with human immunodeficiency virus (HIV) infection. Azithromycin has a superior pharmacokinetic profile compared with the latter agents because it maintains prolonged intracellular concentrations (long half-life). As a result, azithromycin can be administered once weekly for prophylaxis of MAC in patients with HIV, whereas clarithromycin must be administered twice daily. Similarly, 3-day and 5-day regimens of azithromycin have been found to be as effective as a 10-day regimen of erythromycin for the treatment of CAP.[36] Telithromycin was approved for the treatment of AECB, acute bacterial sinusitis, and CAP. It may serve as an alternative agent for patients at risk of infection with penicillin-resistant or macrolide-resistant *S. pneumoniae* and in patients with penicillin allergies. Telithromycin is available only in oral formulation.[36]

Adverse Reactions and Precautions

> **KEY POINT**
>
> Clinically significant drug interactions may occur with *erythromycin, clarithromycin, telithromycin,* and other drugs metabolized by the same hepatic enzymes, resulting in potentially life-threatening complications (i.e., arrhythmias and seizures with high serum concentrations of theophylline; bleeding with warfarin).

Clarithromycin, azithromycin, and telithromycin are generally better tolerated than erythromycin. The most common adverse reactions of these agents include gastrointestinal complaints such as nausea, vomiting, abdominal cramps, and diarrhea. The use of intravenous erythromycin is associated with thrombophlebitis. Ventricular tachycardia and Q–T interval prolongation have been reported with the use of the macrolides, azithromycin, and telithromycin. Erythromycin, clarithromycin, and telithromycin are potent inhibitors of the hepatic drug metabolism system known as the *cytochrome P450 (CYP) system*. As a result, these agents can increase the systemic concentrations of drugs metabolized through the CYP system. For drugs with narrow therapeutic indices, such as theophylline, warfarin, and triazolam, this interaction can lead to potential life-threatening complications.[36]

Fluoroquinolones

The *fluoroquinolones* (Table 14-6) are a semisynthetic group of antimicrobials structurally related to nalidixic acid (quinolone), one of the byproducts of chloroquine synthesis. They are widely distributed into most body fluids and tissues (achieving high respiratory tract concentrations). Fluoroquinolones are eliminated primarily through the kidneys and achieve high concentrations in the urine. Agents from this class have variable activity against gram-negative bacteria, gram-positive bacteria, anaerobes, atypical bacteria, and mycobacteria. Ciprofloxacin, levofloxacin, and moxifloxacin are the most commonly used fluoroquinolones in the United States.[38]

KEY POINT

Fluoroquinolones exert their antibacterial effect through inhibition of DNA synthesis and are considered bactericidal agents, showing concentration-dependent killing.

Mechanism of Action

Fluoroquinolones exert their antibacterial effect through inhibition of DNA synthesis. They inhibit topoisomerase II (DNA gyrase) and topoisomerase IV, which are necessary for bacterial replication. They are considered bactericidal agents and exhibit concentration-dependent killing.

Clinical Uses

Most fluoroquinolones have activity against the common respiratory pathogens, including *S. pneumoniae, H. influenzae, M. catarrhalis, C. pneumoniae, M. pneumoniae,* and *L. pneumophila*. These agents have been shown to be effective in the treatment of upper and lower respiratory tract infections, genitourinary tract infections, and skin and skin structure infections. Fluoroquinolones do not penetrate the cerebrospinal fluid to any significant extent. Ciprofloxacin has been shown to have the best in vitro

activity of the fluoroquinolones against *P. aeruginosa* and other gram-negative aerobes. Ciprofloxacin and levofloxacin have been used for the treatment of nosocomial pneumonia.[38]

Adverse Reactions and Precautions

Fluoroquinolones are well tolerated and are considered one of the safest antimicrobial classes. Gastrointestinal side effects such as nausea, vomiting, and diarrhea occur in less than 5% of patients treated with these agents. Prolongation of the Q–T interval (especially in female patients) has been reported. Seizures have been reported with ciprofloxacin in elderly patients and those with diminished renal function. Studies in immature laboratory animals have shown changes in weight-bearing joints after fluoroquinolone exposure. Use of fluoroquinolones in children (18 years old or younger) should be reserved for cases in which the benefits outweigh the risks. Drug interactions between fluoroquinolones and warfarin can increase the potential for bleeding, necessitating close monitoring of patients on warfarin. Dosage adjustment, except for moxifloxacin, is necessary in the presence of renal insufficiency. Concomitant use of antacids and iron supplements reduces the absorption of fluoroquinolones.[38]

Other Antibiotics

The following agents belong to various classes of antimicrobials with different mechanisms of action and spectra of activity. Individual agents are discussed when they represent the clinically used agents of their antimicrobial class.

Chloramphenicol

Chloramphenicol has a broad spectrum of activity against gram-positive, gram-negative, and anaerobic bacteria. Chloramphenicol distributes well into various tissues, including the brain. Use of this antibiotic has declined significantly with the availability of less toxic agents.[39]

Mechanism of action. Chloramphenicol inhibits protein synthesis by reversibly binding to the 50S ribosome subunit and essentially has a bacteriostatic effect. With prolonged exposure, chloramphenicol exhibits bactericidal activity against some organisms by inducing bacterial cell lysis.[39]

TABLE 14-6	Classification and Clinical Uses of Fluoroquinolones[38]		
GENERIC NAME	**BRAND NAME**	**ROUTE**	**COMMON USES (MICROORGANISMS)**
Ciprofloxacin	Cipro	IV, PO	*Pseudomonas aeruginosa,* Enterobacteriaceae, *Neisseria gonorrhoeae, Mycoplasma pneumoniae, Legionella pneumophila*
Ofloxacin	Oflox	IV, PO	*P. aeruginosa,* Enterobacteriaceae, *N. gonorrhoeae, M. pneumoniae, Chlamydrophila pneumoniae, L. pneumophila*
Levofloxacin	Levaquin	IV, PO	*P. aeruginosa,* Enterobacteriaceae, *Streptococcus pyogenes,* MSSA, *Haemophilus influenzae, M. catarrhalis,* penicillin-resistant *Streptococcus pneumoniae, M. pneumoniae, C. pneumoniae, L. pneumophila*
Moxifloxacin	Avelox	PO	Enterobacteriaceae, *S. pyogenes,* MSSA, *H. influenzae, Moraxella catarrhalis,* penicillin-resistant *S. pneumoniae, M. pneumoniae, C. pneumoniae, L. pneumophila*

IV, Intravenous; *MSSA,* methicillin-susceptible *Staphylococcus aureus; PO,* oral.

Clinical uses. Chloramphenicol is highly active against *Salmonella* and has been used for the treatment of gastroenteritis with sepsis and *Salmonella* meningitis. Chloramphenicol has excellent activity against rickettsial diseases, such as scrub typhus, murine typhus, and Rocky Mountain spotted fever. However, these diseases are usually treated with tetracyclines, with chloramphenicol reserved for pregnant patients. Anaerobic infections and mixed anaerobic-aerobic infections, such as peritonitis and aspiration pneumonia, can be treated with chloramphenicol. In addition, chloramphenicol can be used to treat bacteremias caused by *Enterococcus* species, including some isolates that are resistant to vancomycin.[39]

Adverse reactions and precautions. Because of the possibility of irreversible bone marrow suppression that may lead to serious and fatal blood dyscrasias (aplastic anemia), chloramphenicol has little place in the antimicrobial armament at the present time. Aplastic anemia is a life-threatening complication reported in 1 of every 20,000 patients treated with chloramphenicol. Chloramphenicol should not be used in premature and newborn infants, who cannot adequately metabolize this drug. The decreased metabolism of chloramphenicol results in high serum concentrations that can lead to gray baby syndrome (vomiting, pallor, cyanosis, circulatory collapse), which has an attributable mortality of 60%. The prolonged use of chloramphenicol in children with CF has been associated with optic neuritis leading to blindness.[39]

Colistin (Colistimethate)

Colistin, a member of the polymyxin family, was used in the early 1960s for serious gram-negative infections, including infections caused by *P. aeruginosa*. It was approved in 1968 by the U.S. Food and Drug Administration (FDA) but was later abandoned for drugs with similar gram-negative efficacy and more favorable side effect profiles.[32] However, there has been a resurgence in the use of colistin, because of the emergence of MDR gram-negative bacteria including *P. aeruginosa* and *Acinetobacter* species.

Mechanism of action. Colistin is a surface-active, antipathic agent with a mechanism of action similar to that of a detergent. Because colistin has both hydrophilic and hydrophobic portions, it is relatively easy for the molecule to incorporate into bacterial cell membranes, causing disruption. Colistin exhibits bactericidal activity against most gram-negative bacteria.[32]

Clinical uses. Colistin has a broad range of activity against most gram-negative bacteria, including MDR *P. aeruginosa* and *Acinetobacter* species. Use of colistin is often reserved for severe systemic infections, including VAPs. *Proteus* and *Neisseria* species are generally resistant to colistin, along with most anaerobes and gram-positive bacteria. Colistin is administered in an inactive form (colistimethate) intravenously, intramuscularly, or by nebulization. After administration, inactive colistimethate is converted in vivo to the active form colistin.[26] Nebulized colistin is used often in patients with CF who harbor MDR *P. aeruginosa* and *Acinetobacter*.[32]

Adverse reactions and precautions. The most serious side effect associated with intravenously administered colistin is nephrotoxicity, which seems to be dose-related and reversible. Nephrotoxicity has been reported to occur in 20% of patients given colistin. Neuromuscular blockage, seizures, and respiratory paralysis have also been reported and seem to be dose-dependent phenomena as well. Caution should be used when coadministering colistin with other agents capable of causing nephrotoxicity, neuromuscular blockage, or respiratory failure, such as aminoglycosides.[32]

Daptomycin

KEY POINT

Daptomycin is a novel cyclic lipopeptide that has activity against a wide range of gram-positive bacteria, including multidrug-resistant (MDR) staphylococci and enterococci.

Daptomycin is a novel cyclic lipopeptide that has activity against a wide range of gram-positive bacteria, including MDR staphylococci and enterococci. However, daptomycin is inactive against gram-negative bacteria.[40-41]

Mechanism of action. The exact mechanism of daptomycin has not been completely elucidated; however, it is believed to occur by irreversible binding to the cytoplasmic membrane of bacterial cells and subsequent disruption of the membrane potential. This disruption apparently causes leakage of intracellular ions, leading to rapid cell death.[40]

Clinical uses. Daptomycin is currently approved for use in complicated skin and skin structure infections caused by susceptible gram-positive bacteria and *S. aureus* bacteremia. It has excellent activity against resistant staphylococci and enterococci, including vancomycin-resistant strains, although it is not approved for this use. In a phase 3 trial involving daptomycin for the treatment of CAP, daptomycin was inferior to the comparator agent (ceftriaxone), especially in patients with more serious infections. This poor response in pulmonary infections has been attributed to inactivation of daptomycin by pulmonary surfactants. Consequently, daptomycin is not indicated for use in the treatment of pneumonia. It is available only as an intravenous infusion.[40-41] With the increased incidence of MRSA in skin and soft tissue infections, daptomycin use has significantly increased due to efficacy and convenience of a once-daily administration.

Adverse reactions and precautions. In earlier clinical studies involving daptomycin given every 8 to 12 hours, creatine phosphokinase (CPK) elevations and myalgias were noted that resulted in temporary suspension of drug development of this agent in the early 1990s. Once-daily administration of daptomycin has minimized these abnormalities noted in earlier studies. Clinical data have reported CPK elevations as a rare occurrence; however, the manufacturer recommends stopping hydroxymethylglutaryl-coenzyme A (HMG-CoA) reductase inhibitors (Lipitor, Zocor, Crestor, etc.) and other drugs associated with rhabdomyolysis during daptomycin therapy. In addition, daptomycin should be discontinued in patients with myalgias associated with CPK elevations or in asymptomatic patients with CPK elevations greater than 10 times the upper limit of normal.[40-41]

Trimethoprim-Sulfamethoxazole

Sulfamethoxazole belongs to the class of antibiotics known as the *sulfonamides*. Trimethoprim is a *pyrimidine* found to potentiate the activity of sulfamethoxazole. The combination of trimethoprim and sulfamethoxazole (TMP-SMX; Bactrim) was introduced in 1968 and has since gained a place in the treatment of numerous infections. This combination is active against gram-positive bacteria (streptococci, MSSA, MRSA) and gram-negative bacteria (*H. influenzae, Burkholderia cepacia, Stenotrophomonas maltophilia*). In addition, it is active against *Pneumocystis jiroveci* (formerly known as *Pneumocystis carinii*).[42]

Mechanism of action. TMP-SMX exerts antibacterial effects by sequentially blocking bacterial dihydropteroate synthetase and dihydrofolate reductase. These enzymes are responsible for the production of folic acid. Without folic acid, bacteria are unable to synthesize nucleic acid and proteins necessary for growth. TMP-SMX acts synergistically and is considered bacteriostatic.[42]

Clinical uses. TMP-SMX is used for the treatment and prophylaxis of *Pneumocystis* pneumonia (PCP) in patients infected with HIV. TMP-SMX is widely distributed in the body, achieving detectable levels in most tissues. High concentrations are achieved in the urine, making it an ideal agent for the treatment of UTIs. In addition, TMP-SMX has been used for treatment of acute exacerbations of bronchitis, traveler's diarrhea caused by enterotoxigenic *E. coli*, otitis media, and shigellosis. In recent years, bacterial resistance to TMP-SMX has increased, creating controversy over the continued use of this combination as a first-line agent for UTIs. TMP-SMX also displays good activity against MRSA, including community-acquired strains, which gives practitioners an effective oral option for treatment.[42]

Adverse reactions and precautions. TMP-SMX is relatively well tolerated; nausea, vomiting, diarrhea, and hypersensitivity are the most common adverse effects. In addition, sulfamethoxazole has side effects that are common to all sulfonamides, including neutropenia, thrombocytopenia, hemolytic anemia, jaundice, hepatic necrosis, and drug-induced lupus. TMP-SMX should be avoided in all patients with "sulfa" allergies or hypersensitivities. Patients who are deficient in the enzyme glucose-6-phosphate dehydrogenase (G6PD) should not receive TMP-SMX because this combination can increase the risk of hemolytic anemia. TMP-SMX has a significant drug interaction with warfarin, which can increase the risk of bleeding. The daily dosage of TMP-SMX should be reduced in the presence of renal insufficiency because both agents are eliminated through the kidneys. Patients should be advised to take TMP-SMZ with 8 ounces of water to prevent acute interstitial nephritis.[42]

Clindamycin

Clindamycin, a member of the lincosamide class of antibiotics, has activity against gram-positive and anaerobic bacteria. In addition, this agent is active against *Toxoplasma gondii* and *P. jiroveci*.[39,43]

Mechanism of action. Similar to chloramphenicol, clindamycin binds to the bacterial 50S ribosomal subunit to inhibit protein synthesis, resulting in a bacteriostatic effect. This suppression of protein synthesis has been shown to reduce toxin production in certain strains of *S. aureus* (toxic shock syndrome) and *S. pyogenes* (necrotizing fasciitis).[39,43]

Clinical uses. Clindamycin distributes well in body tissues but has minimal penetration into cerebrospinal fluid even in the presence of meningitis. Clindamycin is used as an adjunct to agents with gram-negative activity for intraabdominal, pelvic, and diabetic foot infections, all of which tend to be polymicrobial. Anaerobic infections of the respiratory tract, such as necrotizing pneumonia, lung abscess, empyema, and aspiration pneumonia, are often treated with clindamycin. AIDS-related illnesses, such as *Toxoplasma* encephalitis and PCP, can also be treated with clindamycin. Clindamycin also has significant activity against MRSA, including community-acquired strains.[39,43]

Adverse reactions and precautions. Nausea, vomiting, and diarrhea are the most common side effects associated with clindamycin. Diarrhea may be a consequence of *Clostridium difficile*. Discontinuing the offending antibiotic and initiating oral vancomycin or metronidazole therapy treats this mild to life-threatening diarrhea. Prolongation of the neuromuscular blocking effects of pancuronium with the concomitant use of clindamycin has also been reported.[39,43]

Metronidazole

Metronidazole is a nitroimidazole that was used initially for its antiprotozoal effects against pathogens such as *Trichomonas vaginalis, Giardia lamblia*, and *Entamoeba histolytica*. Its anaerobic properties were discovered after an observation that acute ulcerative gingivitis improved in patients being treated for trichomonal vaginitis.[39]

Mechanism of action. The exact mechanism of action of metronidazole is unknown, although it is thought to have different effects in protozoa versus anaerobic bacteria. It is postulated that the microorganisms convert metronidazole into its reduced form. This reduced form causes a loss of the helic structure of DNA and results in DNA strand breaks. Metronidazole is bactericidal against most anaerobic pathogens such as *B. fragilis*.[39]

Clinical uses. Anaerobic infections have been implicated in abscesses within the brain, lung, and intraabdominal cavity. Metronidazole is often added as an adjunct, especially when surgical drainage of the abscess is impossible. In contrast to clindamycin, metronidazole penetrates well into the central nervous system and is useful for the treatment of brain abscesses. A key anaerobic pathogen, *B. fragilis* is part of the normal enteric flora and can contribute to sepsis in the event of gastrointestinal disease, surgery, or penetrating trauma. Metronidazole is often added to treat polymicrobial infections, especially when *B. fragilis* is suspected. Bacterial vaginosis caused by *Gardnerella*, *Trichomonas*, and *Bacteroides* species is also treated with metronidazole. In addition, diarrhea caused by *C. difficile* can be treated with metronidazole.[39]

Adverse reactions and precautions. An unpleasant metallic taste, nausea, and vomiting are common complaints associated with the use of metronidazole. The prolonged use of metronidazole, especially with high doses, can lead to peripheral neuropathy. In some rare situations, seizures, encephalopathy, and cerebellar dysfunction have also been noted. Metronidazole can interact with warfarin to potentiate its hypoprothrombinemic effect and lead to significant bleeding. In addition, patients should avoid the use of alcohol while taking metronidazole (inhibits alcohol dehydrogenase) because the concomitant use can result in a disulfiram-like reaction.[39]

Glycopeptides

Vancomycin. Vancomycin is a glycopeptide antibiotic with activity against gram-positive bacteria. It is not active against gram-negative bacteria. Its use in recent years has increased as a result of the emergence of MRSA.[41]

> **KEY POINT**
>
> *Vancomycin* is a glycopeptide antibiotic with activity against gram-positive bacteria. It is not active against gram-negative bacteria.

Mechanism of action. Vancomycin inhibits transglycosylation of peptidoglycan by binding to the precursor D-alanine-D-alanine portion. This process prevents the formation of a rigid cell wall structure and results in bacterial cell lysis. Vancomycin is considered bactericidal against gram-positive organisms with the exception of enterococci (bacteriostatic).[41]

Clinical uses. Vancomycin is used for infections caused by MRSA, such as bacteremias, endocarditis, pneumonia, peritonitis, and skin and soft tissue infections. Vancomycin also serves as the alternative agent to penicillin for the treatment of viridans streptococcal endocarditis. Vancomycin does not cross the blood-brain barrier efficiently, even in the presence of acute meningeal inflammation. However, pneumococcal meningitis resistant to penicillin can still be treated by these low concentrations of vancomycin. An oral formulation of vancomycin can be used to treat *C. difficile* diarrhea that is refractory to metronidazole.[41]

Adverse reactions and precautions. A common reaction known as *red man* or *red neck syndrome* has been associated with the rapid infusion of vancomycin (related to histamine release). Increasing the time of infusion can prevent this syndrome of skin itch, flushing, angioedema, and hypotension. Ototoxicity and nephrotoxicity have been noted to occur more frequently in patients who receive vancomycin concomitantly with aminoglycosides. Vancomycin is renally excreted and requires dosage adjustment in patients with renal impairment.[41]

Telavancin. Vibativ (telavancin) is a lipoglycopeptide that is structurally related to vancomycin. Similar to vancomycin, telavancin displays no activity against gram-negative bacteria; however, it has excellent activity against most gram-positive isolates, including those with resistance to vancomycin.[41,44]

Mechanism of action. Similar to vancomycin, telavancin inhibits transglycosylation of peptidoglycan by binding to the precursor D-alanine-D-alanine portion of the gram-positive cell wall. The lipophilic side chain on telavancin also appears to anchor telavancin into the cell wall, which may contribute to its enhanced potency over vancomycin.[41,44]

Clinical uses. Telavancin is used for infections caused by *S. aureus*, enterococci, and streptococci. Unlike vancomycin, telavancin has activity against those isolates with reduced susceptibility to vancomycin, including VRE, VISA, and VRSA. It is approved for use in complicated skin and skin structure infections, as well as in HAP and VAP caused by *S. aureus*. Like vancomycin, it can be used as an alternative agent for gram-positive infections in individuals with β-lactam allergies.[41,44]

Adverse reactions and precautions. Telavancin is generally well tolerated with mild side effects reported to date. Dysguesia (taste disturbances), nausea, and headache were the most commonly reported adverse reactions during clinical trials. Dizziness and infusion site reactions were also observed, but at a similar rate to those receiving vancomycin.[41,44]

Quinupristin and Dalfopristin

Quinupristin and dalfopristin are streptogramins that act synergistically when used together (as in the product Synercid). These agents are active against gram-positive bacteria and are used primarily to treat infections caused by vancomycin-resistant *Enterococcus faecium* (VREF).[41]

Mechanism of action. Dalfopristin blocks peptide bond formation and distorts the ribosome to enhance the binding of quinupristin. The ribosome-bound quinupristin inhibits the binding of aminoacyl-transfer RNA to inhibit protein synthesis. The combination is bactericidal against MRSA but is bacteriostatic against VREF.[41]

Clinical uses. Quinupristin-dalfopristin is used primarily for life-threatening VREF infections, but it is also indicated for skin and soft tissue infections and pneumonias caused by susceptible gram-positive pathogens. Quinupristin-dalfopristin is inactive against most gram-negative bacteria and anaerobes. However, quinupristin-dalfopristin has good in vitro activity against *M. pneumoniae* and *L. pneumophila*.[41]

Adverse reactions and precautions. Quinupristin-dalfopristin is available only as a parenteral formulation and must be administered through a central line (catheter inserted and threaded to the superior or inferior vena cava) because peripheral administration is associated with a high incidence of thrombophlebitis. Arthralgias and myalgias of varying severity have also been reported with the use of these agents in up to 40% of patients. Similar to erythromycin, quinupristin-dalfopristin is an inhibitor of the CYP system. Drugs (metabolized through the CYP system) with a narrow therapeutic index should be used cautiously in patients receiving quinupristin-dalfopristin.[41]

Oxazolidinones

Linezolid. The antibiotic linezolid belongs to a novel class of antibiotics known as the oxazolidinones. Linezolid, similar to quinupristin-dalfopristin, is active against gram-positive bacteria and is approved for the treatment of severe life-threatening VREF infections. In contrast to vancomycin and quinupristin-dalfopristin, linezolid is available as an oral formulation that is completely absorbed from the gastrointestinal tract.[41] Tedizolid is a new oxazolidinone agent with similar activity to linezolid, but with activity against some linezolid-resistant strains of gram-positive bacteria. Currently it has only been used in skin and skin structure infections.

Mechanism of action. Linezolid prevents RNA translation by binding to the 23S ribosomal RNA of the 50S subunit to prevent the formation of a functional 70S initiation complex. Use of this novel antimicrobial target for the inhibition of protein synthesis has not been previously exploited.[41]

Clinical uses. Linezolid is indicated for the treatment of VREF infections, including cases with concurrent bacteremia. Nosocomial pneumonias and complicated skin and skin structure infections caused by *S. aureus*, including MRSA, may be treated with linezolid. Linezolid has activity against some mycobacterial species; however, it lacks significant activity against gram-negative bacteria.[41]

Adverse reactions and precautions. The most common adverse events reported with linezolid include diarrhea, nausea, and headaches. Thrombocytopenia has been reported with the use of linezolid but is associated with prolonged use of the antibiotic (2 weeks or more). Linezolid is a reversible, nonselective inhibitor of monoamine oxidase and has the potential to interact with adrenergic agents (e.g., dopamine, norepinephrine) and serotoninergic agents (e.g., selective serotonin reuptake inhibitors).[41]

ANTIMYCOBACTERIALS

Tuberculosis has received heightened attention largely because of the increase in cases attributed to the HIV epidemic. Each year, millions of individuals are exposed to tuberculosis, many through casual contact. More than one third of the world's population has contracted tuberculosis. The U.S. Centers for Disease Control and Prevention (CDC) makes annual recommendations for the prevention and treatment of tuberculosis infection. Nosocomial transmission can be prevented by placing patients with suspected or confirmed tuberculosis in respiratory isolation (negative-pressure room) until they are (1) determined not to have tuberculosis, (2) discharged from the hospital, or (3) confirmed to be noninfectious. Other measures such as use of fitted respiratory masks (by health care personnel) can prevent transmission of *M. tuberculosis* by aerosolization to caregivers.

Treatment consists of multiple antibiotic regimens for 6 to 12 months in duration. Single-agent regimens should never be used for treatment because the likelihood of developing resistance is high. Treatment failures often result from poor patient compliance and from resistance to antibiotics. Drugs used in the treatment of tuberculosis can be categorized as either first- or second-line agents, depending on their efficacy and side effect profiles. Initial therapy generally involves a combination of isoniazid (INH), pyrazinamide, rifampin, and ethambutol. Table 14-7 summarizes clinically used antimycobacterial agents, doses, routes of administration, and side effects. Addition or subtraction of agents from this regimen is usually based on culture and sensitivity data, along with patient response to treatment. Guidelines for the treatment of active pulmonary tuberculosis are provided in Table 14-8.

KEY POINT

The most commonly used antimycobacterials in the treatment of tuberculosis include *isoniazid (INH)*, *rifampin*, *rifabutin*, *pyrazinamide*, *ethambutol*, and *streptomycin*.

TABLE 14-7   Dose, Route, and Side Effect Profile of Commonly Used Antimycobacterials[45-47]

ANTIMYCOBACTERIAL	ADULT DOSAGE	ROUTE	SIDE EFFECTS
Isoniazid	5 mg/kg/day; maximum 300 mg/day	PO, IM	Hepatotoxicity (symptoms include nausea, loss of appetite, abdominal pain), peripheral neuritis, rash, fever, anemia
Rifampin	10 mg/kg/day; maximum 600 mg/day	PO, IV	Hepatotoxicity, flulike symptoms, discolorations of body secretions to an orange color
Rifabutin	300 mg/day	PO	
Rifapentine	600 mg once or twice per week	PO	
Pyrazinamide	15-30 mg/kg/day; maximum 2000 mg/day	PO	Hepatotoxicity, arthralgia, hyperuricemia
Ethambutol	15-25 mg/kg/day; maximum 2500 mg/day	PO	Optic neuritis (greater incidence in patients receiving >15 mg/kg/day)
Streptomycin	15 mg/kg/day; maximum 1000 mg/day	IM	Ototoxicity (high-frequency hearing loss, vertigo), nephrotoxicity

IM, Intramuscular; *IV*, intravenous; *PO*, oral.

TABLE 14-8   Guidelines for Treatment of Active Pulmonary Tuberculosis[48]

CLINICAL SCENARIO	TREATMENT REGIMEN
1. INH resistance rate <4%	INH + RIF (or RFB) + PZA + B$_6$ daily for 2 mo, then INH + RIF (or RFB) + B$_6$ daily for additional 4 mo
2. INH resistance rate >4%	INH + RIF (or RFB) + PZA + ETB or SM + B$_6$ daily for 2 mo, then INH + RIF or unknown (or RFB) + B$_6$ daily for additional 4 mo
3. Noncompliant or unreliable patient	Requires DOT INH + RIF (or RFB) + PZA + ETB + B$_6$ or SM daily for 2 wk, then 2-3 times/wk for 6 wk, then INH + RIF (or RFB) + B$_6$ 2-3 times/wk for 6 mo
4. Patient known to be INH-resistant or unable to tolerate INH	DOT RIF (or RFB) + PZA + ETB daily for 6 mo
5. Patient known to be RIF-resistant or unable to tolerate RIF	INH + FQN + ETB + B$_6$ daily for 12-18 mo; supplement with PZA first 2 mo
6. Pregnancy	INH + RIF + ETB daily for 9 mo
7. HIV infection or AIDS	Treatment as in clinical scenarios 1 and 2 for the first 2 mo, then extend INH + RIF (or RFB) + B$_6$ daily for additional 7 mo

AIDS, Acquired immunodeficiency syndrome; *B$_6$,* pyridoxine; *DOT,* directly observed therapy; *ETB,* ethambutol; *FQN,* fluoroquinolone; *HIV,* human immunodeficiency virus; *INH,* isoniazid; *PZA,* pyrazinamide; *RFB,* rifabutin; *RIF,* rifampin; *SM,* streptomycin.

Data from American Thoracic Society, CDC, Infectious Diseases Society of America: Treatment of tuberculosis, *MMWR Recomm Rep* 52(RR-11):1-77, 2003.

Isoniazid

INH is well absorbed orally and is distributed throughout the body, especially in the cerebrospinal fluid. INH is metabolized by the liver, and its metabolite is eliminated by the kidneys.[46]

Mechanism of Action

INH inhibits cell wall synthesis by inhibiting synthesis of mycolic acid, a primary component of the mycobacterial cell wall. This agent is bactericidal against replicating tuberculosis bacilli and bacteriostatic against nonreplicating organisms.[46]

Adverse Reactions and Precautions

An elevation in liver enzymes has been reported in patients receiving INH and is reversible with discontinuation of the drug. Rare cases of serious hepatitis and death also have been reported. Hepatotoxicity usually occurs between the fourth and eighth weeks of treatment but may occur at any time. Tests used to measure hepatocellular injury should be performed and include monitoring liver transaminases such as alanine aminotransferase (ALT) and aspartate aminotransferase (AST). In addition, patients should be monitored for the development of symptoms of hepatitis, such

as nausea, loss of appetite, and abdominal pain. Neurotoxicity has also been reported and occurs more frequently in patients receiving higher dose therapy. Supplementation with pyridoxine (vitamin B$_6$) has been shown to reduce the frequency of this adverse reaction. Rare miscellaneous reactions, such as rash, anemia, and fever, also have been reported.[46]

Rifampin, Rifabutin, and Rifapentine

Rifampin, rifabutin, and rifapentine are semisynthetic antibiotics referred to as *rifamycins.* Rifampin and rifabutin have similar structures and spectra of activity. They are well absorbed orally, with good penetration into most tissues. These agents do not penetrate the central nervous system well in the absence of inflammation. Rifampin is extensively metabolized through the liver and is an inducer of the CYP system. Rifabutin and rifapentine are also metabolized hepatically; however, they are considered weaker enzyme inducers than rifampin. CYP induction is known to decrease plasma concentrations of drugs hepatically metabolized; therefore dosage adjustments of agents metabolized by this system are necessary.[47]

Mechanism of Action

Rifamycins inhibit bacterial DNA-dependent RNA polymerase. They are bactericidal against actively dividing bacteria.

Adverse Reactions and Precautions

Hepatotoxicity is the major adverse reaction associated with rifamycins. Elevations of liver transaminases are commonly reported and are usually reversible on discontinuation of the drug. Patients with preexisting liver damage are more prone to rifamycin-induced hepatotoxicity. Rifamycins are known to change the color of body fluids to a deep orange hue. Patients should be warned that urine, feces, tears, saliva, sputum, and semen might turn an orange color. Uveitis (inflammation of the iris), which manifests as blurry vision, has also been reported. Rarely, flulike symptoms such as fever, chills, nausea, and vomiting have been reported during rifamycin therapy.[47]

Pyrazinamide

Pyrazinamide is a nicotinic acid derivative that is well distributed into most tissues, including the cerebrospinal fluid. Pyrazinamide is hepatically metabolized and excreted by the kidneys.[46]

Mechanism of Action

The precise mechanism of action is unknown. Mycobacteria convert pyrazinamide to pyrazinoic acid. It is speculated that pyrazinoic acid accumulates in macrophages to decrease the intracellular pH and increase the antimycobacterial activity of macrophages in combination with pyrazinamide. Pyrazinamide is bactericidal against mycobacteria when tested in an acidic environment.[46]

Adverse Reactions and Precautions

Nausea and vomiting are the most common side effects with pyrazinamide treatment. Hepatotoxicity has also been reported in patients receiving pyrazinamide; therefore liver transaminases should be monitored frequently. Patients with preexisting liver abnormalities should be monitored closely. Pyrazinamide is not known to induce or inhibit the CYP system to any significant extent.[46]

Ethambutol

Ethambutol is a synthetic, orally administered agent that distributes extensively throughout the body, including the cerebrospinal fluid. Most of it is eliminated unchanged in the urine.[46]

Mechanism of Action

Ethambutol decreases the synthesis of cell wall polysaccharides such as arabinogalactan to inhibit mycobacterial cell growth. It is a bacteriostatic agent.

Adverse Reactions and Precautions

Optic neuropathy is the major toxicity associated with ethambutol. Patients usually complain of blurred vision in conjunction with altered color (red-green) perception. Optic neuritis is usually seen with the use of high doses of ethambutol and is slowly reversible on discontinuation of the drug. Baseline optometric evaluation, followed by periodic examinations, is advisable to help monitor for visual changes during treatment. The dosage of ethambutol should be adjusted in patients with renal insufficiency.[46]

Streptomycin

Streptomycin is an aminoglycoside antibiotic that has been in use since the 1940s for the treatment of tuberculosis. It is available for use intravenously and intramuscularly and is indicated as an add-on agent in patients with documented or suspected drug-resistant tuberculosis.[31-34,46]

Mechanism of Action

Streptomycin has a mechanism of action similar to other aminoglycosides.

Adverse Reactions and Precautions

Streptomycin, similar to other aminoglycosides, is associated with nephrotoxicity and ototoxicity. It is eliminated unchanged in the urine, and dosage adjustment is required in patients with renal insufficiency.[31-34]

ANTIFUNGALS

KEY POINT

Use of *antifungals*, such as *polyenes*, *azoles*, and *echinocandins*, is increasing with the number of immunocompromised patients.

The incidence of fungal infections has increased dramatically. *Candida* species are now the fourth most commonly isolated bloodstream pathogens. Candidemia has a mortality rate of 40%. The number of patients immunocompromised as a result of AIDS, cancer chemotherapy, and organ transplantation has been increasing. These patient populations have diminished cell-mediated immunity and are predisposed to numerous fungal pathogens that vary in incidence geographically. The treatment of choice for most fungal infections has been the polyene amphotericin B. The high incidence of nephrotoxicity associated with this agent served as the impetus for the development of the azoles. Ketoconazole was the first agent of this class, but it has largely been replaced by the triazoles fluconazole and itraconazole. Newer triazoles with improved activity against molds are being developed. In addition, a new class of antifungals known as the *echinocandins* is now available. Systemically used antifungals, including route and clinical uses, are summarized in Table 14-9.

Polyenes

Polyenes include amphotericin B and nystatin. Amphotericin B has been available for more than 50 years and remains the drug of choice for most systemic fungal infections. More recently, amphotericin B has been formulated into lipid-based products. These lipid-based products alter the distribution of amphotericin B, resulting in a higher uptake of the agent into the reticuloendothelial system (liver, spleen, lymphatics) relative to the kidneys. The net effect of this shift in distribution has been shown to reduce the incidence of nephrotoxicity.[49]

Mechanism of Action

Polyenes bind to ergosterol (a type of cholesterol) in the fungal cell membrane, creating pores that increase cell membrane permeability. Intracellular potassium and other components escape through the pores, resulting in cell death (fungicidal).

Clinical Uses

The fungicidal activity of amphotericin B has made it the first-line agent for several pathogens causing pulmonary infections, including aspergillosis, blastomycosis, coccidioidomycosis, histoplasmosis, and cryptococcosis. These infections are associated with a high mortality, especially in patients who are neutropenic. Consequently, preventive measures such as amphotericin B prophylaxis and high-dose treatment (through the use of lipid-based formulations) have been sought. However, the optimal dose and treatment duration have been difficult to define because the successful outcome of a systemic fungal infection depends largely on recovery of the host immune system.[49]

Adverse Reactions and Precautions

Parenteral administration of amphotericin B is associated with two major types of toxicity. The first is infusion-related and includes flushing, fever, and chills. Pretreating patients

TABLE 14-9 Classification of Systemically Used Antifungals[49]

ANTIFUNGAL CLASS AND GENERIC NAME	BRAND NAME	ROUTE	COMMON USES (MICROORGANISM)
Polyenes			
Amphotericin B	Fungizone	IV, PO*	*Candida* spp., *Aspergillus* spp., *Cryptococcus neoformans, Histoplasma capsulatum, Blastomyces dermatitidis, Coccidioides immitis*
Amphotericin B colloidal dispersion	Amphotec	IV	*Candida* spp., *Aspergillus* spp., mucormycosis, *C. neoformans*
Amphotericin B lipid complex	Abelcet	IV	*Candida* spp., *Aspergillus* spp., mucormycosis, *C. neoformans*
Liposomal amphotericin B	AmBisome	IV	*Candida* spp., *Aspergillus* spp., mucormycosis, *C. neoformans,* leishmaniasis
Azoles			
Ketoconazole	Nizoral	PO, TOP	*Candida* spp.,† *C. neoformans, H. capsulatum, B. dermatitidis*
Fluconazole	Diflucan	IV, PO	*Candida* spp., † *C. neoformans*
Itraconazole	Sporanox	PO, TOP	*Candida* spp., † *Aspergillus* spp., *C. neoformans, H. capsulatum, B. dermatitidis, C. immitis, Sporothrix schenckii*
Voriconazole	Vfend	IV, PO	*Candida* spp., † *Aspergillus* spp., *C. neoformans, C. immitis, H. capsulatum, B. dermatitidis, Fusarium* spp., *Scedosporium* spp.
Posaconazole	Noxafil	PO	*Candida* spp., † *Aspergillus* spp., *C. neoformans, C. immitis, H. capsulatum, B. dermatitidis, Fusarium* spp., *Scedosporium* spp.
Echinocandins			
Caspofungin	Cancidas	IV	*Aspergillus* spp., *Candida* spp.
Micafungin	Mycamine	IV	*Aspergillus* spp., *Candida* spp.
Anidulafungin	Eraxis	IV	*Aspergillus* spp., *Candida* spp.
Other Antifungals			
Flucytosine	Ancobon	PO	*Aspergillus* spp., *Candida* spp., *C. neoformans*

IV, Intravenous; *PO*, oral; *TOP*, topical.
*The oral form of amphotericin B is not absorbed through the gastrointestinal tract.
†*Candida krusei* is intrinsically resistant to all azoles.

who manifest these symptoms with antipyretics and antihistamines may minimize these effects. The second major toxicity is renal impairment, thought to be a result of diminished renal perfusion. Hydrating the patient with normal saline boluses before and after amphotericin B infusion has been attempted to prevent this toxicity. The liposomal products, such as amphotericin B lipid complex and liposomal amphotericin B, have been shown to be less nephrotoxic than the traditional product and allow the administration of higher doses of amphotericin B.[49]

Azoles

Systemically used azoles include ketoconazole, fluconazole, itraconazole, voriconazole, and posaconazole. Ketoconazole was the first oral agent available to treat systemic fungal infections. This agent is poorly absorbed from the gastrointestinal tract (when an acidic environment is not present) and has potential for substantial toxicity. As a result, ketoconazole has largely been replaced by the newer triazoles fluconazole, itraconazole, and voriconazole. Fluconazole is available in oral and intravenous formulations, is widely distributed into the tissues, and is relatively nontoxic. Compared with ketoconazole, it has a narrow

spectrum of activity. Itraconazole has an enhanced spectrum of activity compared with fluconazole but slightly less than that of voriconazole. Voriconazole is also available in oral and intravenous forms. Posaconazole was approved more recently for prophylaxis of invasive aspergillosis and disseminated candidiasis in severely immunocompromised hosts and for the treatment of refractory oropharyngeal candidiasis. Use of posaconazole is intended for patients failing or refractory to other therapies and has been documented to be active against Zygomycetes (*Rhizopus* species, *Absidia* species, and Mucor species).[49]

Mechanism of Action

Fungal cell growth is impaired because of the reduced production of ergosterol. Azoles prevent the conversion of lanosterol to ergosterol by inhibiting the fungal CYP system and therefore produce a fungistatic effect.

Clinical Uses

Ketoconazole has largely been replaced by the more potent and better tolerated triazoles. The primary indication for fluconazole is for candidiasis (nonneutropenic patients) and as suppressive therapy for patients with cryptococcal meningitis, but it may also be used to treat coccidioidomycosis. Itraconazole is considered the drug of choice for the treatment of cutaneous and lymphangitic sporotrichosis. Itraconazole is also used as prophylaxis and suppressive therapy for pulmonary aspergillosis, histoplasmosis, blastomycosis, cryptococcosis, coccidioidomycosis, paracoccidioidomycosis, and candidiasis. Voriconazole is considered the drug of choice as primary therapy for invasive aspergillosis and has been approved for the management of candidemia and infections caused by rare pathogens such as *Fusarium* and *Scedosporium apiospermum*. Candidiasis caused by *Candida krusei* (which lacks the CYP system) may be intrinsically resistant to this class of agents, although in vitro activity has been documented with voriconazole and posaconazole.[49]

Adverse Reactions and Precautions

Fluconazole is well tolerated and has minimal side effects. Common adverse effects with ketoconazole, itraconazole, and voriconazole are anorexia, nausea, and vomiting. In addition, transaminase and bilirubin elevations have been reported. Impotence, decreased libido, and gynecomastia are also known to occur with ketoconazole and are attributed to its inhibition of sex steroid synthesis, and consequently it is used clinically for certain endocrine disorders. Voriconazole can cause visual disturbances such as photopsia and chromatopsia, which can occur in 30% of patients. Ketoconazole, itraconazole, and voriconazole are metabolized in the liver and are potent inhibitors of the CYP 3A4 system, so each has a significant potential for drug interactions. Conversely, fluconazole does not undergo significant hepatic metabolism and has the lowest drug interaction potential of the triazoles. Fluconazole is, however, eliminated unchanged in the urine and so dosage adjustment is required in patients with impaired renal function. Renal function is also important when administering the intravenous formulations of itraconazole and voriconazole. These drugs should be avoided in patients with creatinine clearance values less than 30 mL/min to prevent the accumulation of cyclodextrin, an intravenous solubilizing agent. Cyclodextrin is also used to formulate oral itraconazole solution and has been cited as the cause of the high incidence of adverse gastrointestinal intolerance relative to itraconazole capsules, which do not contain this agent.[49]

Echinocandins

Caspofungin was the first echinocandin to receive FDA approval in early 2001. Micafungin and anidulafungin received FDA approval in 2004 and 2006, respectively. These agents have similar pharmacokinetic and pharmacodynamic properties. They have poor gastrointestinal absorption, and all require parenteral administration.[49]

Mechanism of Action

Echinocandins inhibit fungal cell wall synthesis by inhibiting $(1,3)$-β-D-glucan synthase.[49]

These agents may be either fungicidal or fungistatic against fungi depending on the isolate.

Clinical Uses

All echinocandins have shown in vitro and in vivo (animal studies) activity against *Candida* and *Aspergillus* species. Caspofungin is currently indicated for the treatment of febrile neutropenia, candidemia, esophageal candidiasis, and aspergillosis in patients refractory or intolerant to amphotericin B, lipid-based amphotericin B, and itraconazole. Micafungin is indicated only for esophageal candidiasis treatment and prophylaxis after hematopoietic stem cell transplants. Anidulafungin, the most recently approved agent, is indicated for the treatment of candidemia, non-neutropenic candidiasis, and esophageal candidiasis. All echinocandins are considered ineffective against *Cryptococcus* species because these organisms lack $(1,3)$-β-D-glucan in their cell walls.[49]

Adverse Reactions and Precautions

Echinocandins seem to be well tolerated, although most of the safety data are for caspofungin and micafungin. In most studies, common adverse reactions were infusion-related and included fever, rash, flushing, and thrombophlebitis. Infusion-related reactions were approximately 10% for caspofungin and slightly less for micafungin. Anidulafungin has produced infusion-related reactions in 15% of patients. Nausea and vomiting were also frequently reported for all three agents. Elevations in liver transaminase (AST and ALT) levels and hyperbilirubinemia were noted with echinocandins, but these were mild and reversible on drug discontinuation. Echinocandins are not metabolized through the CYP system, reducing the potential for drug interactions. All echinocandins can increase the area under the curve (AUC) of cyclosporine when coadministered, with caspofungin creating the most significant changes in AUC. The mechanism of this interaction is unknown. Concurrent use of cyclosporine and echinocandins may warrant careful monitoring.[49]

Flucytosine

Flucytosine acts as an antimetabolite and is used primarily as adjunctive therapy for susceptible fungal pathogens. It is active against *Candida*, *Cryptococcus*, and *Aspergillus*.[49]

Mechanism of Action

Flucytosine is converted to fluorouracil and competes with uracil during the formation of fungal RNA. Inhibition of RNA formation decreases protein synthesis and prevents cell growth (fungistatic).

Clinical Use

Resistance to flucytosine develops rapidly when it is used as a single agent for systemic fungal infections. As a result, flucytosine has been used in combination with amphotericin B for the treatment of cryptococcal meningitis and aspergillosis.[49]

Adverse Reactions and Precautions

The most common adverse event associated with flucytosine is bone marrow suppression leading to anemia, leukopenia, and thrombocytopenia. This toxicity usually results when serum concentrations exceed 100 mcg/mL. Dosage reduction in patients with renal impairment is imperative to prevent this serious complication.

ANTIVIRAL AGENTS

 KEY POINT

Antivirals (excluding antiretrovirals) mimic nucleosides and inhibit DNA synthesis.

Several agents are available for treating viral infections (Table 14-10). All of these agents act by inhibiting steps involved in viral replication; none of the agents inhibit nonreplicating viruses. *Antivirals* (excluding antiretrovirals) mimic nucleosides and inhibit DNA synthesis.[50,51] Agents used to treat HIV are not discussed here.

Acyclovir and Valacyclovir

Acyclovir is available in intravenous, oral, and topical formulations. Oral acyclovir is not readily absorbed and requires a frequent daily regimen. Valacyclovir, a prodrug of acyclovir, was developed to improve gastrointestinal absorption of acyclovir. Valacyclovir is available only in oral formulation.[50]

Mechanism of Action

Acyclovir is a nucleoside analog that is phosphorylated and inserted into the replicating viral DNA. Once inserted in the growing chain, viral replication is terminated. Valacyclovir is converted to the active drug acyclovir by enzymatic hydrolysis in the liver and intestine.

Clinical Uses

Acyclovir and valacyclovir are effective against members of the herpesvirus family. They are most effective against herpes simplex virus (HSV)-1 and HSV-2. They also have activity against Epstein-Barr virus (EBV), cytomegalovirus (CMV), and varicella-zoster virus (VZV). Acyclovir and valacyclovir are clinically used for the treatment of genital infections caused by HSV and VZV.[51]

Adverse Reactions and Precautions

Acyclovir is eliminated unchanged in the urine; therefore dosage adjustment is required for acyclovir and valacyclovir in patients with renal impairment. Cases of nephropathy secondary to acyclovir have been reported in individuals with renal impairment. This adverse event occurs primarily in patients taking high doses of acyclovir. Keeping patients well hydrated can prevent nephropathy. The oral formulations are generally well tolerated.[51]

Penciclovir and Famciclovir

Penciclovir and famciclovir are similar in structure and activity to acyclovir. Famciclovir, the prodrug of penciclovir, is converted to its active form (penciclovir) in the gastrointestinal tract. Famciclovir is available in oral formulation, and penciclovir is available only in a 1% topical cream. Penciclovir and famciclovir seem to have greater in vitro activity against HSV and VZV than acyclovir.

Mechanism of Action

Penciclovir and the prodrug famciclovir are guanine nucleoside analogs, which exert their antiviral effects by incorporating into growing DNA chains, subsequently interfering with viral DNA synthesis and replication.[50]

Clinical Uses

Penciclovir has activity against viruses from the herpes family. It is effective against HSV-1, HSV-2, and VZV. Similar

TABLE 14-10	Classification of Antivirals[50,51]		
GENERIC NAME	**BRAND NAME**	**ROUTE**	**COMMON USES (MICROORGANISM)**
Acyclovir	Zovirax	IV, PO, TOP	HSV-1, HSV-2, HZV, VZV
Valacyclovir	Valtrex	PO	HSV-1, HSV-2, HZV, VZV
Famciclovir	Famvir	PO	HSV-1, HSV-2, HZV, VZV
Ganciclovir	Cytovene	IV, PO	CMV
Valganciclovir	Valcyte	PO	CMV
Cidofovir	Vistide	IV	CMV
Foscarnet	Foscavir	IV	HSV-1, HSV-2, VZV, CMV that are suspected to be resistant to acyclovir and ganciclovir
Amantadine	Symadine	PO	Influenza A
Rimantadine	Flumadine	PO	Influenza A
Oseltamivir	Tamiflu	PO	Influenza A and B
Zanamivir	Relenza	IH	Influenza A and B

CMV, Cytomegalovirus; *HSV-1, -2*, herpes simplex virus types 1 and 2; *HZV*, herpes zoster virus; *IH*, inhaled; *IV*, intravenous; *PO*, oral; *TOP*, topical; *VZV*, varicella-zoster virus.

to acyclovir, it is less effective against EBV and CMV. In vitro studies have shown some activity against hepatitis B virus (HBV). Penciclovir and famciclovir are clinically used for the treatment of genital infections caused by HSV and VZV.

Adverse Reactions and Precautions

Penciclovir and famciclovir are considerably well tolerated. Use of famciclovir has been associated with nausea, vomiting, diarrhea, and headaches. Rare cases of neutropenia have been reported. Penciclovir is eliminated through the kidneys; therefore dosage adjustment of famciclovir is required in patients with moderate to severe renal insufficiency.[50]

Ganciclovir and Valganciclovir

Ganciclovir is a guanine nucleoside analog with a mechanism of action similar to acyclovir. Valganciclovir is a newly approved prodrug of ganciclovir that improves ganciclovir absorption. Ganciclovir has a higher affinity for DNA transferase than acyclovir, which increases the intracellular half-life of the drug and allows a less frequent regimen. Valganciclovir is available only in oral formulation; ganciclovir is available in oral, intravenous, and intraocular (eye implant) formulations.[50,51]

Mechanism of Action

Ganciclovir and the prodrug valganciclovir are guanine nucleoside analogs. They have a similar mechanism of action as acyclovir. Both agents incorporate into growing DNA chains, consequently terminating viral DNA synthesis and replication.[50,51]

Clinical Uses

Ganciclovir resembles acyclovir in its activity against members of the herpes virus family and VZV. It has much higher activity against CMV in vitro and in vivo. Ganciclovir is indicated for the treatment and long-term suppression of CMV retinitis and prevention of CMV disease in AIDS and posttransplantation patients.[50,51]

Adverse Reactions and Precautions

The most common adverse reaction associated with the use of ganciclovir is bone marrow suppression. In patients with AIDS, the incidence of thrombocytopenia and neutropenia may be 20% (thrombocytopenia) and 40% (neutropenia). Dosages should be reduced in the presence of renal insufficiency. In addition to the side effects of myelosuppression, headache, nausea, rash, fever, and liver transaminase elevations have been reported.[50,51]

Cidofovir

Cidofovir is an acyclic phosphonate nucleoside analog that has potent antiviral activity against a wide variety of viruses. In contrast to the guanine nucleoside analogs, cidofovir has enhanced activity against HSV, EBV, VZV, and CMV. Cidofovir is available only in intravenous formulation.[50,51]

Mechanism of Action

Cidofovir exerts its mechanism of action by inhibition of viral replication. Cidofovir is phosphorylated and inserted into the growing DNA chain. Once inserted, viral replication is terminated by inhibition of viral polymerases.

Clinical Uses

Cidofovir has potent activity against members of the herpesvirus family, EBV, and CMV. It is indicated for use in patients with CMV who failed previous treatments with ganciclovir or foscarnet. It has been used extensively in the treatment of CMV retinitis in patients with AIDS.[50,51]

Adverse Reactions and Precautions

Severe dose-dependent nephrotoxicity has been associated with the use of cidofovir. It is contraindicated in individuals with renal insufficiency. Saline infusions before and concomitant probenecid administration during cidofovir treatment have been used to help reduce nephrotoxicity. In addition to nephrotoxicity, neutropenia, fever, headache, emesis, rash, and diarrhea have been reported with cidofovir use.[50,51]

Foscarnet

Foscarnet is a pyrophosphonate nucleoside analog that has potent antiviral activity against HSV, EBV, VZV, and CMV. In addition, foscarnet has shown activity against HBV and influenza viruses. It is poorly absorbed, and it is available only in intravenous formulation.[50,51]

Mechanism of Action

Because foscarnet is a pyrophosphate analog, it does not require phosphorylation to become active. Foscarnet works by reversibly blocking viral polymerase phosphorylation, which inhibits viral replication.[50,51]

Clinical Uses

Foscarnet has activity against herpesviruses, including VZV and EBV, and influenza A and B. Foscarnet is used mainly to treat CMV retinitis in patients with AIDS who are unable to tolerate ganciclovir therapy. It is also used for treatment of CMV infections in other immunosuppressed individuals (organ transplantation). In addition, foscarnet has been used to treat HSV and VZV infections that are resistant to acyclovir and ganciclovir. Ganciclovir or acyclovir may act synergistically with foscarnet against some strains of CMV.[50,51]

Adverse Reactions and Precautions

Nephrotoxicity is a relatively common side effect that occurs in approximately 25% of patients treated. Adequate hydration during foscarnet infusion may reduce the incidence of nephrotoxicity. Dosage reduction is required in individuals with renal insufficiency. Other adverse reactions include fever, nausea, electrolyte imbalances, vomiting, diarrhea, and headache.[50,51]

Amantadine and Rimantadine

Amantadine and rimantadine are closely related antiviral agents with activity against influenza A only. Both agents are well absorbed from the gastrointestinal tract and are suitable for oral administration.[50]

Mechanism of Action

Amantadine and rimantadine act by inhibiting viral replication and viral assembly. It is also thought that these agents inhibit the influenza virus from uncoating and entering the mucosal cells of the respiratory tract.

Clinical Uses

Amantadine and rimantadine have a narrow spectrum of activity because they are active against influenza A virus only. Both agents may be used prophylactically in high-risk (i.e., immunocompromised) patients who are unable to tolerate or benefit from influenza vaccination. They may also be used in conjunction with vaccination in the same high-risk patient populations. To be effective, these agents should be initiated within the first 48 hours of onset of symptoms.[50]

Adverse Reactions

Amantadine and rimantadine are well tolerated. Central nervous system side effects such as tremor, insomnia, light-headedness, seizure, cardiac arrhythmias, and agitation have been reported with both drugs (more often with amantadine) and seem to be related to higher serum concentrations of these agents. A dosage adjustment of amantadine, but not rimantadine, is required in the presence of renal insufficiency.[50]

Oseltamivir and Zanamavir

Oseltamivir and zanamavir belong to the class of antivirals known as *neuraminidase inhibitors*. Oseltamivir is a prodrug that is converted to its active form (oseltamivir carboxylate) after it is absorbed. It is available only as an oral formulation. Zanamavir is structurally related to oseltamivir; however it is administered by oral inhalation only.[50]

Mechanism of Action

Oseltamivir and zanamavir specifically inhibit influenza A and B neuraminidase, which prevents influenza viruses from leaving the host cell to infect other cells.[50]

Clinical Uses

Neuraminidase inhibitors are effective only for the treatment of influenza A and B infection. They have been shown clinically to reduce the duration of influenza infection. However, therapy must be initiated within 40 hours of the initiation of symptoms to be effective.[50]

Adverse Reactions and Precautions

Oseltamivir and zanamavir are well tolerated; nausea and vomiting are reported as the most frequent adverse reactions. These symptoms usually occur on the first 2 days of therapy. Bronchospasm has been seen more frequently with zanamivir and appears to be related to the route of administration. Dosage adjustment is required in patients with renal insufficiency.[50]

RESPIRATORY CARE ASSESSMENT OF ANTIBIOTIC THERAPY

Before Treatment

- Assess the effectiveness of drug therapy on the basis of indications for the agent (i.e., virus or bacteria).

During Treatment and Short Term

- Consider susceptibility testing.
- Assess the effectiveness of the current agents.

Long Term

- Monitor response to therapy.
- Consider combination of agents.

General Contraindications

- Antimicrobials should not be used unless a specific pathogen is known or suspected to avoid the development of drug resistance.

SELF-ASSESSMENT QUESTIONS

Answers can be found in Appendix A.

1. What is the difference between bacteriostatic and bactericidal antimicrobial agents?
2. Give an example of a class of antimicrobials that kill in a concentration dependent AND concentration independent manner.
3. Describe at least three parameters that may indicate antibiotic failure in a patient.
4. Why is combination antibiotic therapy useful? (Be specific.)
5. Describe the mechanism of action of penicillin antibiotics. Name at least two additional antibiotic classes with similar mechanisms of action.
6. Which β-lactam antibiotic is least likely to cause an allergic reaction in a patient with a penicillin allergy?
7. Name three antimicrobial agents that would be useful in the treatment of community-acquired pneumonia (CAP).
8. What is the antimicrobial agent of choice for treatment of *Pneumocystis* pneumonia (PCP)?
9. What agents are considered first-line therapy for treatment of pulmonary tuberculosis?

SELF-ASSESSMENT QUESTIONS—cont'd

10. Which antimicrobial agents are useful for the treatment of nosocomial pneumonia caused by *Pseudomonas aeruginosa?*

CLINICAL SCENARIO

Answers can be found in Appendix A.

Chief Complaint

Jackson Daniels is a 64-year-old white male who presented to the Community Hospital with complaints of fever, cough, and shortness of breath. He states that he has been coughing up "thick, greenish mucus."

History of Present Illness

Mr. Daniels states that he has been feeling bad for over a week, but that his symptoms had gotten much worse a couple of days ago. He had gone to an Urgent Care Center and they gave him azithromycin, guaifenesin, and an albuterol inhaler; however, his symptoms did not improve and he was still having fevers and productive cough, and the inhaler was not helping his breathing.

Past Medical History

- Chronic alcohol abuse, with several admissions in the past for alcohol withdrawal (delirium tremors)
- Chronic obstructive pulmonary disease (COPD) with multiple hospital admissions for COPD exacerbation
- Recurrent pneumonia, including methicillin-resistant *Staphylococcus aureus* (MRSA) pneumonia
- Gastroesophageal reflux disease (GERD)

Social History

- Divorced with no children; unable to work because of poor health

Tobacco/Alcohol/Substance Use

- Tobacco history: 1 pack per day (ppd) for over 40 years
- Alcohol: 6 to 8 cans of beer daily
- Substance use: Denies use of illicit drugs.

Allergies

- Penicillin (rash), sulfa (rash and GI upset)

Home Medications

- Azithromycin 500 mg PO daily for 1 day, then 250 mg PO daily for 4 days (2 tabs remaining)
- Guaifenesin ER 1200 mg PO twice daily
- Albuterol MDI 2 puffs PRN q4-6h
- Prilosec OTC 20 mg PO twice daily (GERD)
- Duonebs (albuterol-ipratropium) inhaled QID (COPD)

Physical Examination

- General: Breathing fast; appears in moderate to severe respiratory distress
- Head, ears, eyes, nose, throat (HEENT): Pupils equally round and reactive to light and accommodation (PERRLA), denies headache, no sore throat or nasal discharge
- Cardiovascular: Tachycardic with a regular rhythm. No murmurs, rubs, or gallops
- Pulmonary: Bilateral crackles, worse on left side; decreased breath sounds over lower left lobe
- GI, GU, musculoskeletal, skin, neurologic: Unremarkable

Vital Signs

- Temperature (T) 102.2° F
- Blood pressure (BP) 150/85 mm Hg
- Heart rate (HR) 105 beats/min
- Respiratory rate (RR) 29 breaths/min
- Oxygen saturation by pulse oximetry (SpO_2) 90% on 2 L O_2, 82% on room air
- Weight 185 lb
- Height 70 inches

Laboratory/Radiographic Tests

- White blood cell (WBC) count 18.4×10^3 cells/mm³
- Liver function tests (AST, ALT): Moderately elevated
- Sputum gram stain: Many white blood cells, few epithelial cells, many gram-positive cocci in clusters
- Sputum culture: Pending
- Chest x-ray film (CXR): Left lower lobe infiltrate
- *Using the SOAP method, assess this clinical scenario.*

REFERENCES

1. Bartlett JG: Diagnostic tests for agents of community-acquired pneumonia. *Clin Infect Dis* 52(S4):S296–S304, 2011.
2. Jorgensen JH, Ferraro MJ: Antimicrobial susceptibility testing: A review of general principles and contemporary practices. *Clin Infect Dis* 49:1749–1755, 2009.
3. Jenkins SG, Schuetz AN: Current concepts in laboratory testing to guide antimicrobial therapy. *Mayo Clin Proc* 87(3):290–308, 2012.
4. Leekha S, Terrell CL, Edson RS: General principles of antimicrobial therapy. *Mayo Clin Proc* 86(2):156–167, 2011.
5. Lynch TJ: Choosing optimal antimicrobial therapies. *Med Clin N Am* 96:1079–1094, 2012.
6. Lee GC, Burgess DS: Antimicrobial regimen selection. In DiPiro JT, Talbert RL, Yee GC, et al, editors: *Pharmacotherapy: A pathophysiologic approach*, ed 9, New York, 2014, McGraw Hill.
7. Mandell LA, Wunderink RG, Anzueto A, et al: Infectious Diseases Society of America/American Thoracic Society consensus guidelines on the management of community-acquired pneumonia in adults. *Clin Infect Dis* 44(2):S27–S72, 2007.
8. Bonten MJ, Chastre J, Craig WA, et al: Guidelines for the management of adults with hospital-acquired, ventilator-associated, and healthcare-associated pneumonia. *Am J Respir Crit Care Med* 171:388–416, 2005.
9. Wunderink RG, Waterer GW: Community-acquired pneumonia. *N Engl J Med* 370:543–551, 2014.

10. Moran GJ, Rothman RE, Volturo GA: Emergency management of community-acquired bacterial pneumonia: what is new since the 2007 Infectious Diseases Society of America/American Thoracic Society guidelines. *Am J Emerg Med* 31:602–612, 2013.

11. Chow AW, Benninger MS, Brook I, et al: IDSA clinical practice guideline for acute bacterial rhinosinusitis in children and adults. *Clin Infect Dis* 54(8):e72–e112, 2012.

12. Russell PT, Bekeny JR: Oral antibiotics and the management of chronic sinusitis: What do we know? *Curr Opin Otolaryngol Head Neck Surg* 22:22–26, 2014.

13. Tackett KL, Atkins AA: Evidence-based acute bronchitis therapy. *J Pharm Pract* 25(6):586–590, 2012.

14. Kim V, Criner GJ: Chronic bronchitis and chronic obstructive pulmonary disease. *Am J Respir Crit Care Med* 187(3):228–237, 2013.

15. Falcone MF, Blasi F, Menichetti F, et al: Pneumonia in frail older patients: an up to date. *Intern Emerg Med* 7:415–424, 2012.

16. Freifeld AG, Bow EJ, Sepkowitz KA, et al: Clinical practice guideline for the use of antimicrobial agents in neutropenic patients with cancer: 2010 update by the Infectious Diseases Society of America. *Clin Infect Dis* 52(4):e56–e93, 2011.

17. Mulanovich VE, Kontoyiannis DP: Fungal pneumonia in patients with hematologic malignancies: current approach and management. *Curr Opin Infect Dis* 24:323–332, 2011.

18. Waybright RA, Coolidge W, Johnson TJ: Treatment of clinical aspiration: A reappraisal. *Am J Health Syst Pharm* 70:1291–1300, 2013.

19. Ciofu O, Hansen CR, Hoiby N: Respiratory bacterial infections in cystic fibrosis. *Curr Opin Pulm Med* 19:251–258, 2013.

20. Desai H, Agrawal A: Pulmonary emergencies: Pneumonia, acute respiratory distress syndrome, lung abscess, and empyema. *Med Clin N Am* 96:1127–1148, 2012.

21. Wright AJ: The penicillins. *Mayo Clin Proc* 74:290, 1999.

22. Preston SL, Drusano GL: Penicillins. In Yu VL, Edwards G, McKinnon PS, et al, editors: *Antimicrobial therapy and vaccines, vol 2: antimicrobial agents*, ed 2, Pittsburgh, PA, 2005, ESun Technologies, LLC.

23. McKinnon PS, Freeman C: Beta-lactam and beta-lactamase inhibitor combinations (amoxicillin/clavulanic, ampicillin/ sulbactam, piperacillin/tazobactam, ticarcillin/clavulanic). In Yu VL, Edwards G, McKinnon PS, et al, editors: *Antimicrobial therapy and vaccines, vol 2: antimicrobial agents*, ed 2, Pittsburgh, PA, 2005, ESun Technologies, LLC.

24. Capitano B, Kaya MB: Cephalosporins. In Yu VL, Edwards G, McKinnon PS, et al, editors: *Antimicrobial therapy and vaccines, vol 2: antimicrobial agents*, ed 2, Pittsburgh, PA, 2005, ESun Technologies, LLC.

25. Bazan JA, Martin SJ, Kaye KM: Newer beta-lactam antibiotics: doripenem, ceftobiprole, ceftaroline, and cefepime. *Infect Dis Clin North Am* 23:983–996, 2009.

26. Frampton JE: Ceftaroline fosamil: A review of its use in the treatment of complicated skin and soft tissue infections and community-acquired pneumonia. *Drugs* 73:1067–1094, 2013.

27. Anne S, Relsman RE: Risk of administering cephalosporin antibiotics to patients with histories of penicillin allergy. *Ann Allergy Asthma Immunol* 74:167, 1995.

28. Norrby SR: Side effects of cephalosporins. *Drugs* 34(Suppl 2):105, 1987.

29. Zhanel GG, Wiebe R, Dilay L, et al: Comparative review of the carbapenems. *Drugs* 67:1027–1052, 2007.

30. Asbel LE, Levison ME: Cephalosporins, carbapenems, and monobactams. *Infect Dis Clin North Am* 14:435, 2000.

31. Gilbert DN: Aminoglycosides. In Mandell GL, Bennet JE, Dolin R, editors: *Mandell, Douglas and Bennett's principles and practices of infectious disease*, vol 1, ed 7, New York, 2010, Churchill Livingstone.

32. Chen LF, Kaye D: Current use for old antibacterial agents: polymyxins, rifamycins, and aminoglycosides. *Infect Dis Clin North Am* 23:1053–1075, 2009.

33. Jackson J, Chen C, Buising K: Aminoglycosides: how should we use them for the 21st century? *Curr Opin Infect Dis* 26(6):516–525, 2013.

34. Poulikakos P, Falagas ME: Aminoglycoside therapy in infectious diseases. *Expert Opin Pharmacother* 14(12):1585–1597, 2013.

35. Smilack JD: The tetracyclines. *Mayo Clin Proc* 74:727, 1999.

36. Zuckerman JM, Qarnar F, Bono BR: Macrolides, ketolides, and glycylcyclines: azithromycin, clarithromycin, telithromycin, tigecycline. *Infect Dis Clin North Am* 23:997–1026, 2009.

37. Stein GE, Babinchak T: Tigecycline: an update. *Diagn Microbiol Infect Dis* 75:331–336, 2013.

38. Bolon MK: The new fluoroquinolones. *Infect Dis Clin North Am* 23:1027–1051, 2009.

39. Kasten MJ: Clindamycin, metronidazole, and chloramphenicol. *Mayo Clin Proc* 74:825, 1999.

40. Schriever CA, Fernandez C, Rodvold KA, et al: Daptomycin. *Am J Health Syst Pharm* 62:1145, 2005.

41. Nailor MD, Sobel JD: Antibiotics for gram-positive bacterial infections: vancomycin, teicoplanin, quinupristin/dalfopristin, oxazolidinones, daptomycin, dalbavancin, and telavancin. *Infect Dis Clin North Am* 23:965–982, 2009.

42. Smilack JD: Trimethoprim-sulfamethoxazole. *Mayo Clin Proc* 74:730, 1999.

43. Akins RL, Coyle EA, Levison ME, et al: Clindamycin. In Yu VL, Edwards G, McKinnon PS, et al, editors: *Antimicrobial therapy and vaccines, vol 2: antimicrobial agents*, ed 2, Pittsburgh, PA, 2005, ESun Technologies.

44. Guskey MT, Tsuji BT: Comparative review of the lipoglycopeptides: oritavancin, dalbavancin, and telavancin. *Pharmacother* 30(1):80–94, 2010.

45. American Thoracic Society: Targeted tuberculin testing and treatment of latent tuberculosis infection. *MMWR Recomm Rep* 49(RR–6):1, 2000.

46. Van Scoy RE, Wilkowske CJ: Antimycobacterial therapy. *Mayo Clin Proc* 74:1038, 1999.

47. Peloquin CA, Vernon AA: Rifamycins for mycobacterial infections. In Yu VL, Edwards G, McKinnon PS, et al, editors: *Antimicrobial therapy and vaccines, vol 2: antimicrobial agents*, ed 2, Pittsburgh, PA, 2005, ESun Technologies.

48. American Thoracic Society, CDC, Infectious Diseases Society of America: Treatment of tuberculosis. *MMWR Recomm Rep* 52(RR–11):1, 2003.

49. Russell RE: Current concepts in antifungal pharmacology. *Mayo Clin Proc* 86(8):805–817, 2011.

50. Razonable RR: Antiviral drugs for viruses other than human immunodeficiency virus. *Mayo Clin Proc* 86(10):1009–1026, 2011.

51. Vigil KJ, Adachi JA, Chemaly RF: Viral pneumonias in immunocompromised adult hosts. *J Intensive Care Med* 25:307–326, 2010.

Cold and Cough Agents

Douglas S. Gardenhire

OBJECTIVES

After reading this chapter, the reader will be able to:

1. Define key terms that pertain to cold and cough agents
2. Differentiate between the common cold and the flu
3. Differentiate between the specific types of cold and cough agents

4. Discuss the mechanism of action for each specific cold and cough agent

KEY TERMS AND DEFINITIONS

Antihistamines Drugs that reduce the effects mediated by histamine, a chemical released by the body during allergic reactions. Antihistamines are often administered to reduce secretions (e.g., runny nose and sneezing), but they can cause drowsiness and impaired responses. *Note:* Drying of secretion, whether caused by antimuscarinic or antihistamine action, may suppress a needed defense reaction of the airways. Nocturnal use is indicated more than around-the-clock use.

Antitussives Drugs that suppress the cough reflex. *Note:* Productive coughs should not be suppressed; the logic of an expectorant-antitussive combination is questionable.

Common cold Nonbacterial respiratory tract infection, generally caused by a viral infection of the epithelial layer of the upper airway and characterized by malaise, low-grade fever, cough, sneezing, and a runny nose.

Expectorants Drugs that increase the stimulation of mucus. Many have questionable efficacy in a cold. The best

expectorant, especially with colds, is plain water and juices, avoiding caffeinated beverages, such as tea or colas, and beer or other alcoholic mixtures.

Flu Nonbacterial infection with rapid onset of symptoms, including fever, headache, and fatigue.

Mucokinesis Therapeutic movement of excessive or abnormal secretions from the respiratory tract.

Mucolytic expectorants Agents that facilitate removal of mucus by a lysing, or mucolytic, action. *Example:* dornase alfa.

Stimulant expectorants Agents that increase the production and presumably the clearance of mucus secretions in the respiratory tract. *Example:* guaifenesin.

Sympathomimetics Drugs that partially or completely mimic the effects of the sympathetic nervous system. Note: Tremor, tachycardia, and increased blood pressure can occur with their use, especially when taken orally. Rebound congestion can occur if used for longer than a day.

TABLE 15-1	Differences in Symptoms Between the Common Cold and Influenza	
SIGNS AND SYMPTOMS	**COLD**	**INFLUENZA**
Chills	None	Typical
Cough	Present, hacking	Nonproductive, may be severe
Fatigue	Mild	Early and severe
Fever	Rare	Typical, high
Headache	Rare	Prominent
Myalgia	None or slight	Usual, may be severe
Nasal congestion	Common	Occasional
Sore throat	Common	Occasional
Sneezing	Common	Occasional

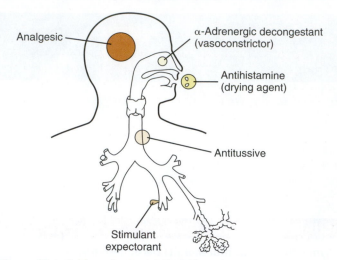

Figure 15-1 Cold medications include four classes of drugs targeted at the symptoms produced by this upper respiratory viral infection, along with analgesics.

TABLE 15-2	Examples of Adrenergic Agents Used as Nasal Decongestants
DRUG	**ROUTE**
Naphazoline (Privine)	Topical
Oxymetazoline (Afrin)	Topical
Phenylephrine (Sudafed PE)	Topical, oral
Pseudoephedrine HCl (Sudafed, various)	Oral
Pseudoephedrine sulfate (Afrinol)	Oral
Tetrahydrozoline (Tyzine)	Topical
Xylometazoline (Otrivin)	Topical

Large numbers of compounds, both prescription and over the counter (OTC), are available for treating symptoms of the common cold. The term "**common cold**" is used to describe nonbacterial upper respiratory tract infections (URIs), usually characterized by a mild general malaise and a runny, stuffy nose. Other symptoms include sneezing, cough, and possibly a sore throat or some chest discomfort. Allergic rhinitis and serious illnesses such as influenza, acute bronchitis, and infections of the lower respiratory tract are not included in this discussion. Influenza, or the "**flu**," is caused by the influenza virus and is associated with symptoms of fever, headache, general muscle ache, and extreme fatigue or weakness. Onset of symptoms is usually rapid. The fever and systemic symptoms of influenza are contrasted with symptoms of the common cold in Table 15-1.

Four classes of agents can be distinguished in cold remedies, used individually or in combination, as follows:

- **Sympathomimetics:** For decongestion
- **Antihistamines:** To reduce (dry) secretions
- **Expectorants:** To increase mucus clearance
- **Antitussives:** To suppress the cough reflex

The previously listed four classes of cold medications target the primary symptoms caused by the cold virus in the respiratory tract; this is illustrated conceptually in Figure 15-1. Each class is discussed subsequently, with representative agents listed. In addition to these four types of ingredients, an analgesic such as acetaminophen may be included in a cold medication, as in Sinutab, which consists of 30 mg of pseudoephedrine (decongestant) and 325 mg of acetaminophen (analgesic).

SYMPATHOMIMETIC (ADRENERGIC) DECONGESTANTS

 KEY POINT

Adrenergic agents act to vasoconstrict and relieve *nasal congestion*.

Sympathomimetic (adrenergic) agents are discussed as bronchodilators in Chapter 6, and the general effects of sympathetic stimulation are outlined in Chapter 5. In cold remedies, sympathomimetics are intended for a decongestant effect, which is based on their α-stimulating property and resulting vasoconstriction.

Sympathomimetics such as pseudoephedrine are found under brand names such as Sudafed and can be taken orally. As a result of changes in the USA PATRIOT Act, single agents or combination drugs using pseudoephedrine are placed behind the counter in pharmacies and regulated sales are documented because the drug has been overpurchased for use in the illegal production of methamphetamines. Manufacturers have turned to phenylephrine as a substitute; however, the 10-mg dose that has been approved by the U.S. Food and Drug Administration (FDA) has little effect on nasal decongestion when used orally because of the drug's high first-pass effect. In a meta-analysis by Hatton and associates,[1] it was found that 10 mg of phenylephrine was no more effective than a placebo. Oxymethazoline, a sympathomimetic used in brand names such as Afrin and Vicks Sinex, can be used topically for the nasal mucosa. Topical applications generally require lower dosages than oral use. Problems can occur with either route of administration. Table 15-2 lists sympathomimetic agents used as nasal decongestants in cold remedies.

Topical Application

Topical sympathomimetic decongestant sprays or drops produce results faster than oral applications. However, repeated use of these agents can cause a vicious cycle of increased secretions and nasal edema as the effect of the agent fades. This condition is referred to as rebound congestion and can cause the patient to become addicted to the agent and use it repeatedly. However, in rebound congestion, nasal vasoconstriction does not occur; the nasal mucosa actually swells.

 KEY POINT

Adrenergic decongestants are useful for nasal clearing, but *rebound congestion* can occur.

Systemic Application

Systemic (in comparison with topical) application has the advantage of giving more extensive decongestant effects involving deeper blood vessels. However, producing nasal vasoconstriction through systemic routes often leads to other systemic effects of sympathomimetics, such as an increase in blood pressure and increased heart rate.

ANTIHISTAMINE AGENTS

Histamine occurs naturally in the body and is contained in tissue mast cells and blood basophils. The role of the mast cell in releasing histamine with allergic asthma is discussed in Chapters 11 and 12.

Effect of Histamine

Histamine is an important mediator of local inflammatory responses that causes effects such as smooth muscle contraction, increased capillary permeability and dilation, itching, and pain. Scraping a tongue depressor or blunt pencil across the sensitive skin of the inner arm can illustrate a local inflammatory reaction at least partly mediated by histamine. The result is a wheal and flare reaction, also called a "triple response" (local redness, welt formation, and a reddish-white border). The redness and wheal (welt) are caused by dilation and leakage of plasma proteins from skin capillaries. The exudation of plasma causes the swelling. The flare, or reddish-white area surrounding the wheal, is probably due to local axon reflexes from sensory fibers causing dilation of neighboring arterioles.

Histamine Receptors

Histamine produces its inflammatory effects by stimulating specific cell surface receptors. Three types of histamine (H) receptors have been discovered. Two of the receptors are distinguished in mediating local inflammatory responses. The three histamine receptors are as follows.

1. H_1 *receptors:* Located on nerve endings and smooth muscle and glandular cells. H_1 receptors are involved in inflammation and allergic reactions, producing wheal and flare reactions in the skin, bronchoconstriction and mucus secretion, nasal congestion and irritation, and hypotension in anaphylaxis.[2]
2. H_2 *receptors:* Located in the gastric region. H_2 receptors regulate gastric acid secretion and feedback control of histamine release.[2]
3. H_3 *receptors:* Located primarily in the central nervous system (CNS). H_3 receptors may be autoreceptors for cholinergic neurotransmission in the airway at the autonomic ganglia, which are involved in CNS functioning and feedback control of histamine synthesis and release.[2,3]

The typical antihistamine found in cold medications is an H_1-receptor antagonist. Examples of these are pyrilamine and chlorpheniramine. H_1-receptor antagonists block the bronchopulmonary and vascular actions of histamine to prevent rhinitis and urticaria.[4] H_2-receptor antagonists are used to block gastric acid secretion when treating ulcers. Examples of H_2-receptor antagonists are cimetidine (Tagamet) or ranitidine (Zantac). Currently H_3 receptors are under investigation, no FDA approved agents are available in the United States.

Antihistamine Agents

 KEY POINT

Antihistamines *dry secretions* through an anticholinergic effect and by blockade of H_1 receptors.

All of the antihistamines discussed in this chapter are H_1-receptor antagonists. These antihistamine agents are classified further into the major groups listed in Table 15-3. The first five groups of antihistamines listed in Table 15-3 all are first-generation agents and can be found in cold preparations. Some of the brand names given may be familiar from OTC preparations readily available in drugstores. Others are found in combination products; these are discussed and listed subsequently. Second-generation antihistamines, which are longer acting and nonsedating, are also listed in Table 15-3.

Effects of Antihistamines

Antihistamines have three major classes of effects: antihistaminic, sedative, and anticholinergic activity. Second-generation agents are selective for H_1 receptors and are less sedating than first-generation agents. Antihistaminic activity blocks the increased vascular permeability, pruritus, and bronchial smooth muscle constriction caused by histamine. These actions are the reason antihistamines are used to treat allergic disorders such as rhinoconjunctivitis, allergic rhinitis, and urticaria.

TABLE 15-3	Major Groups of Antihistamines With Representative Agents by Nonproprietary and Brand Names

GROUP	DRUG
First Generation (Nonselective)	
Alkylamine derivatives	Chlorpheniramine (Chlor-Trimeton)
	Brompheniramine
	Dexchlorpheniramine maleate
Ethanolamine derivatives	Diphenhydramine HCl (Benadryl)
	Clemastine (Tavist)
	Carbinoxamine
Phenothiazine derivatives	Promethazine HCl
Piperazine	Hydroxyzine (Vistaril)
Piperidine derivatives	Cyproheptadine
Second Generation (Peripherally Selective)	
Nonsedating, Long-Acting	
Phthalazinone	Azelastine (Astelin, Astepro)
Piperazine	Cetirizine (Zyrtec)
	Levocetirizine (Xyzal)
	Olopatadine (Patanase)
Piperidines	Loratadine (Claritin)
	Fexofenadine (Allegra)
	Desloratadine (Clarinex)

The sedative effect of antihistamines is thought to be caused by penetration of the agents into the brain, where inhibition of histamine N-methyltransferase and blockage of central histaminergic receptors occurs. There is also antagonism of other CNS receptors, such as serotonin and acetylcholine.[2] The effect of drowsiness with first-generation (older) antihistamines can be a major hazard if alertness is required, such as in operating heavy machinery (e.g., a car) or monitoring a patient. This effect can be so pronounced that diphenhydramine HCl is added to acetaminophen in Tylenol PM, and the compound is described as a nonprescription sleep aid.

Finally, the anticholinergic effect produces considerable upper airway drying, just as would occur with an antimuscarinic agent such as atropine sulfate. In addition, effects seen with cholinergic blockade may occur, including CNS effects of stimulation, anxiety, and nervousness and peripheral effects of dilated pupils, blurred vision, urinary retention, and constipation.[3] These effects are less likely in occasional use with a cold, but they may be significant with greater use (and dose) for allergic rhinitis or other conditions (e.g., urticaria).

!   **KEY POINT**

Antihistamines dry secretions but can cause *impaction of secretions* and possible sinus blockage and should be used sparingly. Use during work should be avoided because of the side effect of *drowsiness*.

The duration of action of older antihistamines is generally 4 to 6 hours. However, newer, second-generation agents, often termed "nonsedating," are effective for 12 hours or more, depending on dose, and lack the sedating and anticholinergic effects. Examples of these newer agents are fexofenadine (Allegra) and cetirizine (Zyrtec) (see Table 15-3). Second-generation agents have little affinity for muscarinic cholinergic receptors and therefore do not cause dry mouth or gastrointestinal side effects. They also lack antiserotonin activity and do not cause appetite stimulation and weight gain, although astemizole and ketotifen may differ in this.[3] These newer drugs may inhibit mediator release from allergic inflammatory cells in addition to blocking the histamine receptor. Allergic symptoms of sneezing and rhinorrhea are equally well controlled with first-generation and second-generation H_1 antagonists.[3]

Structure-Activity Relationships

H_1-receptor antagonists were first discovered in 1937.[4] The chemical structure of histamine, the general structure of H_1-receptor antagonists, and two examples of H_1-receptor antagonists are shown in Figure 15-2. Chlorpheniramine is an antihistamine found in many cold remedies; it represents one of the older, classic H_1-receptor antagonists. Fexofenadine is a newer, nonsedating H_1-receptor antagonist.

The resemblance between histamine and the general formula for the H_1-blocking agents can be seen in the structures shown. In older agents, exemplified by chlorpheniramine, R_1 and R_2 attachments are usually a ring structure connected to an ethylamine (C–C–N) group. The presence of the ring structures and other substitutions on the structure makes older antihistamines lipophilic. As a result, classic first-generation antihistamines readily penetrate into the CNS and produce the effect of sedation and drowsiness previously discussed. Newer, nonsedating agents, such as terfenadine, do not readily cross the blood-brain barrier and therefore do not block central H_1 receptors.[4]

Use With Colds

A beneficial effect of antihistamine use with a cold is the drying of upper airway secretions, which lessens the rhinitis and accompanying sneezing. There is some question whether the drying of secretions is due to histamine antagonism or to the anticholinergic effect of these agents. How much histamine release occurs with colds is debated. In allergic rhinitis, there is no question that histamine causes much of the inflammatory response, and the newer long-acting agents are particularly helpful with this condition. Blockade of H_1 receptors prevents the histamine contribution to the symptoms of nasal itching, congestion, sneezing, rhinorrhea, and ocular irritation.

Regardless of the exact effect, the drying of runny nasal secretions is welcomed by individuals with a cold, and the

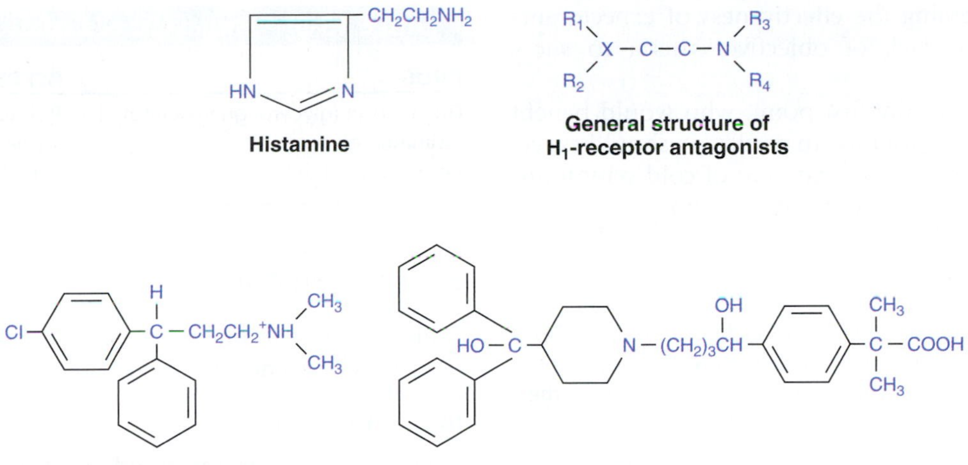

Figure 15-2 Structure of histamine, an inflammatory mediator; the general structure of H_1-receptor antagonists; and the structure of two antihistamines, chlorpheniramine and fexofenadine, are shown. R_1 to R_4 (Ring Structure, 1-4) indicate the sites of attachments, with R_1 and R_2 (Ring Sturcture, 1-2) being ring structures in most H_1 antagonists.

drying of secretions coupled with drowsiness can be useful to produce needed rest and sleep at night. Secretion, however, is a defense mechanism triggered by an upper airway viral infection. Antihistamines may cause harm as a result of suppressed secretion clearance and impacted secretions with sinus blockage.[4] Adequate hydration with a cold is always helpful, with or without use of antihistamines.

An alternative to antihistamines for rhinorrhea in a cold is the anticholinergic nasal spray ipratropium bromide (Atrovent), which is discussed in Chapter 7. Ipratropium has been shown to be effective in reducing nasal discharge in viral infectious rhinitis (colds) and allergic and nonallergic rhinitis.[5] There is no evidence of rebound congestion, mucosal irritation, or significant systemic effects. Ipratropium can be effective for 4 to 8 hours. An anticholinergic agent applied topically offers an attractive alternative to vasoconstricting decongestants and antihistamine H_1 antagonists.

Treatment of Seasonal Allergic Rhinitis

Second-generation H_1-receptor antagonists are more useful in the treatment of seasonal allergic rhinitis and other disorders requiring antihistamine treatment than in the treatment of colds. They are also better tolerated in treating allergic rhinitis than the first-generation agents because side effects of drowsiness are minimal, and duration of action is longer. Agents such as astemizole, loratadine, fexofenadine, and cetirizine are indicated for use in seasonal allergic rhinitis and chronic urticaria. They are intended to relieve symptoms of sneezing; rhinorrhea; itchy nose, palate, and throat; itchy, watery eyes; and pruritus. Table 15-4 lists categories and examples of agents used in the treatment of seasonal allergic rhinitis.[6] Other uses of antihistamines include the treatment of symptoms seen with motion sickness and control of nausea.

TABLE 15-4 Categories of Agents Used to Treat Seasonal Allergic Rhinitis

CATEGORY	EXAMPLE
Anticholinergics	Ipratropium bromide
Corticosteroids	Budesonide, ciclesonide
H_1-receptor antagonists	Cetirizine
Mediator antagonist	Cromolyn sodium
Specific immunotherapy	Standardized extracts
Vasoconstrictors	Pseudoephedrine

EXPECTORANTS

Expectorants are defined as agents that facilitate removal of mucus from the lower respiratory tract. A distinction is made in Chapter 9 between the following types of expectorants:

- **Mucolytic expectorants:** Agents that facilitate removal of mucus by a lysing, or mucolytic, action (*example:* dornase alfa).
- **Stimulant expectorants:** Agents that increase the production and presumably the clearance of mucus secretions in the respiratory tract (*example:* guaifenesin).

Generally, the expectorants considered here are stimulant expectorants, although the action does not always allow clear distinction. An example is guaifenesin, which is thought to reduce the adhesiveness and surface tension of mucus and increase **mucokinesis**—that is, movement and clearance of the secretion.

Efficacy and Use

There is controversy over the effectiveness and use of expectorants. The issue is clouded by the following.

- Difficulty in assessing the effectiveness of expectorants and in particular lack of objective criteria to show effectiveness.
- In conjunction with the first point, who would benefit from the use of expectorants? In particular, should expectorants be included in the treatment of cold symptoms, if a cold involves the upper respiratory tract?

 KEY POINT

Expectorants *stimulate mucus* production, and cough suppressants *depress the cough* reflex. The use of expectorants is questionable in an uncomplicated cold because the lower respiratory tract is not involved.

Use in Chronic Bronchitis

Petty[7] reported the results of a national study evaluating use of the expectorant iodinated glycerol (Organidin). Patients had chronic bronchitis, which is quite different from a common cold. The study concluded that in chronic obstructive bronchitis, iodinated glycerol was safe and effective. Its use improved cough symptoms, chest discomfort, ease in bringing up sputum, and sense of well-being. The duration of acute exacerbations of chronic bronchitis was decreased. It is reasonable that in bronchitis, symptoms and airflow improve and further infection is reduced if mucus clearance can be improved. However, Rubin and associates[8] found no change in lung function or sputum in patients with chronic bronchitis who used expectorants.

Irwin and colleagues[9] published evidence-based guidelines in the diagnosis and management of cough. The guidelines cover acute and chronic cough and specific diseases such as chronic bronchitis and cystic fibrosis (CF). The specific guidelines can be accessed at http://journal.publications.chestnet.org/article.aspx?articleid=1084267.

Mechanism of Action

Stimulant expectorants are thought to work by various means, depending on the agent. The mechanisms include the following:

- Vagal gastric reflex stimulation
- Absorption into respiratory glands to increase mucus production directly
- Topical stimulation with inhaled volatile agents

Guaifenesin, also known as glycerol guaiacolate, is classified as a category I agent, which means it is safe and effective.[10] Ziment[11] reviewed the mechanisms of action with iodides, such as iodinated glycerol. Other agents, such as terpin hydrate, sodium citrate, ammonium chloride, and menthols, have no demonstrated efficacy.[10]

Because mucus incorporates water as it is produced, an adequate intake of plain water or other nondiuresing liquids (milk, fruit juices) can help preserve normal mucus viscosity and clearance, especially with a simple cold.

TABLE 15-5	Partial List of Expectorants
DRUG	**REPRESENTATIVE BRAND**
Guaifenesin (glycerol guaiacolate)	Robitussin, Mucinex
Iodinated glycerol	Iophen, Par Glycerol, R-Gen
Potassium iodide	SSKI, Pima

Expectorant Agents

Table 15-5 lists available expectorant agents. Major agents or groups of agents are briefly characterized.

Iodine Products

Potassium iodide is a very old agent that has been used as an expectorant in asthma and chronic bronchitis.[12] It has a direct mucolytic effect in sufficient concentrations. It also has an indirect effect on mucus viscosity by stimulating submucosal glands to produce new, lower viscosity secretions.

The exact mechanism of action with iodine products is unclear. Iodide appears to distribute to mucous glands, where it is secreted along with increased mucus. Iodide also stimulates the gastropulmonary reflex, has a mucolytic effect, and can stimulate ciliary activity.[11] Iodides are associated with hypersensitivity reactions in some individuals, and a case of pulmonary edema has been reported with its use.[13]

Guaifenesin (Glycerol Guaiacolate)

Guaifenesin taken by inhalation is also considered to be an emollient. In experimental animals, doses larger than those used in humans caused an increase in bronchial secretions. Guaifenesin taken orally is thought to reduce the adhesiveness and surface tension of mucus secretions, enhancing mucus clearance. It is considered safe and effective by the FDA.

Topical Agents

Topical agents usually evoke memories of the heated humidifier (vaporizer) with clouds of steam scented with camphor, menthol, or (in the past) chloroform. These agents may still be found in use, but efficacy as expectorants has not been shown. The burn risk of a hot vaporizer should preclude its use with young or old and debilitated individuals.

Some research has shown that so-called bland aerosols of saline do increase sputum volume, possibly through reflex irritation of the bronchi and with increased secretion clearance as a result of coughing.[14] A particulate suspension may have the potential to function as an irritant to the upper airways.

Parasympathomimetics (Cholinergic Agents)

Using parasympathomimetic agents stimulates mucous gland secretion, but the effect on other muscarinic receptors is too diffuse for practical use as an expectorant. For this reason, a drug such as pilocarpine is not used as an expectorant. Likewise, stimulation of the medulla can increase respiratory tract secretions, but stimulation of the CNS is hazardous (see discussion of CNS stimulants in Chapter 20).

COUGH SUPPRESSANTS (ANTITUSSIVES)

 KEY POINT

Cough suppressants are useful for the treatment of a non-productive, irritating, *dry, hacking cough.*

A fourth category of drugs used with colds and cold symptoms is cough suppressants. Coughing is a defense mechanism to protect the upper airway from irritants such as dust particles, aerosols, liquids, and other foreign objects. This mechanism is a reflex, coordinated by a postulated cough center in the medulla. Detailed guidelines for cough management are provided by Irwin and associates.[9]

Agents and Mechanism of Action

Cough suppressants act by depressing the cough center in the medulla. Narcotics (see Chapter 20) exert powerful depressant effects on the medullary centers, including the carbon dioxide chemoreceptors, and are often used for this purpose. Common agents are codeine or hydrocodone. A commonly used nonnarcotic is dextromethorphan.

Benzonatate (Tessalon), a nonnarcotic, is chemically related to the local anesthetic tetracaine and anesthetizes stretch receptors in the lungs and pleura; this inhibits the cough reflex at its source. There is no inhibitory effect on the CNS. The effect begins in 15 to 20 minutes and lasts 3 to 8 hours.[15] The antihistamine diphenhydramine (Benadryl), available as a syrup, in liquid form, and in combination with other products, may be an effective cough suppressant. Diphenhydramine is becoming more common in products because of increased abuse of dextromethorphan. It should be noted that individuals taking any agent with diphenhydramine should be warned of the effect of drowsiness.

Some cough suppressants, or antitussives, contain codeine. In a dose less than 15 mg, codeine does not produce analgesia in an adult. In the 10- to 20-mg range, there is an antitussive action. At doses greater than 30 mg, codeine produces analgesia. Hydrocodone produces an antitussive effect with a dose of approximately 5 mg. Box 15-1 lists common antitussive agents, many of which are used in cold compounds. Dextromethorphan and codeine

BOX 15-1 Cough Suppressant Drugs

- Benzonatate (Tessalon)
- Codeine sulfate (various brand names)
- Dextromethorphan (Delsym, Trocal, Robitussin Maximum Strength Cough)
- Diphenhydramine (various brand names)
- Hydrocodone (Tussionex Pennkinetic)

are considered to be preferred cough suppressants based on safety and efficacy. However, the need for a prescription antitussive is unusual, especially in a cold, with the availability of OTC preparations. Not long ago codeine was available OTC in some states. As of April 10, 2014 manufacturers can no longer distribute any codeine or dihydrocodeine products that have not been approved by the FDA, which ultimately did away with any codeine products at any strength OTC.

Use of Cough Suppressants

Several principles apply to the use of antitussives, as follows:

- They are helpful and indicated to suppress dry, hacking, nonproductive irritating coughs, especially if the coughing causes sleep loss. A constant nonproductive cough can cause irritation of the trachea, leading to more coughing.
- The cough reflex should not be suppressed in the presence of copious bronchial secretions that need to be cleared. This includes situations of CF and other chronic obstructive lung diseases such as chronic bronchitis. Excess mucus secretions from the lower respiratory tract are not present in an uncomplicated cold (see the definition of a common cold at the beginning of the chapter) and indicate the need for further evaluation and possible treatment with an antibiotic.
- The combination of an expectorant and an antitussive in a cold medication is questionable. This combination suppresses the clearance mechanism, while also stimulating secretions to be cleared. Use of a single-entity cough preparation, such as Benylin DM (10 mg dextromethorphan per 5 mL) or Robitussin Pediatric (7.5 mg dextromethorphan per 5 mL), to treat a dry, irritating cough is recommended.

The combination of expectorant and antitussive is based on the rationale that a dry, hacking, frequent cough can be better replaced by a less frequent but productive cough. It can be questioned whether this is needed in an uncomplicated cold. Also, many cold compounds combine an antihistamine to dry secretions with an expectorant to stimulate mucus production. The rationale for this is questionable.

COLD COMPOUNDS

Table 15-6 lists selected cold remedies, with the classes of agents included in the compounds. Table 15-6 includes single-ingredient products, such as Sudafed, and examples of compounds with multiple drug classes, such as Sudafed PE Sinus and Allergy. Some preparations in elixir form use significant amounts of alcohol as a solvent. NyQuil Cold/Flu liquid contains 10% alcohol; however, you can find it alcohol free. Another confusing aspect of cold remedies is the variation in ingredients of formulas that are all under the same basic brand name with suffixed initials to indicate substituted or deleted ingredients. For example, Robitussin, Robitussin Cough & Allergy liquid, Robitussin

TABLE 15-6   Categories of Ingredients Found in Selected Cold Medications

TRADE NAME	ADRENERGIC	ANTIHISTAMINE	EXPECTORANT	ANTITUSSIVE
Claritin 24-Hour Allergy		Loratadine, 10 mg		
Cheratussin AC expectorant cough suppressant			Guaifenesin, 100 mg	Codeine, 10 mg
Mucinex D	Pseudoephedrine, 60 mg		Guaifenesin, 600 mg	
Neo-Synephrine	Phenylephrine, 1%			
Robitussin			Guaifenesin, 100 mg/5 mL	
Robitussin Cough & Allergy liquid	Phenylephrine, 5 mg	Chlorpheniramine, 2 mg		Dextromethorphan, 10 mg
Robitussin DM liquid			Guaifenesin, 100 mg	Dextromethorphan, 10 mg
Sudafed tablets	Pseudoephedrine, 30 and 60 mg			
Sudafed PE Sinus & Allergy tablets	Phenylephrine, 10 mg	Brompheniramine, 4 mg		
Vicks 44 Cough Relief				Dextromethorphan, 10 mg/5 mL
Robitussin Cold, Cough & Congestion	Pseudoephedrine, 30 mg		Guaifenesin, 200 mg	Dextromethorphan, 10 mg
Robitussin DAC	Pseudoephedrine, 30 mg		Guaifenesin, 100 mg	Codeine, 10 mg

Cold, Cough & Congestion, and Robitussin DAC all vary in ingredients (see Table 15-6). Because these compounds change fairly rapidly, no list remains current in terms of what is on the market. The basic principle of using the typical four classes of combination compounds remains, however, and new compounds can be evaluated for particular uses by considering the effects of these four classes of agents.

Many compounds are available as OTC preparations, thus requiring no prescription. The possibilities of overdose and abuse by combining prescribed compounds and OTC compounds are real. Often OTC preparations have the same classes of ingredients but in lower concentrations.

Treating a Cold

There is no cure for the common cold, and the four classes of drugs used in cold remedies treat only symptoms. Their potentially undesirable effects should be considered:

- *Sympathomimetics:* Tremor, tachycardia, and increased blood pressure can be seen, especially when these agents are used orally. Rebound congestion can occur if used for longer than a day.
- *Antihistamines:* These agents can cause drowsiness and impaired responses. Drying of secretions, whether caused by antimuscarinic or antihistamine action, may suppress a needed defense reaction of the airways. Nocturnal use is indicated more than around-the-clock use.
- *Expectorants:* Many of these agents have questionable efficacy in a cold. The best expectorant, especially with colds, is plain water and juices, avoiding caffeinated beverages, such as tea or colas, and beer or other alcoholic mixtures.

- *Antitussives:* These agents are useful in the presence of an irritating, persistent, nonproductive cough. Productive coughs should not be suppressed, and the logic of an expectorant-antitussive combination is questionable.

A combination of all four classes of drugs in one compound does not allow acute or occasional use of the sympathomimetic for decongestion, nocturnal use of antihistamines, and separate use of an expectorant or antitussive, as indicated by symptoms. Single-entity cold medications, such as Sudafed for decongestion or Delsym for cough suppression, are available to treat specific symptoms based on the principles outlined. Fluids and rest remain a basic and rational approach to managing colds and preventing spread of the rhinovirus, but this approach is probably the least feasible for current lifestyles.

RESPIRATORY CARE ASSESSMENT OF COLD AND COUGH AGENTS

Respiratory care assessment of cold and cough agents is directed primarily at cardiac and pulmonary side effects. Many of the agents discussed are over-the-counter (OTC) preparations, so education of the patient is imperative.

Before Treatment

- Determine whether the patient is febrile. If so, this is a distinguishing feature of flu versus a cold.
- Monitor vital signs, including blood pressure, because cold and cough agents can easily affect changes in cardiovascular status.

- Ensure the patient is not in need of transportation; some agents may cause drowsiness.
- If selecting a combination agent, determine what is needed to relieve symptoms. Combination agents frequently include agents that are not needed.

During Treatment and Short Term

- Monitor for any changes in vital signs.
- Agents treat only symptoms.

Long Term

- These agents are for short-term use only. Do not overuse or overdose on these agents.

General Contraindications

- Decongestant agents can lead to an increase in blood pressure and heart rate. If a patient is being treated for cardiovascular problems, notifying the physician is warranted.
- A patient with a productive cough should not have it suppressed by an antitussive agent.

? SELF-ASSESSMENT QUESTIONS

Answers can be found in Appendix A.

1. Identify the four classes of ingredients found in cold medications.
2. For each of the following agents, identify the category (e.g., adrenergic, antitussive): codeine, chlorpheniramine, phenylephrine, dextromethorphan, pseudoephedrine.
3. What is the intended purpose of α-adrenergic agents in cold medications?
4. What is the intended effect of antihistamines (H_1 blockers) in cold medications?
5. Are antihistamines in cold remedies H_1 or H_2 blockers?
6. You drink several beers at a friend's house after taking a dose of Benadryl. Should you drive home, and why or why not?
7. Identify the most common expectorant in over-the-counter (OTC) cold remedies.
8. Briefly explain how guaifenesin stimulates mucus production.
9. List some specific fluids you would recommend to someone with a cold.
10. Differentiate a "cold" from the "flu."

CLINICAL SCENARIO

Answers can be found in Appendix A.

A 24-year-old respiratory therapy student approaches you after class. He is a previously healthy man, of normal weight, and with mild but irregular physical activity. He complains of mild malaise, a runny stuffy nose, sneezing, and a slight sore throat. In response to questioning, he denies headache or muscle ache, describes the malaise as a very mild fatigue, and states that he noticed a gradually increasing rhinitis over a period of hours, with sneezing beginning during the first 6 hours of these symptoms. He has no fever.

Using the SOAP method, assess this clinical scenario.

REFERENCES

1. Hatton RC, Winterstein AG, McKelvey RP, et al: Efficacy and safety of oral phenylephrine: systematic review and meta-analysis. *Ann Pharmacother* 41:381–390, 2007.
2. Simons FE, Simons KJ: Histamine and H(1)-antihistamines: celebrating a century of progress. *J Allergy Clin Immunol* 128(6):1139–1150, 2011.
3. Du Buske LM: Clinical comparison of histamine H_1-receptor antagonist drugs. *J Allergy Clin Immunol* 98:S307, 1996.
4. Mahdy AM, Webster NR: Histamine and antihistamines. *Anaesth Intensive Care Med* 15(5):250–255, 2014.
5. Meltzer EO: Intranasal anticholinergic therapy of rhinorrhea. *J Allergy Clin Immunol* 90:1055, 1992.
6. Bousquet J, Chanez P, Michel FB: Pathophysiology and treatment of seasonal allergic rhinitis. *Respir Med* 84(Suppl A):11, 1990.
7. Petty TL: The National Mucolytic Study: results of a randomized, double-blind, placebo-controlled study of iodinated glycerol in chronic obstructive bronchitis. *Chest* 97:75, 1990.
8. Rubin BK, Ramirez O, Ohar JA: Iodinated glycerol has no effect on pulmonary function, symptom score, or sputum properties in patients with stable chronic bronchitis. *Chest* 109:348, 1996.
9. Irwin RS, Baumann MH, Bolser DC, et al, American College of Chest Physicians (ACCP): Diagnosis and management of cough executive summary: ACCP evidence-based clinical practice guidelines. *Chest* 129:1S, 2006.
10. Covington TR: OTC cough suppressants/expectorants. *Facts Comp Drug Newsl* 10:4, 1991.
11. Ziment I: Inorganic and organic iodides. In Braga PC, Allegra L, editors: *Drugs in bronchial mucology,* New York, 1989, Raven Press.
12. Alstead S: Potassium iodide and ipecacuanha as expectorants. *Lancet* 2:932, 1939.
13. Huang T, Peterson GH: Pulmonary edema and iododerma induced by potassium iodide in the treatment of asthma. *Ann Allergy* 46:264, 1981.
14. Donaldson SH, Bennett WD, Zeman KL, et al: Mucus clearance and lung function in cystic fibrosis with hypertonic saline. *N Engl J Med* 354:241–250, 2006.
15. *Drug facts and comparisons,* St. Louis, 2014, Facts & Comparisons, Wolters Kluwer Health.

CHAPTER **16**

Selected Agents of Pulmonary Value

Douglas S. Gardenhire, Lynda T. Goodfellow

CHAPTER OUTLINE

OBJECTIVES

After reading this chapter, the reader will be able to:

1. Define key terms and definitions pertaining to selected agents of pulmonary value
2. Discuss the indication for α₁-proteinase inhibitor therapy
3. Recognize α₁-proteinase inhibitor deficiency in a patient
4. List available α₁-proteinase inhibitors
5. List three types of formulations for nicotine replacement
6. Recognize the advantages and disadvantages of nicotine replacement

7. Discuss the indication for nitric oxide
8. Describe the effect of inhaled nitric oxide on a patient
9. List the two toxic products of nitric oxide
10. List the two inhaled prostacyclin analogs available in the United States
11. Name the only inhaled insulin product available in the United States

Chapter 16 presents three groups of drugs that are used for the direct treatment or prevention of respiratory disease: α_1-*proteinase inhibitors (α_1-PI, APIs)*, used in the treatment of congenital α_1-antitrypsin (α_1-AT) deficiency; *nicotine replacement* and other agents used in smoking cessation; and *pulmonary vasodilators,* used for pulmonary hypertension states in newborns and for acute respiratory distress syndrome (ARDS) in adults. Two inhaled *synthetic analogs of prostacyclin (PGI$_2$)* for the treatment of pulmonary hypertension and inhaled insulin for the treatment of diabetes are described as well.

α_1-PROTEINASE INHIBITOR (HUMAN)

KEY POINT

α_1-Proteinase inhibitor (α_1-PI, API) is given intravenously to individuals with *congenital α_1-antitrypsin (α_1-AT) deficiency* and who exhibit panacinar emphysema at a young age.

α_1-Proteinase inhibitor (α_1-PI, API) is also known as **α_1-antitrypsin (α_1-AT)** and is intended for therapy of congenital α_1-AT deficiency, which leads to emphysema. The product is prepared from pooled human plasma from normal donors, with purification and treatment to remove potentially infectious agents. The disease state is usually termed α_1-*antitrypsin deficiency,* and the deficient protein is termed α_1-*proteinase inhibitor.* The terms α_1-*antitrypsin* and α_1-*proteinase inhibitor* are used interchangeably, and refer to the same protein.

α_1-Antitrypsin Deficiency

α_1-AT deficiency is a genetic defect that can lead to the development of severe panacinar emphysema. This autosomal recessive disorder is characterized by serum API levels less than 35% of normal and manifests as panacinar emphysema at age 30 to 50 years. API deficiency is estimated to account for approximately 2% of all cases of emphysema in the United States. It is estimated that there are 60,000 to 100,000 Americans with severe α_1-AT deficiency.[1,2] Studies done in the United States vary in their estimates of the prevalence among newborns of α_1-AT deficiency, ranging from 1 in 2857 to 1 in 5097.[3] Among whites, the genetic disorder α_1-AT deficiency is as common as cystic fibrosis.[4] In about 50% of emphysema cases that result from API deficiency there is accompanying chronic bronchitis with mucus hypersecretion, perhaps as a result of secretory cell metaplasia caused by unchecked proteases in the epithelial lining fluid.[5] Emphysema caused by API deficiency is worse in the lower lung zones and can be markedly accelerated by cigarette smoking.[1]

The basic pathology of emphysema resulting from API deficiency is an imbalance between proteases (especially neutrophil elastase [NE]) and antiproteases (especially API). The main substrate for API is NE. The pathogenesis of emphysema is described as a process of alveolar wall destruction caused by insufficient protection from the protease NE, an enzyme that can cleave all forms of connective tissue and degrade elastic fiber in the lungs by solubilizing elastin. With inadequate API levels in the lung to balance the protease activity, emphysema occurs at a significantly earlier age than is normally seen. A presentation of severe emphysema at an unexpectedly young age, such as the third or fourth decade, leads to a high suspicion of a genetic defect causing inadequate API levels in the blood and subsequently in the lungs. The main role of another protease inhibitor, secretory leukocyte protease inhibitor (SLPI), which is secreted by bronchial glands and goblet cells, is to protect the airway epithelium against proteolytic injury. However, Wewers and associates[6] provided evidence that API (α_1-AT) is the predominant antiprotease protecting against NE.

KEY POINT

Individuals who are homozygous (have both recessive alleles) for the defective gene that expresses *API* lack this enzyme to balance the action of *neutrophil elastase (NE)*, another enzyme in the lung that solubilizes connective tissue, causing alveolar wall destruction.

Genetics

API is a 54-kDa glycoprotein encoded by a single gene on chromosome 14. The alleles of the API gene can be categorized as follows[5]:

- **API normal**: Normal serum levels of normal-functioning API
- **API deficient**: Lower than normal serum concentrations of API with altered electrophoretic properties
- **API null**: Undetectable API levels in the serum
- **API dysfunctional**: Normal amounts of abnormally functioning API

Persons with normal alleles for API (designated by the letter *M* for the alleles) are termed *PI*MM,* for protease inhibitor with a pair of the normal alleles. They are homozygous for the normal allele. Normal values for serum API are 150 to 350 mg/dL based on comparison with a commercial standard preparation and 20 to 48 μM based on comparison with a purified laboratory standard. The commercially available preparations are about 40% higher in concentration than the purified laboratory standards. Results referenced to the commercial standard are expressed as milligrams per deciliter, whereas comparisons with the highly purified (true) standard are given in micromolar units. Commercial standard values can be converted to true standard values by multiplying the commercial value by 0.71.[5,6]

About 95% of persons in the severely deficient category are homozygous for the Z allele and are designated as PI*ZZ. Serum levels of API in these individuals range from 2.5 to 7 μM, or a mean of about 16% of normal.[5] The Z allele is rare in Asians and African Americans. Alleles that do not express API at all are quite rare, and such individuals are designated as PI type null-null. PI type null-null individuals have an absence of measurable API in the serum. Wewers and colleagues[6] described the treatment of a patient with the null-null phenotype and no measurable API serum levels. They were able to show that intravenously administered augmentation therapy with α_1-AT (API) led to normal API levels in the blood and in the lung epithelial lining fluid.

The major risk factor for developing emphysema among PI*ZZ individuals seems to be cigarette smoking, in which emphysema appears much earlier than in nonsusceptible individuals, as previously noted. Other features seen with airflow obstruction in PI*ZZ individuals include a history of pneumonia, episodes of increased cough and sputum production, and a parental history of emphysema.[2]

Indication for Drug Therapy

API therapy is indicated for long-term replacement therapy in individuals with congenital deficiency of API and clinically demonstrable panacinar emphysema. At present four agents are available: Augmentation therapy and maintenance are indicated only for patients who have established API deficiency.[7] Results from controlled, long-term trials to show that long-term therapy halts the progression of emphysema are unavailable because of inherent difficulties in such trials, including the need for large numbers of patients.[1] API therapy has been provided only to adult subjects. Given the nature of the disease and the action of the drugs, the drugs cannot reverse damage or improve lung function. These drugs are extremely expensive, costing $25,000 to $40,000 per year for therapy. A cost-effectiveness analysis of Prolastin-C concluded that α_1-AT replacement therapy is cost-effective in individuals who have severe α_1-AT deficiency and severe chronic obstructive pulmonary disease (COPD).[8]

The American Thoracic Society (ATS) stated that API augmentation therapy should be used for patients with a serum concentration of API less than 11 μM, or 80 mg/dL.[2,9] API therapy is not indicated for patients with emphysema related to cigarette smoking who have normal or heterozygous phenotypes.[5] It is not indicated for individuals with liver disease associated with API deficiency, unless they also have lung disease. ATS guidelines suggest using augmentation therapy if lung function studies become abnormal and if serial studies show deterioration.

Dosage and Administration

The recommended dosage of API is 60 mg/kg of body weight, given once weekly. The dose is given intravenously at a rate of 0.08 mL/kg/min or greater, depending on patient comfort, and usually takes about 15 to 70 minutes for total infusion. Table 16-1 provides a summary of Aralast NP, Prolastin-C, Zemaira, and Glassia.

Warnings and Adverse Reactions

Because API agents are derived from human plasma, there is a risk of disease transmission. Although there was some variation in reactions to each API agent, fever, exacerbation, and flulike symptoms were most common.

TABLE 16-1	α_1-Proteinase Inhibitors Currently Available
BRAND NAME	**STRENGTH (mg)**
Aralast NP*	400 and 800 (active)
Glassia†	1000
Prolastin-C*	500 and 1000
Zemaira*	1000‡

*Powder form; reconstitution must take place before administration.
†Ready to use liquid; no reconstitution needed.
‡Must be administered through a filter.

RESPIRATORY CARE ASSESSMENT OF THERAPY OF α_1-PROTEINASE INHIBITOR (HUMAN)

Respiratory care assessment of α_1-AT replacement therapy is directed primarily at lung function and the rate of change of airflow obstruction in patients.

Before Treatment

- Pulmonary function testing of flow rates is used to monitor the degree of airflow obstruction over long-term use of the drug.

During Treatment and Short Term

- Smoking status should be monitored, and individuals with α_1-AT deficiency who smoke should receive both education on the effect of smoking with this disease and direction to resources to aid in smoking cessation (drug therapy and behavior modification assistance).

Long Term

- Overall pulmonary health should be assessed based on frequency and severity of respiratory infections, cough, sputum production if present, and hospitalization rate.

General Contraindications

- API agents are derived from human plasma; therefore, disease transmission is possible.

SMOKING CESSATION DRUG THERAPY

KEY POINT

Smoking cessation agents include nicotine as a transdermal patch, chewing gum, nasal spray, or inhaler as substitute therapy for *smoking cessation* in individuals with a strong physical addiction and withdrawal symptoms from nicotine absorbed during smoking. A tapered dose regimen allows withdrawal with minimal symptoms and assists in reducing the craving for cigarettes. *Bupropion,* an antidepressant, and *varenicline* have been found to be helpful in smoking cessation.

Nicotine and lobeline are naturally occurring alkaloids that are capable of stimulating acetylcholine receptors at the autonomic ganglia of the sympathetic and the parasympathetic systems and cholinergic nicotinic receptors at skeletal muscle sites (see Chapter 5) and in the brain. The structures of these two agents are shown in Figure 16-1. The affinity of nicotine for ganglionic and neuromuscular receptor sites led to the use of the term *nicotinic* to distinguish these receptors from *muscarinic* receptors because all of these receptors use acetylcholine as a neurotransmitter.

Lobeline is a plant derivative that has less potency than nicotine but a similar spectrum of action. Nicotine itself has greater affinity for ganglionic receptors than for skeletal

muscle nicotinic receptors. The response to nicotine stimulation involves simultaneous discharge of the sympathetic and parasympathetic systems. The sympathetic effect predominates in the cardiovascular system, with hypertension, tachycardia, and peripheral vasoconstriction. Part of the sympathomimetic effect is mediated by nicotinic stimulation of receptors on the adrenal medulla, leading to release of epinephrine and norepinephrine. Nicotine produces a parasympathetic effect in the gastrointestinal and urinary tracts, with nausea, vomiting, diarrhea, and urination. Response to nicotine is dose-dependent, and increasing or toxic doses can produce a depolarizing blockade of receptors. Stimulation of neuromuscular receptors causes tremor and loss of hand steadiness.

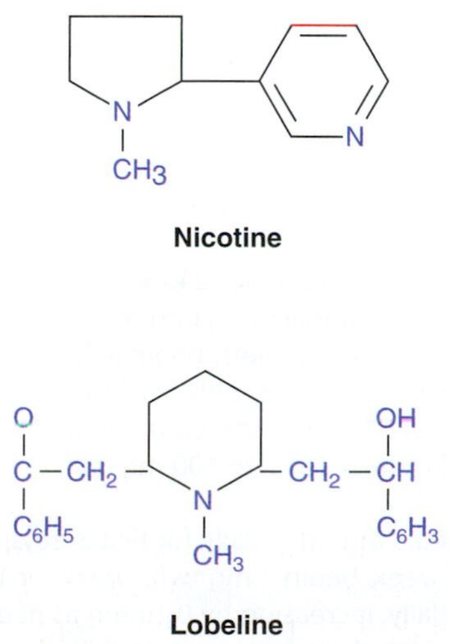

In addition to stimulating nicotinic receptors at the autonomic ganglia, neuromuscular junctions, and adrenal medulla, nicotine binds to receptors in the central nervous system (CNS). This action causes respiratory stimulation, tremors, convulsions, nausea, and emesis. The last two effects are often seen when nicotine is first inhaled as tobacco smoke, although tolerance rapidly occurs. Nicotine is the chief alkaloid in tobacco products, and addiction to nicotine is the basis for tobacco dependence. In a seasoned smoker, within seconds of inhaling from a cigarette, the internal carotid arteries carry a large bolus of nicotine to the brain, where it binds to nicotine receptors.[10] This binding causes secretion of dopamine, which causes a feeling of pleasure and cognitive arousal. Nicotine also increases levels of norepinephrine, β-endorphin, acetylcholine, serotonin, and other substances in the CNS, all of which increases the sensation of euphoria and well-being; enhance concentration, alertness, and memory; and decrease tension and anxiety. Sensitivity and responsiveness to nicotine in the CNS are genetically determined and constitute the basis for forming the physiologic addiction to nicotine. Without the proper genetic substrate, a smoker cannot become nicotine dependent. About 10% of smokers lack this substrate and are not physiologically dependent; 90% have the substrate and are nicotine addicted to various degrees.[10]

Cigarette smoking is a preventable cause of cardiovascular and lung disease. It is well known now that smoking accelerates the rate of decline of lung function that occurs with aging. Aggressive smoking intervention and cessation reduce the age-related decline in forced expiratory volume in 1 second (FEV_1) among middle-aged smokers.[11] Withdrawal from the nicotine in tobacco products is difficult because the stimulatory and reward effects are lost, and physical symptoms occur. The latter include craving for nicotine, nervousness, irritability, anxiety, drowsiness, sleep disturbance, impaired concentration, and increased appetite with attendant weight gain. Nicotine replacement therapy, in various dosing formulations, is intended to aid with smoking cessation by allowing initial replacement and then gradual withdrawal of the nicotine found in tobacco. Because nicotine is well absorbed from the skin and mucosa, a transdermal patch, a chewable gum formulation, a nasal spray, and an inhaler have been developed.

Figure 16-1 Chemical structures of nicotine and lobeline, both of which are nicotinic agonists.

Indication for Use

Nicotine replacement agents are indicated as an aid to smoking cessation to relieve nicotine withdrawal symptoms. Replacement therapy should be used as part of a comprehensive smoking cessation program to increase compliance and reduce relapse. Smokers with signs of strong physical dependence on nicotine may benefit the most from nicotine replacement therapy. Signs of strong physical dependence[10] are listed in Box 16-1.

Drug Formulations

Smoking cessation drug therapy includes various formulations of agents. The U.S. Department of Health and Human Services' Public Health Service 2008 update on guidelines to treat tobacco dependence categorizes pharmacotherapy into first- and second-line agents.[12] First-line medications include nicotine replacement, bupropion (Zyban), and varenicline (Chantix). Second-line agents include clonidine (Catapres) and nortriptyline (Pamelor). Table 16-2 lists pharmaceutical details on the various agents in use at the time of this edition. Goodfellow and Waugh[13] reviewed tobacco prevention and smoking cessation agents. Details on nicotine substitute agents can be found in manufacturers' literature.[14]

BOX 16-1	Signs of Strong Physical Addiction or Dependence on Nicotine

- Smokes more than 15 cigarettes per day
- Prefers brands with nicotine levels above 0.9 mg
- Has habit of inhaling smoke frequently and deeply
- Smokes within 30 minutes of rising
- Finds it difficult to give up the first morning cigarette and smokes more frequently in the morning
- Finds it difficult to refrain from smoking in smoke-free environments
- Smokes even when ill enough to be bedridden

Nicotine Transdermal System

The nicotine transdermal system is a multilayered unit that delivers time-released nicotine for 24 hours after application to the skin. Approximately 68% of the nicotine released from the system enters the circulation. Products may differ in their kinetics. These latex-free transdermal products provide a more consistent level of nicotine than the gum or lozenge. This is an easy, convenient, and inconspicuous method of nicotine replacement delivery. A common side effect is skin irritation at the site, but this is minimized by alternating sites. Any skin site that is clean, dry, and hairless can be used. The largest patch (21 mg) is equal to approximately half a pack of cigarettes per day. Compliance with recommended nicotine replacement transdermal plans leads to higher rates of cessation compared with nicotine polacrilex over-the-counter (OTC) products.[15]

TABLE 16-2	Smoking Cessation Drug Formulations	
CATEGORY	**BRAND NAME**	**DOSAGE**
Nicotine transdermal system	NicoDerm CQ* (OTC)	21 mg/day for first 6 wk, 14 mg/day for next 2 wk, 7 mg/day for last 2 wk
	Nicotrol (available prescription only)	15 mg/day for first 12 wk, 10 mg/day for next 2 wk, 5 mg/day for last 2 wk
Nicotine polacrilex (Nicotine Resin Complex)	Nicorette (gum)	2 mg if <25 cigarettes/day: 9 pieces/day, maximum 24 pieces/day; 4 mg if ≥25 cigarettes/day: 9 pieces/day, maximum of 24 pieces/day
	Commit (lozenge)	2 mg and 4 mg, no more than 5 lozenges in 6 hr, maximum 20 lozenges/day
	Nicotrol NS	0.5 mg/spray, one in each nostril (1 mg); 1 or 2 doses/hr (2 sprays with nasal spray, 1 each nostril, is 1 dose), up to 5 doses/hr, or 40 doses/day
	Nicotrol Inhaler	4 mg/use; recommended dosage 24-64 mg (6-16 cartridges)/day, up to 12 wk, with gradual reduction over 12 wk
Nonnicotine—antidepressant	Zyban SR, XL (Generic-Bupropion)	150-mg sustained-release tablets; begin at 150 mg/day for 3 days; increase to 150 mg/day bid, with maximum of 300 mg/day, interval of 8 hr between doses; continue treatment for 7-12 wk
	Aventyl, Pamelor (Generic- Nortriptyline)	25-mg tablet daily, increasing to 100 mg daily
Nonnicotine—nicotinic receptor agonist	Chantix (Generic- Varenicline)	1-wk titration of 0.5 mg once daily for first 3 days, twice daily for remainder of week; begin 1 mg twice daily for 11 wk
Nonnicotine— antihypertensive agent	Catapres (Generic- Clonidine)	0.10-mg tablet daily, increasing by 0.10 mg as needed; 0.10-mg transdermal patch daily, increasing to 0.20-mg patch as needed

OTC, Over-the-counter.
*Committed quitters.

Nicotine Polacrilex (Nicotine Resin Complex)

Nicotine polacrilex, a resin complex, is available as a chewing gum, lozenge, nasal spray, and inhaler. *Nicotine polacrilex gum* contains nicotine bound to an ion-exchange resin in a chewing gum base. The gum can be difficult to chew, causing jaw ache, and has a bad taste. Absorption of the active nicotine can be inconsistent, although it is faster than with the transdermal patch. Absorption of nicotine is reduced if acidic beverages such as coffee, soda, or orange juice are taken simultaneously. Users are instructed to chew the gum until malleable, then "park" it between the cheek and gum, repeating this every few minutes each time the taste is gone. Chewing slowly titrates the dose of nicotine received. Intermittent rather than continuous chewing slows the buccal absorption of the nicotine released; this also slows the amount of nicotine swallowed, which is not well absorbed from the stomach and can cause gastrointestinal irritation. Each piece of gum (2 or 4 mg) delivers about 50% of its nicotine.

The *nicotine lozenge* is a hard resin complex that is bound with nicotine. The lozenge is placed in the user's mouth to dissolve slowly, with occasional transfer from side to side until dissolved. Users should refrain from drinking liquids 15 minutes before or during use and should not chew or swallow the lozenge.

The *nicotine nasal spray* offers the advantage of producing rapid peak plasma levels of nicotine by delivering the spray directly to the nasal membranes, which may help to reduce or control cravings to smoke. Irritant effects with the nasal spray may include runny nose and nasal irritation, sneezing, cough, and watery eyes. Although rapid relief may be obtained, administration is more obtrusive than with the patch or the gum formulations.

The *nicotine inhaler* offers smokers a "simulated cigarette"; the kit contains a 10-mg/cartridge unit dose, which delivers 4 mg/use; a mouthpiece; blister trays of nicotine cartridges; and a plastic case. The use of a mouthpiece resembling a cigarette holder allows delivery of the nicotine in a manner similar to smoking a cigarette, with oral gratification. This system delivers less nicotine than the other systems. All of the nicotine is absorbed across the oropharyngeal membranes.[10] The inhaler may be most useful in a smoker with low dependency, as an adjunct to the patch to treat sudden cravings, or in combination with bupropion.

Bupropion (Zyban)

Bupropion is an antidepressant found in Wellbutrin; it is also a nonnicotine aid to smoking cessation. The drug is a relatively weak inhibitor of neuronal uptake of norepinephrine, serotonin, and dopamine, which is the basis for its antidepressant effect. The exact mechanism by which bupropion aids in smoking cessation is unknown. Bupropion (Zyban) may relieve nicotine withdrawal by slowing the normal reuptake of dopamine or preventing its breakdown in the CNS. It has been shown that mood and emotional state are related to the need for smoking and nicotine, although bupropion is effective in smoking cessation even if the smoker is not depressed.[10] Symptoms of nicotine dependence among smokers are correlated with the magnitude of symptoms of depression. Subjects who are negative or depressed are less likely to be able to quit smoking. This finding would indicate that the antidepressant effect of bupropion assists in smoking cessation. Jorenby and associates[16] found little difference between a placebo group and a nicotine patch group in smoking cessation at 12 months (15.6% versus 16.4%). A group receiving bupropion alone achieved a 30.3% cessation rate, and the combination of bupropion and nicotine patch gave the highest cessation rate of 35.5%. This study suggests that bupropion added to nicotine substitutes in a program of smoking cessation is helpful. Only about 6% of smokers succeed in quitting with no replacement therapy.[16]

Use of bupropion is associated with a dose-dependent risk of seizure. Doses less than 300 mg/day are generally safer and have a risk of about 0.1% for seizure. If a patient has not made significant progress toward abstinence from smoking by week 7, it is unlikely that the effort will be successful, and bupropion should be discontinued for that attempt. Dose tapering for discontinuation is not required.

Coadministration of bupropion with a monoamine oxidase inhibitor (MAOI) or other medications containing bupropion is contraindicated. The drug should not be used by individuals with seizure disorders or with bulimia or anorexia nervosa, which have a higher incidence of seizures.

Varenicline (Chantix)

Varenicline is a selective $\alpha_4\beta_2$ nicotinic acetylcholine receptor partial agonist developed for explicit use in smoking cessation. Varenicline (Chantix) works by attaching to $\alpha_4\beta_2$ receptors, inhibiting the activation of this receptor by nicotine. The sensation produced by smoking is blocked, breaking the cycle of nicotine addiction.[17] Varenicline is administered in a 12-week-long treatment process that begins with a 1-week titration process. The most common adverse reactions with use of varenicline were nausea, insomnia, constipation, and vomiting.

In clinical trials, varenicline produced a 39% quit rate compared with 20% for bupropion and 11% for placebo after 12 weeks.[18] In another study, varenicline produced quit rates of 44% and 49%, respectively, at lower and higher doses of the drug compared with a placebo (12%).[19] Current clinical trials are investigating combination therapy of varenicline with other drug therapies such as naltrexone and bupropion. Ebbert and colleagues[20] found that participants taking a combination of varenicline and bupropion SR at 52 weeks achieved a 31% prolonged abstinence rate in a randomized multicenter controlled trial. Another study of heavy drinkers combined varenicline with naltrexone (used for treatment of alcohol dependence) and found this combination more effective than a placebo and monotherapy in reducing consumption of both cigarettes and alcohol.[21]

Precautions

Individuals receiving nicotine replacement therapy should be informed that the replacement formulations do contain active nicotine. If nicotine replacement products are used while still using tobacco products, potentially toxic concentrations of nicotine can occur in the blood. Individuals should stop smoking when initiating therapy. Transference of nicotine dependency from the tobacco product to the replacement product can occur. Use within a program of smoking cessation is encouraged to achieve complete withdrawal. Replacement formulations should be gradually withdrawn and stopped by 3 months. Use of nicotine replacement therapy should be carefully weighed in patients with cardiovascular disease, including coronary artery disease, cardiac arrhythmias, or vasospastic disease, and in patients with hypertension.

Health care workers should avoid handling active nicotine products, such as patches, because nicotine is easily absorbed through the skin. Washing with soap increases absorption; it is recommended to only use water. Used products must be disposed of properly so that children or pets are not exposed.

Clonidine (Catapres)

Clonidine (Catapres) is an antihypertensive agent that has been prescribed to reduce symptoms of opioid and alcohol withdrawl.[12] At present clonidine is not approved by the U.S. Food and Drug Administration (FDA) for use as a smoking cessation aid. It can be taken orally or is available as a transdermal patch. Common side effects include drowsiness, fatigue, depression, nausea, and weight gain. More importantly, this agent should not be stopped abruptly; this can cause nervousness, tremors, headache, and increased blood pressure.

Nortriptyline (Aventyl, Pamelor)

Nortriptyline is a tricyclic antidepressant approved by the FDA to treat depression. It is not FDA approved for use as a smoking cessation aid. However, similar to bupropion, it is thought to have an effect on tobacco dependence because of its antidepressant mode of action.[11] As with other antidepressants, common side effects include dizziness, insomnia, and blurred vision.

RESPIRATORY CARE ASSESSMENT OF SMOKING CESSATION DRUG THERAPY

The primary outcome of interest with smoking cessation drug therapy is success in quitting over the long term.

Before Treatment

- Patient must be willing to quit. The higher the willingness, the more successful the outcome.

During Treatment and Short Term

- Monitor abstinence rates at intervals of 3, 6, or 12 months.
- Monitor for symptoms of nicotine overdosage (possible if subjects continue smoking while using nicotine substitutes), such as nausea, salivation, abdominal pain, vomiting, diarrhea, cold sweat, headache, dizziness, disturbed vision and hearing, mental confusion, or marked weakness.
- Assess bupropion use for improvement in emotional attitude, including reduction in irritability, anxiety, difficulty in concentrating, or depression.
- Assess varenicline use for improvement in nicotine withdrawal symptoms.
- Assess clonidine and nortriptyline for possible use as smoking cessation aids.
- Monitor clonidine for adverse actions related to cardiovascular status.
- Monitor nortriptyline for change in emotional state.

Long Term

- Assess patients for weight gain, and encourage an exercise program to prevent relapse caused by desire for appetite control.
- Continue to provide counseling and support throughout treatment for smoking cessation.

General Contraindications

- Nicotine replacement agents contain nicotine. Continue monitoring for nicotine overdose.
- Avoid smoking with concurrent use of nicotine replacement agents.
- Mental status should be considered with use of nonnicotine agents.

NITRIC OXIDE

KEY POINT

Nitric oxide (NO) is approved for pulmonary vascular relaxation and is used in the treatment of persistent pulmonary hypertension in newborns and investigationally in acute respiratory distress syndrome (ARDS) in adults.

Nitric oxide (NO) is a product of endothelial cells that acts as a nitrovasodilator. It was investigated for its ability to reduce pulmonary vascular resistance in various disease states, such as persistent pulmonary hypertension of the newborn (PPHN) and ARDS. Furchgott and Zawadzki[22] showed that endothelial cells in blood vessels elaborate a short-lived vasodilator, which was termed *endothelium-derived relaxing factor (EDRF)*. The neurotransmitter acetylcholine, which can normally dilate blood vessels, has no effect or vasoconstricts if applied to blood vessels without endothelium. Subsequently, the substance EDRF was identified by Palmer and colleagues[23] and Ignarro and colleagues[24] as NO. This endogenously produced vasodilator can be inhaled as a gas to cause pulmonary vasodilation.[25]

Indication for Use

NO is approved for use in neonates with hypoxic respiratory failure to reduce pulmonary artery pressure and to increase oxygenation in newborns with pulmonary hypertension and hypoxia. Off-label use of NO in adults with ARDS has been reported; however, data on its effectiveness are conflicting.[14]

Nitric oxide (INOmax) is used in conjunction with ventilatory support and other critical care measures in the treatment of term and near-term (>34 weeks) neonates with hypoxic respiratory failure associated with clinical or echocardiographic evidence of pulmonary hypertension. Off-label uses of NO include reduction of pulmonary vascular resistance and pulmonary artery pressure during neonatal cardiac surgery, treatment of hypoxemia or pulmonary hypertension after lung transplantation, and treatment of ARDS. NO has been approved with an orphan drug designation.

Dosage and Administration

NO, supplied in two sizes of gas cylinder, is available at 100 ppm and 800 ppm. The recommended dose is 20 ppm. The treatment should be maintained up to 14 days or until the underlying oxygenation problem has resolved and the neonate can be successfully weaned from NO. In the Neonatal Inhaled Nitric Oxide Study (NINOS) trial, most patients who failed to improve on 20 ppm and whose dose was increased to 80 ppm had no response at the higher concentration.[27] The risk of methemoglobinemia and elevated nitrogen dioxide (NO_2) levels increases significantly at doses greater than 20 ppm, as discussed subsequently.

The safety and effectiveness of NO were established in patients receiving other critical care support for hypoxic respiratory failure, including vasodilators, intravenous fluids, bicarbonate therapy, and mechanical ventilation. Additional therapies might be needed to maximize oxygen delivery, such as surfactant administration and high-frequency oscillatory ventilation. Information about the effectiveness of NO therapy in infants older than 14 days or adults is unavailable.

In clinical trials of NO, the delivery system used was the INOvent system (Ikaria, Clinton, N.J.), which gives a constant concentration of NO during the respiratory cycle with minimal NO_2 generation. The following summarizes guidelines for the safe administration of NO, based on several sources listed in the references, including a statement by the American Academy of Pediatrics[3,26,27]:

- Blending and delivery systems should be designed and tested for accurate NO delivery, minimum NO_2 production, and capability of administering NO in constant concentration ranges in parts per million or less throughout the respiratory cycle.
- The delivery system should be calibrated using a precisely defined mixture of NO and NO_2.
- Sample gas for analysis should be drawn before the Y-piece, proximal to the patient.
- Inhaled NO and NO_2 should be monitored continuously, using chemiluminescence or electrochemical analyzers.
- Oxygen levels in the inspired gas should be measured.
- Blood methemoglobin levels should be measured frequently.
- The minimal effective concentration of NO should be used.
- Weaning from NO should be gradual to prevent arterial desaturation and pulmonary hypertension.
- Because inhaled NO is used in respiratory failure, institutions that offer NO therapy generally should have extracorporeal membrane oxygenation (ECMO) capability in the event NO therapy fails. Alternatively, a plan for timely transfer of infants to a collaborating ECMO center should be established prospectively, and transfer should be accomplished without interruption of NO therapy.

The second-to-last point is particularly significant in the clinical use of NO to manage pulmonary hypertension. When withdrawing NO, rebound hypertension occurs; this can be severe and cause oxygen desaturation. Rebound pulmonary hypertension may be due to a downregulating effect on endogenous NO production in the pulmonary endothelium. The vasodilating effect of inhaled NO ends with the removal of the gas because of its short half-life (as subsequently described), which is a result of its binding to hemoglobin. An increase in the fractional concentration of oxygen in inspired gas (FIO_2) up to 1.0 may be needed as the inhaled NO is terminated. FIO_2 can be reduced over the next few hours as pulmonary hemodynamics restabilize. Close monitoring of arterial oxygenation is crucial when weaning from NO.

KEY POINT

NO is administered as an inhaled gas; it readily diffuses into the vascular endothelium, where it *stimulates guanylyl cyclase* in the cell, *increases cyclic guanosine monophosphate (cGMP)*, and produces *smooth muscle relaxation*. NO also quickly diffuses into the bloodstream, where it is *inactivated by binding to hemoglobin*, producing methemoglobin. NO has a *short half-life* of less than 5 seconds because it is quickly bound by hemoglobin. In the presence of oxygen, NO is converted to *nitrogen dioxide*, a nitrite toxic to the lung.

Pharmacology of Nitric Oxide

The formation, mode of action, and fate of endogenous NO are diagrammed in Figure 16-2. NO is formed endogenously in vascular endothelial cells of the respiratory tract from the precursor amino acid L-arginine by several isoforms of the enzyme nitric oxide synthase (NOS). NOS requires the cosubstrates nicotinamide adenine dinucleotide phosphate (NADPH) and oxygen (O_2). In the reaction, nitrogen is contributed by the arginine; oxygen, by the

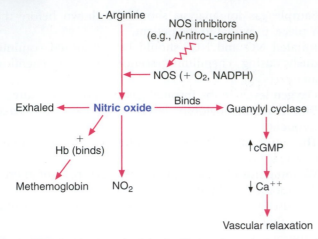

Figure 16-2 Production, physiologic effect, and metabolism of endogenous nitric oxide. *cGMP,* cyclic guanosine 3',5'-monophosphate; *Hb,* hemoglobin; *NADPH,* nicotinamide adenine dinucleotide phosphate; *NO₂,* nitrogen dioxide; *NOS,* nitric oxide synthase.

oxygen molecule; and a free electron, by NADPH. NOS is categorized as constitutive NOS (cNOS), including that found in endothelial cells (ecNOS) and in neurons (nNOS), and as inducible NOS (iNOS).[26] The vascular relaxation caused by acetylcholine is due to stimulation of cNOS, which results in an increase in NO. Histamine, leukotrienes, and bradykinin are other mediators that increase cNOS-mediated NO and promote vasodilation and lowering of blood pressure.

Proinflammatory cytokines, such as interferon-γ (IFN-γ), tumor necrosis factor-α (TNF-α), and interleukin-1 (IL-1), can induce iNOS to increase endogenous levels of NO. Glucocorticoids block the induction of iNOS and inhibit the formation of NO.[22] NO is the active form of nitrovasodilators such as nitroglycerin and sodium nitroprusside.[24] NO has also been identified as at least one of the neurotransmitters in the nonadrenergic, noncholinergic (NANC) inhibitory nervous system[26] (see Chapter 5). The endogenous production of NO can be inhibited by L-arginine analogs, which inhibit NOS—for example, N-nitro-L-arginine. The NO molecule is small and lipophilic, and it has a very short duration of action of 0.1 to 5 seconds in physiologic systems.[24,28]

NO is generated in vascular endothelial cells and diffuses rapidly into myocytes in the endothelium, binding to guanylyl cyclase. Guanylyl cyclase (also termed *guanylate cyclase*) stimulates the production of cyclic guanosine-3',5'-monophosphate (cGMP), which causes a decrease in intracellular calcium and consequent vascular or nonvascular smooth muscle relaxation. The NO-induced increase in cGMP within the cells also inhibits platelet adherence and aggregation and polymorphonuclear leukocyte chemotaxis.[27] NO readily diffuses into the blood vessel itself and into endothelial cells and enters the red blood cells to bind rapidly with hemoglobin, forming methemoglobin and becoming inactivated in the process. NO is also converted in the red blood cells to nitrate, and some endogenous NO is exhaled from the lung.[29] Because NO diffuses so readily

into the bloodstream and is inactivated by being bound to hemoglobin, its action is limited to the pulmonary vascular endothelium, whether generated endogenously within the lung or inhaled as an exogenous gas. It is a selective pulmonary vasodilator. The end products of NO that enter the systemic circulation are predominantly methemoglobin and nitrate. Nitrite is the predominant NO metabolite excreted in the urine, accounting for more than 70% of the inhaled dose. Aranda and Pearl[30] published a more detailed review of the biology of NO.

Effect on Pulmonary Circulation

With normal pulmonary hemodynamics (normal vascular resistance), inhalation of NO produces no effect on pulmonary arterial pressure or gas exchange.[22] However, Frostell and associates[31] reported that hypoxic pulmonary vasoconstriction caused by breathing 12% oxygen in healthy adults increased mean pulmonary arterial pressure from 14.7 ±0.8 mm Hg to 19.8 ±0.9 mm Hg.[29] This increase in pulmonary arterial pressure was reversed by adding 40 ppm of NO to the gas mixture. No change occurred in systemic vascular resistance because NO was inactivated locally by hemoglobin. Taylor and associates[32] found that 5 ppm of NO successfully improved oxygenation in the short term for patients with acute lung injury.

In persistent PPHN, pulmonary vascular resistance is elevated, which causes right-to-left shunting through the patent ductus arteriosus and foramen ovale. Inhaled NO dilates pulmonary blood vessels in regions of the lung where ventilation is delivered; this redistributes pulmonary blood flow from areas of low ventilation to areas with better ventilation. The improved ventilation-perfusion matching leads to an improved partial pressure of oxygen in arterial blood (PaO₂). Because NO is rapidly and locally inactivated by hemoglobin, no systemic vasodilation or hypotension occurs.[33]

Toxicity

Toxicity with exposure to NO can be caused by the NO itself, by the formation of the nitrite, NO₂, and the formation of methemoglobin. NO can be a mediator of lung injury, for example, with paraquat poisoning, in which inhibition of NOS reduces the amount of lung injury.[34] NO₂ is a strong oxidizer that causes lipid peroxidation in cells. The amount of NO₂ produced depends on the amount of NO and the amount of surrounding O₂. The higher the FIO₂, the greater the amount of oxidation of NO to NO₂. Similarly, the higher the concentration of NO, the shorter the time to achieve oxidation to NO₂. The lethal effect of NO₂ is due to pulmonary edema, and short-term exposure to more than 150 ppm of NO₂ is usually fatal.[29] In the usual doses of NO, such as 0.5% to 4%, methemoglobinemia is not usually a problem, although this should be monitored.

It is unknown whether NO can cause fetal harm when given to pregnant women, and the manufacturer notes that it is not intended for adults. It is unknown whether NO is excreted in human milk. Occupational exposure to NO is set by the Occupational Safety and Health Administration (OSHA) at 25 ppm, and exposure to NO_2 is set at 5 ppm (manufacturer's literature).

Contraindications

Nitric oxide should not be used in neonates who are known to be dependent on right-to-left shunt.

RESPIRATORY CARE ASSESSMENT OF NITRIC OXIDE

Before Treatment

- Because NO is administered in conjunction with ventilatory support, the usual measures of critical care assessment and in particular ventilator monitoring should be followed.

During Treatment and Short Term

- Evaluate therapy for a reduction in the oxygenation index (OI = mean airway pressure in cm H_2O × FIO_2/ PaO_2).
- Evaluate the effect of NO and monitor the PaO_2 and the overall level of ventilatory support (FIO_2, inspiratory pressure and time, end-expiratory pressure, rate).
- Monitor preductal and postductal pulse oximetry (SpO_2) to evaluate shunting.
- If available, review the echocardiogram to evaluate right-to-left shunting.
- Monitor inspired NO and NO_2, along with methemoglobin.
- Monitor cardiovascular status and stability, including the level of intravenous fluids and vasoactive medications needed.

Long Term

- Continue assessment of O_2, NO, NO_2, and methemoglobin levels.

General Contraindications

- NO should not be used in neonates who are dependent on a right-to-left-shunt.

SYNTHETIC ANALOGS OF PROSTACYCLIN

At present, two inhaled forms of synthetic prostacyclins (PGI_2s)are FDA approved to help decrease shortness of breath in individuals with pulmonary hypertension. The two agents available in the United States are iloprost (Ventavis) and treprostinil (Tyvaso). However, epoprostenil sodium (Flolan) has been prescribed off-label for inhalation to adults and children.

Iloprost (Ventavis)

> **! KEY POINT**
>
> Iloprost is an inhaled prostacyclin (PGI_2) available in the United States.

Iloprost is a synthetic analog of PGI_2. The drug Ventavis is made available as an inhalation solution that is delivered via one of two novel aerosol delivery devices: the I-neb AAD (adaptive aerosol delivery) system or the Prodose AAD system. Ventavis dilates systemic and pulmonary arterial vascular beds.

Indication for Use

Ventavis is indicated for the treatment of pulmonary arterial hypertension in patients with New York Heart Association (NYHA) class III or IV symptoms. NYHA is a functional and therapeutic classification of physical activity in patients with cardiac dysfunction. The classification, I through IV, describes the limitations of physical activity; NYHA III and IV are higher and pose considerable restriction on patient activity. Ventavis is not intended for pediatric use; it is intended for adults 18 years old and older. In clinical studies, Ventavis has been shown to improve NYHA functional class, improve exercise capacity, and increase walking distance.[35]

Dosage and Administration

Ventavis is supplied in 1-mL ampules with two concentrations available—10 mcg/mL and 20 mcg/mL. An initial dose of 2.5 mcg should be administered and evaluated for tolerability. If tolerated, increasing the dose to 5 mcg is acceptable. Ventavis should be administered six to nine times daily during waking hours. Doses should be given more than 2 hours apart. Ventavis is an inhalation solution. This agent should be nebulized only with the intended aerosol devices.

Precautions

Ventavis has not been studied in patients with underlying lung disease (e.g., asthma, COPD). Ventavis can cause bronchospasm. It should not be mixed with any other agents; however, patients with underlying lung disorders may benefit from pretreatment with a β agonist.

Treprostinil (Tyvaso)

> **! KEY POINT**
>
> Tyvaso is an inhaled PGI_2 vasodilator used for the treatment of pulmonary hypertension.

Treprostinil was first approved by the FDA as an injectable form in 2002. Since that time, research has been ongoing to create and test an inhaled version.[36] Inhaled treprostinil (Tyvaso) was approved for use in the United States in 2009. Tyvaso is a PGI_2 analog that causes vasodilation of the pulmonary and systemic arterial vascular beds and inhibits platelet aggregation. It is administered using the Tyvaso Inhalation System (United Therapeutics Corp., Silver Spring, Md.), which is an ultrasonic, pulsed-delivery device.

Indication for Use

Tyvaso is indicated for the treatment of pulmonary arterial hypertension to increase walking distance in patients with NYHA class III symptoms. Tyvaso is not intended for use in patients younger than 18 years.

Dosage and Administration

Tyvaso is available in a 2.9-mL ampule, which contains 1.74 mg of treprostinil (0.6 mg/mL). It is nebulized in the Tyvaso Inhalation System. The ampule is dumped into the medication cup of the nebulizer and is used for the entire day.

The patient nebulizes the prescribed amount of drug in four separate, equally spaced treatment sessions per day during waking hours. Each breath delivers 6 mcg of treprostinil. The initial dose is 3 breaths (18 mcg) per treatment session. If not tolerated, the dose may be reduced to 1 to 2 breaths per session and then increased to 3. Tyvaso should be increased by 3 breaths every 1 to 2 weeks until 9 breaths (54 mcg) per treatment session is reached.

Precautions

Tyvaso has not been studied in patients with underlying lung disease (e.g., asthma, COPD). Tyvaso may cause bronchospasm. This agent should not be mixed with any other agents.

RESPIRATORY CARE ASSESSMENT OF SYNTHETIC ANALOGS OF PROSTACYCLIN

Respiratory care assessment of prostacyclin (PGI$_2$) agents is directed primarily at lung function. These agents are capable of causing bronchospasm. Assessment of the lungs for the frequency and severity of bronchospasm is the most important.

Before Treatment

- Assess walking distance.

During Treatment and Short Term

- Monitor ventilatory and cardiovascular status.

Long Term

- Monitor effects of agents on improvement in walking distance.

General Contraindications

- PGI$_2$ agents have not been tested in patients with underlying pulmonary disorders.

INSULIN HUMAN (rDNA ORIGIN)

Insulin Human (Afrezza)

 KEY POINT

Afrezza is an inhaled from of insulin and is not recommended for use in patients with lung disease.

Individuals diagnosed with diabetes had two common formulations to regulate insulin production and control sugar: oral medications or injectable insulin. Several years ago Exubera, an orally inhaled insulin, was made available; however, Pfizer voluntarily removed it from the market in 2007 because of poor sales. Pfizer lost $2.8 billion in the research, development, and launch of the product. In 2014 the U.S. FDA approved Afrezza, an inhaled human insulin utilizing a dry powder cartridge from the Afrezza Inhaler. Although this is not a respiratory medication, side effects such as bronchospasm and reduction in lung function are possible. The respiratory therapist should be aware of its use and inhaled formulation.

Indication for Use

Afrezza is indicated to improve glycemic control in adult patients with diabetes mellitus. Afrezza is not a replacement for long-acting insulin and should be used in combination in patients with type 1 diabetes.

Dosage and Administration

Afrezza is available in 4- and 8-unit inhaled dosages. It should be used before meal time. Dosage will be individualized and should be adjusted when switching from another form of insulin.

Precautions

Afrezza has not been tested in patients who smoke or those who have lung disease. Therefore patients with a history of smoking and lung disorders should not use this form of insulin.

RESPIRATORY CARE ASSESSMENT OF INHALED INSULIN

Respiratory care assessment of inhaled insulin therapy is directed primarily at lung function. Afrezza may cause bronchospasm and exacerbate patients with a history of lung disease. In patients that were not known to have pulmonary dysfunction a decline in pulmonary function was noted.[37] Assessment of the lungs for the frequency and severity of bronchospasm is the most important.

Before Treatment

- Assess lung health; does patient have lung disease?
- Smoking status should be monitored; patients who smoke should not take the drug.

During Treatment and Short Term

- Monitor airway status; listen for abnormal breath sounds.

Long Term

- Monitor effects of agents on lung function.
- Overall pulmonary health should be assessed on the basis of frequency and severity of respiratory infections, cough, bronchospasm, and pulmonary function.

General Contraindications

- Patients with a history of smoking and lung disorders should not use this form of insulin.

 SELF-ASSESSMENT QUESTIONS

Answers can be found in Appendix A.

1. For which disease state is an α_1-proteinase inhibitor (API) indicated?
2. What is the route of administration for an API?
3. What is the mode of action of APIs in treating emphysema associated with inadequate API levels?
4. Is treatment with an API indicated for age-related emphysema or in general for individuals who smoke and have emphysema later in life?
5. Identify three pharmaceutical formulations of nicotine that are used as smoking cessation aids.
6. What is the usual effect of nicotine, whether in a smoking cessation aid or in cigarettes, on blood pressure?
7. Name two nonnicotine agents used in the treatment of smoking cessation.
8. What is the effect of inhaled nitric oxide?
9. Identify two potentially toxic byproducts of inhaled nitric oxide.
10. What is the usual dose of inhaled nitric oxide?
11. Identify two disease states in which nitric oxide has been used to reverse pulmonary hypertension.
12. What is the greatest hazard in terms of pulmonary health with the delivery of Ventavis?
13. What is the initial dose of Tyvaso?
14. What is the trade name of the only inhaled insulin on the market?
15. What patient population should avoid use of inhaled insulin?

 CLINICAL SCENARIO

Answers can be found in Appendix A.

A 42-year-old white woman with complaints of shortness of breath on exertion and increasing fatigue during her usual activities was referred by her family physician to a pulmonologist. On questioning, she reported that she had an uncle who had died "many years previously" in middle age with lung disease, but he had also smoked cigarettes. She admitted that she had been a heavy smoker (around a pack per day) for 5 or 6 years but had quit more than 8 years ago. She denied any use of alcohol. She described having several attacks of "bronchitis" in the past year, for which her family physician had prescribed antibiotics, with subsequent resolution each time. She also described a small but increasing production of sputum during the past year, usually clear unless she had an episode of bronchitis. She currently has a cough, with occasional production of a slight amount of greenish sputum. Her medications include albuterol by metered dose inhaler (MDI), prescribed by her family physician last year.

On physical examination, she appears well developed and well nourished and exhibits mild respiratory distress. Auscultation of the chest reveals expiratory wheezing, diminished breath sounds bilaterally, and a prolonged expiratory phase. There is no digital clubbing, cyanosis, pedal edema, or jugular distention. Her vital signs are as follows: temperature (T) of 37.1° C, blood pressure (BP) of 110/76 mm Hg, pulse (P) of 76 beats/min, and respiratory rate (RR) of 24 breaths/min and regular. Pulse oximetry on room air is 91%. Other findings include a mild elevation of white blood cell count (WBC) ($13.1 \times 10^3/mm^3$), normal hemoglobin and hematocrit, and normal electrolytes. Pseudomonas and normal flora were found in her sputum. A chest radiograph showed some hyperlucency; hyperinflation with moderately lowered, flattened hemidiaphragms on full inspiration; and an infiltrate in the right lower lobe. Arterial blood gas (ABG) values on room air were as follows: pH at 7.35, $PaCO_2$ of 54 mm Hg, PaO_2 of 66 mm Hg, HCO_3^- of 30 mEq/L, and SaO_2 of 92%. Pulmonary function tests showed forced expiratory volume in 1 second (FEV_1) at 60% of predicted, elevated residual volume (RV) and RV/total lung capacity (TLC) ratio, increased TLC above predicted, and decreased DL_{CO} (diffusing capacity of the lung for CO).

Using the SOAP method, assess this clinical scenario.

REFERENCES

1. Wewers MD, Casolaro MA, Sellers SE, et al: Replacement therapy for α_1-antitrypsin deficiency associated with emphysema. *N Engl J Med* 316:1055, 1987.
2. Stoller JK: Clinical features and natural history of severe α_1-antitrypsin deficiency. *Chest* 111:123S, 1997.
3. American Thoracic Society, European Respiratory Society: Standards for the diagnosis and management of individuals with alpha-1 antitrypsin deficiency. *Am J Respir Crit Care Med* 168:818, 2003.
4. Memorandum: α_1-Antitrypsin deficiency: memorandum from a WHO meeting. *Bull World Health Organ* 75:397, 1997.
5. Snider GL: α_1-Protease inhibitor deficiency and the preventive therapy of emphysema. In Leff AR, editor: *Pulmonary and critical care pharmacology and therapeutics*, New York, 2000, McGraw-Hill.
6. Wewers MD, Casolaro MA, Crystal RG: Comparison of alpha-1-antitrypsin levels and antineutrophil elastase capacity of blood and lung in a patient with the alpha-1-antitrypsin

phenotype null-null before and during alpha-1-antitrypsin augmentation therapy. *Am Rev Respir Dis* 135:539, 1987.

7. Kohnlein T, Welte T: Alpha-1 antitrypsin deficiency: pathogenesis, clinical presentation, diagnosis, and treatment. *Am J Med* 121:3–9, 2008.

8. Alkins SA, O'Malley P: Should health-care systems pay for replacement therapy in patients with α_1-antitrypsin deficiency? *Chest* 117:875, 2000.

9. American Thoracic Society: Guidelines for the approach to the patient with severe hereditary alpha-1-antitrypsin deficiency. *Am Rev Respir Dis* 140:1494, 1989.

10. Lillington GA, Leonard CT, Sachs DPL: Smoking cessation: techniques and benefits. *Clin Chest Med* 21:199, 2000.

11. Anthonisen NR, Connett JE, Kiley JP, et al: Effects of smoking intervention and the use of an inhaled anticholinergic bronchodilator on the rate of decline of FEV_1: the Lung Health Study. *JAMA* 272:1497, 1994.

12. Fiore MC, Jaen CR, Baker TB, et al: *Treating tobacco use and dependence: 2008 update*, Washington, DC, 2008, U.S. Department of Health and Human Services, Public Health Service.

13. Goodfellow LT, Waugh JB: Tobacco treatment and prevention: what works and why. *Respir Care* 54:8, 2009.

14. *Drug facts and comparisons*, St. Louis, 2014, Facts & Comparisons, Wolters Kluwer Health.

15. Hajek P, West R, Foulds J, et al: Randomized comparative trial of nicotine polacrilex, a transdermal patch, nasal spray, and an inhaler. *Arch Intern Med* 159:17, 1999.

16. Jorenby DE, Leischow SJ, Nides MA, et al: A controlled trial of sustained-release bupropion, a nicotine patch, or both for smoking cessation. *N Engl J Med* 340:685, 1999.

17. Hays JT, Ebbert JO: Varenicline for tobacco dependence. *N Engl J Med* 359:2018, 2008.

18. Nides M, Oncken C, Gonzales D, et al: Smoking cessation with varenicline, a selective $\alpha_4\beta_2$ nicotinic receptor partial agonist. *Arch Intern Med* 166:1561, 2006.

19. Oncken C, Gonzales D, Nides M, et al: Efficacy and safety of the novel selective nicotinic acetylcholine receptor partial agonist, varenicline, for smoking cessation. *Arch Intern Med* 166:1571, 2006.

20. Ebbert JO, Hatsukami DK, Croghan IT, et al: Combination varencline and bupropion SR for tobacco-dependence treatment in cigarette smokers: a randomized trial. *JAMA* 311:2, 2014.

21. Ray LA, Courtney KE, Ghahremani DG, et al: Varenicline, low dose naltrexone, and their combination for heavy-drinking smokers: human laboratory findings. *Psychopharmacology (Berl)* 2014. [Epub ahead of print].

22. Furchgott RF, Zawadzki JV: The obligatory role of endothelial cells in the relaxation of arterial smooth muscle by acetylcholine. *Nature* 288:373, 1980.

23. Palmer RMJ, Ferrige AG, Moncada S: Nitric oxide release accounts for the biological activity of endothelium-derived relaxing factor. *Nature* 327:524, 1987.

24. Ignarro LJ, Buga GM, Wood KS, et al: Endothelium derived relaxing factor produced and released from artery and vein is nitric oxide. *Proc Natl Acad Sci U S A* 84:9265, 1987.

25. Neonatal Inhaled Nitric Oxide Study Group: Inhaled nitric oxide in full-term and nearly full-term infants with hypoxic respiratory failure. *N Engl J Med* 336:597, 1997.

26. Zapol WM, Rimar S, Gillis N, et al: Nitric oxide and the lung. *Am J Respir Crit Care Med* 149:1375, 1994.

27. American Academy of Pediatrics Committee on Fetus and Newborn: Use of inhaled nitric oxide. *Pediatrics* 106:344, 2000.

28. Barnes PJ, Kharitonov SA: Exhaled nitric oxide: a new lung function test. *Thorax* 51:233, 1996.

29. Mizutani T, Layon AJ: Clinical applications of nitric oxide. *Chest* 110:506, 1996.

30. Aranda M, Pearl RG: The biology of nitric oxide. *Respir Care* 44:156, 1999.

31. Frostell CG, Blomqvist H, Hedenstierna G, et al: Inhaled nitric oxide selectively reverses human hypoxic pulmonary vasoconstriction without causing systemic vasodilation. *Anesthesiology* 78:427, 1993.

32. Taylor RW, Zimmerman JL, Dellinger RP, et al: Inhaled Nitric Oxide in ARDS Study Group: Low dose inhaled nitric oxide in patients with acute lung injury. *JAMA* 291:1603, 2004.

33. Palevsky HI: Treatment of pulmonary hypertension. In Leff AR, editor: *Pulmonary and critical care pharmacology and therapeutics*, New York, 2000, McGraw-Hill.

34. Martin WJ, Rehm S: Toxic injury of the lung parenchyma. In Leff AR, editor: *Pulmonary and critical care pharmacology and therapeutics*, New York, 2000, McGraw-Hill.

35. Olschewski H, Simonneau G, Galie N, et al: Aerosolized Iloprost Randomized Study Group: Inhaled iloprost for severe pulmonary hypertension. *N Engl J Med* 347:322, 2002.

36. Channick RN, Olschewski H, Seeger W, et al: Safety and efficacy of inhaled treprostinil as add-on therapy to bosentan in pulmonary arterial hypertension. *J Am Coll Cardiol* 48:1433, 2006.

37. Rosenstock J, Bergenstal R, Defronzo RA, et al: Efficacy and safety of technosphere inhaled insulin compared with technosphere powder placebo in insulin-naïve type 2 diabetes suboptimally controlled with oral agents. *Diabetes Care* 31:2177–2182, 2008.

CHAPTER 17

Neonatal and Pediatric Aerosolized Drug Therapy

Diana Marcela Serrato, Ruben D. Restrepo

OBJECTIVES

After reading this chapter, the reader will be able to:

1. Define key terms that pertain to neonatal and pediatric drug therapy
2. Explain off-label use of aerosolized medications
3. List and describe the most important factors affecting neonatal and pediatric aerosol drug delivery
4. Describe the clinical response of neonatal and pediatric patients to aerosolized drugs
5. Describe special circumstances related to selection of delivery devices for neonatal and pediatric patients
6. Explain the most relevant factors to select the appropriate aerosol delivery device according to age group
7. Describe the implications of compliance and cooperation on the efficiency of aerosol delivery
8. List some of the novel inhaled therapies under investigation for pediatric patients
9. Explain lung deposition of inhaled drugs in pediatric and neonatal intubated patients

KEY TERMS AND DEFINITIONS

Emitted dose Dose released by aerosol device.

Infant Child between 1 month and 1 year of age.

Inhaled (delivered) dose Dose reaching the patient's mouth or artificial airway.

Lung dose Dose reaching the trachea and beyond.

Neonatal Refers to period of time between birth and first month of life.

Nominal dose Dose in delivery device.

Off-label Use of drugs with no U.S. Food and Drug Administration (FDA)–approved labeled use.

Pediatric Refers to period of time between 1 month and 18 years of age.

BOX 17-1   Terms and Age Ranges Defining Periods from Birth to Adult

Premature neonate	Less than 37 weeks of gestational age
Neonate	First month of postnatal life
Infant	1-12 months
Child	1-12 years
Adolescent	12-18 years
Adult	Older than 18 years

Effective administration of aerosol therapy to neonates and pediatric patients is challenging. Inherent anatomic, physiologic, pathophysiologic, and behavioral factors make this age group a unique subpopulation.[1-3] The lack of **neonatal** and **pediatric** dose labeling for many drugs given by inhaled aerosol complicates determining proper doses of aerosol drugs. The number of studies on clinical deposition of aerosols in the neonatal population is very limited because of the inability to use radiolabeled aerosols. Labeling aerosol particles with radioactive agents makes it possible to quantify deposition dose and distribution in the respiratory tract. The few available lung deposition studies in infants are strikingly similar with only 2% to 5% deposition.[4,5] Results of studies on therapeutic aerosols and their lung deposition cannot simply be extrapolated from adult data. The differences between aerosol drug delivery as a form of topical administration and systemic administration of drugs are not appreciated in many instances, causing aerosol doses to be modified in neonates and children as if they were given systemically. Neonates and toddlers cannot perform an inhalation maneuver; they are usually nasal breathers and often get distressed during the administration of aerosol therapy.

Both the prescribing physician and the respiratory therapist need to be aware that a good understanding of the anatomic and physiologic characteristics associated with this age group has to be matched to selection of the proper device. When an optimal device has been selected, factors such as crying, lack of cooperation, and presence of leaks around the aerosol masks dramatically decrease lung deposition. Identification of the determinants of efficient aerosol delivery and the specific challenges of aerosol delivery to infants and young children can facilitate a systematic approach to optimize aerosol delivery to this population. All considerations in this chapter relate to inhaled aerosols used for the treatment of pulmonary disorders and not for systemic treatment. The data cited are based largely on traditional aerosol delivery devices. New, highly efficient delivery systems may lead to different results in the future. Terms used for different age ranges are given in Box 17-1.

OFF-LABEL USE OF DRUGS IN NEONATAL AND PEDIATRIC PATIENTS

KEY POINT

Pediatric patients are the most common group in which off-label use medications are prescribed.

The term **off-label** is used to refer to drugs lacking U.S. Food and Drug Administration (FDA)–approved dosage information for a specific age group or condition.[6] Off-label prescribing is a commonly used and accepted medical practice. Although these drugs do have FDA approval, the approval is for a different use. Aspirin has been a common pain reliever for more than 100 years; in 1988, physicians began prescribing it to prevent heart attacks. Use of aspirin for the prophylaxis of heart attack is considered an off-label use. It has been estimated that nearly half of all prescriptions today are written for off-label uses. Infants, children, and pregnant women are the most common groups in which off-label use medications are prescribed. The introduction of pediatric regulations in 1994 that required a sponsor to review available pediatric data to determine whether existing data were adequate to support pediatric labeling was a move in the right direction. However, no clinical studies were required. The FDA Modernization Act (FDAMA) of 1997 created pediatric exclusivity incentives for the sponsors of certain products based on Written Request (WR) from the U.S. FDA, but required that sponsors provide sufficient data and information to support direction of pediatric use for the claimed indications. In 1994 the Center for Drug Evaluation and Research of the FDA issued guidelines encouraging pediatric testing of drugs.[6] A subsequent FDA ruling mandated that drugs submitted for FDA approval after December 2000 be evaluated in children. Waivers can be given if the drug has no meaningful application in children or is likely to be unsafe or ineffective in pediatric patients.[6] There is a substantial cost associated with additional studies to document safety and efficacy in pediatric patients. The creation of the "pediatric rule" has provided the pharmaceutical companies that carry out studies with pediatric patients an economic incentive by allowing extended time of marketing before generic formulations of the product are marketed.[7] The FDA cannot, by law, regulate how a drug is used medically or "interfere with the practice of medicine."[8] FDAMA was replaced by the Best Pharmaceuticals for Children Act (BPCA) in 2002 (FDA, 2002), which renewed the FDA's authority to grant 6 months of marketing exclusivity to sponsors who conduct and submit studies in response to a WR from the agency. The Pediatric Research Equity Act (PREA) of 2003 (FDA, 2003) made the pediatric assessment of certain applications of drug and biologic products mandatory, unless the requirement was waived or deferred by the FDA. The act required pediatric assessment for application containing a new ingredient, a new indication, a new dose form, a new dosage regimen, or a new route of drug administration. Few years ago, more than 80% of the entire *Physicians' Desk Reference (PDR)* entries had either no existing dosage information for pediatric patients or specific statements that the safety and efficacy in children had not been determined. Today, more than 50% of all currently marketed drug products include pediatric information on the product labeling.[6] Additionally, not only medications but also medical devices need to be approved for pediatric use. That is why in September 2007, the United States Congress passed Title III of the FDA Amendments Act, The Pediatric Medical Device

Safety and Improvement Act, requiring that new applications or protocols submitted to the FDA for the use and approval of a medical device must include a description of any pediatric subpopulation that suffers from the condition that the device will treat, diagnose, or cure.[9]

Although it is legal for physicians to prescribe off-label use of drugs, determining drug dose becomes more problematic when standardized dose guidelines have not been previously developed during drug clinical trials. Generally, drug dosage regimen with inhaled aerosols for neonatal and pediatric patients is not based on body size and blood level but rather based on a target effect strategy with avoidance of toxicity. Aerosol doses to neonates or children are "self-limiting" because of differences between pediatric and adult airways. Even though the drug labeling often states that safety and efficacy in children have not been determined, many of the inhaled aerosol drugs reviewed in this text have clinical indications and uses in neonatal and pediatric patients. Virtually all inhaled β agonists and corticosteroid formulations have been approved by the FDA in patients older than 12 years.

Table 17-1 lists inhaled aerosol drugs and leukotriene modifiers that have an approved age labeling for pediatric use at the time of this edition. Drugs that are not listed in Table 17-1 do not have labeling for pediatric use. In March 2004, the U.S. Patent and Trademark Office (USPTO) issued a patent covering AccuNeb, the only FDA-approved (in 2001) lower concentration, unit-dose albuterol sulfate for the treatment of asthma in children 2 to 12 years old.

FACTORS AFFECTING NEONATAL AND PEDIATRIC AEROSOL DRUG DELIVERY

 KEY POINT

Although a smaller fraction of the aerosol reaches the pediatric lower airway compared with an adult, the need for age adjustment of aerosol doses based on body weight has been clinically debated.

The same mechanisms of aerosol penetration and deposition in the lung that were outlined in Chapter 3 apply to aerosol therapy in neonatal and pediatric patients. However, the airway environment differs in neonatal and pediatric subjects compared with adults. Newborns, infants, and small children have a smaller airway diameter. Besides cooperation, ability to hold a mouthpiece, and avoidance of mouth breathing, obvious limitations of inspiratory flows can greatly affect aerosol delivery and deposition. They are either obligate or preferential nose breathers, have a proportionally larger tongue, and have smaller and incompletely developed airways. These differences produce flow characteristics different from adults. Table 17-2 outlines functional and structural features of the infant lung that may affect aerosol delivery and deposition.

Although it may seem obvious that aerosol therapy in infants and young children is quite different from that of

adults, much more research is required to confirm the differences in aerosol drug delivery. Some in vitro studies have suggested that the increasing upper airway geometry in adults may explain the higher amount of aerosol deposition reaching the lower airway compared with neonatal and pediatric patients.[10] The nose may filter out 75% of the dose received by mouth breathing in adults and children. A smaller fraction of the **nominal dose** of an aerosol reaches the lower airways with the child-size oropharynx compared with an adult-size oropharynx.[11] The oral route has been considered superior to the nasal route for aerosol delivery to the lower respiratory tract (LRT) in adults and children. However, this may not be the case in infants. Amirav et al recently used radio-labeled (99mDTPA) normal saline solution aerosol generated by a soft-mist inhaler and aerosol delivered via a valved holding chamber (VHC) and an air-tight mask to a simulated 5- to 20-month-old airway model. They found that nasal delivery to the LRT exceeded that of oral delivery in the 5- and 14-month models and was equivalent to oral delivery in the 20-month model, and that differences between nasal and oral delivery diminished with "age"/size.[12] The smaller diameter of neonatal and pediatric lower airways, added to the effects of bronchoconstriction, inflammation, secretions, and the possible presence of an endotracheal tube, dramatically decreases aerosolized drug deposition in the lungs.[13] Some other variables associated with the reduction in **lung dose** in infants and young children are discussed subsequently.

Effect of Age on Aerosol Lung Dose

Systemic side effects, rather than local side effects caused by treatment in the lung, have been the basis for aerosol dose adjustment for age, which is usually based on body weight. However, the need for age adjustment of aerosol doses based on body weight has been clinically debated.[14] Available data suggest that the actual dose of an inhaled aerosol drug could be between 0.1% and 1% in neonates and infants[15-17] and around 2.5% in young children compared with 8% to 22% in adults.[17,18] Although a smaller percentage of the aerosol deposits in the lungs, small patients may receive a considerably higher rate of drug per kilogram of body weight than adults. However, the lower deposition may provide a comparable safety and efficacy profile to that of adults.[19]

Wildhaber and colleagues[20,21] studied children 2 to 9 years of age with stable asthma inhaling radiolabeled salbutamol from a nebulizer and a pressurized metered dose inhaler (pMDI) through a nonstatic holding chamber. Mean (absolute dose) total lung deposition expressed as a percentage of the nebulized dose was 5.4% (108 mcg) in younger children (<4 years) and 11.1% (222 mcg) in older children (>4 years). Mean (absolute dose) total lung deposition expressed as a percentage of the metered dose was 5.4% (21.6 mcg) in younger children and 9.6% (38.4 mcg) in older children. The authors reported equivalent percentages of total lung deposition of radiolabeled salbutamol aerosolized by either a nebulizer or a pMDI with holding chamber within each age group. However, the delivery rate

TABLE 17-1	Pediatric Drug Labeling for Inhaled Aerosols and Leukotriene Modifiers*	
DRUG NAME	**FORMULATION**	**AGE LABELING (FDA APPROVED)**
β-Adrenergic Agents		
Albuterol	MDI	*≥4 yr:* 2 inhalations q4-6h
	SVN	*2-12 yr:* 1.25-2.5 mg tid-qid[†]
Formoterol	DPI	*≥5 yr:* 1 inhalation (12-24 mcg) bid
Levalbuterol	MDI	*≥4 yr:* 2 inhalations (90 mcg) q4-6h
	SVN	*6-11 yr:* 0.31 mg tid; maximum 0.63 mg tid
Metaproterenol	SVN	*≥6 yr:* 0.1-0.2 mL of 5% solution tid-qid
Racemic epinephrine	SVN	*≥4 yr:* 0.5 mL of 2.25% solution in 3 mL diluent; q3-4h
Salmeterol	DPI	*≥4 yr:* 1 inhalation (50 mcg) bid
Corticosteroids		
Beclomethasone	MDI	*≥5 yr:* 40-80 g twice daily
Budesonide	DPI	*≥6 yr:* 180-360 mcg bid
	SVN	*12 mo-8 yr:* 0.5 mg total daily dose given once or twice daily in divided doses; maximum 1 mg total daily given once or 0.5 mg twice daily
Flunisolide	MDI	*6-11 yr:* 1 puff daily, no more than 2 puffs daily
Fluticasone	DPI	*≥4 yr:* 50 mcg twice daily up to 100 mcg twice daily
	MDI	*4-11 yr:* 88 mcg bid
Fluticasone propionate/ salmeterol	DPI	*≥4 yr:* 100 g fluticasone/50 g salmeterol, 1 inhalation twice daily, about 12 hr apart
Mometasone furoate	DPI	*4-11 yr:* 110 mcg daily
Mucoactive Agent		
Dornase alfa	SVN	Safety and efficacy in children <5 yr have not been studied; usual dose 2.5 mg once daily
Nonsteroidal Antiasthma Agent		
Cromolyn sodium	SVN	*≥2 yr:* 20 mg tid-qid
Inhaled Antiinfectives		
Aztreonam	SVN (altera)	75 mg TID, alternate 28 days on, 28 days off
Ribavirin	SPAG	*Infants and young children:* a 20 mg/mL solution nebulized for 12-18 hr/day for 3-7 days
Tobramycin	SVN	*≥6 yr:* 300 mg bid, alternate 28 days on, 28 days off
Leukotriene Modifiers		
Montelukast	PO	*12-23 mo:* one packet of 4-mg oral granules daily in the evening
		2-5 yr: one 4-mg chewable tablet daily in evening or one packet of 4-mg oral granules daily in the evening
		6-14 yr: one 5-mg chewable tablet daily in evening
Zafirlukast	PO	*5-11 yr:* one 10-mg tablet bid
Zanamivir	DPI	*≥5 yr:* 2 inhalations bid for 5 days
Bronchial Challenge		
Mannitol	DPI	*>6 yr*

DPI, Dry powder inhaler; *MDI,* metered dose inhaler; *PO,* by mouth; *SPAG,* small particle aerosol generator; *SVN,* small volume nebulizer.
*Additional detail on dosing for adults can be found in previous chapters. Manufacturers' information and other sources on drug administration and dosing should be consulted before use. Drug labeling is current at the time of this edition.
[†]Most frequent administration is not recommended. Patients 6 to 12 years of age with more severe asthma (baseline FEV$_1$ <60% predicted), patients with weight greater than 40 kg, or patients 11 to 12 years of age may achieve a better initial response with higher dose.

per minute and the total dose of salbutamol deposited were significantly higher for the nebulizer.

Anhoj and associates[22] found that a pMDI of budesonide with a 250-mL steel NebuChamber (Astrazenica, London, UK) having less than 2 mL of dead space delivered the *same* approximate dose to a range of ages from 2 to 41 years. A facemask was used for children 2 to 3 years of age, and a mouthpiece was used for older subjects. Although the resulting plasma concentration of drug was the same in

children and adults (Figure 17-1), the **inhaled (delivered) dose** and the dose reaching the lung were not the same. Because the holding chamber eliminated oropharyngeal and stomach loss and there is high first-pass metabolism of budesonide, plasma drug levels reflect the dose in the lung. If the same dose went to the lungs in adults as in 2-year-olds, higher plasma levels would be observed in younger subjects, who have smaller circulating blood volumes. This report suggests that inhaled doses need not be adjusted for

TABLE 17-2	Comparison of Neonatal and Adult Respiratory Parameters

PARAMETER	NEONATE	ADULT
Tracheal diameter	≈4 mm	≈20 mm
Tracheal length	5-6 cm	10-12 cm
Tidal volume	6 mL/kg	6 mL/kg
Respiratory rate	30-40/min	12-14/min
Minute ventilation	200-300 mL/kg/min	6 L/min
Dead space	0.75 mL/lb	1.0 mL/lb
Inspiratory flow rate	≤100 mL/sec	≈500 mL/sec

From Kacmarek R, Stoller JK, Heuer AH, editors: *Egan's fundamentals of care,* ed 10, St Louis, 2013, Mosby.

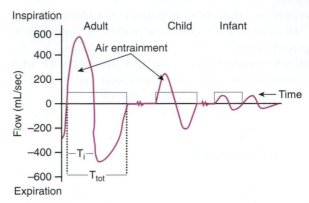

Figure 17-2 Illustration of the amount of nebulizer output inspired with varying inspiratory patterns (volumes, flow rates, times), indicating a smaller fraction of output inspired with low tidal volumes and flow rates in infants compared with adults. T_i, Inspiration time; T_{tot}, total cycle time. (From Collis GG, Cole CH, Le Souef PN: Dilution of nebulised aerosols by air entrainment in children, *Lancet* 336:341, 1990.)

Effect of Small Tidal Volumes, Short Respiratory Cycles, and Low Flow Rates

Small pediatric patients have low tidal volumes, low vital capacities, short respiratory cycles, and low inspiratory flow rates. Children inhale a smaller percentage of the **emitted dose** from either a small volume nebulizer (SVN) or a pMDI with a reservoir device (holding chamber or spacer). The aerosol deposition is reduced because of a short residence time for small particles in the airways. These factors can significantly alter the inhaled dose and the lung dose of patients younger than 6 months of age.[18,24]

Effect on Small Volume Nebulizer

If we assume a 6 L/min power gas, an adult with inspiratory flow of 500 mL/sec (30 L/min) and a tidal volume of 500 mL (500 mL/sec × 1 or 2 seconds) would completely inhale all of a nebulizer output. However, an **infant** with inspiratory flow of less than 100 mL/sec (less than 6 L/min) and a tidal volume less than 100 mL would not completely inhale all of the nebulizer output during the inspiratory phase (Figure 17-2).

Collis and associates[25] studied the fraction of nebulizer output inspired by infants 1 to 12 months old, children 3 to 16 years old, and adults 20 to 23 years old. Infants were sedated with chloral hydrate, and tidal breathing was recorded by facemask and pneumotachygraph. The fraction of nebulizer output inspired was lower in infants younger than age 6 months, then reached a plateau and remained constant in subjects older than 6 months. Wildhaber and colleagues[20,21] also found that inhaled aerosol dose from an SVN attached to a mask increased with weight in infants 4 to 12 months old and was lower in smaller infants.

Several hazards, in addition to bacterial contamination, are associated with using an ultrasonic nebulizer (USN). The high-density aerosol from USNs has been associated with bronchospasm, increased airway resistance, and irritability in a substantial portion of the population. Overhydration may occur when using a USN for prolonged treatment

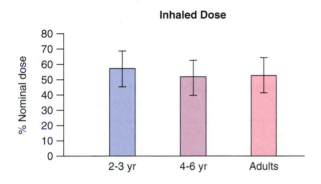

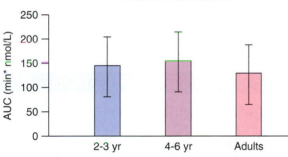

Figure 17-1 Mean values (with 95% confidence interval) for inhaled dose of budesonide from a metered dose inhaler and steel chamber (NebuChamber) and area under the curve *(AUC)* of corresponding plasma drug levels for three age ranges. Inhaled dose (dose reaching the patient) is equivalent for various age groups. Blood levels from lung absorption remain the same in younger subjects, indicating that the dose reaching the lung is proportionately less for younger, smaller subjects. (Data from Anhoj J, Thorsson L, Bisgaard H: Lung deposition of inhaled drugs increases with age, *Am J Respir Crit Care Med* 162:1819, 2000.)

age to reduce systemic levels and possible toxicity. When a fixed dose of 2.5 mg by nebulizer was compared with a dose of 0.1 mg/kg body weight in children 4 to 12 years of age with acute asthma, there was no difference between the two dose protocols in either clinical improvement measured by flows, oxygen saturations, clinical score, or cardiovascular and tremor side effects. The fixed dose of 2.5 mg by nebulizer was efficacious and safe.[23]

of a neonate, small child, or patient with renal insufficiency. The structure of the medication may be disrupted by acoustic power output rated greater than 50 W/cm^2.[26,27] Several ventilator manufacturers have provided USNs for administration of aerosols during mechanical ventilation. Disadvantages may be the weight of the USN in the ventilator circuit, a tendency to heat up over time, and the potential for reduced therapeutic efficacy of medications.

Effect on Reservoir Dose

The same effect of low tidal volumes would theoretically reduce the amount of volume and drug mass inhaled from a reservoir chamber[28] (Figure 17-3). The amount of reduction is proportional to the chamber volume for a given infant tidal volume. For a 50-mL tidal volume, approximately one third (33%) of a 150-mL chamber and one fifth (20%) of a 250-mL chamber would be inhaled. Even assuming no redistribution of aerosol in the chamber volume, gravitational settling would reduce the available dose further within seconds of pMDI actuation into the chamber. The ideal volume for a spacer device is small enough to allow drug inhalation with few breaths for infants with low tidal volumes (less than 50 mL).

This theoretical prediction is supported by data from Everard and colleagues.[29] Delivery (not lung deposition) of pMDI cromolyn sodium by reservoir and facemask with tidal volumes of 25, 50, and 150 mL was measured in vitro using various sizes of chambers. Smaller tidal volumes were associated with decreased inhaled drug mass. Higher aerosol concentrations in a smaller chamber enhanced drug delivery with tidal volumes less than 150 mL. Introduction of dead space between the chamber outlet and the filter col-

lecting inspired drug reduced the dose deposited by 50% or more.[2] The results are summarized in Table 17-3.

In contrast, Wildhaber and colleagues found that 17 children with asthma between ages 2 and 9 had equivalent percentages of total lung deposition of radiolabeled salbutamol aerosolized by either a nebulizer or a pMDI and holding chamber.[20] However, the delivery rate per minute and the total dose of salbutamol deposited were significantly higher for the nebulizer. Mean (absolute dose) total lung deposition expressed as a percentage of the nebulized dose was 5.4% (108 mcg) in younger children (<4 years) and 11.1% (222 mcg) in older children (>4 years). Mean (absolute dose) total lung deposition expressed as a percentage of the metered dose was 5.4% (21.6 mcg) in younger and 9.6% (38.4 mcg) in older children.[21] Turpeinen and colleagues[30] compared the same reservoir devices and found that inhaled mass of budesonide did increase with increasing height, weight, and tidal volume with the Babyhaler but not with the NebuChamber. One of the most recent evaluations of aerosol deposition in children was conducted by Ditcham et al. They measured lung deposition of (99m)Tc-radiolabeled albuterol delivered through a pMDI and antistatic spacer with facemask or mouthpiece in 12 children with stable asthma and found that mean (SD) lung deposition (% total dose) was 18.1 (9.1)% with the facemask and 22.5 (7.9)% with the spacer mouthpiece (p >0.05).[31]

Such variation in study results indicates that testing conditions, type of drug, and choice of reservoir device can affect inhaled dose, although not necessarily the lung dose. Box 17-2 lists factors in reservoir devices that may affect the inhaled dose for neonates, infants, and small children.

NEBULIZED DRUG DISTRIBUTION

It might be obvious to the respiratory clinician that outcomes of aerosol therapy in young children are quite different from that in adults, and that much more research is required to confirm the differences in aerosol drug delivery. The most definitive data for answering the question of how much aerosol drug reaches the lungs of neonates and pediatric patients are actual measures of lung deposition. However, most radiolabeled substances used to estimate lung deposition may be harmful to children, which limits the scope of measurements.[25] Some available data indicate that the lung dose of an aerosol drug does in fact decrease with age. Anhoj and associates[22] found that blood levels of

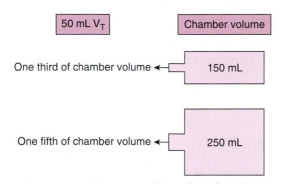

Figure 17-3 Conceptual illustration of the effect of small tidal volumes (V_T) on chamber evacuation with different-sized reservoir chambers.

TABLE 17-3	Effect of Inspired Tidal Volumes on Mean (Range) Inhaled Aerosol Dose in Two Reservoir Devices		
	TIDAL VOLUME (mL)		
DEVICE	**25**	**50**	**150**
AeroChamber (150 mL)	0.33 mg (0.29-0.35 mg)	1.15 mg (1.08-1.24 mg)	1.41 mg (1.33-1.46 mg)
Nebuhaler (750 mL)	0.29 mg (0.26-0.32 mg)	0.93 mg (0.91-0.97 mg)	1.55 mg (1.48-1.61 mg)

Data from Everard ML, Clark AR, Milner AD: Drug delivery from holding chambers with attached facemask, *Arch Dis Child* 67:580, 1992.

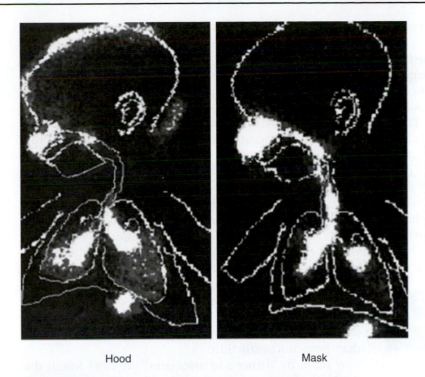

Hood   Mask

Figure 17-4 Scan of patient obtained during hood and mask treatments showing deposition of aerosolized medication in the upper respiratory tract (URT) and gastrointestinal (GI) system. Notice considerably higher URT and GI deposition with mask treatment. (From Amirav I, Balanov I, Gorenberg M, et al: Nebuliser hood compared to mask in wheezy infants: aerosol therapy without tears, *Arch Dis Child* 88:719-723, 2003.)

BOX 17-2   Factors That May Affect Dose Inhaled From a Reservoir Chamber in Neonatal and Pediatric Patients

Mechanical and Design Factors
- Chamber volume
- Electrostatic charge on plastic devices
- Shape of aerosol plume relative to chamber size
- Design of inspiratory and expiratory valves, if present
- Presence of inspiratory valve
- Amount of dead volume in mouthpiece

Patient Factors
Anatomic
- Larger tongue in proportion to oral airway
- Smaller airway diameter
- Smaller number of alveoli

Breathing Pattern
- Nasal breathing
- Inability to hold mouthpiece

Inspiratory Flow Rate
- Tidal volume

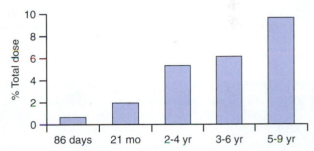

Figure 17-5 Data from four separate studies giving the percent of total aerosol dose that reaches the lungs of infants and children of varying ages. In each study, aerosol dose was delivered using a metered dose inhaler with reservoir device and a face mask in subjects younger than 4 years of age. Studies shown are Fok and colleagues[15] for 86 days, Tal and colleagues[34] for 21 months, Wildhaber and colleagues[21] for 2 to 4 years and 5 to 9 years, and Agertoft and colleagues[31] for 3 to 6 years.

---

drug, reflecting the dose reaching the lungs, were constant in younger and older subjects, despite the smaller circulating volume of younger patients.

It has been hypothesized that the greater the infant's distress, the lower the lung deposition and the higher the upper respiratory tract and gastrointestinal tract deposition. Evaluation of distribution of nebulized bronchodilators in wheezy infants has shown an average of 10% to 12% adherence to the patient's face, 7.8% ± 4.9% deposition in the upper respiratory and gastrointestinal tracts, and 1.5% ± 0.7% deposited in the lungs[32,33] (Figure 17-4).

Figure 17-5 summarizes data on lung deposition with inhaled aerosols compiled from four studies. All of the studies used a pMDI with a reservoir device and a facemask for delivery in subjects younger than 4 years. Values represent the percentage of total dose from the device. Fok and colleagues[15] found that 0.67% (standard error of the mean [SEM] 0.17) of the total dose of albuterol reached the lungs of infants with a mean age of 86 days (range 25-187 days).

Tal and associates[34] found a mean (SD) of 1.97% (1.4) as a lung dose of albuterol in patients with a mean age of 21 months (range 3 months to 5 years). Wildhaber and colleagues[21] found 5.4% (SD 2.1) and 9.6% (SD 3.9) of albuterol reached the lungs of 2- to 4-year-olds and 5- to 9-year-olds. Agertoft and coworkers,[35] using indirect measures of plasma levels, found 6.1% of a budesonide dose reached the lungs of 3- to 6-year-olds. Similar data have been reported for aerosol delivery with nebulizers (see Chapter 3, Table 3-4).

If the amount of aerosolized albuterol reaching the lungs of infants and children in the study by Tal and colleagues[34] is used, it can be shown that the self-limiting effect of younger ages on lung dose results in the same dose per amount of body weight in children as in adults (Table 17-4). The equivalence of dose per body weight illustrated in Table 17-4 and based on lung deposition data argues strongly against the need to adjust the nominal dose of an aerosol drug for age or body size with current aerosol delivery devices. Age and size have a self-limiting effect on lung dose, producing a natural titration of dose. This conclusion may need to be revised pending more efficient aerosol delivery devices.

CLINICAL RESPONSE TO AEROSOLIZED DRUGS IN NEONATAL AND PEDIATRIC PATIENTS

 KEY POINT

Crying and distress, even with the best-designed facemask, seriously affect the efficiency of aerosol administration in young children.

TABLE 17-4	Calculation of Dose per Kilogram of Aerosolized Albuterol for Children and Adults Based on Lung Deposition Data (1.75%) Showing Equivalence of Dose per Body Size

	ADULT	CHILD
Weight	60 kg	10 kg
Lung deposition	20%*	2%
Nominal dose	200 mcg	200 mcg
Dose to lung	40 mcg	4 mcg
Per kilogram dose	0.5 mcg/kg	0.4 mcg/kg

Data from Tal A, Golan H, Grauer N, et al: Deposition pattern of radiolabeled salbutamol inhaled from a metered-dose inhaler by means of a spacer with mask in young children with airway obstruction, *J Pediatr* 128:479, 1996.
*Percentage lung disposition measured by Tal and colleagues in two adult volunteers in the same study.

The lung deposition data reviewed in the previous section argue that aerosolized drugs reach the lungs of infants and do so in a self-regulating amount. The question of clinical response to aerosol drugs in infants and pediatric patients is not determined by lung deposition data. The most commonly studied drug class—one of great interest in neonates and infants—is the adrenergic bronchodilator group. Compared with corticosteroids, the clinical response to bronchodilator occurs within minutes and is more feasible to study in young subjects.

Commonly cited studies from the late 1970s concluded that response to inhaled bronchodilators was lacking in infants and children younger than 18 months of age.[36,37] These studies found no change in respiratory resistance with phenylephrine, epinephrine, or salbutamol (albuterol) in infants and children 7 to 18 months of age using a forced oscillation technique. The authors of the studies speculated that there was either poor development of smooth muscle in children younger than 18 months of age or the bronchial obstruction was due to secretions and airway edema rather than bronchoconstriction.

A study by Turner and associates[38] in 1993 found that the level of response to a bronchodilator increases significantly with increasing age in young asthmatics 3 to 9 years of age. However, studies of ventilated and nonventilated preterm infants have shown dose-related changes in respiratory mechanics, including airway resistance, and compliance with aerosolized bronchodilators.[39] Table 17-5 lists several studies and the outcomes measured that have documented clinical efficacy of aerosolized bronchodilators in infants.

SELECTION OF DELIVERY DEVICES

The current methods to deliver therapeutic aerosols can be classified in three categories: nebulizers (jet or ultrasonic); pMDIs that can be used with a press-and-breathe technique, as a breath actuated device, or in combination with a VHC or spacer; and dry powder inhalers (DPIs). Table 17-6 gives the age guidelines for use of current aerosol delivery devices in infants and children, based on the 2007 National Asthma Education and Prevention Program (NAEPP) guidelines.[43] Either a jet nebulizer or an MDI can be used with suitable auxiliary devices attached. An evidence-based review by the American College of Chest Physicians determined that for

TABLE 17-5	Results of Studies Examining Clinical Response to Aerosolized Albuterol in Infants

REFERENCE	AGE	DELIVERY	OUTCOME MEASURED
Rotschild, 1989[40]	1-4 wk	SVN via ETT	*Improved:* respiratory resistance and dynamic compliance
Sivakumar, 1999[41]	12 ±8 days	MDI/spacer via ETT Versus SVN via ETT	*Improved:* respiratory resistance and dynamic compliance*
Modl, 2005[39]	8.5 ±4.2 mo	SVN	*Improved:* oxygen saturation, respiratory distress
Hyvarinen, 2006[42]	14.1 ±6.1 mo	Not specified	*Improved:* oxygen saturation, respiratory distress

ETT, Endotracheal tube; *MDI*, metered dose inhaler; *SVN*, small volume nebulizer
*MDI delivery resulted in significantly better dynamic compliance than SVN delivery, with no difference between delivery systems in respiratory resistance.

TABLE 17-6	Age Guidelines for Use of Current Aerosol Delivery Devices

DELIVERY DEVICE	AGE RECOMMENDED (yr)
SVN with mask	≤3
SVN with mouthpiece	≥3
pMDI with spacer/VHC and mask	<4
pMDI with spacer/VHC	≥4
DPI	≥4
pMDI	≥5
Breath-actuated MDI	≥5
Breath-actuated nebulizers	≥5

Data from National Asthma Education and Prevention Program; *Expert Panel Report III: guidelines for the diagnosis and management of asthma*, Bethesda, Md., 2007, National Institute of Health.

DPI, Dry powder inhaler; *ETT*, endotracheal tube; *MDI*, metered dose inhaler; *pMDI*, pressurized metered dose inhaler; *SVN*, small volume nebulizer; *VHC*, valved holding chamber.

most patients with asthma, SVNs, DPIs, and MDIs are equally effective in delivering short-acting β agonists.[44,45] Nebulizer systems and the pMDI plus spacer are the most suitable aerosol delivery systems for young children because they only require tidal breathing to inhale the aerosol. Even in acute asthma attacks, delivery of bronchodilators by a pMDI plus spacer is equally effective as nebulizers.[3] Nebulizers could be considered as an alternative if the child appears very distressed during the administration of a pMDI. Studies cited in Chapter 3 (see Table 3-4) showing equivalent clinical response between jet nebulizers and the MDI-reservoir systems, with or without a mask as needed by age, have been validated in young children.[46]

Nebulizers

Jet nebulizers used to be the mainstay of aerosol therapy in infants and young children. However, they require a pressurized gas source, bulky equipment, a long treatment period, and additional preparation and cleaning time. A significant disadvantage of nebulizer therapy in children is the poor tolerance often exhibited because of noise of operation and the need for a tight-fitting mask.[29] Although nebulizers may not routinely be used as compared with pMDIs, nebulizers are preferred by numerous patients and parents. They are also the preferred delivery device for emerging therapies, such as aerosolized surfactants[47,48] and antibiotics[49] currently under investigation. With a deposition estimated to be less than 1% in small children and infants, only 25 mcg of a 2.5-mg (2500-mcg) dose will be delivered to the lung.

Although the use of breath-actuated nebulizers (BANs) in adults has been associated with greater aerosol deposition, results in pediatric in vivo and in vitro studies are still controversial. Lin and Huang compared the therapeutic effects of a BAN and a constant-flow nebulizer (CFN) on 72 asthmatic patients, aged 5 to 15. They found that all the

spirometric parameters, including forced expiratory volume in 1 second (FEV_1), peak expiratory flow (PEF), and forced expiratory flow 25%-75% (FEF 25%-75%) and arterial oxygen saturation (SaO_2) at various time points of both groups significantly improved. For between-group comparison, the BAN group had greater improvement in all the data of spirometric parameters and SaO_2 at various time points, but only reached statistical significance at some time points in PEF, FEF 25%-75%, and SaO_2. The pulse rate of the BAN group was significantly higher than that of the CFN group beginning 5 minutes after treatment.[50]

On the other hand, Lin et al modeled toddler breathing patterns and found that the use of a mechanical BAN was associated with a substantial reduction in inhaled dose compared with conventional constant output nebulizers.[51] A recent randomized trial of a BAN versus continuous 1-hour nebulization and/or a small-volume constant-output nebulizer in 149 pediatric asthma patients reported that the admission rate using BAN was significantly lower (38% vs. 57%). Time in the emergency department was not statistically different (BAN, 102 minutes; standard therapy, 125 minutes), but the BAN group had a significantly greater improvement in clinical asthma score (1.9 ±1.2 vs. 1.2 ±1.4) and respiratory rate. There was no difference in adverse effects.[52]

Large volume nebulizers (LVNs) are sometimes used in newborns or children using incubators and hoods. Because LVNs produce significant levels of noise, alternative methods to deliver oxygen therapy may be required to reduce the sleep disruption and stress caused by noise levels above 58 decibels (dB). Additional caution needs to be exercised to prevent the use of high fractional inspired oxygen (FIO_2) to power nebulizers in premature newborns to avoid adverse effects associated with oxygen therapy at this early age.

Pressurized Metered Dose Inhalers

The pMDIs are the method of choice in infants and children younger than 5 years of age only when used in combination with an appropriate spacer or VHC.[53] A pMDI should not be used without a spacer or VHC, even in children 8 years of age or older, because most patients are unable to coordinate actuation of the pMDI with the breathing maneuver. An additional advantage of the pMDI and spacer combination is that it considerably reduces the oropharyngeal deposition, which could be as high as 80%, by reducing the velocity of the aerosol jet,[17] allowing time for evaporation of the propellants and for the particles to "age" before impacting on a surface. The pMDI delivery system has the advantage of smallness, portability, and shorter treatment time, even with an increased number of actuations. However, drug delivery to the lungs using pMDIs can vary greatly, depending on the formulation used and the age of the child. Children 4 to 8 years of age should be encouraged to use a mouthpiece along with the pMDI whenever possible, whereas a mask attached to the spacer is typically recommended in children younger than 4 years. Similar issues regarding leaks around the mask already mentioned for nebulizers apply to the pMDI-spacer-mask interface.[54,55] The use of a pMDI autohaler may be a sound alternative to the pMDI with spacer in children with asthma who are older than 8 years.

There are different types of spacers: plastic or metal, with large or small volumes. For children with small tidal volumes, the volume of a spacer is crucial because of the time it takes to empty the spacer. The less time it takes to empty the spacer, the higher the concentration of aerosol.

As mentioned in Chapter 3, immediately after the aerosol cloud is released from the pMDI, gravitational forces result in sedimentation of aerosol particles onto the spacer wall. This effect is more pronounced when a plastic spacer is used with electrostatic charge. A metal spacer could deliver to the mouth twice the amount of drug as a plastic spacer. However, although the electrostatic charge is totally eliminated with the use of a metal chamber, the simple act of coating a plastic spacer with household detergent minimizes the electrostatic charge and substantially increases lung deposition.[20] The improvement in lung deposition associated with elimination of the electrostatic charge could be seriously compromised by a suboptimal facemask seal, as previously shown by Smaldone and colleagues.[56]

VHCs also reduce the need to coordinate breathing with actuation. They should be used with infants, small children, and any child taking steroids because they can reduce the pharyngeal dose of aerosol from the pMDI 10- to 15-fold over administration without a holding chamber.[57-59]

Dry Powder Inhalers

DPIs are usually not appropriate for children younger than 6 years of age because they are driven by peak inspiratory flows much greater than those required by pMDIs.[60]

Even if some young children are able to generate the 30 to 120 L/min range of inspiratory flow required by most inhaled corticosteroids (ICSs) to disperse adequate mass and particle size, it is questionable whether or not children can generate reproducible inspiratory flow patterns.[61,62] In addition, competence and good understanding will be necessary from a child to perform the steps required to take full advantage of the device. If for example a child exhales into a DPI, condensation will form inside the device and can prevent optimal dispersion of the powder into the mouthpiece.[63]

USE OF SELECTIVE AGENTS IN NEONATAL AND PEDIATRIC PATIENTS

Although a wide variety of aerosol devices have been made available to deliver aerosol for therapeutic purposes, a very limited number of the newer drugs and those in development are approved by the FDA for use in the neonatal and pediatric population. However, research on pediatric and adult models has helped in clarifying the role of some novel therapies summarized subsequently.

Antibiotics

Aerosolization has been known to deliver a high concentration of antibiotic to the airway with minimal systemic absorption, side effects, and toxicity. The first commercially available antibiotic for aerosol administration was tobramycin solution for inhalation (or TOBI), approved for the therapy of cystic fibrosis (CF) lung disease. Currently available aerosolized antibiotics include TOBI, aztreonam, colistin, and several antiviral agents. Some other antimicrobials being developed for aerosol use include quinolones (ciprofloxacin and levofloxacin), aminoglycosides (gentamicin and neomycin), and antifungal agents. These agents are designed to target pulmonary infections that include ventilator-associated pneumonia (VAP), tuberculosis, and seasonal influenza.

Mucoactive Agents

These agents are designed to influence mucus secretion or mucus clearance. Dornase alfa is the only approved peptide mucolytic for the treatment of CF and has been available for more than a decade. Actin depolymerizers, such as thymosin agents and β-4, are synergistic with dornase alfa and appear to act not only as a mucolytic but may have antiinflammatory properties.[64]

Expectorants and mucokinetics that have been evaluated in small children include hypertonic saline and dry powder mannitol. These medications act by increasing ion and water transport across the epithelium, altering the mucus rheology, inducing mucin secretion, and stimulating ciliary beating: more than simply acting as "airway hydrators."[65] The Australian National CF Hypertonic Saline study showed fewer pulmonary exacerbations and a significant improvement in FEV$_1$ in subjects with CF compared with normal saline.[66] Small studies suggest that hypertonic saline may not be as effective as dornase alfa in improving FEV$_1$ in persons with CF.[67] Because hypertonic saline can irritate the airway and cause bronchospasm, it is usually administered along with a β$_2$-adrenergic agent such as albuterol. Inhaled dry powder mannitol has been shown to be effective in improving pulmonary function and reducing exacerbations in patients with CF, and appears to be tolerated at least as well as hypertonic saline.[68] The improvement in pulmonary function with mannitol appears to be sustained for at least 18 months.[69] Unfortunately, bronchoconstriction and cough have been largely responsible for the high attrition rate observed in few clinical trials and the improvement in pulmonary function does not appear superior to the administration of dornase alfa.[70-72] Although the combination of inhaled mannitol and dornase alfa does not provide any additional improvement in pulmonary function of patients with CF,[70] combining inhaled mannitol as a therapeutic carrier with bronchodilators and antibiotics may benefit patients with pulmonary hypersecretion and infection.[73] Despite the positive results obtained with nebulized N-acetylceisteine in 100 children (2 months to 24 months of age) with acute bronchiolitis in a very recent study, the use of this agent is still controversial.[74,75]

Aerosol Surfactants

Some of the neonatal and pediatric diseases that are characterized by surfactant inactivation include CF, acute respiratory distress syndrome (ARDS), meconium aspiration, and severe asthma. Surfactant works as a mucokinetic or adhesive medication and may have antiinflammatory properties. Delivery of liquid surfactant in a nebulized form has been shown to be challenging because of its high viscosity and formation of foam at high-velocity airflows. In vitro and animal studies suggest that surfactant and perfluorocarbons can be aerosolized using an inhalation catheter.[76-78] Degradation of airway surfactant in the CF airway can impair mucociliary clearance. Surfactant can reduce sputum stickiness, and the aerosolization of surfactant has been shown to improve pulmonary function in patients with chronic obstructive pulmonary disease (COPD).[79] In addition, use of inhaled surfactants may improve antibiotic distribution within the lungs.[80]

Antiinflammatory Drugs and Antibiotics

Although ICSs are the most commonly used antiinflammatory medications for the treatment of asthma, a number of other drugs have been studied as aerosols in the pediatric population affected with CF. Recombinant secretory leukoprotease inhibitor, antineutrophil elastase, and α-1 antiproteases can decrease the activity of neutrophil elastase in the chronically inflamed airway.[81] Aerosolized glutathione is currently being studied as adjuvant therapy for the treatment of CF lung disease.[82]

Cyclosporine analogs can be efficiently nebulized and may protect against the airway inflammation and allergic challenge present in patients with asthma.[40] Aerosolized cyclosporine appears to ameliorate important pulmonary function parameters in lung transplant recipients compared with an aerosol placebo and historical control patients.[83]

Patients with CF are known to be affected by recurrent bacterial infections. It is in this group of patients where most clinical trials have evaluated the use of nebulized antimicrobials. Dry powder tobramycin and colistine can be substituted for the same drug delivered by nebulization. Nebulized aztreonam needs more studies to determine its place.[84]

Aerosolized Peptides and Proteins

Peptides have been delivered as aerosols both to treat pulmonary diseases such as CF and systemic diseases like diabetes.[85] In the particular case of CF, large peptides might include gene-transfer therapy using complimentary DNA delivered as an aerosol in a vector package to the affected cells.[86]

Prostacyclin Analogs for Pulmonary Hypertension

The prostacyclin analogs epoprostenol and iloprost are well accepted as nebulized medications for treating severe pulmonary hypertension,[87] including the setting of respiratory distress syndrome of the neonate[88] and after surgery to correct congenital heart disease.[89,90] Inhaled iloprost showed greater safety than the intravenous preparation with preferential vasodilatation in the pulmonary circulation. A drawback of inhaled iloprost is the short hemodynamic effect, which requires frequently given doses. Prostacyclin analogs with a longer half-life (e.g., treprostinil) and controlled-release formulations are in clinical development.[91,92]

COMPLIANCE AND COOPERATION DURING AEROSOL THERAPY

KEY POINT

Aerosolized bronchodilators change respiratory mechanics in ventilated and nonventilated infants.

The most important factor to consider in the administration of aerosol therapy in infants and young children is their compliance. Two practical issues are important when dealing with young children, particularly infants: facemask and crying. The interaction between crying and the facemask is complex. It is very likely that crying and distress, even with the best-designed facemask, explain the poor seal that seriously affects the efficiency of aerosol administration in young children.[93]

Effects of Crying and Facemask Fitting on Aerosol Delivery

It is widely accepted that delivery devices that produce small particles are less flow dependent. This characteristic may be of critical importance for less cooperative children. Crying is associated with high inspiratory flows, high dose variability, and almost no lung deposition.[94-97] A typical pediatric patient does not tolerate a mask applied to the face, and agitation and crying are frequently observed. The efficacy of aerosol therapy administered to a combative or crying toddler is known to be negligible because of the changes in respiratory patterns during nebulization. Amirav and associates[27] have shown that the more distress infants were in during the treatment, the more aerosol was deposited extrathoracically. This finding should alert clinicians to the potential for increased systemic absorption and greater risk for side effects.

Although theoretically the poor aerosol delivery associated with crying could make aerosol administration during sleep an attractive alternative, the positive results of in vitro studies[70] have not been consistently reported in vivo. Almost 70% of children wake up when aerosol is given during sleep and become distressed, resulting in similar lung deposition found with crying. However, a very recent study by Amirav et al on 13 infants using the SootherMask revealed that all infants received the treatment during sleep without difficulty and that mean lung deposition averaged 1.6% ± 0.5% in the lung.[98] Because crying may be inevitable, the caregiver may have to find creative ways to prepare the child for the facemask at a time when the child does not need the treatment.[99,100] This strategy would apply to maintenance therapy and not to the emergency setting or transport, where distracting and comforting the child may be the only available options to improve compliance. Dose variability seems to be independent of facemask design and more dependent on cooperation[101] (Figure 17-6).

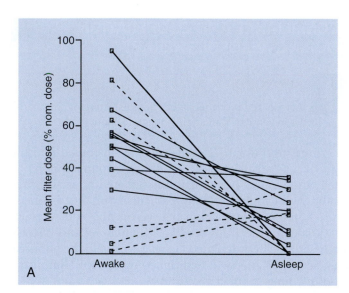

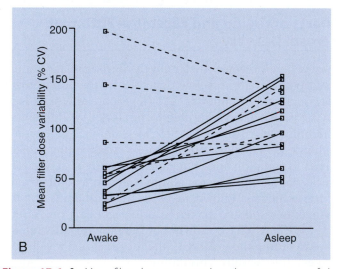

Figure 17-6 **A,** *Mean filter dose,* expressed as the percentage of the nominal *(nom)* dose, during awake administration and during sleep administration for children who slept through the administration procedure. **B,** *Mean filter dose variability (%CV)* during awake administration and during sleep administration for children who slept through the administration procedure. *Straight line* = Cooperative child; *dotted line* = uncooperative child during awake administration. (From Esposito Festen JE, Ijsselstijn H, Hop WCJ, et al: Aerosol therapy by pMDI-spacer in sleeping young children: to do or not to do? *Chest* 130:487-492, 2006.)

Mask-Fit-to-Face and Mask Design

Because children must be about 3 years of age before they fully understand how to use a mouthpiece, younger children must use a mask. Efficient aerosol therapy requires the mask to fit to the face tightly and still be comfortable. The absence of a tight seal between the mask and the patient's face results in a decrease in the amount of medication available for inhalation.[55] Many parents are forced to hold the facemask near the face to avoid struggling with the child. This technique is well known as "blow-by." However, it has been clearly documented in numerous studies that even a 0.5-cm gap in the facemask can drastically reduce the efficiency of drug delivery up to 50% in a lung model or spontaneously breathing children.[102]

To evaluate the effect of mask-fit and crying on aerosol delivery, Erzinger et al studied eight recurrently wheezy children, age 18 to 36 months, for the administration of radiolabelled salbutamol with either a vent-assisted nebulizer or a pMDI attached to a holding chamber. Lung deposition expressed as a percentage of the total dose (metered dose and nebulizer fill, respectively) was 0.2% and 0.3% in children who inhaled with a nontightly fitted facemask. Lung deposition was 0.6% and 1.4% in screaming children with a tightly fitted facemask, and between 4.8% and 8.2% in patients breathing normally. Overall mask deposition was between 0.8% and 5.2%. Overall face deposition was between 2.6% and 8.4%.[103]

Development of more efficient, more acceptable, and friendlier facemask interfaces has been evaluated as an option to improve the inhaled drug mass. More recent reports comparing the standard aerosol pediatric mask with other proprietary masks have shown that the newly designed masks significantly increase the inhaled drug mass[4,95,104] (Figure 17-7). The first facemask interfaces had several shortcomings, most notably large mask dead space and chamber volumes making it difficult for infants to clear with normal tidal breathing. Other devices[4,105,106] made improvements by decreasing dead space, reducing electrostatic charge, and improving mask fit. The Soother-Mask (InspiRx, Somerset, New Jersey) is one of the newest devices, and is designed for the facial structure of infants and children. It allows aerosol delivery during nasal breathing so an infant can continue to use a preferred oral pacifier during treatments.[107] A scintigraphy study by Amirav et al with this device showed that aerosol deposition in the lungs of infants was comparable to that of a standard nebulizer mask.[100] The mask is held in place mostly by the difference between atmospheric pressure and the infant's suction, so very little external pressure is needed. The InspiraMask (InspiRx, Somerset, New Jersey) is intended for older children, and does not allow the use of a pacifier. Both devices can be paired either with a VHC or nebulizer. Despite the level of innovation obtained with these facemasks, it is recommended that children be switched to a mouthpiece as soon as they are old enough to inhale through the mouth voluntarily.

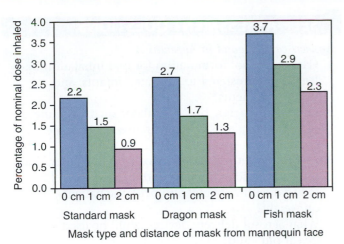

Figure 17-7 Mean values of inhaled drug mass for all face masks at varying distances from the inhalation filter. The differences between the Fish facemask and both the standard and the Dragon facemasks were significant at all distances. There was a significantly higher inhaled drug mass for all masks at 0 cm compared with 2 cm. *P* <.001, all masks compared at 0 cm versus 2 cm. *P* <.001, Fish facemask compared with standard and Dragon facemasks at all distances. (From Lin H-L, Restrepo RD, Gardenhire DS: An in vitro investigation of nebulized albuterol delivery by pediatric aerosol facemasks to spontaneously breathing infants, *Respir Care* 50:1551, 2005.)

Nebulizer Hood

Because it is very difficult to hold a mask snugly fitted to the face, particularly with infants, other alternatives have been explored. The nebulizer hood was designed as an attempt to develop more acceptable and patient-friendly interfaces. Janssens and co-workers,[69,93] and Amirav[33] all reported much greater aerosol delivery with a hood than the mask in vivo and in vitro. Hoods seem to reduce crying in infants significantly because nothing comes in contact with the infant's face (Figure 17-8).

AEROSOL ADMINISTRATION IN INTUBATED NEONATAL AND PEDIATRIC PATIENTS

KEY POINT

Although several aerosolized drugs have been used in the treatment of neonatal respiratory illnesses, an optimized aerosol drug delivery system for mechanically ventilated infants still does not exist. A number of variables, including particle size, aerosol flows, nebulizer choice, and placement of the aerosol generator represent a significant challenge in this age group. For example, an externally powered nebulizer may interfere with patient-triggered modes of ventilation, may cause increases in airway pressures and unexpected positive end-expiratory pressure (PEEP), and may result in variable FIO_2 levels.

Aerosol delivery seems to be less efficient in pediatric intubated patients than in spontaneously breathing patients.[108,109] Nebulizers producing aerosol particles with a mass median

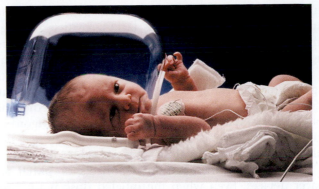

Figure 17-8 Infant oxygen hood nebulizer. (Courtesy Utah Medical Products, Inc., Midvale, Utah.)

aerodynamic diameter (MMAD) of 0.5 to 3 μm are more likely to achieve greater deposition in the LRT of small children undergoing mechanical ventilation.[17]

It is important to consider changes associated with the use of jet nebulizers in-line on pediatric, and particularly neonatal, ventilated patients because unexpected changes in volume and pressure may have deleterious effects. An externally powered nebulizer increases volume and pressure during volume-targeted ventilation, creates a bias flow in the ventilator circuit that may interfere with patient-triggered modes of ventilation, may result in increased airway pressure and unexpected positive end-expiratory pressure (PEEP), and may result in variable fractional inspired oxygen (FIO_2) levels. Constant flow during expiration seriously limits the concentration of the inspired aerosol. Other nebulizer designs, such as vibrating mesh/membrane systems, do not require a gas source to operate and do not affect airway pressures during operation as usually seen with externally gas-powered nebulizers.[110,111] If rapid respiratory rates are used, the ventilator duty cycle may be inadequate for the aerosol cloud to develop in the circuit and may seriously decrease aerosol deposition.[112]

The respiratory clinician should also be aware that aerosol delivery may be less effective with manual ventilation versus mechanical ventilation. Placement of the aerosol delivery device in an intubated infant requires the clinician's attention. Although most studies show a slightly higher lung deposition with the pMDI when inserted between the Y-piece and the endotracheal tube, when an SVN is placed in the inspiratory limb away from the Y-piece, lung deposition also averages 1% of the nominal dose.[113] In pediatric patients, a pMDI and spacer with a one-way valve is associated with a significantly larger amount of inhaled drug mass.[114] No difference has been found between in vitro and in vivo studies. It has been suggested that the pMDI be actuated before inspiration to improve lung deposition.[115,116]

SUMMARY

Efficient aerosol therapy in young children is a challenge. Although the advantages with inhaled drugs to treat pulmonary problems in neonates and pediatric patients support their use, consensus is lacking in determining a suitable dose for this population. More recent research suggests that age has a dose-regulating effect on the amount of aerosol drug reaching the lungs, with less drug reaching the lungs of younger subjects. Safety profile, therapeutic efficacy, and efficiency of routinely aerosolized medications delivered to infants and children need to be rigorously studied. With patients at less than 6 months of age, tidal volumes and inspiratory flow rates can reduce the amount of aerosol drug inhaled from nebulizers or pMDI and spacer devices. Even when the inhaled dose is the same for pediatric and adult patients, data indicate that the lung dose decreases for younger patients. Neonatal and pediatric patients should be assessed for adverse systemic effects with aerosol drug administration because of inefficient drug absorption from the lung and the presence of large extrathoracic deposition when masks are not tightly applied.

There is no difference in clinical effect for bronchodilators between pMDI and nebulizer administration. The pMDI dose may need to be adjusted upward for neonatal, pediatric, or adult use because the pMDI nominal dose is usually lower than the nebulizer dose. Neonates and very young pediatric patients show a clinical response to aerosolized bronchodilator administration. How to determine doses for aerosolized drugs delivered to neonatal and pediatric patients is not completely understood. Despite the differences in drug action between adults and children, the ability to control particle size by selecting the optimal aerosol delivery, placement of the aerosol device, and understanding patterns of aerosol generation are the key elements to improve efficiency of aerosol administration. Identifying the ability of the patient, rather than specific age, is also essential to selecting the most appropriate device in any population.[117]

It needs to be remembered that optimal aerosol administration requires matching patient characteristics with the aerosol delivery system. Infants and young children are a special group of patients with different anatomic, physiologic, and behavioral characteristics that dramatically affect outcomes of pharmacotherapy. Physicians, respiratory therapists, and nurses need to know how to select the right aerosol delivery device appropriately for children of different ages. Lack of coordination, inadequate inspiratory flows, limited cooperation, and crying are factors in infants and young children that greatly affect the efficiency of aerosol therapy in this age group. Because of the seriousness of treatment and possible errors in the inhalation technique, it is recommended that caregivers be reassessed at each patient encounter and that instructions be written in a manner the caregivers can understand. The development of in vitro models that better replicate not only the anatomy but also realistic breathing patterns may allow a better prediction of in vivo lung deposition of aerosols in neonatal and pediatric patients.[118]

 SELF-ASSESSMENT QUESTIONS

Answers can be found in Appendix A.

1. Can an aerosol formulation for oral inhalation be legally administered to neonates, infants, and pediatric patients?
2. Can an adrenergic bronchodilator such as albuterol reduce airway resistance when used in neonates and children?
3. According to the data reviewed in this chapter, does the adult dose of an aerosol drug need to be reduced with neonatal and pediatric patients, based on weight?
4. What aerosol delivery devices could be used with a 2-year-old child?

 CLINICAL SCENARIO

Answers can be found in Appendix A.

A 24-month-old boy, who was born premature at 27 weeks' gestation, presents to the emergency department in respiratory distress. His medical history is significant for bronchopulmonary dysplasia. Vital signs are temperature of 37.5° C, pulse of 175 beats/min, respiratory rate at 76 breaths/min, blood pressure of 85/55 mm Hg, and SpO_2 at 85% on room air. The physical examination reveals the presence of intercostal retractions, increased anteroposterior diameter, nasal flaring, and bilateral diffuse expiratory wheezing. The patient is administered oxygen and admitted to the pediatric intensive care unit. The attending physician orders a 1.25-mg unit dose of albuterol via a small volume nebulizer. While receiving the aerosol, the patient's pulse rate increases to 220 beats/min, and he becomes cyanotic despite the O_2 used to nebulize the drug. The patient is promptly intubated and mechanically ventilated. The patient receives albuterol throughout his hospital course and is discharged home 2 weeks later with a prescription for albuterol syrup.

Using the SOAP method, assess this clinical scenario.

REFERENCES

1. Everard ML: Aerosol delivery to children. *Pediatr Ann* 35(9):630–636, 2006.
2. Everard ML: Inhaler devices in infants and children: challenges and solutions. *J Aerosol Med* 17(2):186–195, 2004.
3. Ahrens RC: The role of the MDI and DPI in pediatric patients: "Children are not just miniature adults". *Respir Care* 50(10):1323–1328, discussion 1328–1330, 2005.
4. Amirav I: Evidence based design of face masks for infants. *Int J Pharm* 457(1):342–346, 2013.
5. Everard ML: Ethical aspects of using radiolabelling in aerosol research. *Arch Dis Child* 88(8):659–661, 2003.
6. Gupta A, Khan MA: Challenges of pediatric formulations: a FDA science perspective. *Int J Pharm* 457(1):346–348, 2013.
7. Tauer CA: Central ethical dilemmas in research involving children. *Account Res* 9(3–4):127–142, 2002.

8. Blumer JL: Off-label uses of drugs in children. *Pediatrics* 104(3 Pt 2):598–602, 1999.

9. America, O.h.t.C.o.T.U.S.o., *Title III—Pediatric Medical Device Safety and Improvement Act of 2007*. 2007, pp 37–44.

10. Olsson B: Aerosol particle generation from dry powder inhalers: can they equal pressurized metered dose inhalers? *J Aerosol Med* 8(Suppl 3):S13–S18, discussion S19, 1995.

11. Silverman M: Aerosol therapy in the newborn. *Arch Dis Child* 65(8):906–908, 1990.

12. Amirav I, et al: Nasal versus oral aerosol delivery to the "lungs" in infants and toddlers. *Pediatr Pulmonol* 2014.

13. Dolovich M: Aerosol delivery to children: what to use, how to choose. *Pediatr Pulmonol Suppl* 18:79–82, 1999.

14. Christensen ML, Helms RA, Chesney RW: Is pediatric labeling really necessary? *Pediatrics* 104(3 Pt 2):593–597, 1999.

15. Fok TF, et al: Efficiency of aerosol medication delivery from a metered dose inhaler versus jet nebulizer in infants with bronchopulmonary dysplasia. *Pediatr Pulmonol* 21(5):301–309, 1996.

16. Dolovich MB: Assessing nebulizer performance. *Respir Care* 47(11):1290–1301, discussion 1301–1304, 2002.

17. Rubin B, Fink J: Aerosol therapy for children. *Respir Care Clin N Am* 7(2):100–108, 2001.

18. Rubin BK, Fink JB: Aerosol therapy for children. *Respir Care Clin N Am* 7(2):175–213, 2001.

19. Fink JB: Aerosol delivery to ventilated infant and pediatric patients. *Respir Care* 49(6):653–665, 2004.

20. Wildhaber JH, et al: High-percentage lung delivery in children from detergent-treated spacers. *Pediatr Pulmonol* 29(5):389–393, 2000.

21. Wildhaber JH, et al: Inhalation therapy in asthma: nebulizer or pressurized metered-dose inhaler with holding chamber? In vivo comparison of lung deposition in children. *J Pediatr* 135(1):28–33, 1999.

22. Onhoj J, Thorsson L, Bisgaard H: Lung deposition of inhaled drugs increases with age. *Am J Respir Crit Care Med* 162(5):1819–1822, 2000.

23. Oberklaid F, et al: A comparison of a bodyweight dose versus a fixed dose of nebulised salbutamol in acute asthma in children. *Med J Aust* 158(11):751–753, 1993.

24. Rubin BK, Fink JB: The delivery of inhaled medication to the young child. *Pediatr Clin North Am* 50(3):717–731, 2003.

25. Collis GG, Cole CH, Le Souef PN: Dilution of nebulised aerosols by air entrainment in children. *Lancet* 336(8711):341–343, 1990.

26. Doershuk CF, et al: Evaluation of jet-type and ultrasonic nebulizers in mist tent therapy for cystic fibrosis. *Pediatrics* 41(4):723–732, 1968.

27. Boucher RM, Kreuter J: The fundamentals of the ultrasonic atomization of medicated solutions. *Ann Allergy* 26(11):591–600, 1968.

28. Mudd SS, et al: Pediatric asthma and the use of metered dose inhalers with valve holding chambers: barriers to the implementation of evidence-based practice. *J Emerg Nurs* 2014.

29. Everard ML, Clark AR, Milner AD: Drug delivery from holding chambers with attached facemask. *Arch Dis Child* 67(5):580–585, 1992.

30. Turpeinen M, et al: Metered dose inhaler add-on devices: is the inhaled mass of drug dependent on the size of the infant? *J Aerosol Med* 12(3):171–176, 1999.

31. Ditcham W, et al: Lung deposition of (99m)tc-radiolabeled albuterol delivered through a pressurized metered dose inhaler and spacer with facemask or mouthpiece in children with asthma. *J Aerosol Med Pulm Drug Deliv* 27(Suppl 1):S63–S75, 2014.

32. Amirav I, et al: Beta-agonist aerosol distribution in respiratory syncytial virus bronchiolitis in infants. *J Nucl Med* 43(4):487–491, 2002.

33. Amirav I, et al: Nebuliser hood compared to mask in wheezy infants: aerosol therapy without tears! *Arch Dis Child* 88(8):719–723, 2003.

34. Tal A, et al: Deposition pattern of radiolabeled salbutamol inhaled from a metered-dose inhaler by means of a spacer with mask in young children with airway obstruction. *J Pediatr* 128(4):479–484, 1996.

35. Agertoft L, et al: Systemic availability and pharmacokinetics of nebulised budesonide in preschool children. *Arch Dis Child* 80(3):241–247, 1999.

36. Lenney W, Milner AD: Alpha and beta adrenergic stimulants in bronchiolitis and wheezy bronchitis in children under 18 months of age. *Arch Dis Child* 53(9):707–709, 1978.

37. Lenney W, Milner AD: At what age do bronchodilator drugs work? *Arch Dis Child* 53(7):532–535, 1978.

38. Turner DJ, Landau LI, LeSouef PN: The effect of age on bronchodilator responsiveness. *Pediatr Pulmonol* 15(2):98–104, 1993.

39. Modl M, et al: Does bronchodilator responsiveness in infants with bronchiolitis depend on age? *J Pediatr* 147(5):617–621, 2005.

40. Rotschild A, et al: Increased compliance in response to salbutamol in premature infants with developing bronchopulmonary dysplasia. *J Pediatr* 115(6):984–991, 1989.

41. Sivakumar D, Bosque E, Goldman SL: Bronchodilator delivered by metered dose inhaler and spacer improves respiratory system compliance more than nebulizer-delivered bronchodilator in ventilated premature infants. *Pediatr Pulmonol* 27(3):208–212, 1999.

42. Hyvarinen MK, et al: Responses to inhaled bronchodilators in infancy are not linked with asthma in later childhood. *Pediatr Pulmonol* 41(5):420–427, 2006.

43. Gupta RS, Weiss KB: The 2007 National Asthma Education and Prevention Program asthma guidelines: accelerating their implementation and facilitating their impact on children with asthma. *Pediatrics* 123(Suppl 3):S193–S198, 2009.

44. Rubin BK, Fink JB: Optimizing aerosol delivery by pressurized metered-dose inhalers. *Respir Care* 50(9):1191–1200, 2005.

45. Dolovich MB, et al: Device selection and outcomes of aerosol therapy: Evidence-based guidelines: American College of Chest Physicians/American College of Asthma, Allergy, and Immunology. *Chest* 127(1):335–371, 2005.

46. Deerojanawong J, et al: Randomized controlled trial of salbutamol aerosol therapy via metered dose inhaler-spacer vs. jet nebulizer in young children with wheezing. *Pediatr Pulmonol* 39(5):466–472, 2005.

47. Donn SM, Sinha SK: Aerosolized lucinactant: a potential alternative to intratracheal surfactant replacement therapy. *Expert Opin Pharmacother* 9(3):475–478, 2008.

48. Mazela J, Merritt TA, Finer NN: Aerosolized surfactants. *Curr Opin Pediatr* 19(2):155–162, 2007.

49. Tamma PD, Lee CK: Use of colistin in children. *Pediatr Infect Dis J* 28(6):534–535, 2009.

50. Lin YZ, Huang FY: Comparison of breath-actuated and conventional constant-flow jet nebulizers in treating acute asthmatic children. *Acta Paediatr Taiwan* 45(2):73–76, 2004.

51. Lin HL, et al: Influence of nebulizer type with different pediatric aerosol masks on drug deposition in a model of a spontaneously breathing small child. *Respir Care* 2012.

52. Sabato K, et al: Randomized controlled trial of a breath-actuated nebulizer in pediatric asthma patients in the emergency department. *Respir Care* 56(6):761–770, 2011.

53. Nikander K, Berg E, Smaldone GC: Jet nebulizers versus pressurized metered dose inhalers with valved holding chambers: effects of the facemask on aerosol delivery. *J Aerosol Med* 20(Suppl 1):S46–S55, discussion S55–S58, 2007.

54. Esposito-Festen JE, et al: Effect of a facemask leak on aerosol delivery from a pMDI-spacer system. *J Aerosol Med* 17(1):1–6, 2004.

55. Amirav I, Newhouse MT: Aerosol therapy with valved holding chambers in young children: importance of the facemask seal. *Pediatrics* 108(2):389–394, 2001.

56. Smaldone GC, Berg E, Nikander K: Variation in pediatric aerosol delivery: importance of facemask. *J Aerosol Med* 18(3):354–363, 2005.

57. Toogood JH, et al: Use of spacers to facilitate inhaled corticosteroid treatment of asthma. *Am Rev Respir Dis* 129(5):723–729, 1984.

58. Salzman GA, Pyszczynski DR: Oropharyngeal candidiasis in patients treated with beclomethasone dipropionate delivered by metered-dose inhaler alone and with Aerochamber. *J Allergy Clin Immunol* 81(2):424–428, 1988.

59. Rubin BK: Pressurized metered-dose inhalers and holding chambers for inhaled glucocorticoid therapy in childhood asthma. *J Allergy Clin Immunol* 103(6):1224–1225, 1999.

60. Pedersen S: Delivery options for inhaled therapy in children over the age of 6 years. *J Aerosol Med* 10(Suppl 1):S41–S44, 1997.

61. Engel T, et al: Peak inspiratory flow and inspiratory vital capacity of patients with asthma measured with and without a new dry-powder inhaler device (Turbuhaler). *Eur Respir J* 3(9):1037–1041, 1990.

62. Pedersen S, Hansen O, Fuglsang G: Influence of inspiratory flow rate upon the effect of a Turbuhaler. *Arch Dis Child* 65:308, 1990.

63. Newhouse M, Kennedy A: Rapid temperature change from 25 C to 15 C impairs powder deaggregation in Bricanyl Turbuhaler. *J Aerosol Med* 12:113, 1999.

64. Rubin BK, Kater AP, Goldstein AL: Thymosin beta4 sequesters actin in cystic fibrosis sputum and decreases sputum cohesivity in vitro. *Chest* 130(5):1433–1440, 2006.

65. Kishioka C, et al: Hyperosmolar solutions stimulate mucus secretion in the ferret trachea. *Chest* 124(1):306–313, 2003.

66. Elkins MR, et al: A controlled trial of long-term inhaled hypertonic saline in patients with cystic fibrosis. *N Engl J Med* 354(3):229–240, 2006.

67. Suri R, et al: Comparison of hypertonic saline and alternate-day or daily recombinant human deoxyribonuclease in children with cystic fibrosis: a randomised trial. *Lancet* 358(9290):1316–1321, 2001.

68. Hurt K, Bilton D: Inhaled mannitol for the treatment of cystic fibrosis. *Expert Rev Respir Med* 6(1):19–26, 2012.

69. Wills PJ: Inhaled mannitol in cystic fibrosis. *Expert Opin Investig Drugs* 16(7):1121–1126, 2007.

70. Minasian C, et al: Comparison of inhaled mannitol, daily rhDNase and a combination of both in children with cystic fibrosis: a randomised trial. *Thorax* 65(1):51–56, 2010.

71. Burness CB, Keating GM: Mannitol dry powder for inhalation: in patients with cystic fibrosis. *Drugs* 72(10):1411–1421, 2012.

72. Hart A, et al: Inhaled hyperosmolar agents for bronchiectasis. *Cochrane Database Syst Rev* (5):CD002996, 2014.

73. Ong HX, et al: Combined inhaled salbutamol and mannitol therapy for mucus hyper-secretion in pulmonary diseases. *AAPS J* 16(2):269–280, 2014.

74. Naz F, et al: Effectiveness of nebulized N-acetylcysteine solution in children with acute bronchiolitis. *J Coll Physicians Surg Pak* 24(6):408–411, 2014.

75. Li X, et al: Design, characterization, and aerosol dispersion performance modeling of advanced spray-dried microparticulate/nanoparticulate mannitol powders for targeted pulmonary delivery as dry powder inhalers. *J Aerosol Med Pulm Drug Deliv* 27(2):81–93, 2014.

76. Murgia X, et al: Surfactant and perfluorocarbon aerosolization by means of inhalation catheters for the treatment of respiratory distress syndrome: an in vitro study. *J Aerosol Med Pulm Drug Deliv* 24(2):81–87, 2011.

77. Murgia X, et al: Surfactant and perfluorocarbon aerosolization during different mechanical ventilation strategies by means of inhalation catheters: an in vitro study. *J Aerosol Med Pulm Drug Deliv* 25(1):23–31, 2012.

78. Walther FJ, et al: Synthetic surfactant containing SP-B and SP-C mimics is superior to single-peptide formulations in rabbits with chemical acute lung injury. *PeerJ* 2:e393, 2014.

79. Anzueto A, et al: Effects of aerosolized surfactant in patients with stable chronic bronchitis: a prospective randomized controlled trial. *JAMA* 278(17):1426–1431, 1997.

80. Corcoran TE, et al: Imaging the postdeposition dispersion of an inhaled surfactant aerosol. *J Aerosol Med Pulm Drug Deliv* 25(5):290–296, 2012.

81. Brand P, et al: Lung deposition of inhaled alpha1-proteinase inhibitor in cystic fibrosis and alpha1-antitrypsin deficiency. *Eur Respir J* 34(2):354–360, 2009.

82. Snyder AH, et al: Acute effects of aerosolized S-nitrosoglutathione in cystic fibrosis. *Am J Respir Crit Care Med* 165(7):922–926, 2002.

83. Groves S, et al: Inhaled cyclosporine and pulmonary function in lung transplant recipients. *J Aerosol Med Pulm Drug Deliv* 23(1):31–39, 2010.

84. Dubus JC, et al: Inhaled treatments in cystic fibrosis: what's new in 2013? *Rev Mal Respir* 31(4):336–346, 2014.

85. Rubin BK: Experimental macromolecular aerosol therapy. *Respir Care* 45(6):684–694, 2000.

86. Laube BL: The expanding role of aerosols in systemic drug delivery, gene therapy, and vaccination. *Respir Care* 50(9):1161–1176, 2005.

87. Moreno-Galdo A, et al: Use of inhaled iloprost in children with pulmonary hypertension. *Pediatr Pulmonol* 2014.

88. Yilmaz O, et al: Inhaled iloprost in preterm infants with severe respiratory distress syndrome and pulmonary hypertension. *Am J Perinatol* 31(4):321–326, 2014.

89. Xu Z, et al: Iloprost for children with pulmonary hypertension after surgery to correct congenital heart disease. *Pediatr Pulmonol* 2014.

90. Vorhies EE, et al: Use of inhaled iloprost for the management of postoperative pulmonary hypertension in congenital heart surgery patients: review of a transition protocol. *Pediatr Cardiol* 2014.

91. Buckley MS, et al: Clinical utility of treprostinil in the treatment of pulmonary arterial hypertension: an evidence-based review. *Core Evid* 9:71–80, 2014.

92. Enderby CY, et al: Transition from intravenous or subcutaneous prostacyclin therapy to inhaled treprostinil in patients with pulmonary arterial hypertension: a retrospective case series. *J Clin Pharm Ther* 2014.

93. Janssens HM, Tiddens HA: Facemasks and aerosol delivery by metered dose inhaler-valved holding chamber in young children: a tight seal makes the difference. *J Aerosol Med* 20(Suppl 1):S59–S63, discussion S63–S65, 2007.

94. Iles R, Lister P, Edmunds AT: Crying significantly reduces absorption of aerosolised drug in infants. *Arch Dis Child* 81(2):163–165, 1999.

95. Lin HL, Restrepo RD, Gardenhire DS, Rau JL: Effect of face mask design on inhaled mass of nebulized albuterol, using a pediatric breathing model. *Respir Care* 52(8):1021–1026, 2007.

96. Rubin BK: Air and soul: the science and application of aerosol therapy. *Respir Care* 55(7):911–921, 2010.

97. Everard ML: Trying to deliver aerosols to upset children is a thankless task. *Arch Dis Child* 82(5):428, 2000.

98. Amirav I, et al: Feasibility of aerosol drug delivery to sleeping infants: a prospective observational study. *BMJ Open* 4(3):e004124, 2014.

99. Amirav I, Newhouse MT: Deposition of small particles in the developing lung. *Paediatr Respir Rev* 13(2):73–78, 2012.

100. Amirav I, et al: Lung aerosol deposition in suckling infants. *Arch Dis Child* 97(6):497–501, 2012.

101. Esposito-Festen J, et al: Aerosol therapy by pressured metered-dose inhaler-spacer in sleeping young children: to do or not to do? *Chest* 130(2):487–492, 2006.

102. Restrepo RD, Dickson SK, Rau JL, Gardenhire DS: An investigation of nebulized bronchodilator delivery using a pediatric lung model of spontaneous breathing. *Respir Care* 51(1):56–61, 2006.

103. Erzinger S, et al: Facemasks and aerosol delivery in vivo. *J Aerosol Med* 20(Suppl 1):S78–S83, discussion S83–S84, 2007.

104. Amirav I, et al: Redesigned face mask improves "real life" aerosol delivery for Nebuchamber. *Pediatr Pulmonol* 37(2):172–177, 2004.

105. Blake K, et al: Bioavailability of inhaled fluticasone propionate via chambers/masks in young children. *Eur Respir J* 39(1):97–103, 2012.

106. Voeurng V, et al: A new small volume holding chamber for asthmatic children: comparison with Babyhaler spacer. *Pediatr Allergy Immunol* 17(8):629–634, 2006.

107. Amirav I, et al: Design of aerosol face masks for children using computerized 3d face analysis. *J Aerosol Med Pulm Drug Deliv* 27(4):272–278, 2014.

108. Di Paolo ER, Pannatier A, Cotting J: In vitro evaluation of bronchodilator drug delivery by jet nebulization during pediatric mechanical ventilation. *Pediatr Crit Care Med* 6(4):462–469, 2005.

109. Mazela J, Polin RA: Aerosol delivery to ventilated newborn infants: historical challenges and new directions. *Eur J Pediatr* 170(4):433–444, 2011.

110. Dhand R: New frontiers in aerosol delivery during mechanical ventilation. *Respir Care* 49(6):666–677, 2004.

111. Dhand R: Basic techniques for aerosol delivery during mechanical ventilation. *Respir Care* 49(6):611–622, 2004.

112. Dhand R: Inhalation therapy in invasive and noninvasive mechanical ventilation. *Curr Opin Crit Care* 13(1):27–38, 2007.

113. Fok TF, et al: Delivery of salbutamol to nonventilated preterm infants by metered-dose inhaler, jet nebulizer, and ultrasonic nebulizer. *Eur Respir J* 12(1):159–164, 1998.

114. Mandhane P, et al: Albuterol aerosol delivered via metered-dose inhaler to intubated pediatric models of 3 ages, with 4 spacer designs. *Respir Care* 48(10):948–955, 2003.

115. Ari A, et al: Influence of nebulizer type, position, and bias flow on aerosol drug delivery in simulated pediatric and adult lung models during mechanical ventilation. *Respir Care* 55(7):845–851, 2010.

116. Ari A, Areabi H, Fink JB: Evaluation of aerosol generator devices at 3 locations in humidified and non-humidified circuits during adult mechanical ventilation. *Respir Care* 55(7):837–844, 2010.

117. Ari A, Restrepo RD: American Association for Respiratory, Aerosol delivery device selection for spontaneously breathing patients: 2012. *Respir Care* 57(4):613–626, 2012.

118. Mitchell JP: Appropriate face models for evaluating drug delivery in the laboratory: the current situation and prospects for future advances. *J Aerosol Med Pulm Drug Deliv* 21(1):97–112, 2008.

UNIT THREE

Critical Care, Cardiovascular, and Polysomnography Agents

CHAPTER 18

Skeletal Muscle Relaxants (Neuromuscular Blocking Agents)

Douglas S. Gardenhire

CHAPTER OUTLINE

OBJECTIVES

After reading this chapter, the reader will be able to:

1. Define terms that pertain to skeletal muscle relaxants
2. Define neuromuscular blocking agents (NMBAs)
3. List the uses of NMBAs
4. Describe the physiology of the neuromuscular junction
5. Describe the makeup of nondepolarizing agents
6. Describe the makeup of depolarizing agents
7. Describe uses of NMBAs and mechanical ventilation
8. Identify methods of monitoring neuromuscular blockade

KEY TERMS AND DEFINITIONS

Acetylcholinesterase (AchE) Enzyme that breaks down the neurotransmitter acetylcholine (Ach) at the synaptic cleft so that the next nerve impulse can be transmitted across the synaptic gap.

Amnestic properties Having the ability to cause total or partial loss of memory.

Aspiration Accidental inhalation of food particles, fluids, or gastric contents into the lungs.

Fasciculation Involuntary contractions or twitching of groups of muscle fibers.

Myasthenia gravis Autoimmune neuromuscular disorder characterized by chronic fatigue and exhaustion of muscles.

Nerve cell (neuron) A basic functional unit of the nervous system that is specialized to transmit electrical nerve impulses and carry information from one part of the body to another. A neuron consists of a cell body, axons, and dendrites.

Neuromuscular blocking agents (NMBAs) Substances that interfere with the neural transmission between motor neurons and skeletal muscles.

Neurotransmitter Chemical that is released from a nerve ending to transmit an impulse from a nerve cell to another nerve, muscle, organ, or other tissue.

Nosocomial pneumonia Pneumonia that is acquired in a health care setting.

Sedation Production of a restful state of mind, particularly by the use of drugs that have a calming effect, relieving anxiety and tension.

Somatic motor neurons Part of the nervous system that controls muscles that are under voluntary control.

Status asthmaticus Exacerbation of asthma that does not respond to standard treatment.

Status epilepticus At least 30 minutes of continuous seizure activity without full recovery between seizures.

Neuromuscular blocking agents (NMBAs), also termed paralytics or muscle relaxants, are drugs that cause skeletal muscle weakness or paralysis, preventing movement. These agents produce this effect at the neuromuscular junction by interfering with the action of the neurotransmitter acetylcholine (Ach). NMBAs either depolarize the presynaptic and postsynaptic membrane receptors or compete with Ach for binding of the Ach receptors at the neuromuscular junction.

KEY POINT

Neuromuscular blocking agents (NMBAs) are used for skeletal muscle paralysis in several clinical situations, including *intubation, surgery,* and *facilitation of ventilation* in certain critically ill patients.

NMBAs are divided into two types: depolarizing agents and nondepolarizing agents. Depolarizing agents bind to Ach receptors and cause a sustained postsynaptic membrane depolarization. By preventing repolarization of the nerve ending, the postsynaptic ending becomes refractory and unexcitable, resulting in flaccid muscles. At present, succinylcholine is the only available agent in this class. Nondepolarizing agents produce paralysis and muscle weakness by competing with Ach for binding at the Ach receptors. By preventing the binding of Ach, nondepolarizing agents block the depolarizing effects of Ach, thereby preventing muscle contraction.

KEY POINT

The two types of NMBAs are *nondepolarizing* and *depolarizing*. Nondepolarizing agents, such as pancuronium, *competitively block* the cholinergic nicotinic receptor on the postsynaptic muscle fiber, preventing Ach from depolarizing the muscle fiber. Depolarizing agents, such as succinylcholine, act by first depolarizing the muscle fiber and then *prolonging the depolarized state* to prevent repolarization and further stimulation.

USES OF NEUROMUSCULAR BLOCKING AGENTS

The clinical uses of NMBAs are as follows:

- To facilitate endotracheal intubation
- To obtain muscle relaxation during surgery, particularly of the thorax and abdomen
- To enhance patient-ventilator synchrony
- To reduce intracranial pressure in intubated patients with uncontrolled intracranial pressure
- To reduce oxygen consumption
- To terminate convulsive **status epilepticus** and *tetanus* in patients refractory to other therapies
- To facilitate procedures or diagnostic studies
- To paralyze selected patients who must remain immobile (e.g., trauma patients)

NMBAs are usually given intravenously and exhibit a dose-related response on muscles. The primary use of NMBAs in the operating room is for anesthesia induction before endotracheal intubation. In the intensive care unit (ICU), NMBAs are used primarily for management of mechanical ventilation.

KEY POINT

The most common examples of *ventilated patients requiring muscle relaxation* are patients with severe asthma, reduction of oxygen consumption in difficult to manage patients, such as patients with acute respiratory distress syndrome (ARDS) and patients requiring "uncomfortable" modes of ventilation, such as pressure-controlled inverse ratio ventilation.

PHYSIOLOGY OF THE NEUROMUSCULAR JUNCTION

The autonomic nervous system consists of the central nervous system (CNS) and the peripheral nervous system (PNS). The CNS consists of the brain and the spinal cord, and the PNS includes all the nerves outside of the CNS. The PNS is divided further into the **somatic motor neurons**, sensory afferent neurons, and autonomic motor neurons. The somatic motor neurons include all the peripheral nerves that control skeletal muscle over which humans have control of "voluntary" movement. Examples of skeletal muscles include the quadriceps, biceps, diaphragm, and accessory muscles of ventilation, which are responsible for motor functions such as movement, lifting, and breathing. The autonomic motor neurons include peripheral nerves that control smooth muscle (e.g., wall of the digestive system, vascular smooth muscle), cardiac muscle (rate and force of contraction), and glands (e.g., adrenal medulla, sweat glands, exocrine glands of the pancreas). For a review, refer to Chapter 5.

The basic **nerve cell**, or **neuron**, consists of a *cell body, axons,* and *dendrites* (Figure 18-1). The cell bodies of somatic motor neurons, which are located in the spinal cord, stimulate skeletal muscles via the axons running through the peripheral nerves. These axons are large myelinated nerve fibers extending from the peripheral nerve cell bodies to the muscle fibers. A single peripheral nerve branches and innervates many different muscle fibers as a *motor unit*. The area between the nerve and muscle, or *synapse*, is specialized into a *motor end plate*. This area between the axon and the skeletal muscle fiber is also termed the *neuromuscular junction* (Figure 18-2).

The transmission of nerve signals in the skeletal muscle is chemically mediated by the **neurotransmitter** Ach. When a nerve impulse reaches the end of the motor neuron, Ach is released from the presynaptic membrane into the synaptic cleft. Ach diffuses across the synaptic space and interacts with specific Ach receptors on the postsynaptic muscle fiber membrane, resulting in a contractile response by the muscle fiber. During the short period that Ach is in contact with the receptor on the postsynaptic (muscle fiber) membrane, a nerve action potential, or nerve impulse, is initiated in the postsynaptic membrane. Ach is broken down and inactivated by the enzyme **acetylcholinesterase (AchE)**, allowing the muscle fiber to repolarize.

On the basis of the neuromuscular physiology described, muscle contraction may be blocked in the following two ways:

1. *Competitive inhibition:* The binding and blocking of the Ach receptors without depolarization; this is the action of the *nondepolarizing* agents
2. *Prolonged occupation and persistent binding of the Ach receptors:* Resulting in sustained depolarization of the neuromuscular junction; this is the action of the *depolarizing* agents

Both depolarizing and nondepolarizing agents resemble the neurotransmitter Ach. Table 18-1 reviews both types of NMBA, including major chemical classification, duration of action, and elimination route.

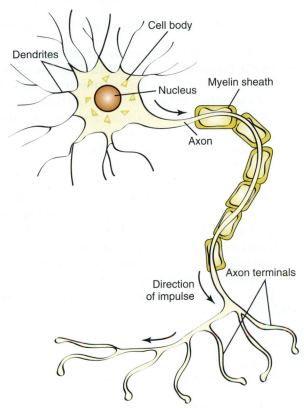

Figure 18-1 Schematic drawing of a nerve cell.

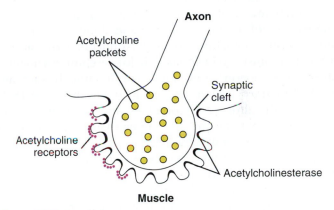

Figure 18-2 Schematic description of the anatomy of the motor end plate.

TABLE 18-1	Classification of Neuromuscular Blocking Agents (NMBAs)				
AGENT	**CHEMICAL CLASS**	**PHARMACOLOGIC PROPERTIES**	**TIME OF ONSET (min)**	**CLINICAL DURATION (min)**	**MODE OF ELIMINATION**
Depolarizing NMBAs					
Succinylcholine (Anectine, Quelicin)	Dicholine ester	Ultra-short duration	1-1.5	10-15	Hydrolysis by plasma cholinesterases
Nondepolarizing NMBAs					
Atracurium	Benzylisoquinoline ester	Intermediate duration; competitive	2-4	30-60	Hofmann degradation; hydrolysis by plasma esterases; renal elimination
Cisatracurium (Nimbex)	Benzylisoquinoline ester	Intermediate duration; competitive	2-3	40-60	Hofmann degradation; hydrolysis by plasma esterases; renal elimination
Pancuronium	Ammonio steroid	Long duration; competitive	4-6	120-180	Renal elimination
Rocuronium (Zemuron)	Ammonio steroid	Intermediate duration; competitive	1-2	30-60	Liver metabolism
Vecuronium	Ammonio steroid	Intermediate duration; competitive	2-4	60-90	Liver metabolism and clearance; renal elimination

NONDEPOLARIZING AGENTS

The earliest groups of NMBAs used clinically were agents such as curare. These agents paralyze skeletal muscle by simple competitive inhibition of Ach at muscle receptor sites. This group is referred to as nondepolarizing because they block the Ach receptors without activating them. Chemically, nondepolarizing NMBAs are either steroid-structured agents (vecuronium, rocuronium, and pancuronium) or benzylisoquinoline esters (atracurium and cisatracurium). The differences between the structures are important regarding complications and side effects.

Mechanism of Action

Nondepolarizing agents cause muscle paralysis by affecting the postsynaptic cholinergic receptors at the neuromuscular junction. By either blocking the channel externally, occupying the channel pore, or affecting the receptor from the internal side of the muscle membrane, these agents reduce the frequency of channel opening. Nondepolarizing agents compete against endogenous Ach for receptor occupancy. Muscle contraction does not occur if enough sites are blocked by these agents. This is illustrated in Figure 18-3, in which the drug (ND) occupies and then blocks the postsynaptic site at the neuromuscular junction. With nondepolarizing agents, depolarization of the postsynaptic membrane becomes a function of the amount of drug and the amount of Ach located around the receptor. In other words, because nondepolarizing agents act by competitive inhibition, their effect is dose related: Larger doses over-come the effects of Ach and block more receptors. The receptor blockade by nondepolarizing agents can be reversed by making more Ach available to compete for receptor sites. Inhibitors of AchE, an enzyme that breaks down Ach, can be used to reverse the competitive blockade. Neostigmine is an example of a cholinesterase inhibitor.

Pharmacokinetics of Nondepolarizing Agents

Nondepolarizing NMBAs chemically resemble Ach. These agents have a positively charged quaternary ammonium group (NH_4^+) that binds to the negatively charged Ach receptor. Nondepolarizing agents are poorly lipophilic and do not penetrate well into fat tissue or across the blood-brain barrier. Also, these agents are poorly absorbed from the gastrointestinal tract and therefore must be given intravenously to allow for rapid onset of neuromuscular blockade.

The onset of paralysis and the duration of action of nondepolarizing blockers vary widely among members of this group of drugs. Pancuronium has the longest duration of action and is considered a long-acting NMBA. Atracurium, cisatracurium, vecuronium, and rocuronium are redistributed more rapidly and have shorter durations of action. These agents are considered intermediate-acting NMBAs.[1]

> **! KEY POINT**
>
> Nondepolarizing agents have a longer duration of action than the depolarizing agent succinylcholine.

As previously noted, the magnitude of effect, rate of onset of maximum blockade, and duration of action of NMBAs are dose-dependent; this is illustrated in Table 18-2 for the drug rocuronium when used in adults. Factors such as advanced age generally increase the length of neuromuscular blockade activity. Hepatic or renal failure can cause decreased clearance, increased blood levels, and prolonged duration of action for agents metabolized and eliminated by the liver and kidney.

Metabolism

Neuromuscular blockade diminishes and transmission is restored after a single bolus dose once the agent is cleared

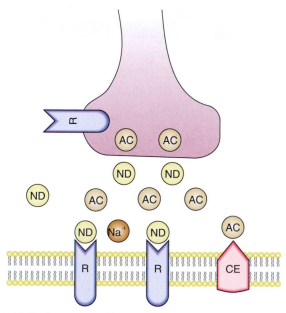

Figure 18-3 Competitive blocking agents, or nondepolarizers (ND), occupy but do not activate acetylcholine receptors (R). Acetylcholine (AC) is prevented from occupying receptors and muscle contraction fails to occur. Released acetylcholine is rapidly metabolized by membrane cholinesterase (CE). Nondepolarizers can also bind to prejunctional acetylcholine receptors and modify acetylcholine release. Na+, Sodium.

TABLE 18-2	Dose-Dependent Effects of Rocuronium in Adults	
DOSE (mg/kg)	**TIME TO MAXIMUM BLOCK (min)**	**CLINICAL DURATION (min)**
0.45	3	22
0.6	1.8	31
0.9	1.4	58
1.2	1	67

Data from *Drug facts and comparisons*, St Louis, 2014, Facts & Comparisons, Wolters Kluwer Health.

off the receptor site via redistribution to the rest of the body. When normal conduction returns, 75% of Ach receptors may still be occupied by a blocker; this explains why additional boluses of NMBA seem more potent and have a markedly prolonged duration of action. After prolonged infusion or repeated boluses, metabolism and excretion provide the mechanism for removal of the blocking agent from the neuromuscular junction.

Pancuronium is eliminated primarily by the kidneys. Pancuronium also undergoes some hepatic metabolism with production of an active metabolite that is eliminated by the kidneys.

Alternatively, vecuronium is an agent metabolized primarily by the liver. The metabolite of vecuronium also has activity and relies on the kidneys for excretion. All of these agents can accumulate in renal failure and cause prolonged paralysis when given in sufficient doses.

Atracurium and cisatracurium differ from other NMBAs regarding route of elimination. These agents are partly inactivated by a spontaneous degradation mechanism that is dependent on the pH of blood and temperature of the body. This nonenzymatic breakdown is termed *Hofmann degradation*. In addition to Hofmann degradation, these agents are rapidly converted to less active metabolites by circulating plasma esterases that cause hydrolysis of the compounds. Because of the lack of liver and kidney elimination, atracurium and cisatracurium are optimal choices for patients with hepatic or renal failure.

Atracurium further differs from cisatracurium because it has a breakdown product of Hofmann degradation called *laudanosine*. Laudanosine, which is eliminated primarily by the kidneys and is slowly metabolized by the liver, has a long half-life and can cross the blood-brain barrier. Laudanosine has been associated with neurostimulatory effects. CNS excitation and seizures should be considered as a possible complication, especially in patients receiving atracurium who have impaired renal function or liver failure.[2] Cisatracurium has less laudanosine production than atracurium and is considered more potent. The risk of further brain injury from seizures in patients with poor intracranial compliance (e.g., severe head injury) may make these drugs poor choices in these patients.[3] These agents, which complicate assessment of the patient, might mask seizure activity. The effects of organ failure on NMBA duration are illustrated in Table 18-3.

Adverse Effects

Cardiovascular Effects

It is important to understand that the nondepolarizing NMBAs also competitively block Ach receptors at the autonomic ganglia, producing cardiovascular side effects on heart rate and blood pressure. They may cause a vagolytic effect, which produces tachycardia, and an increase in mean arterial pressure by promoting an increase in norepinephrine, a potent vasoconstrictor.[3] Pancuronium has the greatest potential to cause cardiovascular side effects, especially tachycardia and hypertension. Agents such as vecuronium and cisatracurium have minimal effects on heart rate and blood pressure.

Histamine Release

All of the nondepolarizing agents have a tendency to release histamine from mast cells. However, the potential for adverse cardiac effects varies among the different agents. Clinically, histamine release can cause hypotension secondary to direct vasodilation, reflex tachycardia, and bronchospasm, leading to increased airway resistance. The vasodilatory effect may also give the appearance of skin flushing. The degree of histamine release for several NMBAs is shown in Table 18-4. Atracurium has been reported to stimulate the most histamine release, which could cause bronchoconstriction. It is recommended that this agent be given at a reduced rate or at lower doses to avoid these effects. Antihistamines may also be administered as pretreatment to avoid such effects.

Inadequate Ventilation

Muscle paralysis of the diaphragm and the intercostals results in an inadequate respiratory function. Adequate

TABLE 18-3   Major Metabolic Pathways of Neuromuscular Blockers and Effect on Duration of Action Caused by Organ Failure

AGENT	PROLONGATION OF EFFECT WITH RENAL FAILURE	PROLONGATION OF EFFECT WITH HEPATIC FAILURE	ALTERNATIVE METABOLISM
Atracurium	0	0	Hofman degradation, ester hydrolysis
Cisatracurium	0	0	Hofman degradation, ester hydrolysis
Pancuronium			
Rocuronium	++	0	
Succinylcholine	0	0	Plasma cholinesterase*
Vecuronium	++†	+	

0, No effect; + through ++++, degree of effect.
*Atypical pseudocholinesterase may prolong relaxant effect dramatically.
†Metabolic product is one third as potent as the parent compound and is entirely removed by renal excretion.

TABLE 18-4	Comparison of Side Effects of Neuromuscular Blocking Agents			
AGENT	HISTAMINE RELEASE	BLOCKADE OF AUTONOMIC GANGLIA	BLOCKADE OF VAGAL RESPONSE	VAGAL STIMULATION
Atracurium	++	0	0	0
Cisatracurium	+	0	0	0
Pancuronium	+	++	++	0
Rocuronium	+	0	+	0
Succinylcholine	+	0	0	+++
Vecuronium	0	0	0	0

0, No effect; + through ++++, degree of effect.

airway control and ventilatory support are required until muscle recovery is adequate for spontaneous ventilation. Close patient and machine monitoring are essential in the ICU to prevent hypoventilation and hypoxemia.

Reversal of Nondepolarizing Blockade

Muscle paralysis caused by nondepolarizing NMBAs can be reversed by use of cholinesterase inhibitors such as neostigmine. Neostigmine inhibits the cholinesterase that would normally break down Ach. This action allows for more Ach to be available at the neuromuscular junction to compete with and displace the blocker from receptor sites. Other cholinesterase inhibitors include edrophonium and pyridostigmine. Edrophonium is rapid-acting but also has the shortest duration of action. Pyridostigmine has a slower onset and is the longest acting; it is often used to treat **myasthenia gravis** and can be given orally. Neostigmine is intermediate in onset and duration of action. Table 18-5 summarizes these agents with recommended doses to reverse neuromuscular blockage produced by the nondepolarizing agents.[4]

KEY POINT

The effects of nondepolarizing agents can be reversed with an indirect-acting cholinergic agent (*cholinesterase inhibitor*) such as neostigmine. There is no reversal agent for succinylcholine.

Because the reversing agents increase the levels of Ach, they also increase the effects of Ach at parasympathetic ganglia, producing cholinergic autonomic side effects. Major side effects of these agents include severe bradycardia and salivation. To reduce these adverse effects, agents such as atropine or glycopyrrolate are also given in conjunction with cholinesterase inhibitors. As vagolytic and anticholinergic agents, atropine and glycopyrrolate, respectively, prevent bradycardia, increased salivation, and hyperperistalsis associated with excessive Ach.[5]

KEY POINT

Myasthenia gravis is caused by an immune response to *acetylcholine receptors (AchRs)*, which are found on nerve and muscle cells. In this disease, the body produces antibodies that attack AchRs, preventing signals from reaching the muscles.

TABLE 18-5	Agents Used for Reversal and Antimuscarinic Effects With Nondepolarizing Blocking Agents	
AGENT	DOSE (mg/kg)	TIME FOR EFFECT
Reversal Agents		
Edrophonium	0.3-1.0	Rapid onset, short acting
Neostigmine	0.01-0.035	Intermediate onset and duration
Pyridostigmine	0.1-0.25	Slowest onset, longest acting
Antimuscarinic Agents		
Atropine	0.008-0.018	Rapid onset, short acting
Glycopyrrolate	0.002-0.016	Rapid onset, short acting

Data from Buck ML, Reed MD: Use of nondepolarizing neuromuscular blocking agents in mechanically ventilated patients, *Clin Pharm* 10:32, 1991.

DEPOLARIZING AGENTS

Depolarizing agents have a different mechanism of action from nondepolarizing agents; they are shorter acting, and there are no agents that reliably reverse their blockades. Succinylcholine is the only available agent in this group. An intravenous dose of 1 to 1.5 mg/kg causes total muscle paralysis in 60 to 90 seconds that lasts 10 to 15 minutes. Because of the quick onset and brief duration of action of succinylcholine, it is an ideal agent for patients requiring intubation.

Mechanism of Action

The initial action of depolarizing NMBAs is to open sodium channels and depolarize the postsynaptic muscle membrane in the same manner as Ach. Depolarizing agents are resistant to the effects of AchE, allowing for a persistent and longer duration at the neuromuscular junction. Because depolarization lasts longer, the membrane is unable to repolarize, resulting in flaccid muscles.[5] This is illustrated in Figure 18-4, in which molecules of succinylcholine *(S)* have occupied two Ach receptors, each opening a pore and allowing the local membrane to become permeable to sodium. If enough receptors are activated, depolarization

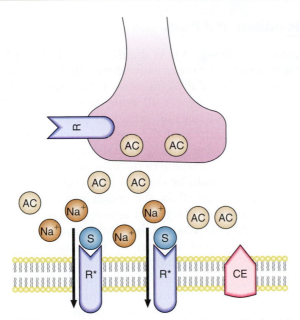

Figure 18-4 Succinylcholine produces a depolarizing block. Molecules of succinylcholine *(S)* occupy and activate the acetylcholine receptors *(R*)*, permitting sodium entry and an initial action potential. Continued occupancy prevents repolarization and the next action potential from released acetylcholine *(AC)*. Activation of prejunctional acetylcholine receptors can modify acetylcholine release. *CE,* Cholinesterase; *Na⁺,* sodium; *R,* prejunctional receptor.

occurs and is maintained until succinylcholine leaves the receptors. Further stimulation and contraction of the muscle fiber is impossible until the drug is removed by redistribution and metabolism.

In contrast to any agent discussed so far, succinylcholine has a unique feature of blockade activity. On initial bolus dose, succinylcholine depolarizes the membrane, similar to Ach. The initial depolarization causes uncoordinated skeletal muscle contractions, referred to as **fasciculation.** Because succinylcholine remains at the neuromuscular junction longer than Ach, depolarization is prolonged, and flaccid paralysis occurs. This is referred to as *phase I block.* After prolonged use or large doses of succinylcholine, the type of blocking activity changes. Instead of showing depolarization characteristics, activity resembles the block produced by the nondepolarizing agents. This is referred to as *phase II block* or *desensitization block.* Phase II block involves a "fading" phenomenon in which stimulation of the motor neuron is poorly sustained and paralysis is prolonged. Although cholinesterase inhibitors can reverse phase II block, they may decrease the clearance of succinylcholine and enhance further blockade. The occurrence of a desensitization block must be considered as a possibility in patients with prolonged paralysis after succinylcholine administration. The fear of this "dual" mechanism limits the use of succinylcholine in repeated doses or as a continuous infusion.

Metabolism

Succinylcholine has a very short duration of action; this is mostly due to its rapid hydrolysis by plasma cholinesterase

in blood. Succinylcholine is metabolized to succinylmonocholine, which provides weak nondepolarizing activity. Succinylmonocholine is thought to account for some of the reason why repeated doses of succinylcholine produce prolonged blockade.

Reversal

No agents are available for the reversal of succinylcholine. Use of cholinesterase inhibitors such as neostigmine may delay the elimination of succinylcholine, resulting in an even more prolonged depolarization and slower recovery of muscle activity.

Adverse Effects

Succinylcholine produces many side effects, several of which can be life-threatening. The significance of these side effects may be of more concern in the ICU than during routine operating room use. Most adult patients have a sympathomimetic response causing tachycardia and an increase in blood pressure. Repeated bolus doses of succinylcholine may produce vagal responses, including bradycardia and hypotension. This side effect is seen more often in children. Succinylcholine also provokes histamine release, resulting in bronchospasm and hypotension in susceptible individuals.[5]

Muscle pain and soreness similar to myalgias are common after the administration of succinylcholine. A relationship between the pain and muscle fasciculations has been implicated but not confirmed. Some practitioners administer a small dose of a nondepolarizing blocker (e.g., 10% of the intubating dose) before giving succinylcholine to reduce fasciculations and pain.[6] This pretreatment is often referred to as *defasciculation.* In patients receiving a nondepolarizing agent to prevent fasciculations, higher doses of succinylcholine are needed for complete paralysis because pretreatment reduces the effectiveness of succinylcholine. This practice is considered controversial because increased doses of succinylcholine are required, and pretreatment may cause partial paralysis, necessitating urgent intubation under nonideal conditions.[7] Muscle fasciculations can also cause an increase in serum potassium and creatinine phosphokinase, an effect that is also reduced but not totally eliminated by pretreatment.

Succinylcholine can cause an efflux of potassium from muscle cells, causing serum potassium to increase by 0.5 to 1 mEq/L in normal individuals.[6] Patients with spinal cord injury or upper motor neuron lesions, thermal injuries, and severe trauma, including closed head injury, are at a higher risk of developing life-threatening hyperkalemia if succinylcholine is administered. Effects of severe hyperkalemia include arrhythmias and cardiac arrest.

Succinylcholine-induced fasciculations can increase intraocular pressure and intragastric pressure. Patients are at risk of extrusion of intraocular contents and aspiration of gastric contents. These conditions may be partially prevented by defasciculation.

Succinylcholine can dangerously increase intracranial pressure in patients with cerebral edema and head trauma by a mechanism that is not well understood.[6] One of the most serious complications that can occur with succinylcholine is malignant hyperthermia. Malignant hyperthermia is caused by a genetic defect of muscle metabolism. It is a potentially fatal hypermetabolic state of skeletal muscles. An uncontrolled release of calcium from the sarcoplasmic reticulum of muscles occurs, resulting in a host of harmful effects. The clinical features can manifest as intractable spasm of the jaw muscles, rigidity, increased oxygen demand, severe hyperthermia, metabolic acidosis, and tachycardia. Malignant hyperthermia is treated with dantrolene, an agent that blocks the release of intracellular calcium from the sarcoplasmic reticulum. Early recognition and treatment are key to ensuring a full recovery.[8]

Sensitivity to Succinylcholine

As mentioned, succinylcholine is metabolized by plasma cholinesterase, which is also called *pseudocholinesterase.* Patients with abnormal or deficient pseudocholinesterase do not metabolize succinylcholine effectively and experience a prolonged recovery from paralysis. In these patients, prolonged mechanical ventilation support is warranted. A family history of prolonged paralysis after surgery may suggest an abnormality in the enzyme. Laboratory tests are also available to determine the existence of abnormal cholinesterase.[9]

NEUROMUSCULAR BLOCKING AGENTS AND MECHANICAL VENTILATION

An indication for use of NMBAs in patients receiving mechanical ventilation is to improve ventilator-patient synchrony. Ventilator dyssynchrony can cause increased intrathoracic pressure, decreased alveolar ventilation, and increased work of breathing for the patient. The desired goal with these drugs is to improve ventilation and oxygenation and to reduce ventilation pressures. Disease states in which neuromuscular blockade may be beneficial include the following:

- Acute respiratory distress syndrome (ARDS)
- Status asthmaticus, severe bronchospasm
- Certain modes of ventilatory support (e.g., pressure-controlled inverse ratio ventilation, high-frequency oscillatory ventilation)
- Status epilepticus or other intractable convulsive activity
- Neuromuscular toxins (e.g., strychnine poisoning)
- Tetanus

Patients with **status asthmaticus** and those with ARDS requiring pressure-controlled ventilation with or without inverse ratio ventilation to limit peak airway pressure are at highest risk of ventilator dyssynchrony.

Precautions and Risks

All patients receiving NMBAs should receive additional care measures to decrease the negative effects that can be associated with the use of these agents. Proper eye care should be a standard of care for all patients receiving NMBAs. Normally, eye blinking lubricates and cleans the corneas. NMBAs cause paralysis of the eyelid muscles, which can result in corneal drying and ulceration. Appropriate eye lubrication and light taping of the eyes can prevent corneal abrasions. Eyes should be checked frequently.

With complete paralysis, the cough reflex is inhibited. Frequent suctioning along with appropriate sedation and analgesia to prevent pain and discomfort during suctioning is necessary. Retention of secretions is thought to increase the incidence of **nosocomial pneumonia** in patients receiving neuromuscular blockade for a prolonged period. Elevating the head can reduce the risk of **aspiration**, which is a risk factor for ventilator-associated pneumonia (VAP).

Support equipment must be closely monitored, including constant observation for extubation and ventilator malfunction. Alarm systems to detect hypoventilation and hypoxemia are the standard of care when NMBAs are used.

Patients receiving prolonged therapy with NMBAs are at risk for developing prolonged skeletal muscle weakness that persists long after the NMBA is discontinued. Myopathy, which may take months to resolve, may be associated more often with steroid-structured agents, such as vecuronium and pancuronium (see Table 18-1 for classification), especially when they are combined with corticosteroids, such as prednisone. Daily physical therapy with range of motion exercises may lessen the potential for muscle atrophy or wasting in patients receiving prolonged NMBA therapy. Patients given an NMBA should also be turned frequently to prevent the formation of pressure sores and decubitus ulcers. The risk of developing a deep vein thrombosis (DVT) is increased in these patients because of their immobility, making DVT prophylaxis imperative.

Use of Sedation and Analgesia

Of all adjunctive therapies patients may receive, it is essential to provide adequate **sedation** and analgesia for ventilated patients receiving a blocking agent. NMBAs cause muscle paralysis without affecting consciousness or the perception of pain. In 1947 a classic experiment that established this fact was performed by Smith and colleagues,[10] in which Smith allowed himself to be paralyzed with tubocurarine, an NMBA that is no longer marketed in the United States. He reported full awareness during the paralysis, including sensations of choking while he was unable to swallow and shortness of breath even though he was being adequately ventilated. Neuromuscular blockade is unthinkable without proper sedation and pain control to prevent the nightmare of paralysis with full consciousness and sensory perception. Although many sedative and analgesia agents can cause hemodynamic instability, it is inappropriate to reduce or discontinue sedation and analgesia while a patient is paralyzed to address hemodynamic instability. Because clinical signs of restlessness, distress, and anxiety are lost with neuromuscular blockade, continuous cardiac monitoring is necessary, and vital signs should be assessed closely. Tachycardia, hypertension, diaphoresis, and lacrimation are physiologic responses that can indicate anxiety caused by inadequate sedation or lack of pain control.

KEY POINT

Paralysis of a conscious patient is torture, and adequate sedation and analgesia are mandatory.

For short procedures including endotracheal intubation, a sedative that has **amnestic properties** should be administered. In surgery, a sedative and an analgesic agent are recommended for all patients. For patients in the ICU, a sedative should be administered on a continuous basis before initiation of neuromuscular blockade. Continuous analgesia should also be used secondary to poor assessment capabilities for pain and the discomfort associated with the constant suctioning and the endotracheal tube itself. Sedatives that have amnestic effects include propofol, lorazepam, and midazolam. It is important to realize that these agents do not provide pain control. Analgesics commonly used for pain control include fentanyl, hydromorphone, and morphine. In many situations, deep sedation with continuously infused sedatives and analgesics may prevent the need for a blocking agent in the ICU. Other suggestions for sedation and analgesia are presented in Chapter 20.

Interactions With Neuromuscular Blocking Agents

Several clinical conditions and medications may alter the effect of an administered NMBA. Because different blocking drugs may act at different locations on the Ach receptor–pore complex (e.g., external, in the pore, intercellular), combination with certain agents may be synergistic and potentiate blockade. Advantage has been taken of this potential to produce a combination of relaxant drugs that gives adequate relaxation with fewer cardiovascular side effects. Examples include combining inhaled anesthetics, such as halothane or isoflurane, with a nondepolarizing NMBA. The inhaled anesthetics decrease the sensitivity of the neuromuscular junction to Ach, potentiating blockade. The dosage of the NMBA can be reduced, perhaps decreasing side effects. The problem with this approach has been the unpredictability of the duration of relaxation, which tends to be extremely prolonged, especially after repeated mixture administrations.

Some classes of drugs and other conditions have neuromuscular blocking effects themselves; these may be additive, antagonistic, or synergistic with NMBAs. Aminoglycoside antibiotics are often administered to critically ill patients in

TABLE 18-6   Drugs and Conditions That Interact With Nondepolarizing Neuromuscular Blocking Agents

POTENTIATING FACTORS	ANTAGONIZING FACTORS
Drugs	
• Potent anesthetic vapors	• Phenytoin
• Antibiotics	• Carbamazepine
• Aminoglycosides	• Theophylline
• Clindamycin	• Anticholinesterase agents
• Vancomycin	• Azathioprine
• Tetracycline	• Ranitidine
• Local anesthetics	
• Antiarrhythmics	
• Procainamide	
• Quinidine	
• Calcium channel blockers	
• β-adrenergic blockers	
• Cyclosporine	
• Dantrolene	
• Cyclophosphamide	
• Lithium	
• Mineralocorticoids	
• Echothiophate	
• Tacrine	
• Metoclopramide	
Conditions	
• Acidosis	• Alkalosis
• Hyponatremia	• Hypercalcemia
• Hypocalcemia	• Demyelinating injuries
• Hypokalemia	• Peripheral neuropathy
• Hypermagnesemia	
• Hypothermia	
• Renal failure	
• Hepatic failure	
• Organophosphate poisoning	
Diseases	
• Myasthenia gravis	• Diabetes mellitus
• Muscular dystrophy	
• Amyotrophic lateral sclerosis	
• Poliomyelitis	
• Multiple sclerosis	
• Eaton-Lambert syndrome	

Data from Feldman S, Karalliedde L: Drug interactions with neuromuscular blockers, *Drug Saf* 15:261, 1996.

the ICU. Aminoglycosides produce blockade by inhibiting the release of Ach from presynaptic nerve endings and, to a lesser extent, by blocking the postsynaptic receptor. Agents such as phenytoin, azathioprine, and theophylline antagonize neuromuscular blockade.

Clinical factors such as acidosis, hypokalemia, hyponatremia, hypocalcemia, and hypermagnesemia all potentiate neuromuscular blockade. Alkalosis and hypercalcemia are known to inhibit the effects of blockade. Factors affecting the activity of NMBAs are listed in Table 18-6.

Choice of Agents

Characteristics of the perfect NMBA (not yet developed) include the following:

- Nondepolarizing block
- Rapid onset of action
- Predictable and controllable duration of action
- Hemodynamic stability at all levels of block and rate of administration
- No histamine release
- Predictable kinetics independent of age, gender, and organ dysfunction
- No active metabolites or toxicity
- Inexpensive

To date, there is no NMBA that exhibits all these ideal characteristics. Selection of an appropriate NMBA depends on the situation. Several factors must be taken into account when choosing an agent, including duration of procedure (consider duration of action), the need for quick endotracheal intubation (consider onset of action), adverse-effect profile (hemodynamic stability, histamine release), route of elimination (especially in patients with renal or hepatic insufficiency), concurrent medications and other drug interactions, and cost. The depolarizing agent succinylcholine is well suited only for intubation because of its rapid onset and short duration of action. Rocuronium may be the most reasonable alternative to succinylcholine with a better side effect profile. Rocuronium has a quick onset of action but longer duration of effect than succinylcholine. For patients requiring prolonged paralysis, nondepolarizing blocking agents are more suitable. The kinetics of nondepolarizing agents allow for a longer duration of action, more gradual onset and offset of block, and fewer hemodynamic changes. They can be administered by continuous infusion, and the blockade can be reversed if necessary with cholinesterase inhibitors.

The choice of agent for continuous paralysis involves clinical judgment and preference. Currently available nondepolarizing agents can be compared with one another in regard to adverse-effect profile (histamine release and cardiovascular instability), route of elimination, drug interactions, and cost-effectiveness to guide drug choice for paralysis of ventilated patients. Tables 18-3 and 18-4 compare some of these factors for several NMBAs.

Most nondepolarizing agents release histamine from mast cells. Pancuronium is thought to provoke the smallest release of histamine. Agents such as vecuronium, rocuronium, and cisatracurium are similar to pancuronium and have minimal histamine release relative to the other agents. Atracurium has been shown to induce more histamine release than pancuronium. Flushing is the most common effect of histamine release after atracurium administration. Histamine release by these drugs can be minimized by administering a bolus dose slowly over 60 seconds, administering several smaller boluses, or giving the agent by slow continuous infusion.

Vecuronium, atracurium, and cisatracurium have minimal effects on heart rate and blood pressure. Pancuronium often produces a transient increase in blood pressure and heart rate. Rocuronium seems to cause little systemic cardiovascular effect, but an increase in pulmonary vascular resistance has been seen. Caution is recommended in using this agent in patients with pulmonary hypertension or valvular heart disease.

The method of drug elimination (e.g., renal or hepatic) is a very important factor in selecting an agent for patients with multiorgan dysfunction syndrome requiring mechanical ventilation. Agents that depend on the liver and kidney for elimination are poorly suited for patients with disease or failure of these organs. The potential effects of organ failure on each agent are described in Table 18-3. In patients with hepatic or renal failure, atracurium and cisatracurium have the advantage of plasma metabolism and do not rely on hepatic metabolism or renal excretion. The metabolite laudanosine, created from atracurium metabolism, may be of concern in patients with kidney or liver failure. Cisatracurium results in less laudanosine than does atracurium.

Patients in the ICU have clinical conditions and are often receiving medications that can affect blockade with an NMBA. As discussed earlier, myopathy can occur in patients receiving NMBAs. The potential is increased in patients receiving concomitant corticosteroids. Agents such as vecuronium, pancuronium, and rocuronium are steroid-structured and may prolong muscle weakness further. Nonsteroid-structured agents such as atracurium or cisatracurium may be better suited for patients requiring high-dose corticosteroids.

Finally, cost is an important consideration in choosing an agent. Many hospitals limit the number of NMBAs available on formulary because of economic issues. Newer, shorter-acting agents are very expensive, especially if used for a prolonged period in the ICU. Most hospitals restrict their use to procedures of short duration. Guidelines for blockade use in the ICU have been published and suggest that cost-effective relaxation can be provided with bolus dosing or continuous infusions of pancuronium (if tachycardia is not a concern) or vecuronium in patients with ischemic cardiovascular issues.[2] For patients with hepatic and renal dysfunction, cisatracurium or atracurium is the best option. The clinician is advised to reassess the need for continuous paralysis on a daily basis.

Pancuronium provides the least expensive option for prolonged paralysis of patients who are hemodynamically stable with no organ dysfunction. For unstable patients, vecuronium produces the least amount of histamine release and fewest cardiovascular effects. Atracurium and cisatracurium offer alternative choices for ventilator management, with these agents having the advantage of alternative metabolic pathways but at a higher cost.

 KEY POINT

Nondepolarizing agents are preferred for paralysis of ventilated patients because of the predictability, longer duration of action, and manageable side effects of these agents. Specific agents should be selected on the basis of potential for histamine release and cardiovascular effects, patient-specific metabolic pathways, and cost.

MONITORING OF NEUROMUSCULAR BLOCKADE

Patients receiving NMBAs require constant monitoring with frequent physical assessment and regularly scheduled evaluations of laboratory studies because clinical signs and symptoms of acute disease can be masked by muscle paralysis. Alarm systems to detect accidental disconnection from the ventilator are mandatory and alarms to detect hypoventilation and hypoxemia are the standard of care when neuromuscular blockade is employed.

Before initiating neuromuscular blockade of an agitated patient, ventilator malfunction must first be ruled out as the cause of agitation, or muscle paralysis could cause death in the face of inadequate machine volume or oxygen delivery. Patients receiving paralytics can be assessed by visual, tactile, and electronic methods to evaluate muscle tone and depth of neuromuscular blockade. Direct observation of muscle activity provides the simplest means of monitoring adequacy of blockade. The sequence of paralysis of the skeletal muscles can be monitored physically: first, small, rapid-moving muscles such as the eyelids; then the face, neck, extremities, abdomen, and intercostals; and finally, the diaphragm. Recovery of paralysis is in reverse order, with recovery of the diaphragm and respiratory muscles occurring first. The sensitivity of individual muscles to paralysis is related to the number of fibers innervated by each motor neuron and by regional blood flow, with areas receiving a greater blood flow having more drug delivery and therefore a quicker onset of paralysis.

The majority of experience with NMBAs occurs in the operating room. The time course of relaxant effect and rate of recovery is not the same when these drugs are used for prolonged periods in patients in the ICU. During brief periods of paralysis, the depth of blockade or the adequacy of recovery of neuromuscular function can be assessed by simple measures of voluntary muscular functions. These include subjective assessments, such as handgrip strength or the ability to lift the head off the bed for 5 seconds. Objective assessments include measurement of vital capacity, negative inspiratory force, and spontaneous respiratory rate. Patients requiring prolonged paralysis are not as easy to evaluate because of issues such as heavy sedation. Although clinical signs may be helpful in these patients, a more physiologic and objective evaluation of neuromuscular blockade can be achieved by using electronic methods such as peripheral nerve stimulation. Examples of modes of peripheral nerve stimulation include single twitch, double burst, train-of-four (TOF), and tetanic and posttetanic count.

Peripheral nerve stimulation or "twitch monitoring" is used as a monitoring tool for efficacy and toxicity in surgical and ICU patients. In peripheral nerve stimulation, a stimulator is applied to a peripheral nerve, and the response of the corresponding muscle is observed. The ulnar nerve, which innervates the adductor pollicis muscle of the thumb, is the most commonly used area. Another nerve is the facial nerve, which innervates the orbicularis oculi muscle of the eye. The nerve response to electrical stimulation depends on the current applied, the duration for which the current is applied, and placement of the electrodes. For ulnar nerve stimulation, two small conducting pads are placed on the forearm over the nerve tract, several inches apart. A single electrical stimulus is discharged from a nerve stimulator to the ulnar nerve; the responses or twitches of the thumb that occur are then measured. As the amount of paralysis increases, the strength and degree of movement of the twitch decrease.

The most commonly used technique for monitoring blockade is the TOF evaluation. In TOF, a supramaximal stimulus at a frequency of 2 Hz is applied to the nerve over 2 seconds. The nonpainful stimuli are delivered as four pulses, one every 0.5 second. The number of twitches that occur, ranging from zero (100% blockade) to four (less than 75% blockade), are measured. Comparison of the strength of the fourth twitch and first twitch predicts the degree of receptor occupancy (Table 18-7). Clinically, the degree of block can be determined by counting the number of twitches seen. Four equal twitches indicate that less than 75% of the receptors are occupied with a blocker. If only three twitches are seen, approximately 80% of receptors are blocked; if only one or two are seen, 90% to 95% are blocked.

TABLE 18-7	Receptor Occupancy Associated With Various Measurements of Neuromuscular Blockade		
RECEPTORS OCCUPIED (%)	**TWITCH HEIGHT (%)**	**TRAIN-OF-FOUR**	**CLINICAL OBSERVATIONS**
100	0	0	Total paralysis, no voluntary movement of any muscle; no PTF
98-99	0	0	Diaphragm may move; PTF present
95-98	1-5	1 or 2 twitches	Diaphragm can move minimally; PTF and fade present
90-95	10-25	2 or 3 twitches	Breathing inadequate
75-90	10-25	4 twitches, 1st > 4th	Tidal volume restored, voluntary movement apparent, can sustain head lift for 5 seconds (75%-80% occupancy), NIP >55 cm H_2O, vital capacity 60%-70% of normal
50-75	100	4 equal twitches	Normal strength and movement, cough strength decreased; double burst suppression abnormal
<30	100	4 equal twitches	No apparent deficits, double burst suppression normal

NIP, Negative inspiratory pressure; *PTF*, posttetanic facilitation.

Proper placement of the conducting pads is essential to proper assessment of the TOF. TOF evaluates the conduction of an impulse across the neuromuscular junction. If the pads are placed directly on the muscle, the patient falsely exhibits inadequate paralysis, which leads to the administration of higher than necessary doses of paralytic. Although TOF is the most common method used, changes in patient condition (e.g., third spacing, anasarca) limit the utility of this test, and alternative means must be sought.

TOF monitoring allows for an accurate assessment of neuromuscular blockade depth with or without baseline control. To avoid overdosing of patients, the NMBA (bolus or infusion) should be titrated to produce the minimal blockade required to maintain the desired clinical response. Predefined goals, such as decreased oxygen requirements, peak inspiratory pressure, and positive end-expiratory pressure (PEEP) reduction should be assessed frequently. If the response is adequate, a TOF count of at least one twitch to two or four stimulations is recommended. It is possible that lesser degrees of blockade may achieve the clinical goal of ventilator synchrony or improved oxygenation. In the ICU, the depth of blockade should be assessed every 2 to 3 hours on initiation until a stable dose is maintained. Thereafter, TOF assessment may occur every 8 to 12 hours. If there is no twitch response or the clinical response is achieved at a higher twitch, the dose of the NMBA should be decreased by 10%. If three or four twitches occur without adequate response, the dose can be increased by 10%. The need for continued paralysis of a patient in the ICU should be assessed daily, and if appropriate, paralysis should be discontinued as soon as possible.[7]

KEY POINT

Titration of drug dose and monitoring of reversal are performed with a *peripheral nerve stimulator* and train-of-four (TOF) stimulation.

FUTURE OF NEUROMUSCULAR BLOCKING AGENTS AND REVERSAL

Research is continuing in an effort to develop an ideal NMBA. At the present time, gantacurium has promise as a new agent. Still in the research phase, gantacurium is a nondepolarizing agent with rapid-onset and short-acting properties. Its organ-independent inactivation is ideal in patients with organ dysfunction. Histamine release has been found to occur, resulting in tachycardia and hypotension. The histamine release seems to be less compared with the histamine release produced by the benzylisoquinolines.[11] Although gantacurium offers a promising alternative to currently available NMBAs, it may have drawbacks that have not yet been discovered and requires further evaluation in larger trials.

At present, the method of reversing NMBAs involves the use of AchE inhibitors, such as neostigmine, which increase the levels of Ach in the synaptic cleft to compete with NMBA for receptor sites. Sugammadex, an agent currently under study, provides a newer approach to NMBA reversal. The novel mechanism of action involves the actual inactivation and removal of the NMBA from the neuromuscular junction and the body. Sugammadex functions by encapsulating the NMBA to form a complex that can no longer bind to the receptors. The kidneys excrete the stable complex that is formed. Sugammadex has been shown to reverse only rocuronium and vecuronium effectively. It is much less effective for reversal of pancuronium, succinylcholine, and the benzylisoquinolines. Adverse effects are mild and include nausea, dry mouth, cough, and taste perversions.[12]

SELF-ASSESSMENT QUESTIONS

Answers can be found in Appendix A.

1. List four general uses of skeletal muscle relaxants.
2. What are the two classifications of neuromuscular blocking agents?
3. Identify each of the following agents by classification type: vecuronium, succinylcholine, and pancuronium.
4. Which type of neuromuscular blocker can be reversed?
5. What type of drug would you use to reverse vecuronium?
6. Identify another drug that you would want to give before you reverse vecuronium.
7. Briefly explain why you might need to paralyze a patient receiving mechanical ventilation.
8. Neuromuscular blocking agents do not block consciousness; what two types or classes of drugs would be indicated in a paralyzed patient on mechanical ventilation?
9. Identify at least two neuromuscular blocking agents that would be preferred for paralysis in a patient receiving mechanical ventilation (assume normal renal and hepatic function).
10. You are called to the recovery room to set up a ventilator for an elderly patient who has just undergone a total hip replacement and has failed to breathe after a single dose of succinylcholine. What might the problem be?
11. What would you do first to assess a ventilated patient who is restless and "fighting" the ventilator before using a paralyzing agent?

CLINICAL SCENARIO

Answers can be found in Appendix A.

A 64-year-old white woman comes to the emergency department with a complaint of shortness of breath and congestion along with fatigue and lethargy over the last 3 days. Her problem list includes a history of diabetes mellitus, hypertension, and chronic obstructive pulmonary disease (COPD) secondary to smoking. She has had

CLINICAL SCENARIO—cont'd

a cough productive of greenish yellow sputum and states she has had fever and chills over the past several days. Her current medications include metformin, glyburide, lisinopril, ipratropium inhaler, albuterol inhaler as needed, and Advair inhaler.

On physical examination, her vital signs are as follows: pulse (P) of 130 beats/min, blood pressure (BP) of 100/72 mm Hg, temperature (T) of 38.5° C, and respiratory rate (RR) of 30 breaths/min with a moderate amount of respiratory distress. On auscultation, breath sounds are diminished bilaterally.

An electrocardiogram shows sinus tachycardia. Pulse oximetry shows 80% saturation on room air. A chest radiograph shows bilateral interstitial infiltrates. Her white blood cell count (WBC) is $23.7 \times 10^3/mm^3$ with 35% bands; hemoglobin is 11.2 g/dL; hematocrit is 33.2%; and electrolytes are normal except for glucose, which is 250 mg/dL.

After approximately 3 hours of intense treatment with intravenous fluids, antibiotics, and albuterol and ipratropium nebulizations, the patient continues to be short of breath. She is anxious and exhibits labored breathing. Her heart rate (HR) ranges from 126 to 154 beats/min, RR is 32 to 40 breaths/min, BP is 85/60 mm Hg, and her mental status has deteriorated. Arterial blood gas values on a 100% nonrebreather mask are as follows: pH of 7.2, arterial carbon dioxide pressure ($PaCO_2$) of 50 mm Hg, arterial oxygen pressure (PaO_2) of 55 mm Hg, and arterial oxygen saturation (SaO_2) of 82%.

Using the SOAP method, assess this clinical scenario.

REFERENCES

1. Hibbs RE, Zamon AC: Agents acting at the neuromuscular junction and autonomic ganglia. In Brunton LL, Chabner BA, Knollman BC, editors: *Goodman & Gilman's the pharmacological basis of therapeutics*, ed 12, New York, 2011, McGraw-Hill.
2. Society of Critical Care Medicine and American Society of Health-System Pharmacists: Clinical practice guidelines for sustained neuromuscular blockade in the adult critically ill patient. *Am J Health Syst Pharm* 59:179, 2002.
3. McManus MC: Neuromuscular blockers in surgery and intensive care, part 1. *Am J Health Syst Pharm* 58:2287, 2001.
4. *Drug facts and comparisons*, St Louis, 2014, Facts & Comparisons, Wolters Kluwer Health.
5. Wheeler AP: Sedation, analgesia, and paralysis in the intensive care unit. *Chest* 104:566, 1993.
6. Fisher DM: Clinical pharmacology of neuromuscular blocking agents. *Am J Health Syst Pharm* 56(Suppl):S4, 1999.
7. McManus MC: Neuromuscular blockers in surgery and intensive care, part 2. *Am J Health Syst Pharm* 58:2381, 2001.
8. Simon HB: Hyperthermia. *N Engl J Med* 329:483, 1993.
9. Davis L, Britten JJ, Morgan M: Cholinesterase: its significance in anaesthetic practice. *Anaesthesia* 52:244, 1997.
10. Smith SM, Brown HO, Toman JEP, et al: The lack of cerebral effects of d-tubocurarine. *Anesthesiology* 8:1, 1947.
11. Belmont MR, Lien CA, Tjan J, et al: Clinical pharmacology of GW280430A in humans. *Anesthesiology* 100:768, 2004.
12. Adam JM, Bennett DJ, Bom A, et al: Cyclodextran-derived host molecules as reversal agents for the neuromuscular blocker rocuronium bromide: synthesis and structure-activity relationships. *J Med Chem* 45:1806, 2002.

CHAPTER **19**

Diuretic Agents

Ruben D. Restrepo

CHAPTER OUTLINE

OBJECTIVES

After reading this chapter, the reader will be able to:

1. Define terms pertaining to diuretic agents
2. Describe renal function, filtration, reabsorption, and acid-base balance
3. List and describe the various groups of diuretics
4. List some indications for diuretic therapy
5. List the most common adverse effects associated with the use of diuretics
6. Describe special situations related to diuretic therapy

KEY TERMS AND DEFINITIONS

Congestive heart failure (CHF) Failure of the heart to pump the blood adequately, resulting in lung congestion and tissular edema.

Diuretics Substances or drugs that promote the production of urine.

Edema Swelling caused by abnormal accumulation of fluid in intercellular spaces of the body.

Glomerular filtration Mechanism whereby fluid in the blood is filtered across the capillaries of the glomerulus to be eliminated through the renal ducts.

Hypovolemia Physiologic state characterized by a decrease in total blood volume.

Nephrocalcinosis Disorder in which there is excessive accumulation of calcium in the kidney parenchyma and tubules.

Nephron Microscopic structural and functional unit of the kidney, responsible for regulating concentration of water and electrolytes and maintaining fluid balance; each kidney has approximately 2 million nephrons.

Ototoxicity Damage to the hearing or balance functions of the ear caused by drugs or chemicals.

Reabsorption Return to the blood of most of the water, sodium, amino acids, and sugar that were removed during filtration; occurs mainly in the proximal tubule of the nephron.

Synergistic effect Effect of two chemicals on an organism is greater than effect of either chemical individually.

Urine output Amount of urine produced in 24 hours; normal urine output averages 30 to 60 mL/hr.

The main purpose of **diuretics**, or agents that increase **urine output**, is to eliminate excess fluid from the body. Introduced into medicine in 1958, diuretics are drugs that increase the excretion of solutes and water by directly increasing urine output. Generally, the primary goal of diuretic therapy is to reduce extracellular fluid volume (ECFV) to decrease blood pressure or to rid the body of excess interstitial fluid. Chapter 19 summarizes the essentials of the clinical pharmacology of diuretics, briefly reviewing renal function with an emphasis on acid-base balance. The major groups of diuretics, their mechanisms of action, and common interactions and side effects are summarized. These groups include osmotic diuretics, carbonic anhydrase inhibitors (CAIs), thiazides, loop diuretics, and potassium-sparing agents.

RENAL STRUCTURE AND FUNCTION

The kidneys are paired retroperitoneal organs found on either side of the spinal cord at the level of the umbilicus. In an adult, each kidney weighs approximately 160 to 175 g and is 10 to 12 cm long. The renal artery provides perfusion to the kidneys. Kidneys receive the highest blood flow per gram of organ weight in the body. Approximately 22% of the cardiac output, or about 1.1 L/min in a normal 70-kg adult, flows through the kidneys. Similar to the heart and brain, the kidney is an active organ (not a passive filter) with high oxygen consumption. For this reason, impaired circulation can cause renal failure or damage.

Figure 19-1 illustrates the kidney and a **nephron**, which is the functional unit of the kidney. The nephron is composed of the glomerulus, proximal tubule, loop of Henle, distal tubule, and collecting duct. Nearly 75% of the almost 1 million nephrons may need to be compromised before renal disease is apparent. The renal artery branches into the afferent arteriole, which enters and forms the capillary tuft of the glomerulus. This blood flow leaves in the efferent arteriole, which forms the capillary network around the tubules and loop of Henle. This capillary network rejoins to form the renal vein.

The glomerulus is supported and surrounded by an epithelial-lined capsule named the *Bowman capsule*. The glomerular capsule is actually the beginning of the proximal tubule, and filtration of fluid from the blood to the tubule occurs in the glomerulus. This fluid is the glomerular filtrate, which empties into the proximal tubule, goes through the descending and ascending loops of Henle, goes into the distal tubule, and later goes into the collecting duct. Each of the nearly 250 collecting ducts collects urine from about 4000 nephrons. The collecting ducts merge to form larger ducts that eventually empty into the renal papillae and finally empty into the ureter to be stored in the bladder.

The principal function of the nephron is to maintain homeostasis or equilibrium between the internal volume and electrolyte status and the influences of the environment, diet, and intake. This mission is accomplished by almost 2 million nephrons through the processes of glomerular ultrafiltration, tubular reabsorption, and tubular secretion. The kidney cannot regenerate new nephrons.

Renal injury, disease, and aging are associated with a gradual decrease in the number of nephrons. The body maintains blood pressure at the expense of ECFV. Control of ECFV is achieved by adjusting sodium chloride (NaCl) and water (H_2O) excretion.

Glomerular Filtration

Glomerular filtration begins in the glomerulus, the nephron forms a cell-free ultrafiltrate with a relatively small

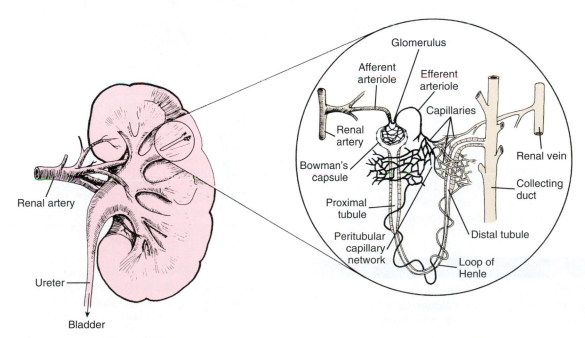

Figure 19-1 Basic structure of the kidney, with a detailed view of the nephron.

amount of protein, which has the same ionic concentration (e.g., sodium [Na^+], chloride [Cl^-], bicarbonate [HCO_3^-]) as plasma. Of the total blood flow that goes through the nephron, 20%, or about 130 mL/min, is filtered through the glomerulus. More than 99% of this *glomerular filtrate* is reabsorbed in the tubules, and less than 1% of the fluid is excreted as urine. The total urine output for an adult is approximately 0.5 to 1 mL/min, or about 30 to 60 mL/hr. Because diuretics interfere with the **reabsorption** of water in the tubules of the nephron, they increase the urine output.

Electrolyte Filtration and Reabsorption

The ions listed in Box 19-1 are filtered and exchanged in the tubules.

- *Sodium:* About 70% of Na^+ in the filtrate is reabsorbed in the proximal tubules; 20%, in the loops of Henle; and about 10%, in the distal tubules. There is an exchange of Na^+ for hydrogen (H^+) or potassium (K^+) in the distal tubules.
- *Potassium:* Most filtered K^+ is reabsorbed in the proximal tubules. K^+ found in the urine is that secreted by the distal tubule.
- *Chloride and bicarbonate:* Cl^- and HCO_3^- are passively reabsorbed in the proximal and distal tubules.

KEY POINT

Urine output more than 100 mL/day but less than 400 mL/day in adults and less than 0.5 mL/kg/hr in children is known as *oliguria*. Urine output greater than 60 mL/hr is known as *polyuria*. Oliguria and *anuria* (less than 50 mL/day) are often signs of renal failure.

Water is also passively reabsorbed or excreted, depending on the concentration of electrolyte, primarily Na^+, in the filtrate. By inhibiting sodium reabsorption, diuretics cause less water to be retained and more is excreted in the filtrate.

Aldosterone, a mineralocorticoid secreted by the adrenal cortex, increases sodium and water reabsorption in the distal tubule. Spironolactone is a diuretic that increases sodium and water loss by inhibiting aldosterone.

Acid-Base Balance

Because a fundamental function of the kidney is the control of buffering substances, especially HCO_3^-, diuretics may cause acid-base imbalances to occur as they increase water loss. Figure 19-2 illustrates the hydrogen and bicarbonate

pathways that regulate pH. The filtration and reabsorption of Na^+, Cl^-, and HCO_3^-, described previously, can be seen in Figure 19-2.

The important exchange for acid-base balance is that of Na^+. Na^+ is reabsorbed in the tubules by several means, as follows:

- Reabsorption with *chloride* to preserve electrical neutrality
- Exchange of Na^+ for H^+ or K^+, also to preserve neutrality

Either low chloride (hypochloremia) or low potassium (hypokalemia) forces Na^+ to exchange for H^+, producing a loss of H^+ and metabolic alkalosis:

$$\left.\begin{array}{l} \text{Hypochloremia} \\ \text{Hypokalemia} \end{array}\right\} \rightarrow \text{Metabolic alkalosis}$$

Finally, preventing HCO_3^- in the *filtrate* from forming carbon dioxide (CO_2) and water leads to a loss of bicarbonate buffer in the urine and metabolic acidosis.

DIURETIC GROUPS

The primary therapeutic goal of diuretic use is to reduce the ECFV. NaCl output *must* exceed NaCl intake. Diuretics primarily prevent Na^+ entry into the tubule cell. Diuretics need to access the tubule fluid to exert their action. Once in the

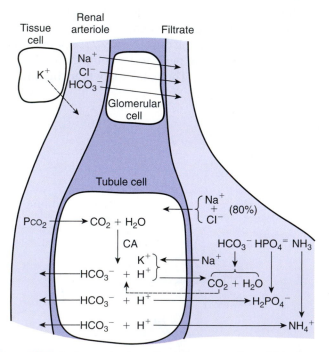

Figure 19-2 Basic mechanisms for kidney retention of bicarbonate with hydrogen ion buffering. Sodium exchange with chloride and for hydrogen is also indicated. *CA,* Carbonic anhydrase; *Cl⁻,* chloride ion; *CO₂,* carbon dioxide; *H⁺,* hydrogen ion; *H₂O,* water; *H₂PO₄⁻,* dihydrogen phosphate ion; *HCO₃⁻,* bicarbonate ion; *HPO₄⁼,* hydrogen phosphate ion; *K⁺,* potassium ion, *Na⁺,* sodium ion; *NH₃,* ammonia; *NH₄,* ammonium; *Pco₂,* partial pressure of carbon dioxide.

BOX 19-1	Common Electrolytes
• Sodium (Na^+)	• Hydrogen (H^+)
• Potassium (K^+)	• Calcium (Ca^{++})
• Chloride (Cl^-)	• Magnesium (Mg^{++})
• Bicarbonate (HCO_3^-)	

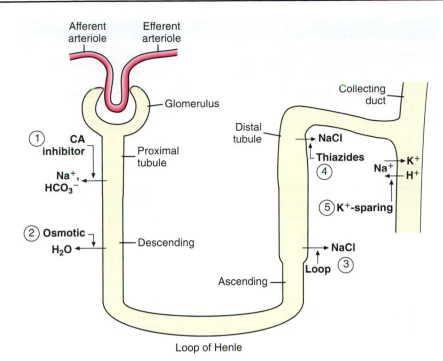

Figure 19-3 Illustration of the nephron, from glomerulus to collecting duct, showing various sites of action for diuretic groups. *CA*, Carbonic anhydrase; *H⁺*, hydrogen ion; *H₂O*, water; *HCO₃⁻*, bicarbonate ion; *K⁺*, potassium ion; *Na⁺*, sodium ion; *NaCl*, sodium chloride. *1-5*, Points at which the five major groups of diuretics exert their effects.

tubule fluid, the nephron site at which the diuretic acts determines its effect. The site of action also determines which electrolytes, other than Na⁺, are affected. All diuretics except spironolactone exert their effects from the luminal side of the nephron.[1]

Five major groups of diuretics are described in this chapter. Figure 19-3 illustrates the site of action, and Table 19-1 summarizes the mechanism of action and the indications for use of each of the five major groups of diuretics.[2,3]

Because hypertension affects one third of adults in the United States,[4] the diuretics of most immediate relevance to respiratory and critical care clinicians are those used to treat hypertension and **congestive heart failure (CHF)**. There is evidence that diuretic-based therapy is effective in reducing morbidity and mortality among elderly hypertensive patients.[5,6] Diuretics are also used to aid in the treatment of other conditions associated with fluid retention, such as corticosteroid therapy and certain renal and liver diseases.

KEY POINT

Diuretic agents are important in reducing the morbidity and mortality of cardiovascular patients with fluid retention.

Osmotic Diuretics

Osmotic diuretics (Table 19-2) are freely filtered at the glomerulus but are not reabsorbed. These agents remain in the tubule lumen and impair the ability of the proximal tubule and thick ascending limb of Henle to reabsorb NaCl. The net result is that osmotic substances are potent diuretics

that lead to increased excretion of water and NaCl. The resultant increased delivery of sodium and chloride to the distal tubule results in increased exchange of Na⁺ for K⁺, producing a net potassium loss in urine.

Of the four currently available osmotic diuretics (glycerin, isosorbide, mannitol, and urea), mannitol is the typically selected agent because of its lower toxicity. Mannitol has a relatively short half-life and has a rapid onset and quick offset of action. To maintain a continued diuretic action, the drug is frequently administered via continuous infusion. Mannitol (Aridol) is also available in dry powder inhaler form (DPI). Aridol is used to assess bronchial hyperresponsiveness in patients 6 years of age or older who do not have clinically diagnosed asthma. Osmotic diuretics are often used in the management of traumatic brain injury with cerebral **edema**.[7,8]

Carbonic Anhydrase Inhibitors

The primary site of action of CAIs is within the proximal tubule. Carbonic anhydrases are enzymes that catalyze the hydration of carbon dioxide and the dehydration of bicarbonate: $CO_2 + H_2O \leftrightarrow HCO_3^- + H^+$. CAIs prevent the normal breakdown of carbonic acid and therefore decrease bicarbonate reabsorption.

CAIs inhibit transport of bicarbonate into the interstitium from the proximal convoluted tubule. Therefore less sodium is reabsorbed, causing greater sodium, bicarbonate, and water loss in the urine, resulting in a net increased flow of alkaline urine (Figure 19-4). The potential for metabolic acidosis coupled with their weak diuretic properties limit the use of CAIs as the first-line treatment for patients who require more aggressive management of their hypervolemic status.

TABLE 19-1 Site and Mechanism of Action, Main Indications, and Other Uses of Diuretics

DIURETIC CLASS (MECHANISM OF ACTION)	MAIN INDICATIONS	OTHER USES
Osmotic Diuretics		
Freely filtered, nonreabsorbable osmotic agents such as mannitol, glycerol, and urea: Reduction of reabsorption of H_2O and solutes, including NaCl, primarily in proximal tubule and descending loop of Henle	To treat or prevent ARF	To reduce intracranial or intraocular pressure Bronchial challenge
Carbonic Anhydrase Inhibitors		
Acetazolamide, methazolamide, and dichlorphenamide: Inhibition of carbonic anhydrase in luminal membrane of proximal tubule, reducing proximal sodium and bicarbonate reabsorption	To reduce intraocular pressure in glaucoma; to lower HCO_3^- in mountain sickness; to increase urine pH in cystinuria	Periodic paralysis; adjunctive therapy in epilepsy; hydrocephalus
Loop Diuretics		
Furosemide, bumetanide, torsemide, and ethacrynic acid: Inhibition of $Na^+/K^+/Cl^-$ reabsorption in thick ascending limb of Henle	Hypertension, CHF (in the presence of renal insufficiency or for immediate effect); ARF; CRF, ascites, and nephrotic syndrome	Acute pulmonary edema; to enhance urinary excretion of chemical toxins; hypercalcemia; nonobstructive oliguria; renal transplant; autism
Thiazide Diuretics		
Chlorothiazide, hydrochlorothiazide, chlorthalidone, hydroflumethiazide, methyclothiazide, bendroflumethiazide, polythiazide Thiazide-like diuretics: metolazone, indapamide, chlortalidone Inhibition of NaCl reabsorption in early DT	Hypertension; CHF; idiopathic hypercalciuria (renal calculi)	Nephrogenic diabetes insipidus (prevent further urine dilution from taking place in DT); CRF
K^+-Sparing Diuretics		
Spironolactone and Eplerenone: Competitively blocks actions of aldosterone on CCDs	Chronic liver disease: To treat secondary hyperaldosteronism caused by hepatic cirrhosis complicated by ascites	Primary hyperaldosteronism (Conn syndrome); acne; alopecia; hirsutism
Amiloride and triamterene: Inhibition of the Na^+/K^+ pump by reducing Na entry across luminal membrane of CCDs	CHF: To counteract hypokalemic effect of other diuretics	

ARF, Acute renal failure; *CCDs,* cortical collecting ducts; *CHF,* congestive heart failure; *CRF,* chronic renal failure; *DT,* distal tubule; *HCO_3^-,* bicarbonate concentration.

Other, more common uses of CAIs include treatment of glaucoma, metabolic alkalosis, and altitude sickness. Carbonic anhydrase is an important enzyme in the formation of intraocular fluid. CAIs effectively decrease intraocular pressure and are used to treat glaucoma. Short-term CAIs may also correct metabolic alkalosis as a result of the acidosis they produce. Finally, CAIs have been shown to be useful against altitude sickness, although the exact mechanism of action is unknown. The most common adverse effect of CAIs is hypokalemia resulting from the increased amount of sodium presented to the collecting duct, which is reabsorbed in exchange for potassium excretion.

KEY POINT

Although carbonic anhydrase inhibitors (CAIs) are considered to be very weak diuretics, they are commonly used in patients with glaucoma, metabolic alkalosis, and altitude sickness.

Loop Diuretics

Loop diuretics (see Table 19-2) are often called "high ceiling" diuretics because they can cause up to 20% of the filtered load of NaCl and water to be excreted in the urine. They inhibit the $Na^+/K^+/Cl^-$ cotransporter in the thick ascending limb of Henle, where about 20% of filtered NaCl is usually reabsorbed.[2] Use of loop diuretics leads to increased Na^+, K^+, Cl^-, and water excretion.

KEY POINT

Osmotic diuretics are often used in the management of patients with traumatic brain injury with cerebral edema.

TABLE 19-2 Characteristics of Diuretics

DRUG	ROUTE	ONSET (min)*	PEAK (hr)	DURATION (hr)	HALF-LIFE (hr)	ORAL BIOAVAILABILITY (%)	TYPICAL DOSAGE
Osmotic							
Glycerin	PO	10-30	1-1.5	4-5	0.5-0.75	ND	1-2 g/kg
Isosorbide	PO	10-30	1-1.5	5-6	5-9.5	ND	1-3 g/kg
Mannitol	IV	30-60	1	6-8	0.25-1.5	NA	50-100 g
Urea	IV	30-45	1	5-6	NA	NA	1-1.5 g/kg
Loop							
Bumetanide	PO	30-60	1-2	4-6	1-1.5	72-96	0.5-2.0 mg
	IV	5	0.25-0.5	0.5-1	1-1.5	72-96	0.5-2.0 mg
Ethacrynic acid	PO	30	2	6-8	1	100	50-100 mg
	IV	5	0.25-0.5	2	1	100	50-100 mg
Furosemide	PO	60	1-2	6-8	2	60-64	20-80 mg
	IV	5	0.5	2	2	60-64	20-80 mg
Torsemide	PO	60	1-2	6-8	3.5	80	5-20 mg
	IV	10	<1	6-8	3.5	80	5-20 mg
Thiazide							
Bendroflumethiazide	PO	120	4	12-16	3-4	100	5 mg
Benzthiazide	PO	120	4-6	16-18	ND	ND	50-100 mg/day
Chlorothiazide	PO	120	4	12-16	0.75-2	10-21	0.5-2.0 g/day
	IV	15	0.5	12-16	0.75-2	10-21	0.5-2.0 g/day
Chlorthalidone	PO	120-180	2-6	24-72	40	64	50-100 mg/day
Hydrochlorothiazide	PO	120	4-6	12-16	50.6-14.8	65-75	50-200 mg/day
Hydroflumethiazide	PO	120	4	12-16	17	50	25-200 mg/day
Indapamide	PO	60-120	<2	36	14	93	1.25-5 mg/day
Methylclothiazide	PO	120	6	24	ND	ND	5 mg
Metolazone	PO	60	2	12-24	ND	65	5-20 mg/day
Polythiazide	PO	120	6	24-48	25-37	ND	2-4 mg/day
Quinethazone	PO	120	6	18-24	ND	ND	50-100 mg/day
Trichlormethiazide	PO	120	6	24	2.3-7.3	ND	2-4 mg/day
Potassium Sparing							
Amiloride	PO	2 hr	6-10	24	6-9	30-90	5-20 mg/day
Spironolactone	PO	24-48 hr	48-72	48-72	20	73	25-400 mg/day
Triamterene	PO	2-4 hr	6-8	12-16	3	30-70	200-300 mg/day

IV, Intravenous; *NA,* not applicable; *ND,* no data; *PO,* oral.
*Unless otherwise indicated.

When administered intravenously, loop diuretics produce an acute hemodynamic effect independent of their diuretic properties.[2,9] Within 5 minutes of the administration of intravenous loop diuretics to cardiac patients, an acute vasodilatory effect is observed.[10] This effect is manifested by a decrease in pulmonary capillary wedge pressure (PCWP), blood pressure, and systemic vascular resistance. The effect seems to be derived from the renal release of vasodilating prostaglandins.[11,12]

Because the diuretic effect of intravenous loop diuretics is typically not seen for 15 to 20 minutes after administration, patients with acute pulmonary edema may derive a clinical benefit from intravenous loop diuretics before the onset of diuresis. The hemodynamic effect is short-lived, with all measurements returning to baseline once diuresis has begun.

The acute hemodynamic effect has also been reported to activate the sympathetic nervous system, resulting in an adverse hemodynamic profile characterized by increased afterload and diminished cardiac function before the onset of diuresis.[11] This effect is also short-lived and dissipates with the onset of diuresis. Because the diuretic effect may last several hours, several doses per day may be required to maintain a net diuretic effect for 24 hours. Patients requiring frequent bolus doses may benefit from continuous infusion.

KEY POINT

Loop diuretics produce a hemodynamic effect characterized by acute vasodilation and manifested by a decrease in pulmonary capillary wedge pressure (PCWP), blood pressure, and systemic vascular resistance.

Administration of loop diuretics to patients with renal dysfunction results in less total drug reaching the site of action within the nephron, and the administration of larger doses is required to achieve a therapeutic effect.[13,14] In these

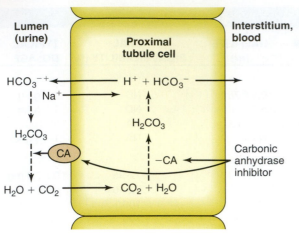

Figure 19-4 Effect of carbonic anhydrase inhibitor diuretics, such as acetazolamide, which block the availability of hydrogen to exchange for sodium in the proximal tubule, causing a loss of sodium, bicarbonate, and water, along with reduced bicarbonate reabsorption into the cell and the blood. *CA,* Carbonic anhydrase; *CO₂,* carbon dioxide; *H⁺,* hydrogen ion; H_2CO_3, bicarbonate; H_2O, water; HCO_3^-, bicarbonate ion; *Na⁺,* sodium ion.

patients, differences exist among the effects of furosemide, bumetanide, and torsemide. Furosemide may have a more prolonged effect in patients with renal dysfunction. However, patients may be resistant to furosemide compared with bumetanide. Because loop diuretics are the most potent diuretics, they are effective at very low creatinine clearance levels (a low creatinine clearance level indicates kidney disease). Loop diuretics as single agents should be considered as first-line therapy in patients with creatinine clearance values less than 40 mL/min. If this dose is inadequate to produce diuresis within 20 minutes, the dose can be doubled every 20 minutes until a response occurs or until a maximum dose is reached. Various studies have reported a ceiling effect to furosemide of approximately 250 mg. Increasing the dose above this ceiling dose may not produce an increased response.[15]

Although patients with renal dysfunction require larger doses to deliver diuretics into the urine, the remaining nephrons in these patients continue to function normally. Overall, sodium excretion may be limited as a result of diminished sodium filtration. To overcome this relative resistance, an effective response may occur by administering a large enough effective dose several times a day. Certain disease states result in a diminished response that does not improve by administering larger doses. Although the mechanism for this effect is unknown, it has been reported in patients with CHF, cirrhosis, and nephrotic syndrome.[15] In these patients, multiple doses should be given rather than larger single doses. This finding implies a modest ceiling dose of loop diuretics in patients with CHF and cirrhosis.

Thiazide Diuretics

Thiazide diuretics (see Table 19-2) block NaCl reabsorption at the distal tubule.[3] Thiazide diuretics are of moderate potency because only about 5% to 10% of filtered NaCl is reabsorbed in the distal tubule. However, they are considered the first line of therapy for mild hypertension. Thiazide diuretics are effective to a creatinine clearance of approximately 30 mL/min. Thiazide diuretics have a limited dose-response curve compared with loop diuretics. This limited dose-response curve results in a narrow difference between maximal and minimal effective doses. Doses greater than 50 mg may not produce greater diuresis, but they may predispose the patient to increased toxicity.

Doses greater than 50 mg may, however, be useful in the treatment of hypertension. The use of thiazide diuretics in the treatment of hypertension produces an effect initially as a result of diuresis-induced decreases in blood volume. Long-term benefits of thiazide diuretics in hypertension are most likely not due to a diuretic response. One proposed mechanism is decreased peripheral vascular resistance.

> ### ! KEY POINT
>
> Thiazide diuretics are considered the first line of therapy for mild hypertension.

Potassium-Sparing Diuretics

Potassium-sparing diuretics increase urine output by interfering with the Na⁺ and K⁺ exchange in the distal convulated tubule *(Amiloride* and *triamterene)* or by acting as an antagonist at the aldosterone receptor *(spironolactone)* (see Table 19-2). On the basis of its mechanism of action, spironolactone is specifically used for conditions known to have elevated aldosterone concentrations, such as hyperaldosteronism (primary and secondary), cirrhosis and ascites, adrenal hyperplasia, and renal artery stenosis. The most common use is in patients with cirrhosis and ascites. Because the duration of effect of spironolactone is 1 or more days, the dose should be increased every 3 or 4 days until the desired level of diuresis is attained.

In the distal tubule, sodium is typically exchanged for potassium and hydrogen. Blocking this exchange is what makes these agents *potassium-sparing diuretics.* Although frequently used in combination with thiazide diuretics to produce better diuresis and to diminish potassium loss, the rationale for this is controversial. Only about 5% of patients receiving thiazide diuretics become potassium depleted.[16] In addition, potassium-sparing agents may produce hyperkalemia, which is a more life-threatening situation than potassium depletion.

Triamterene is a short-acting agent requiring multiple doses per day. Triamterene must be converted to an active metabolite by the liver, and this agent may be a poor choice in patients with liver dysfunction.[17]

Amiloride has a moderately long half-life and does not require metabolic activation. Coadministration of potassium supplements, angiotensin-converting enzyme inhibitors, and nonsteroidal antiinflammatory agents, as well as renal dysfunction, may predispose patients receiving potassium-sparing diuretics to develop hyperkalemia.[17]

DIURETIC COMBINATIONS

Various diuretic combinations may be used in an attempt to obtain an additive or **synergistic effect** in patients who respond poorly to one agent. By using agents with different sites of action within the nephron, the diuretic response may be enhanced. The most common combination is of a loop diuretic and a thiazide. Although not consistently effective, combinations occasionally may result in pronounced diuresis.

DRUG INTERACTIONS

Because diuretics are commonly prescribed in combination with other medications, knowledge of drug interaction plays an important role in the selection of the diuretic agent. Clinicians who prescribe diuretics need to be informed of associated comorbidities, such as diabetes, renal disease, hepatic disease, or gout. Table 19-3 summarizes some of the most common drug interaction side effects associated with diuretic agents.

ADVERSE EFFECTS

Although diuretics have been used successfully for more than 40 years, they have the potential to cause adverse effects (Table 19-4). Most complications associated with diuretic use can be anticipated as an extension of their pharmacologic activity, with hypovolemia and electrolyte and acid-base abnormalities being the most common. Rare side effects that need immediate medical attention include the following:

- Black, tarry stools
- Blood in the urine or stools
- Cough or hoarseness
- Falls[18]

- Fever or chills
- Joint pain
- Lower back or side pain
- Painful or difficult urination
- Pinpoint red spots on the skin
- Ringing or buzzing in the ears
- Any loss of hearing
- Skin rash or hives
- Severe stomach pain with nausea and vomiting
- Unusual bleeding or bruising
- Yellow eyes or skin
- Yellow vision

Other adverse effects are even rarer or idiosyncratic and cannot be anticipated or prevented. There is a particular concern with the suggested association between long-term diuretic therapy and the risk of developing renal cell carcinoma.

TABLE 19-3	Drug Interactions and Their Potential Side Effects Associated With Use of Diuretics
INTERACTING DRUG	**POTENTIAL SIDE EFFECT**
Angiotensin-converting enzyme inhibitors *AND* K⁺-sparing diuretics	Hyperkalemia and cardiac irritability
Aminoglycosides *AND* loop diuretics	Ototoxicity and nephrotoxicity
Digoxin *AND* thiazide and loop diuretics	Hypokalemia
β Blockers *AND* thiazide diuretics	Hyperglycemia, hyperlipidemia, hyperuricemia
Steroids *AND* thiazide and loop diuretics	Increased risk of hypokalemia
Carbamazepine or chlorpropamide *AND* thiazide diuretics	Increased risk of hyponatremia

TABLE 19-4	Common Side Effects of Diuretic Therapy
DRUG	**EFFECT**
Osmotic diuretics	Acute expansion of ECFV and increased risk of pulmonary edema
	Acute hyperkalemia
	Nausea and vomiting; headache
Loop diuretics	*Depletions:* Hypokalemia; hypomagnesemia; hyponatremia; hypovolemia
	Retention: Hyperuricemia
	Metabolic: Hyperglycemia (insulin resistance)
	Metabolic alkalosis (partly secondary to ECFV reduction)
	Ototoxicity and diarrhea (mainly with ethacrynic acid)
Thiazide diuretics	*Depletions:* Hypokalemia, hyponatremia, hypovolemia
	Retentions: Hyperuricemia secondary to enhanced urate reabsorption; hypercalcemia secondary to enhanced Ca⁺⁺ reabsorption
	Metabolic alkalosis (hypochloremia)
	Metabolic: Hyperglycemia (insulin resistance), hyperlipidemia
	Hypersensitivity (fever, rash, purpura, anaphylaxis)
	Interstitial nephritis
K⁺-sparing diuretics	*Spironolactone:* Hyperkalemia, gynecomastia, hirsutism, menstrual irregularities, testicular atrophy (with prolonged use)
	Amiloride: Hyperkalemia, glucose intolerance in diabetic patients
	Triamterene: Hyperkalemia; megaloblastic anemia in patients with liver cirrhosis
Carbonic anhydrase inhibitors	Metabolic acidosis (secondary to HCO_3^- depletion)
	Drowsiness, fatigue, CNS depression, paresthesia

CNS, Central nervous system; *ECFV,* extracellular fluid volume.

Hypovolemia

Because diuretics promote sodium and fluid excretion, elimination may exceed intake, resulting in **hypovolemia**. Hypovolemia should be suspected if dizziness, extreme thirst, excessive dryness of the mouth, decreased urine output, dark-colored urine, or constipation is observed. Certain situations may predispose a patient to hypovolemia (Box 19-2). Diuretic-induced hypovolemia should be treated by discontinuation of the diuretic. Mild cases of hypovolemia may respond to liberalization of sodium intake, whereas more severe cases require intravenous volume replacement.

Hypokalemia

Preserving potassium balance has emerged as one of the most important factors in the management of hypertension. Potassium is exchanged for sodium in the distal convoluted tubule and collecting duct. Any diuretic that increases sodium delivery to these regions may potentially induce hypokalemia. In addition to a direct potassium loss, diuretic-induced volume depletion produces reabsorption of sodium via release of aldosterone in the distal tubule in an effort to bolster intravascular volume. This additional sodium reabsorption also contributes to potassium excretion. Dietary sodium intake and chloride depletion may also influence potassium excretion.

Diuretic-induced hypokalemia apparently is dose-related, with loop diuretics having a lower incidence than thiazide diuretics.[19,20]Although studies have tried to identify the incidence of diuretic-induced hypokalemia, it is impossible to predict whether a particular patient will develop hypokalemia. The issue of potassium supplementation is also controversial. Who to treat, when to treat, and how to treat hypokalemia all are unresolved questions. At the center of this unresolved issue is whether hypokalemia poses a risk for arrhythmias or sudden cardiac death. Supplemental potassium should be considered in patients with a history of cardiac disease, patients with symptoms indicating hypokalemia, patients with a serum potassium level less than 3 mEq/L, and patients receiving digitalis therapy.

Potassium-sparing diuretics may induce a hyperkalemic state in 8.6% of patients receiving spironolactone and in 23% of patients receiving a potassium-sparing diuretic and potassium supplementation.

Acid-Base Disorders

With diuresis and volume depletion, hypokalemia and hypochloremia may result. This state may cause metabolic alkalosis, which is responsive to potassium and chloride replacement therapy. Exceptions are CAIs, the use of which may result in metabolic acidosis.

Glucose Changes

Thiazides are also known to be the antihypertensive drugs with the strongest diabetogenic activity.[21] The average increase in serum glucose is 6.5 to 9.6 mg/dL, although cases of diabetic ketoacidosis have also been reported. The severity of glucose elevation in these reports was related to the dose of diuretic used and to the decrease in potassium levels. Although the cause of hyperglycemia is not completely understood, several possible etiologies have been postulated, including decreased pancreatic insulin release and insulin resistance with impaired uptake of glucose in response to insulin.[22,23]

Ototoxicity

Loop diuretics may cause a dose-related **ototoxicity** consisting of tinnitus and clinical or subclinical hearing loss. Ototoxicity results from anatomic and chemical abnormalities produced within the inner ear. Ototoxicity is related to the blood level of these agents. Rapid infusion and drug accumulation with large parenteral doses in renal failure both predispose patients to ototoxicity. Reducing the infusion rate or administering the drug orally may alleviate the hearing loss.[24,25] Most ototoxicity is reversible; however, cases of irreversible hearing loss have occurred. Ethacrynic acid has a higher likelihood of causing irreversible hearing loss. Limited data on bumetanide indicate that it may have a lower incidence of ototoxicity than furosemide and ethacrynic acid.[26]

To minimize diuretic-induced ototoxicity, ethacrynic acid should be avoided. In addition, long-term doses greater than 500 mg in patients with advanced renal disease and repetitive dosing in patients with acute renal failure and rapid infusions should be avoided.

BOX 19-2 Causes of Volume Depletion With Diuretics

- Initiation of treatment or increased dose
- Improved compliance
- Reduced dietary sodium intake
- Development of diarrhea
- Ingestion of drugs that impair diuretic administration
- Improved underlying disease state not requiring diuretics

SPECIAL SITUATIONS

Pregnancy, Lactation, and Children

Diuretics are not recommended for pregnant women because the effects of the drug on the fetus are unknown. Because many diuretics pass into breast milk, diuretics are not recommended to breastfeeding women because of the risk of dehydration in the infant.

TABLE 19-5	Pediatric Dosages of Commonly Prescribed Diuretics		
DRUG	**AGE OF PATIENT**	**ROUTE**	**TYPICAL DOSAGE**
Furosemide	Neonates	PO	1-4 mg/kg/dose once or twice daily
		IV/IM	1-2 mg/kg/dose q12-24h
	Children	PO/IV/IM	1-2 mg/kg/dose q6-12h
Bumetanide	<6 mo	PO/IV/IM	ND
	>6 mo	PO/IV/IM	0.015 mg/kg/dose qd or qod; maximum 0.1 mg/kg/dose
Hydrochlorothiazide	<6 mo	PO	2-3.3 mg/kg/day divided bid
	>6 months	PO	2 mg/kg/day divided bid
Chlorothiazide	<6 mo	PO	20-40 mg/kg/day divided bid
		IV	2-8 mg/kg/day divided bid
	>6 mo	PO	20 mg/kg/day, divided bid
		IV	4 mg/kg/day
Metolazone	Children	PO	0.2-0.4 mg/kg/day, divided q12-24h
Spironolactone	Children	PO	1.5-3.5 mg/kg/day, divided q6-24h

Modified from Bestic M, Reed M: Pharmacology review: common diuretics used in the preterm and term infant, *Neoreviews* 6:392, 2005.[29]
IM, Intramuscular; *IV,* intravenous; *N/D,* no data; *PO,* oral.

Children can safely take diuretics because the side effects are similar to the side effects in adults. However, they may require smaller doses of the drug (Table 19-5). Furosemide is one of the most effective and least toxic diuretics used in pediatric practice. However, long-term use of loop diuretics in children should be carefully evaluated because of the risk of **nephrocalcinosis** and potential decrease in bone mass density.[27,28]

Acute Respiratory Distress Syndrome

A pathophysiologic landmark of acute respiratory distress syndrome (ARDS) is the presence of protein-rich, noncardiogenic pulmonary edema. The inflammatory process associated with ARDS explains the increase of the endothelial permeability that causes intravascular water leakage into the interstitial and alveolar spaces. Although balancing the risks of increased pulmonary edema versus the risks of decreased vital organ perfusion has proven to be a difficult task for clinicians, a reduction in PCWP has been associated with increased survival in ARDS patients.[30] The ARDS Network published the results of the Fluid And Catheter Treatment Trial (FACTT),[31] in which patients who were not in shock and who were managed with a protocolized fluid management plus furosemide (conservative fluid management arm) had significantly more ventilator-free days, more ICU-free days, and lower mortality than those in the liberal fluid management arm. Nevertheless, a recent report showed a potential worse long-term cognitive function in a subset of the trial survivors.[32] In general, fluid administration should be titrated to resolution of hypoperfusion states. Diuretics should be limited to restore euvolemia in hemodynamically stable patients who received higher amounts of fluids in the resuscitation phase of their illness. Because most patients with severe ARDS require high mean airway pressures for oxygenation, hypovolemia may worsen hypoxemia by causing an increase in the intrapulmonary shunt.[33]

Chronic Lung Disease in Preterm Infants

Diuretics are one of the most frequently administered medications in the neonatal ICU. They are often given to infants with oxygen-dependent chronic lung disease (CLD) because it is often complicated by the presence of pulmonary edema. Several trials have evaluated the use of loop diuretics to treat respiratory distress syndrome (RDS) and reduce the need for mechanical ventilatory support.[34-38] The most recent meta-analysis concluded that in preterm infants older than 3 weeks diagnosed with CLD, administration of a single dose of aerosolized furosemide may transiently improve pulmonary mechanics.

Several studies have examined the short-term and long-term effects of furosemide in infants with bronchopulmonary dysplasia (BPD) because the agent seems to inhibit induced bronchoconstriction.[39,40]

Nevertheless, routine or sustained use of aerosolized loop diuretics in infants with (or developing) CLD cannot be recommended based on existing evidence.[41]

Furosemide and Fluid Overload

Diuretics are used in the neonatal population for treatment of several fluid retention states, including renal dysfunction, postoperative management, and during treatment with extracorporeal membrane oxygenation (ECMO). To avoid acute fluctuations in intravascular volume associated with bolus administration of loop diuretics, the use of continuous intravenous administration has been proposed. In cardiac postoperative patients less than 6 months of age, urinary output can be significantly greater when receiving continuous furosemide compared with intermittent dosing.[42] However, using an adjustable dosing of furosemide based on clinical parameters can also result in a higher urine production in the intermittent time period compared with continuous group and required a significantly smaller total daily dose of the drug.[43] In neonates treated with ECMO, no observed benefit of continuous treatment has been shown over intermittent furosemide administration.[44]

? SELF-ASSESSMENT QUESTIONS

Answers can be found in Appendix A.

1. What is a diuretic?
2. Identify the five major groups of diuretics used clinically.
3. If an agent such as one of the loop diuretics causes a loss of potassium, how would this lead to a metabolic alkalosis?
4. Which diuretics would preserve potassium?
5. What is the potential effect of a carbonic anhydrase inhibitor on acid-base balance?
6. Explain how a diuretic such as furosemide can be helpful in acute congestive heart failure with pulmonary and vascular edema.
7. Which diuretic agent has a vasodilatory effect when used for long-term treatment?
8. In an otherwise healthy adult with mild hypertension, what diuretic agent should be considered as the first line of treatment?
9. Which diuretic agent has been successfully used in the management of ARDS?
10. Match each of the following sets of drugs on the left with the most likely interaction on the right.

Gentamicin *PLUS* furosemide	Hyperglycemia
Hydrochlorothiazide *PLUS* prednisone	Ototoxicity and nephrotoxicity
Spironolactone *PLUS* enalapril	Hyperkalemia
Hydrochlorothiazide *PLUS* carbamazepine	Hyponatremia

CLINICAL SCENARIO

Answers can be found in Appendix A.

A 73-year-old white man presents to the emergency department with a chief complaint of severe dyspnea that began about 8 hours before presentation. The patient's history is significant for long-standing hypertension and coronary artery disease. He had an inferior myocardial infarction in 1995 and had another myocardial infarction of unknown location in 1999. After this, he underwent a coronary artery bypass graft procedure. His left internal mammary artery was used to bypass the left anterior descending artery, a saphenous vein graft was placed to the posterior descending artery, and a sequential saphenous vein graft was placed to the first and second obtuse marginal arteries.

Cardiac catheterization revealed inferior wall akinesis with global hypokinesis of the remaining walls. His left ventricular ejection fraction was estimated to be 40%. Since his bypass surgery, he has not had any further angina or infarctions, but he has had two admissions for acute pulmonary edema. Both episodes were believed to have been precipitated by medical noncompliance, but this could not be confirmed. At this presentation, the patient again denies chest pain. He states that he began feeling dyspneic the night before presentation and then awoke about 5 AM severely dyspneic and coughing up white, foamy phlegm. When queried about his compliance with his medicines, he admits that he sometimes forgets to take his clonidine.

The patient has chronic renal insufficiency and has had right inguinal hernia repair. He denies any allergies.

The patient is taking the following medications: clonidine, 0.1 mg PO bid; atenolol, 50 mg PO hs each night; aspirin, 325 mg PO qd; transdermal nitroglycerin, 0.4 mg qh (he places a patch on in the morning and takes it off at bedtime); and furosemide, 40 mg PO q AM

Physical examination reveals an elderly white man in obvious respiratory distress. He is afebrile; other vital signs are as follows: pulse (P) of 120 beats/min and regular, respiratory rate (RR) at 32 breaths/min, and blood pressure (BP) of 230/140 mm Hg. His neck shows positive jugular venous distention. Heart auscultation reveals a regular rate, with a systolic ejection murmur (I/VI), negative S_3, and positive S_4. His lungs show bibasilar inspiratory crackles half of the way up the thorax. His abdomen is flat, and bowel sounds are present; no tenderness or masses are identified. His extremities are slightly cool, and pulses are felt in all extremities but are thready.

The patient's laboratory results are as follows: Na^+ of 138 mEq/L, K^+ of 3.6 mEq/L, blood urea nitrogen (BUN) of 40 mg/dL, and creatinine of 2.8 mg/dL. His electrocardiogram (ECG) shows sinus tachycardia, with inferior Q waves and lateral Q waves of questionable significance. A chest radiograph shows mild cardiomegaly with bilateral infiltrates consistent with pulmonary edema.

Using the SOAP method, assess this clinical scenario.

REFERENCES

1. Roush GC, Kaur R, Ernst ME: Diuretics: a review and update. *J Cardiovasc Pharmacol Ther* 19(1):5–13, 2014.
2. Tamargo J, Segura J, Ruilope LM: Diuretics in the treatment of hypertension. Part 2: loop diuretics and potassium-sparing agents. *Expert Opin Pharmacother* 15(5):605–621, 2014.
3. Tamargo J, Segura J, Ruilope LM: Diuretics in the treatment of hypertension. Part 1: thiazide and thiazide-like diuretics. *Expert Opin Pharmacother* 15(4):527–547, 2014.
4. Vital signs: awareness and treatment of uncontrolled hypertension among adults—United States, 2003–2010. *MMWR Morb Mortal Wkly Rep* 61:703–709, 2012.
5. Messerli FH: Antihypertensive therapy: beta-blockers and diuretics-why do physicians not always follow guidelines? *Proc (Bayl Univ Med Cent)* 13(2):128–131, discussion 131–4, 2000.
6. Chobanian AV, et al: The seventh report of the Joint National Committee on Prevention, Detection, Evaluation, and Treatment of High Blood Pressure: the JNC 7 report. *JAMA* 289(19):2560–2572, 2003.

7. Lazaridis C, et al: High-osmolarity saline in neurocritical care: systematic review and meta-analysis. *Crit Care Med* 41(5):1353–1360, 2013.

8. Grande PO, Romner B: Osmotherapy in brain edema: a questionable therapy. *J Neurosurg Anesthesiol* 24(4):407–412, 2012.

9. Palazzuoli A, et al: Short and long-term effects of continuous versus intermittent loop diuretics treatment in acute heart failure with renal dysfunction. *Intern Emerg Med* 2014.

10. Alqahtani F, et al: A meta-analysis of continuous vs intermittent infusion of loop diuretics in hospitalized patients. *J Crit Care* 29(1):10–17, 2014.

11. Rossignol P, Zannad F: Loop diuretics and ultrafiltration in heart failure. *Expert Opin Pharmacother* 14(12):1641–1648, 2013.

12. Reyes AJ: Loop diuretics versus others in the treatment of congestive heart failure after myocardial infarction. *Cardiovasc Drugs Ther* 7(6):869–876, 1993.

13. Rudy DW, et al: Loop diuretics for chronic renal insufficiency: a continuous infusion is more efficacious than bolus therapy. *Ann Intern Med* 115(5):360–366, 1991.

14. Voelker JR, et al: Comparison of loop diuretics in patients with chronic renal insufficiency. *Kidney Int* 32(4):572–578, 1987.

15. DiNicolantonio JJ: Should torsemide be the loop diuretic of choice in systolic heart failure? *Future Cardiol* 8(5):707–728, 2012.

16. Wile D: Diuretics: a review. *Ann Clin Biochem* 49(Pt 5):419–431, 2012.

17. Rorive G, Bovy P: Pharmacology of potassium-sparing diuretics: amiloride and triamterene. *Coeur Med Interne* 17(2):207–215, 1978.

18. Zang G: Antihypertensive drugs and the risk of fall injuries: a systematic review and meta-analysis. *J Int Med Res* 41(5):1408–1417, 2013.

19. Sarafidis PA, Georgianos PI, Lasaridis AN: Diuretics in clinical practice. Part I: mechanisms of action, pharmacological effects and clinical indications of diuretic compounds. *Expert Opin Drug Saf* 9(2):243–257, 2010.

20. Sarafidis PA, Georgianos PI, Lasaridis AN: Diuretics in clinical practice. Part II: electrolyte and acid-base disorders complicating diuretic therapy. *Expert Opin Drug Saf* 9(2):259–273, 2010.

21. Wehling M: Morbus diureticus in the elderly: epidemic overuse of a widely applied group of drugs. *J Am Med Dir Assoc* 14(6):437–442, 2013.

22. Shen L, et al: Role of diuretics, beta blockers, and statins in increasing the risk of diabetes in patients with impaired glucose tolerance: reanalysis of data from the NAVIGATOR study. *BMJ* 347:f6745, 2013.

23. Elliott WJ: Effects of potassium-sparing versus thiazide diuretics on glucose tolerance: new data on an old topic. *Hypertension* 59(5):911–912, 2012.

24. De Vecchis R, Ciccarelli A, Cioppa C: Intermittent intravenous infusion of high-dose loop diuretics and risk for iatrogenic ototoxicity: an unresolved issue from the DOSE study. *G Ital Cardiol (Rome)* 13(10):701–702, author reply 702–4, 2012.

25. Martinez-Rodriguez R, et al: Loop diuretics and ototoxicity. *Actas Urol Esp* 31(10):1189–1192, 2007.

26. Kohonen A, Jauhiainen T, Tarkkanen J: Experimental deafness caused by ethacrynic acid. *Acta Otolaryngol* 70(3):187–189, 1970.

27. Seikaly MG, Baum M: Thiazide diuretics arrest the progression of nephrocalcinosis in children with X-linked hypophosphatemia. *Pediatrics* 108(1):E6, 2001.

28. Auron A, Alon US: Resolution of medullary nephrocalcinosis in children with metabolic bone disorders. *Pediatr Nephrol* 20(8):1143–1145, 2005.

29. Bestic M, Reed MD: Pharmacology review: common diuretics used in the preterm and term infant. *Neoreviews* 6:2005.

30. Humphrey H, et al: Improved survival in ARDS patients associated with a reduction in pulmonary capillary wedge pressure. *Chest* 97(5):1176–1180, 1990.

31. Wiedemann HP, et al: Comparison of two fluid-management strategies in acute lung injury. *N Engl J Med* 354(24):2564–2575, 2006.

32. Mikkelsen ME, et al: The adult respiratory distress syndrome cognitive outcomes study: long-term neuropsychological function in survivors of acute lung injury. *Am J Respir Crit Care Med* 185(12):1307–1315, 2012.

33. Silversides JA, Ferguson ND: Clinical review: Acute respiratory distress syndrome - clinical ventilator management and adjunct therapy. *Crit Care* 17(2):225, 2013.

34. Segar JL: Neonatal diuretic therapy: furosemide, thiazides, and spironolactone. *Clin Perinatol* 39(1):209–220, 2012.

35. Stewart AL, Brion LP: Routine use of diuretics in very-low birth-weight infants in the absence of supporting evidence. *J Perinatol* 31(10):633–634, 2011.

36. Stewart A, Brion LP, Ambrosio-Perez I: Diuretics acting on the distal renal tubule for preterm infants with (or developing) chronic lung disease. *Cochrane Database Syst Rev* (9):CD001817, 2011.

37. Stewart A, Brion LP: Intravenous or enteral loop diuretics for preterm infants with (or developing) chronic lung disease. *Cochrane Database Syst Rev* (9):CD001453, 2011.

38. Stewart A, Brion LP, Soll R: Diuretics for respiratory distress syndrome in preterm infants. *Cochrane Database Syst Rev* (12):CD001454, 2011.

39. Patel H, et al: Pulmonary and renal responses to furosemide in infants with stage III-IV bronchopulmonary dysplasia. *Am J Dis Child* 139(9):917–919, 1985.

40. Engelhardt B, Elliott S, Hazinski TA: Short- and long-term effects of furosemide on lung function in infants with bronchopulmonary dysplasia. *J Pediatr* 109(6):1034–1039, 1986.

41. Brion LP, Primhak RA, Yong W: Aerosolized diuretics for preterm infants with (or developing) chronic lung disease. *Cochrane Database Syst Rev* (3):CD001694, 2006.

42. Luciani GB, et al: Continuous versus intermittent furosemide infusion in critically ill infants after open heart operations. *Ann Thorac Surg* 64(4):1133–1139, 1997.

43. Klinge JM, et al: Intermittent administration of furosemide versus continuous infusion in the postoperative management of children following open heart surgery. *Intensive Care Med* 23(6):693–697, 1997.

44. van der Vorst MM, et al: Evaluation of furosemide regimens in neonates treated with extracorporeal membrane oxygenation. *Crit Care* 10(6):R168, 2006.

CHAPTER **20**

Drugs Affecting the Central Nervous System

Douglas S. Gardenhire

OBJECTIVES

After reading this chapter, the reader will be able to:

1. Define key terms pertaining to drugs that affect the central nervous system (CNS)
2. Describe the multiple functions of the CNS
3. Recognize various effects of medications on the CNS and their abilities to modulate neurotransmitters
4. Comprehend psychiatric medications, including classification, use, and side effect profiles
5. Recognize the effects of alcohol on the CNS during acute intoxication, chronic use, and after abrupt withdrawal
6. Distinguish physiologic and psychological bases of pain and the classes of analgesics used to treat pain
7. Recognize indications for the use of both local and general anesthesia
8. Describe the concept of conscious sedation and indications and guidelines for use
9. Distinguish drugs that stimulate the CNS and respiratory system, and describe the indications for application

KEY TERMS AND DEFINITIONS

Analgesics Drugs that provide pain relief. Analgesics can be subdivided into narcotic and nonnarcotic medications. Narcotic drugs are derivatives of opium, such as morphine and codeine. Nonnarcotic medications are useful in treating pain and inflammation. They also have antipyretic activity.

Anesthetics Drugs that depress the nervous system. Anesthetics can be divided into local and general anesthetics. General anesthesia causes total loss of consciousness and reflexes, which results in the absence of pain perception. Local anesthetics are applied to a specific site and decrease pain perception at the specific site and do not affect level of

consciousness. Both types of anesthetics are often used during surgical procedures.

Antidepressants Drugs that can alter levels of certain neurotransmitters within the brain, in particular norepinephrine and serotonin. Depending on the class of antidepressant, they can either inhibit the reuptake of neurotransmitters or decrease their degradation, ultimately allowing for increased levels of neurotransmitter at the nerve terminal.

Antipsychotics Drugs used to treat psychotic disorders, such as schizophrenia. Antipsychotics primarily affect the neurotransmitter dopamine.

KEY TERMS AND DEFINITIONS—cont'd

Anxiolytics Minor tranquilizers. Anxiolytics are drugs used to treat several conditions, including anxiety disorders and insomnia. The most common class of anxiolytics is the benzodiazepines. They bind to the γ-aminobutyric acid (GABA) receptor to increase the inhibitory actions of this neurotransmitter.

Central nervous system (CNS) The brain and spinal cord make up the functional components of the CNS. The spinal cord provides nerve fibers that transport signals to and from the brain. The brain largely comprises three components: cortex, midbrain, and brainstem. Together, these provide for all conscious and subconscious functions of the body.

Cholinesterase inhibitors Drugs that block the activity of cholinesterase, an enzyme that inactivates the neurotransmitter acetylcholine. Acetylcholine is found at nerve terminals in both the CNS and the peripheral nervous system. Cholinesterase inhibitors are used in the treatment of dementia to slow the progression of cognitive decline.

Conscious sedation Method used during certain invasive procedures. The goals of conscious sedation are to decrease the level of consciousness and relieve anxiety and pain while allowing the patient to follow verbal commands. Conscious sedation is achieved through the use of several classes of drugs, including benzodiazepines and narcotic analgesics.

Mood stabilizers Drugs used primarily to treat bipolar disorders.

Neurotransmitter Chemical substance that allows neurons to transmit electrical impulses throughout the CNS and peripheral nervous system. The action of the electrical impulse is determined by the chemical structure of the neurotransmitter and the receptor to which it binds.

Stimulant A drug that increases activity of the brain. Stimulants can be divided into two classes: amphetamines and respiratory stimulants. Amphetamines cause increased wakefulness, improved concentration, and appetite suppression. Respiratory stimulants include doxapram, xanthines, carbonic anhydrase inhibitors, salicylates, and progesterone.

The most widely used drugs, both therapeutic and recreational, are agents affecting the **central nervous system (CNS)**. Humans are intrinsically concerned with and perhaps even defined by the processes of thinking and feeling. These processes originate within the brain. Thoughts and feelings, although poorly understood, reside primarily with neurochemical interactions and balance in the brain. Drugs that affect the CNS are used for their effects on perception and mood. Although the gross anatomy of the brain has been elegantly described, the complex interaction of various brain areas and individual neurons is less well understood.

Generally, the cortex, or outer covering, of the brain is considered to be the location of thought, memory, self-awareness, and personality. Perception of sensation and control of body movement, including speech, are also represented in specific areas of the cortex. The midbrain functions as a relay station for information traveling to and from the cortex. It also integrates and modulates autonomic functions; this function occurs primarily in the hypothalamus. The brainstem, or medulla, contains the control areas for autonomic functions, such as breathing and cardiovascular control, and the area responsible for alertness, the reticular activating system. The spinal cord enters the brain at the brainstem, and the cerebellum, immediately behind the brainstem, affects fine motor control and coordinates movement.

Much of our understanding of brain organization and function comes from removing areas of the brain and identifying resulting deficits in animals. Some information has been acquired by studying humans who have had strokes or destructive brain surgery. These observations have led to a general understanding of functional neuroanatomy and recognition that the brain can recover significant function after damage to important areas.

Individual neurons have a wide array of connections with many different neurons in diverse areas of the brain; this is more complicated than the gross anatomy would suggest. These patterns are different in different individuals and change with time in the same individual. Many functions apparently are represented in multiple ways, making them resistant to damage. Although the number of individual neurons does not increase in adulthood, the brain is able to change and increase the number of connections and complexity of the neuronal circuitry throughout life. Although each neuron releases only a single **neurotransmitter** and occasionally a co-neurotransmitter, the actual effect of these neurotransmitters on the next neuron is modified by additional presynaptic and postsynaptic neurons, which may inhibit or augment the primary neurotransmitter effect.

Several diseases are apparently related to loss of particular neurons with specific neurotransmitters. Parkinson disease is caused by a loss of dopamine-containing neurons in the *substantia nigra* area of the midbrain. This condition is characterized by resting tremor; rigidity; bradykinesia, or slowness in initiating movement; gait disturbances; and postural instability. Treatment of Parkinson disease involves increasing the amount of dopamine contained in and released from the remaining neurons.[1,2] Some forms of depression are believed to be caused by reduced activity of norepinephrine neurons in the brain, particularly neurons in the *locus caeruleus*.[3] There seems to be a decrease in the preganglionic augmentation effects of serotonin and in direct stimulatory effects of norepinephrine. Treatment is to restore more normal activity of the norepinephrine neurons by inhibiting the reuptake of serotonin by modulating neurons, enhancing the amount of norepinephrine released, and increasing the duration of its effects in the synapse.

Because of the diversity of neuronal connections and the plasticity of the CNS, drugs used for CNS therapy have widespread and varying effects. This functional and chemical complexity of the brain and peripheral nervous system explains why side effects and toxicities are common with CNS drug therapy.

KEY POINT

Drugs that affect the *central nervous system (CNS)* are *commonly prescribed*. These drugs exert their effects by interacting with *neurotransmission*; by affecting neurotransmitter *release, metabolism,* or *uptake;* or by acting at primary or modifying receptors or *transport proteins*.

NEUROTRANSMITTERS

KEY POINT

Clinical effects of CNS drugs depend on the localization of specific neurotransmitters in specific brain areas.

KEY POINT

Because the organization of the CNS is complex, the main cause of side effects of CNS drugs is their interaction in diffuse brain areas.

KEY POINT

CNS drugs may increase or decrease individual neuronal activity. The balance of activity of different types of neurons seems to affect brain function and mood. Restoration of this balance is the goal of treatment of mood disorders.

Each neuron releases predominantly one type of neurotransmitter from its axon. If enough receptors are activated on the postsynaptic membrane, electrical depolarization occurs and a signal is passed to the next neuron. The functional anatomy and components of neurotransmission are illustrated in Figures 20-1 and 20-2. Released neurotransmitters are bound to and transported by proteins in the synapse, taken back up by the releasing nerve terminal, repackaged into vesicles, and recycled. Bound neurotransmitters are unavailable for receptor interactions, and alterations in the transport proteins in amount or affinity affect the signal propagation potential. Some of the released neurotransmitter is metabolized by membrane-bound enzymes on the postsynaptic cell membrane. The resulting constituent components are taken up presynaptically and used as precursors for neurotransmitter synthesis. Receptors on both the presynaptic membrane and the postsynaptic membrane specific for the released chemicals and for other chemicals from modulating and neighboring neurons affect the activity of the neuron.

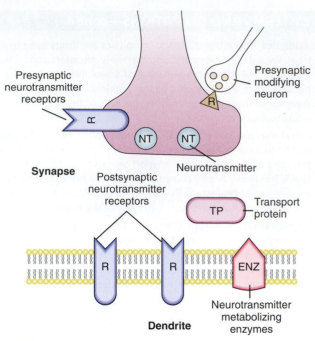

Figure 20-1 Schematic of components of neuron-to-neuron communication. Neurotransmitter *(NT)* is synthesized in the nerve and transported and stored in the nerve terminal. Other components of neurotransmission include transport proteins *(TP)* in the synapse, receptors *(R)* on the postjunctional membrane, receptors *(R)* on the prejunctional membrane, membrane-bound enzymes *(ENZ)*, and modifying neurons.

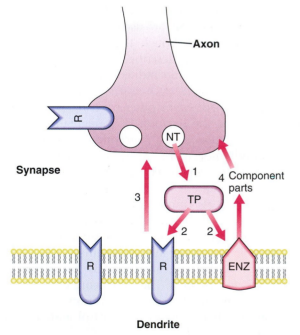

Figure 20-2 Schematic for pathways that neurotransmitters follow after release into the synapse. After axonal depolarization, stored neurotransmitter *(NT)* is released into the synapse *(1)*, where it is bound to the transport or carrier protein *(TP)*. NT is transported to and binds with postjunctional receptors *(2)*, is metabolized by membrane-bound enzymes *(2)*, is actively taken up by the releasing neuron *(3)*, or is released and binds to prejunctional receptors. NT substance that is degraded to its component parts is taken up by the releasing neuron to be resynthesized and reused *(4)*.

TABLE 20-1	Central Nervous System Chemicals That Function as Neurotransmitters

CHEMICAL CLASS	NEUROTRANSMITTER
Biogenic amines	Norepinephrine
	Epinephrine
	Dopamine
	Acetylcholine
	Histamine
	Serotonin (5-hydroxytryptamine)
Amino acids	γ-Aminobutyric acid (GABA)
	Glutamate
	Glycine
	Aspartate
Nucleotides and nucleosides	Adenosine triphosphate
	Adenosine
Peptides	Thyrotropin-releasing hormone
	Enkephalins
	Angiotensin II
	Oxytocin
	Vasopressin
	Bradykinin
	Dynorphin
	Substance P
	Substance K
	Neuropeptide Y
	β-Endorphin
	Luteinizing hormone–releasing factor
	Corticotropin-releasing factor
	Somatostatin
	Secretin
	Melanocyte-stimulating hormone

Chemicals that behave as neurotransmitters are listed in Table 20-1. The effect of the neurotransmitter released is determined by many factors, including the amount of neurotransmitter released, type and quantity of transport proteins, previous release of neurotransmitters, presence of modifying substances, efficiency of reuptake processes, and activities of modulating interneurons. Specifics of this transmission modulation system differ for various brain areas, mental functions, and neurotransmitters. CNS-active drugs may have effects on specific parts of a neurotransmitter system or have generalized effects on brain function. Augmentation or inhibition of neurotransmission can result from drug interaction at any of the sites illustrated in Figures 20-1 and 20-2.

PSYCHIATRIC MEDICATIONS

KEY POINT

Depression is a common *mood disorder*. Several classes of drugs, including *tricyclic antidepressants (TCAs), monoamine oxidase inhibitors (MAOIs),* and *selective serotonin reuptake inhibitors (SSRIs)* are used for this disorder and exhibit a wide range of side effects.

KEY POINT

Other *psychotherapeutic* drugs include *major tranquilizers* and *sedative-hypnotic* drugs.

Antidepressants

Depression is one of the most common psychiatric disorders and a major cause of worldwide disability. In the United States the 12-month prevalence of a major depressive episode has been estimated to involve more than 6% of the population.[4] The Global Burden of Disease Study found unipolar depression accounted for 4.4% of the global disease burden.[5] The prevalence of major depressive disorder may be increasing, and it is predicted that unipolar major depression will be the second leading cause of disability worldwide by 2020.[6]

Depressive disorder has multiple etiologies, including biologic, psychological, and social factors. Serotonin and norepinephrine have been shown to be important neurotransmitters, and their relative deficiency has been linked to depression. For more than a decade, *selective serotonin reuptake inhibitors (SSRIs)* have been the first line of medical treatment for major depressive disorder. These drugs are preferred because they are safer and more tolerable than older medications such as tricyclic antidepressants (TCAs) and monoamine oxidase inhibitors (MAOIs). In addition, newer drugs target both norepinephrine and serotonin; they are called *serotonin norepinephrine reuptake inhibitors.* Depressive disorder agents are listed in Table 20-2.

Mood Stabilizers

Mood stabilizers are used primarily for bipolar disorder. This affective disorder involves alternating episodes of depression and mania or hypomania. Mania is characterized by at least 1 week of elevated or irritable mood and at least three of the following: inflated self-esteem or grandiosity, decreased need for sleep, being more talkative than usual, rapid thoughts or the subjective experience that one's thoughts are racing, distractibility, an increase in goal-directed behavior, or excessive involvement in pleasurable activities that have a high potential for painful consequences.[7] Hypomania is similar to mania but less intense and of shorter duration.[7]

Medical treatment of any degree of bipolar disorder must begin with a mood stabilizer. These drugs include lithium; anticonvulsants such as valproic acid, carbamazepine, gabapentin, and lamotrigine; and **antipsychotics**, which are discussed subsequently. Except for lithium, the main side effect of these drugs is sedation. Lithium has a narrow therapeutic window and consequently must be used judiciously. Lithium can cause tremor, cognitive slowing, hypothyroidism, renal insufficiency, leukocytosis, polyuria, and polydipsia. Lithium toxicity can result in coma.[8] Table 20-3 lists common mood stabilizers.

TABLE 20-2   Drugs Used to Treat Depression

CLASS	GENERIC DRUG	BRAND NAME
Selective serotonin reuptake inhibitors (SSRIs)	Citalopram	Celexa
	Fluoxetine	Prozac, Prozac Weekly, Sarafem, Selfemra
	Fluvoxamine	Luvox, Luvox CR
	Paroxetine	Paxil, Paxil CR, Pexeva, Brisdelle
	Sertraline	Zoloft
	Escitalopram oxalate	Lexapro
Serotonin and norepinephrine reuptake inhibitors	Venlafaxine	Effexor, Effexor XR
	Duloxetine	Cymbalta
	Desvenlafaxine	Pristiq, Khedezla
Serotonin receptor antagonist	Nefazodone	Nefazodone, Serezone
Dopamine reuptake inhibitor	Bupropion	Aplenzin, Forfivo XL, Wellbutrin, Wellbutrin SR, Wellbutrin XL, Zyban
Tricyclic antidepressants (TCAs)	Amitriptyline	Amitriptyline
	Amoxapine	Amoxapine
	Clomipramine	Anafranil
	Desipramine	Norpramin
	Doxepin	Sinequan
	Imipramine HCl	Tofranil
	Imipramine pamoate	Tofranil-PM
	Nortriptyline	Aventyl, Pamelor
	Protriptyline	Vivactil
	Trimipramine	Surmontil
Tetracyclic antidepressants	Maprotiline	Maprotiline
	Mirtazapine	Remeron, Remeron SolTab
Monoamine oxidase inhibitors (MAOIs)	Phenelzine	Nardil
	Tranylcypromine	Parnate
	Isocarboxazid	Marplan
Herbal remedy	St. John's wort (Hypericum perforatum)	St. John's wort
Miscellaneous drugs	Trazodone	Desyrel

CR, Controlled release; *SolTab,* orally disintegrating tablet; *SR,* sustained release (12 hour); *XL,* extra long (extended release 24 hour); *XR,* extended release.

TABLE 20-3   Drugs Used as Mood Stabilizers

GENERIC DRUG	BRAND NAME
Carbamazepine	Tegretol, Tegretol-XR, Epitol, Carbatrol, Equetro, Teril
Lamotrigine	Lamictal, Lamictal XR, Lamictal CD, Lamictal ODT
Lithium	Lithobid, Eskalith
Valproic acid	Depakene, Depakote, Depakote ER, Depakote CP, Stavzor

CD, Chewable; *CP,* delayed release; *ER, XR,* extended release; *ODT,* orally disintegrating.

Antipsychotics

Psychotic disorders are characterized by impaired reality testing. They include schizophrenia spectrum disorders and psychosis associated with depression or mania. Pharmacotherapy is generally used to increase dopamine in the brain. These drugs are most efficacious for active psychotic symptoms, such as hallucinations and abnormal thought processes. Older drugs, such as thorazine, thioridazine, and haloperidol had numerous side effects, which affected compliance. These side effects included extrapyramidal symptoms such as cogwheel rigidity, acute dystonia, oculogyric crisis, and cholinergic side effects. Newer agents, such as risperidone, olanzapine, and quetiapine, are more tolerable. Table 20-4 lists common antipsychotics.

Drugs for Alzheimer Dementia: Cholinesterase Inhibitors

Alzheimer dementia is associated with cognitive deficits secondary to decreased acetylcholine levels within the brain. **Cholinesterase inhibitors** may improve cognition and function in patients with Alzheimer disease. These drugs include donepezil, tacrine, galantamine, and rivastigmine. The use of these drugs is sometimes limited by gastrointestinal side effects, which include nausea, vomiting, diarrhea, and hepatotoxicity, especially with tacrine.[9] These drugs are listed in Table 20-5.

Anxiolytics

 KEY POINT

Hypnotic drugs primarily activate the γ-aminobutyric acid (GABA) receptor–mediated chloride channel, hyperpolarizing the cell and decreasing consciousness, anxiety, and recall.

TABLE 20-4	Drugs Used in Management of Psychotic Disorders	
CLASS	**GENERIC DRUG**	**BRAND NAME**
Phenothiazines	Chlorpromazine	—
	Fluphenazine	—
	Perphenazine	—
	Prochlorperazine	—
	Trifluoperazine	—
Thioxanthene	Thiothixene	Navane
Butyrophenones	Droperidol	Inapsine
	Haloperidol	Haldol
Miscellaneous agents	Clozapine	Clozaril, FazaClo ODT
	Lithium	Lithobid, Eskalith
	Olanzapine	Zyprexa, Zydis
	Pimozide	Orap
	Quetiapine	Seroquel, Seroquel XR
	Risperidone	Risperdal, Consta
	Ziprasidone	Geodon
	Aripiprazole	Abilify
	Paliperidone	Invega
	Iloperidone	Fanapt

ODT, Orally disintegrating; *XR,* extended release.

TABLE 20-5	Drugs Used in Treatment of Dementia	
CLASS	**GENERIC DRUG**	**BRAND NAME**
Cholinesterase inhibitors	Donepezil	Aricept, Aricept ODT
	Galantamine	Razadyne, Razadyne ER
	Rivastigmine	Exelon
	Tacrine	Cognex
	Memantine	Namenda

ER, Extended release; *ODT,* orally disintegrating.

KEY POINT

GABA channel activation may also be important in the production of general anesthesia and sleep. Sleep is a complex activity, and induction of sleep can be pharmacologically influenced by sedative drugs; however, the quality of sleep induced by sedative drugs is poor.

KEY POINT

Antagonism of the *benzodiazepine* receptor site can be accomplished with *flumazenil,* which binds to the receptor site but does not activate the receptor.

Benzodiazepines are agents that have been used to reduce anxiety under a variety of circumstances. **Anxiolytics** are also used as amnestics, preventing conversion of short-term experience into permanent memory. By themselves, they cause no change in respiration; however, these agents may augment the respiratory depression induced by opioids. They have little effect on cardiac function and are very safe agents from this standpoint. Benzodiazepines are excellent induction agents when providing general anesthesia and

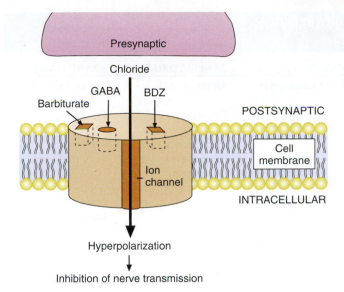

Figure 20-3 Mode of action by which barbiturates and benzodiazepines *(BDZ)* depress central nervous system function; stimulation of receptors on the chloride ion channel facilitates γ-aminobutyric acid *(GABA)*–induced inhibition of neuronal function.

are useful in preventing unpleasant recall during uncomfortable interventions. They may be used as somnifics. These agents are used to terminate seizures, and they elevate seizure threshold. Benzodiazepines exert their effects by binding to benzodiazepine receptors in the γ-aminobutyric acid (GABA) receptor complex on neurons, increasing the GABA chloride channel permeability, which hyperpolarizes the neuron, making depolarization less likely (Figure 20-3). A specific antagonist, flumazenil (Romazicon), can reverse the sedative effects of the benzodiazepines.

Several other drugs are used to treat anxiety and insomnia. Some of these are listed with the benzodiazepines in Table 20-6. Their mechanisms of action are not related to interactions with the benzodiazepine receptor or the GABA system. Some of the drugs listed in Table 20-6 are used to promote sleep; these and other nonrelated sleep-inducing agents are listed in Table 20-7. Although they induce sleep, benzodiazepines and other drug classes interfere with the normal sleep cycles by reducing the amount of time spent in rapid eye movement (REM) sleep.

Barbiturates

The barbiturates, one of the oldest groups of sedative drugs, are derived from barbituric acid. Because of their toxic potential and rapid development of tolerance, barbiturates have largely been replaced by benzodiazepines except for a few specialized uses. Ultra-short-acting barbiturates are used for anesthetic induction (thiopental, thiamylal, and methohexital), as hypnotics (pentobarbital and secobarbital), and for seizure control and prophylaxis (phenobarbital). Use of barbiturates as hypnotics is limited by rapid development of tolerance and reduction in the quality of sleep (decreased amount of REM sleep). They are potent inducers of the cytochrome P450 (CYP) drug-metabolizing

TABLE 20-6   Drugs Used to Treat Anxiety and Insomnia

CLASS	GENERIC DRUG	BRAND NAME
Benzodiazepines	Alprazolam	Xanax, Xanax XR, Niravam
	Clorazepate dipotassium	Tranxene, Gen-Xene
	Chlordiazepoxide	Librium
	Diazepam	Valium, Diastat
	Estazolam	—
	Flurazepam	Dalmane
	Lorazepam	Ativan
	Midazolam	Midazolam
	Oxazepam	—
	Temazepam	Restoril
	Triazolam	Halcion
Benzodiazepine antagonist	Flumazenil	Romazicon
Other anxiolytics	Buspirone HCl	BuSpar
	Doxepin HCl	Sinequan, Zonalon
	Hydroxyzine	Vistaril
	Meprobamate	Meprobamate

XR, Extended release.

TABLE 20-7   Medications Used to Induce Sleep

CLASS	GENERIC DRUG	BRAND NAME
Benzodiazepines	Estazolam	—
	Flurazepam HCl	Dalmane
	Quazepam	Doral
	Temazepam	Restoril
	Triazolam	Halcion
Barbiturates	Secobarbital	Seconal
	Pentobarbital	Nembutal
	Butabarbital	Butisol
Antihistamines	Cyproheptadine	Cyproheptadine
	Diphenhydramine	Benadryl
	Hydroxyzine	Vistaril
Miscellaneous	Chloral hydrate	Somnote
	Dexmedetomidine	Precedex
	Ethanol (alcohol)	
	Eszopiclone	Lunesta
	Ramelteon	Rozerem
	Zaleplon	Sonata
	Zolpidem	Ambien, Ambien CR, Edluar, Intermezzo

CR, Controlled release.

system that can alter the levels of many other drugs. Although many of the therapeutic effects of barbiturates are mediated by a specific receptor at the GABA–mediated inhibitory receptor, they have widespread depressive effects on neuron activity. Intentional or accidental overdose results in respiratory arrest and cardiovascular collapse because of depression of the brain control center. This drug class also carries a high risk of addiction and abuse.

Severe withdrawal symptoms, including seizures, occur after abruptly stopping long-term use of barbiturates.

Other Hypnotics

Difficulty sleeping is a common clinical complaint that frequently results in the prescription of a hypnotic. In addition to the short-acting benzodiazepines and barbiturates mentioned earlier, several other sedatives are used for inducing sleep. All of these agents disrupt sleep patterns and may not improve overall well-being. Hypnotics to induce sleep are generally recommended for brief periods (1 or 2 weeks). However, some patients continue to take these medications for years. A new drug, eszopiclone, is approved for long-term use. Medications used for sleep enhancement are listed in Table 20-7.

ETHYL ALCOHOL

Alcohol is a byproduct of sugar fermentation. It is used as a socially acceptable nonprescription, sedative-hypnotic agent. Ingested to excess, alcohol behaves like a general anesthetic by depressing all brain areas, resulting in loss of voluntary muscle control and consciousness. At toxic levels (400 to 600 mg/dL blood alcohol level), the respiratory center is affected and death as a result of respiratory arrest is likely. The disinhibiting effects of modest alcohol intoxication result from depression of higher cortical behavior control centers, probably by decreasing the GABA receptor effects of endogenous mediators. At higher levels, diffuse membrane-disruptive effects occur, causing generalized neurologic depression. When combined with other sedative-hypnotic drugs, the degree of intoxication is additive.

Chronic alcohol ingestion results in upregulation of GABA receptors and other brain functions, with the development of tolerance to the intoxicating and toxic depression caused by alcohol. Abrupt withdrawal after prolonged use may result in the syndrome of *delirium tremens (DTs)*, characterized by CNS hyperactivity, including hyperthermia, increased blood pressure, muscle twitching, hallucinosis, and seizures. The mortality from DTs is high, ranging from 5% to 10% if seizures occur. The withdrawal syndrome can be prevented or treated with any of the sedative-hypnotic drugs; usually a benzodiazepine is chosen because of its relative safety.

Alcohol is a carbohydrate, and if ingested in large quantities, it replaces many of the dietary calories and decreases appetite. Protein, fat, and vitamin malnutrition are often seen with chronic alcohol abuse. Alcohol is metabolized to CO_2 and H_2O, producing acetaldehyde in the process. Because it is a food, ethyl alcohol saturates the metabolic enzyme system and undergoes first-order elimination kinetics. This means that a constant amount of alcohol is removed per unit of time, rather than a fixed percentage of the blood concentration as with most other drugs. In the average person, this results in about 10 to 12 g of alcohol removed per hour.

PAIN TREATMENT

Pain is common in humans. Because pain is a subjective, unpleasant experience, it is difficult to observe and quantitate objectively. Recognition of the physiologic and psychological consequences of inadequate pain treatment has led to increased attention to pain control in patients. In hospitalized patients, estimation of pain has been elevated to the level of a vital sign, on par with blood pressure, heart rate, respiratory rate, and temperature. Pain is now often referred to as the fifth vital sign.

Besides the difficulty of estimating the amount of pain, many factors alter patient responses to a given degree of discomfort. Physiologic, social, and psychological factors profoundly alter patient perception and tolerance of pain.[10,11] The meaning of pain to the individual can affect the reported pain and the response of the pain to treatment. It is helpful to view the pain experience as composed of at least two components: (1) the sensation of *pain* as mediated by the CNS receiving nociceptive input from peripheral pain receptors and (2) *suffering*, the negative, personal emotional response to the pain experience. The integration and expression of these two components produce the pain behavior, which influences the patient's analgesic requirements. Medications may be directed at the origin, integration, or interpretation of the pain experience. Combinations of medications often are more effective than a single approach to this common problem.

Nonanalgesic drugs also affect perception and tolerance of pain. Sedative drugs such as the barbiturates and benzodiazepines seem to reduce pain tolerance—increasing the amount of pain perceived and reported by patients receiving them. This effect probably occurs by reducing cortical modulation of the pain perception, increasing pain behaviors. These agents, when combined with **analgesics**, however, seem to decrease the painful experience, and enhance analgesia. When interviewed after resolution of the pain episode, patients do not usually report having experienced pain of the extreme magnitude that was perceived by caregivers.

Another factor that must be taken into account when assessing pain is that patients have poor pain memories. With time, the ability to recall the severity and characteristics of pain diminishes; this applies to the effects of treatment as well. Patients asked whether past pain treatment was effective almost always report improvement in pain, even if objective evaluation at the time documents no change or even worsening pain.[12] **Antidepressants** combined with analgesics are used to treat chronic pain states. These agents may be effective by modifying the depressed mood that accompanies chronic discomfort.

Although there are external clues to the presence and magnitude of a person's pain, personal reports are the only way to judge the presence and magnitude of pain. Visual or numeric analog pain scales are the most commonly employed methods for estimating the magnitude of pain. The simplest and most common pain scale employed is an 11-point scale, with 10 being the worst imaginable pain and 0 being totally without pain. Patients are asked to rate their pain from the worst imaginable pain (10) to no pain at all (0). These scales seem to have internal and external validity.[13-15] The numeric rating is convenient and recognizable, and it lends itself to frequent repetition and consistent reporting. In children, a series of smiling and frowning faces, such as the Wong/Baker Rating Scale, may be used to allow the child to report the degree of pain.[16] These scales help in assessing the adequacy of analgesia and create a shorthand way for patients to communicate their need for additional analgesia to the bedside caregiver.

Caregivers must integrate visual or numeric analog pain scale reports, patient pain behaviors, and vital signs with their own biases[17] regarding the degree of pain that should be present to decide whether to administer additional analgesic drugs.[18] Caregivers apparently often deliver inadequate amounts of analgesics.[19] Inappropriate expectations in both the patient and the caregiver regarding the degree of pain contribute to this reluctance to administer potent analgesics. Acute pain remains undertreated in many patients.

Nonsteroidal Antiinflammatory Drugs

KEY POINT

Pain may be relieved by *nonsteroidal antiinflammatory drugs (NSAIDs)*, which modify peripheral inflammation and central integration; by *opiates*, which modify the spinal cord transmission, brainstem processing, and cortical perception of pain; and by local anesthetics, which block sensory transmission.

Nonsteroidal antiinflammatory drugs (NSAIDs) are analgesics frequently used to treat moderate pain (Table 20-8). NSAIDs work by affecting the hypothalamus and by inhibiting the production of inflammatory mediators, primarily prostaglandins, at the peripheral site of the painful stimulus. The salicylates are the oldest member of this class and have been known for more than 100 years for their effects as antipyretics. Aspirin, a salicylate, is a common component of over-the-counter (OTC) analgesics and cold remedies. Aspirin decreases the synthesis of prostaglandin by irreversibly inhibiting two enzymes: cyclooxygenase-1 and cyclooxygenase-2 (COX-1 and COX-2). COX-1 is located primarily on tissues, including the blood vessels, kidney, and gastric mucosa, and COX-2 is associated primarily with inflammation. In contrast to aspirin, others such as ibuprofen and naproxen reversibly inhibit these enzymes. Although selective COX-2 inhibitors are thought to cause fewer gastrointestinal side effects, there are no clinical trials clearly showing this.[20]

Gastric irritation and ulceration are major problems with administering NSAIDs. Renal injury can result from prolonged use and high doses of these medications. NSAIDs also inhibit platelet aggregation, and this compounds the problem of gastrointestinal bleeding. The antiplatelet effects are used therapeutically either after or to prevent cardiac thrombosis. Aspirin use in childhood febrile illness

TABLE 20-8	Nonsteroidal Antiinflammatory Drugs	
CLASS	**GENERIC DRUG**	**BRAND NAME**
Nonspecific Cyclooxygenase Inhibitors		
Salicylates	Aspirin	Bayer
	Choline salicylate	Arthropan
	Diflunisal	Diflunisal
	Magnesium salicylate	
	Salsalate	Amigesic, Disalcid
	Sodium salicylate	
Aniline derivative	Acetaminophen	Tylenol
Indoles	Etodolac	—
	Indomethacin	Indocin, Indocin SR
	Sulindac	Clinoril
Propionic acid derivatives	Ibuprofen	Advil
	Fenoprofen	Nalfon
	Flurbiprofen	Ansaid
	Ketoprofen	—
	Naproxen	Aleve, Anaprox, Naprelan, Naprosyn
	Oxaprozin	Daypro
Piroxicam derivative	Piroxicam	Feldene
Miscellaneous	Diclofenac	Voltaren, Voltaren-XR, Cataflam
	Ketorolac	
	Meclofenamate	
	Mefenamic acid	Ponstel
	Nabumetone	
	Tolmetin	Tolectin
	Ziconotide	Prialt
COX-2 Inhibitors		
	Celecoxib	Celebrex
	Meloxicam	Mobic
	Rofecoxib	Vioxx*
	Valdecoxib	Bextra†

COX-2, Cyclooxygenase-2; *SR*, sustained release; *XR*, extended release.
*Manufacturer voluntarily withdrew agent from the market.
†U.S. Food and Drug Administration removed April 7, 2005.

has been associated with an increased incidence of Reye syndrome, an often fatal increase in intracranial pressure associated with massive hepatic dysfunction.[21,22] Allergic reactions to NSAIDs are common. Rashes, urticaria, angioneurotic edema, asthma, and anaphylaxis have been reported.

Acetaminophen (Tylenol), although a weak inhibitor of the cyclooxygenase system, has no significant antiinflammatory effects but is effective in relieving mild to moderate pain. It does not inhibit platelets or cause gastric ulcers. In large doses, acetaminophen can cause lethal hepatic necrosis. Because it is used in many nonprescription cold preparations, accidental overdose from combining medications during self-medication occasionally occurs. An overdose of acetaminophen can be treated with oral *N-acetylcysteine* as described in Chapter 9.

COX-2 inhibitors have been reevaluated for their potential to cause adverse cardiovascular events. Rofecoxib (Vioxx) and valdecoxib (Bextra) have been withdrawn from the market. Other COX-2 inhibitors are currently undergoing trials to assess their potential to increase cardiovascular risk.

Opioid Analgesics

KEY POINT

Depression of respiratory drive is an important *side effect* of several classes of CNS drugs, including general anesthetics and *opioid analgesics*.

KEY POINT

Opiate effects can be antagonized with *naloxone* or *naltrexone*.

KEY POINT

Naloxone, which is no longer produced under the trade name Narcan, now is produced as Evzio, a new trade-named medication that is available as an automated injection device to be used by laypeople.

Opioids or narcotic analgesics are derivatives of the naturally occurring drug mixture opium, derived from the poppy, *Papaver somniferum*. These agents are used for the treatment of moderate to severe pain. They act by binding to opioid receptors in the brain and spinal cord. They modify pain pathways at the spinal level and profoundly influence the subjective response to pain at the cortical level. Endogenously occurring opioids, the endorphins and enkephalins, are neuromodulators affecting pain perception and mood. Opioids exert their effects and side effects by binding to receptors for these naturally occurring substances.

There are at least three distinct opioid receptors—*mu* (μ), *kappa* (κ), and *delta* (δ)—and several subtypes. Agonist drugs may bind at one or more of these receptors, accounting for some of the differences seen in their effects. Besides pain relief, high enough doses of opioids can result in loss of consciousness and, because of a profound dose-dependent depression of respiratory drive, respiratory arrest. Opioids produce a euphoric effect on mood, making them popular drugs of abuse. Tolerance develops rapidly, and withdrawal is very painful and unpleasant. These factors contribute to the highly addictive potential of the opioids.

The μ receptor is responsible for the analgesic effects in the CNS and spinal cord. It also accounts for respiratory depression, constipation, nausea and vomiting (from the chemotactic trigger zone receptors), and antitussive effects. The κ receptors are located in the spinal cord and, to a lesser extent, in the CNS mediate analgesia. They may be the receptors responsible for the analgesic effects of the mixed agonist-antagonist drugs. The δ receptor is the receptor for the naturally occurring mediator enkephalin; its role in analgesia is unclear. It may be important in the spinal mediation of pain perception. This is just the outline of the opioid receptor system; there are other types and subtypes of receptors. Their actual function in human health is not understood. The effect of various opioids can be explained by their actions at one or more of these receptors.

Opioids are listed in Table 20-9. Some have pure agonist effects, acting as the endogenous mediators at the receptors, and others antagonize the endogenous mediators but have a small agonist effect (mixed drugs or agonist-antagonist drugs). There are several strictly antagonist agents. These drugs are used to reverse the analgesic and respiratory depressive effects of the opioids. The most serious side effect of an opioid agonist is respiratory depression, which is mediated by decreased sensitivity of the respiratory center

to elevations in arterial carbon dioxide pressure ($PaCO_2$). Miosis (small pupils) is pathognomonic for opioid drug administration and is a consequence of effects on the sympathetic nervous system. Constipation results from opioid depression of motility of the stomach and intestines. Nausea and vomiting are a direct effect on the brainstem effectors. Cough suppression results from a direct central effect of the opioid.

Because of their effects on pain perception, narcotics are often used as part of a balanced anesthetic. Doses that cause profound depression of respiration have minimal or no effect on cardiac function; because of this, opioids are the basis for anesthesia for patients with serious cardiovascular compromise. By themselves, opioids have no effect on consciousness or memory. Combined with small doses of benzodiazepines or gaseous **anesthetics**, they can be used to provide surgical anesthesia.

Strong opioid drugs are often referred to as *narcotics*, from the Greek word for stupor. The word *narcotic* has significant legal overtones. For this reason, its use has been avoided in this section. *Opiates* are compounds derived from opium and represent a small number of the drugs discussed in this section. The term *opioids*, as used in this section, implies simply that the agents interact with one or more of the opioid receptors.

Routes of Opioid Administration

KEY POINT

Inadequate pain relief has been identified as a serious problem. Many pain control options are available to hospitalized patients.

KEY POINT

Patient-controlled (opioid) analgesia (PCA), epidural analgesia with local anesthetics and opioids, and combinations of analgesic classes can result in excellent postoperative pain relief.

As discussed previously, pain is a subjective experience. Inadequate analgesia is a common complaint voiced by patients and is especially a problem after surgery. Fear of respiratory depression is often given as the reason caregivers are reluctant to administer more opioids. Novel ways of treating pain have been developed to improve treatment of pain. Patient-controlled analgesia (PCA) is a method by which patients can self-administer a predetermined intravenous bolus of an opioid at a set interval. Use of PCA avoids the delay in getting a dose requested from and later delivered by a nurse.

KEY POINT

More total analgesia drug is needed if pain is allowed to intensify between drug doses. It is more effective to keep control of pain than to regain control of it. Continuous

TABLE 20-9	Opioid Drugs	
EFFECT AT OPIOID RECEPTOR	**GENERIC DRUG**	**BRAND NAME**
Agonist	Morphine	Avinza, Kadian, MS Contin
	Opium	Paregoric
	Codeine	—
	Alfentanil	Alfenta
	Dihydrocodeine	Available only in combination with other agents
	Fentanyl	Sublimaze, Actiq, Duragesic
	Heroin	—
	Hydrocodone	Available only in combination with other agents
	Hydromorphone	Dilaudid
	Levorphanol	Levo-Dromoran
	Meperidine	Demerol
	Methadone	Dolophine, Methadose
	Oxycodone	Roxicodone, OxyContin
	Oxymorphone	Opana, Opana ER
	Propoxyphene	Darvon
	Remifentanil	Ultiva
	Sufentanil	Sufenta
	Tramadol	Ultram, Ultram ER, Ryzolt
Mixed agonist-antagonist	Buprenorphine	Buprenex, Subutex
	Butorphanol	Stadol
	Nalbuphine	
	Pentazocine	Talwin
Antagonist	Naloxone	Evzio
	Naltrexone	ReVia, Vivitrol

ER, Extended release; *MS,* morphine sulfate.

administration of a background opioid rate also may help with this problem. Patients using PCA for postoperative pain use less total opioid and report subjectively less pain than patients receiving scheduled or as-needed opioids delivered by nurses.

Opioid Inhalation

Opioids are occasionally administered by inhalation. Inhaled opioids have been suggested to be more effective than systemic opioids for decreasing the sensation of dyspnea in patients with advanced respiratory failure. Opioid receptors have been found in lung tissue, but their exact function in modifying the sensation of dyspnea has not been determined. Inhaled (nebulized) opioids may affect dyspnea by a central mechanism because these drugs are rapidly absorbed from the lung. No controlled studies have shown improved effectiveness of opioids when administered by inhalation; however, this route may be an alternative when intravenous access is unavailable.[23] Patients with terminal cancer without lung disease have been given systemic doses of analgesics through this route with good clinical effect.

Local Anesthetics

> **KEY POINT**
>
> *Local anesthetics* consist of a *hydrophilic end* connected to an active *amino end* connected by an *amine* or *ester* linkage.

> **KEY POINT**
>
> Local anesthetics block *sodium channels* in axons and abolish neural transmission.

Pain treatment can be achieved by blocking transmission of the pain impulse from the damaged area. Local anesthetics are used to interrupt these nervous signals. Local anesthetics produce nerve conduction block by blocking sodium channels. These are located all along the cell, including the axon. When depolarization occurs, the impulse is propagated down the axon by an abrupt increase in the membrane sodium permeability. When the drug binds to and occludes the channel pore, sodium is unable to enter the cell, and propagation of the electrical impulse is stopped. All local anesthetics consist of a lipophilic part and a hydrophilic, amine part connected by either an amide or ester linkage; this is illustrated in Figure 20-4. Table 20-10 lists several common agents. Sodium channel blockade makes some of these drugs useful in terminating cardiac conduction abnormalities in addition to providing analgesia. Some evidence suggests that systemic administration or inhalation may also enhance bronchodilation in asthma and suppress irritant tracheal cough responses. At toxic levels, CNS excitation occurs, and frank seizures may result. Epinephrine is often added to a local anesthetic for

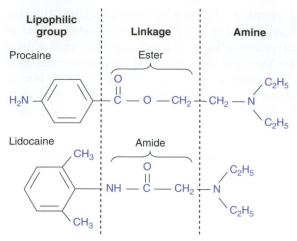

Figure 20-4 Chemical structures of local anesthetics procaine and lidocaine, showing their respective ester and amide linkages, location of the lipophilic group, and ionizable amine group.

TABLE 20-10	Examples of Local Anesthetics	
CLASS	**GENERIC DRUG**	**BRAND NAME**
Esters	Benzocaine	Hurricane, Solarcaine
	Chloroprocaine	Nesacaine
	Procaine	Novocain
Amides	Bupivacaine	Marcaine, Sensorcaine
	Lidocaine	Xylocaine
	Mepivacaine	Carbocaine, Polocaine
	Prilocaine	Citanest
	Ropivacaine	Naropin

vasoconstriction to delay its absorption, prolonging its effect and decreasing blood levels and potential toxicity. Bupivacaine is very cardiotoxic, and a toxic dose may result in profound and prolonged cardiac depression or arrest.

Epidural Analgesia

Continuing epidural infusions for analgesia have improved postoperative pain therapy. There is evidence that patient outcome may also be improved with epidural infusions of local anesthetics, opioids, or both[24,25]; this is especially true for very ill patients.[26-29] The quality of analgesia and the ability to eliminate pain in many body areas are superior with local anesthetic infusion compared with systemic analgesics. Epidural infusions are common in some surgical procedures, especially in the delivery of newborns by cesarean section. Minimal effects on normal sensory and motor function can be achieved with very dilute local anesthetics. Addition of opioids to the mixture permits even less local anesthetic to be infused. If sympathetic blockade produces unacceptable hypotension, local anesthetics can be eliminated completely, with significant analgesia obtained with opioid infusion alone. Pain modulation from epidural opioids occurs at receptors at the spinal cord segmental level. The major side effects of epidural analgesia using local and opioid infusions are listed in Box 20-1.

Combinations of Analgesic Classes

Another strategy to improve analgesia and to reduce the likelihood of opioid overdose is to combine several different classes of analgesics. Prescription combinations of NSAIDs and opioids are widely available (Table 20-11). The concept of attacking pain at several places is useful, but the fixed combinations of drugs with different effects, toxicities, and half-lives make titration to an individual patient's needs difficult with these agents. Use of the separate agents, independently titrated, may improve this problem, but it is more difficult for patients to take numerous medications.

KEY POINT

The U.S. Food and Drug Administration (FDA) set the safe 24-hour dose limit of acetaminophen at 4000 mg per adult. No combination analgesic prescription contains more than 325 mg of acetaminophen per unit dose.

CHRONIC PAIN SYNDROMES

Surgery or trauma causing acute pain can lead to central sensitization and persistence of pain after the peripheral lesion has resolved. It is unknown how frequently this problem leads to a chronic pain syndrome, but data are accumulating suggesting that specific treatment in the acute period may reduce the likelihood of a neuropathic problem later.

Neuropathic pain may start with nerve injury, which results in axon degeneration and regeneration. In animal models, abnormal discharges at the spinal cord level are associated with this process, leading to sensitization, abnormal sensation, phantom pain, and rapid changes in the functional architecture of the pain pathways at the level of the spinal cord and lower brain. *Hyperesthesia* (increased and unpleasant sensitivity to all sensory modalities), *hyperpathia* (increased unpleasant abnormal feeling from mildly uncomfortable stimuli), and *allodynia* (painful feeling from gentle stimuli) can be shown to occur soon after acute painful trauma in some patients, especially after surgery on or near major nerve trunks. In some patients, this process may persist and advance to result in a chronic pain syndrome.

The characteristics of neuropathic pain include evidence of a primary injury; pain involving (but not confined to) a body area with a sensory deficit; a burning, electric, or shooting character to the pain; dysesthesias in the area; pain spreading beyond the cutaneous nerve distribution; sympathetic hyperactivity; and allodynia, hyperpathia, and hyperalgesia. In some complex regional pain syndromes, autonomic deregulation results in skin changes, edema, and nail and hair loss. This syndrome may lead to severe suffering and incapacitation. Once established, neuropathic pain is poorly responsive to analgesic treatment, but the pain may respond to sympathetic interruption or α-receptor blockade.[30] Modification of the initial pain input possibly may decrease the incidence or reduce the severity of the syndrome that develops over time.

Preemptive analgesia is the delivery of adequate and appropriate analgesia before initiation of nociceptive input from the surgical incision. By totally abolishing the painful stimulus, the potential for chronic pain syndromes should be reduced. Although general anesthetics and opioids do modify the central sensitization to some extent, regional analgesia, antiinflammatory agents, central α-receptor blockers, and *N*-methyl-D-(+)-aspartate (NMDA) receptor antagonists, alone or in combination, offer hope of preempting pain and eliminating postoperative pain syndromes.

TABLE 20-11	Examples of Combinations of Nonsteroidal Antiinflammatory Drugs and Opioid Analgesics			
NSAID		**OPIOID**		
AGENT	**DOSE (mg)**	**AGENT**	**DOSE (mg)**	**BRAND NAME**
Acetaminophen	325	Hydrocodone	5	Anexsia 5/325; Norco
Aspirin	325	Oxycodone	4.8335	Percodan
Acetaminophen	325	Oxycodone	5	Roxicet, Percocet
Acetaminophen	300	Codeine	15	Tylenol No. 2
Acetaminophen	300	Codeine	30	Tylenol No. 3
Acetaminophen	300	Codeine	60	Tylenol No. 4
Ibuprofen	200	Hydrocodone	7.5	Vicoprofen

ANESTHESIA

The state of general anesthesia is a drug-induced absence of perception. Stronger stimuli may require deeper anesthesia. Anesthetics are usually administered by inhalation or intravenously because of the more predictable time course of drug actions. Often, combinations of drugs are used to achieve the state of anesthesia. The ideal anesthetic would include the following:

- Pleasant and rapid induction and emergence
- Rapid changes of depth of anesthesia to match surgical demands
- Skeletal muscle relaxation to facilitate surgical exposure
- A wide margin of safety
- No toxic or adverse effects

The first and most common anesthetic agents are gases and volatile liquids (Table 20-12). Dosage and potency are compared by using the concept of minimal alveolar concentration (MAC), which is the amount necessary to achieve the anesthetic state. This is a statistical concept, similar to the ED_{50} (effective dose for 50% of subjects to respond), based on the measured agent concentration in exhaled gas (which is in equilibration with the blood) sufficient to prevent movement on surgical incision in half of the subjects. The mechanisms by which anesthetic gases and vapors exert their effects are poorly understood but may be receptor-mediated (the GABA receptor being a top candidate) or may be a more diffuse, temporary disruption of nerve cell communication. The facts that anesthetic vapor potency is linearly related to fat solubility and that anesthetics can be reversed by high pressures (50 to 100 atmospheres) suggest that cell wall swelling from the agent dissolving in the lipid membrane is an important contributor to the anesthetic state.

Volatile anesthetics by themselves achieve some of the characteristics of the ideal anesthetic in that depth of anesthesia can be changed rapidly, induction and emergence are rapid (with some agents), and there are few toxic concerns. These agents do not reliably provide muscle relaxation. Neuromuscular blockers and other adjuvant drugs are often titrated to create the desired anesthetic state and to prevent potent agent overdose. Neuromuscular blockers are discussed in Chapter 18. Their use in anesthesia includes facilitation of tracheal intubation (often a short-acting agent) and surgical relaxation, which is necessary for intrathoracic, intraabdominal, and other procedures. Pharmacologic reversal of long-acting neuromuscular blocking agents is also discussed in Chapter 18.

Because volatile anesthetics provide little analgesia, narcotic and nonnarcotic analgesics are often a part of the anesthetic mixture. Analgesics may reduce the amount of volatile agent necessary to achieve anesthesia. Induction of general anesthesia is usually facilitated by a rapidly effective sedative-hypnotic agent, although inhalation induction with a newer volatile agent (sevoflurane) is rapid and not unpleasant. Table 20-13 lists commonly used anesthetic induction agents.

KEY POINT

The use of a mixture of agents to achieve the anesthetic state is often referred to as *balanced anesthesia*, in which each element is provided in balance and by a different drug.

Depth of anesthesia is determined by patient response to painful stimuli and is often judged by the sympathetic response—that is, a change in heart rate or blood pressure. Because other factors may influence these signs, determination of anesthetic depth is much more of an art than a science. Monitors are available that are based on the processed electroencephalogram and that are touted to predict depth of anesthesia (bispectral index [BIS] monitor), but these devices are subject to other influences as well. During the course of surgery and anesthesia, the degree of surgical stimulus and the depth of anesthesia vary, and one function of the anesthesiologist is to match these two. Analgesia may be needed intraoperatively and as a part of pain management in the postoperative period. In medically compromised patients, the main activity of the anesthesiologist is to obtain and maintain stability and prevent death; the anesthetic may simply consist of preventing pain and abolishing recall of intraoperative events. The entire cardiovascular armamentarium may be used as part of anesthetic management for these critically ill, unstable patients.

Anesthetic induction agents are used in other areas of care, including the intensive care unit (ICU), the emergency department, and in conscious sedation. Although diazepam, lorazepam, and midazolam are commonly used agents, ketamine, propofol, and fospropofol disodium are

TABLE 20-12	Gases and Volatile Liquids Used to Produce General Anesthesia	
CLASS	**AGENT**	**COMMON OR BRAND NAME**
Gases	Nitrous oxide	Laughing gas
Liquids	Halothane	—
	Isoflurane	Forane
	Enflurane	Ethrane
	Sevoflurane	Ultane
	Desflurane	Suprane

TABLE 20-13	Anesthetic Induction Agents	
CLASS	**GENERIC DRUG**	**BRAND NAME**
Barbiturates	Methohexital	Brevital
Benzodiazepines	Diazepam	Valium
	Lorazepam	Ativan
	Midazolam	Versed
Miscellaneous agents	Etomidate	Amidate
	Ketamine	Ketalar
	Propofol	Diprivan
	Fospropofol disodium	Lusedra

indicated and used in the ICU and in emergency department procedures. These agents may affect patients differently, so close monitoring is indicated. As a respiratory therapist (RT), the monitoring of ventilation and cardiac function are of utmost importance.

Conscious Sedation

KEY POINT

Conscious sedation is a technique using sedatives and analgesics to prevent patient discomfort during invasive procedures. To prevent catastrophe, a *dedicated individual* must *monitor* the progress of sedation and be prepared to correct airway and cardiovascular problems.

KEY POINT

The pain experience, including the physical and emotional components, associated with clinical interventions is unnecessary and may increase morbidity and mortality. For these reasons, minimizing fear and pain is an important part of clinical care.

Fear and pain are frequent side effects of many clinical interventions. Besides general anesthesia, many approaches are available to modify the unpleasant experience of diagnostic and therapeutic procedures. Patient preparation, education, relaxation exercises, hypnosis, and drugs may be useful. **Conscious sedation** is the term applied to pharmacologic modification of painful and frightening experiences during medical procedures. As implied by this term, sedated patients should remain conscious and able to communicate, protect their own airway, and breathe adequately. Improved patient comfort and outcome are the goals of sedation. However, because of variations in patient responses, consciousness and the patient's ability to maintain an unobstructed airway may be lost during sedation.

Institutional standards for safe and effective provision of conscious sedation are required by the Joint Commission on Accreditation of Healthcare Organizations and other regulatory agencies. These standards must be adhered to throughout the institution, whether sedation is provided by a nurse, RT, anesthesiologist, or other health care provider. Many concerned groups have developed guidelines for providing safe conscious sedation. RTs should understand sedative and analgesic pharmacology and may actively participate in provision of conscious sedation.[31-33] Because most of the serious complications of conscious sedation relate to airway compromise, RTs are uniquely qualified to safeguard patients and improve outcomes during conscious sedation.

Standards for Providing Conscious Sedation

Most guidelines for conscious sedation and many clinical reports differentiate several levels of sedation. Often a clear distinction is drawn between conscious and deep sedation.[34] However, the progression from conscious sedation to deep sedation to general anesthesia is difficult to control clinically, and each deeper level implies increased risks and mandates more intensive monitoring and an increased level of support. The definitions of these states and suggested requirements for monitoring are given in Table 20-14.

TABLE 20-14	Levels of Sedation and Recommendations for Monitoring	
LEVEL OF SEDATION	**DEFINITION**	**SUGGESTED MONITORS**
Conscious sedation	Minimally depressed level of consciousness, retaining patient's ability to maintain airway independently and continuously and to respond to physical stimulation and verbal commands	Dedicated monitoring assistant ECG monitoring Pulse oximetry IV access Blood pressure measurement every 15 minutes
Deep sedation	Depressed consciousness accompanied by partial loss of protective reflexes and inability to respond purposefully to verbal command	Skilled airway person Monitoring and recording person IV access Pulse oximetry Continuous ECG monitoring Blood pressure measurement every 5 minutes
General anesthesia	Unconsciousness accompanied by partial or complete loss of protective reflexes and inability to maintain airway independently	Anesthesia personnel Anesthesia assistant IV access Pulse oximetry Carbon dioxide measurement device Continuous ECG monitoring Blood pressure measurement every 5 minutes Other requirements dictated by patient's physiologic condition

ECG, Electroencephalogram; *IV,* intravenous.

All published conscious sedation standards insist on the presence of *more than one* person during the period of sedation (at least the operator and a monitoring assistant). Several guidelines suggest that deep sedation and general anesthesia are *indistinguishable* and that at least three qualified people must be continually present during the sedation period.[35] The standards also suggest that one person must have, *as sole responsibility,* continual monitoring of the patient and recording of vital signs. When providing conscious sedation, it is necessary to assess continuously and ensure oxygenation, ventilation, and temperature maintenance.

Although some conscious sedation guidelines suggest how to monitor these vital functions, the decision to use a particular device and frequency of repeated observations is left to the responsible clinician.[36] What is not left to the discretion of the clinician is the number of personnel necessary and that they must be specially qualified and assigned *only* to monitor one patient's vital functions and the progress of sedation. Resuscitation equipment must be immediately available with individuals trained to use it. Competency in providing conscious sedation requires a didactic understanding of the pharmacology of the drugs discussed in this chapter and a performance-based competency including intravenous therapy, monitor use, and supervised clinical practice.[37]

CENTRAL NERVOUS SYSTEM AND RESPIRATORY STIMULANTS

KEY POINT

CNS-stimulating drugs include *methylxanthines* (caffeine and aminophylline) and doxapram. These agents have little clinical usefulness in treating respiratory failure or drug-induced respiratory depression.

KEY POINT

Specific antagonists for benzodiazepine sedative drugs and opioids are more useful for reversing drug-induced hypoventilation.

In contrast to most of the sedative drugs discussed in this chapter, some drugs can *increase* activity of the brain rather than depress it. Such drugs are termed *analeptic* drugs. If the effects are primarily on the respiratory center, the agent may be a respiratory or ventilatory **stimulant**. Stimulant drugs are used for treatment of narcolepsy, attention-deficit hyperactivity disorder (ADHD), obesity, and, to a lesser extent, respiratory failure. Some of these drugs are listed in Table 20-15. Most stimulant drugs are sympathomimetics, acting directly on α and β receptors. Their abuse potential is great, and their side effects are predictable. They interfere with sleep and are used (and abused) to promote wakefulness and weight loss.

Some drugs can increase ventilation. Doxapram was used in the past as a treatment for acute and chronic respiratory failure. It was given intravenously and caused a transient increase in rate and depth of ventilation. Doxapram is rarely used at the present time because no sustained improvement of respiratory failure has been shown. Methylxanthines, used to promote bronchodilation, also increase catecholamines and increase ventilation. Caffeine, a common component in popular beverages, is used therapeutically in apnea-bradycardia syndromes of premature births. Agents causing metabolic acidosis such as salicylate toxicity, including carbonic anhydrase inhibitor diuretics, can increase ventilation in response to the systemic acidosis that develops. This increase in minute ventilation is not considered therapeutic, however. Progesterone can cause a sustained increase in ventilation and decrease in $PaCO_2$ and is occasionally used to treat

TABLE 20-15	Central and Peripheral Nervous System–Stimulating Drugs		
CLASS	**USE**	**GENERIC DRUG**	**BRAND NAME**
Sympathomimetics	Diet	Benzphetamine	Didrex
		Diethylpropion	Tenuate
		Phendimetrazine	Bontril
		Phentermine	Adipex-P
		Sibutramine	Meridia
	Diet and CNS stimulant	Amphetamine	Adderall
	Diet and CNS stimulant	Methamphetamine	Desoxyn
	CNS stimulant	Dextroamphetamine	Dexedrine
Xanthines	CNS stimulant	Aminophylline	
		Caffeine	
Progestational agent	CNS stimulant	Medroxyprogesterone acetate	Provera
Respiratory stimulant	Peripheral chemoreceptor stimulant	Doxapram	Dopram
Miscellaneous	ADHD	Dexmethylphenidate	Focalin
		Methylphenidate	Ritalin, Methylin, Concerta, Daytrana

ADHD, Attention-deficit hyperactivity disorder; *CNS,* central nervous system.

chronic elevations in CO_2 from advanced obstructive lung disease. Hormonal effects on mood and breast development limit its usefulness.

Respiratory failure resulting from sedative or opioid drug overdose should be treated with specific antagonists flumazenil and naloxone rather than with nonspecific analeptic drugs. Respiratory stimulants have little or no clinical role in treating respiratory failure. Elevated $PaCO_2$ caused by muscle fatigue from increased work of breathing as a result of chronic obstructive pulmonary disease (COPD), acute respiratory distress syndrome (ARDS), or severe bronchospasm would not be expected to improve with catecholamine-stimulating agents. Mechanical ventilation, muscle rest, and bronchodilators are more appropriate approaches.

? SELF-ASSESSMENT QUESTIONS

Answers can be found in Appendix A.

1. What is the difference between sedation and analgesia?
2. Identify the general class (sedative-hypnotic, analgesic, tranquilizer, anesthetic, antipsychotic) of each of the following agents: lorazepam, phenobarbital, doxapram, chloral hydrate, thiopental, midazolam, nitrous oxide, chlorpromazine, halothane, morphine, ibuprofen.
3. You are planning to extubate and remove a patent from the ventilator. However, the nurse administers a large dose of lorazepam (Ativan) for anxiety. What problem may occur if you proceed?
4. What is the most serious side effect of tranquilizers, sedatives, or analgesics (especially opioids)?
5. You have two patients, both of whom have overdosed on central nervous system depressants: *Patient 1 is comatose, cyanotic, with dilated pupils. Patient 2 is comatose, cyanotic, with pinpoint pupils.* Which patient may have taken a barbiturate and which may have taken a narcotic analgesic?
6. Identify your initial priorities as a respiratory therapist in caring for a patient with an overdose of tranquilizers.
7. What is the mode of action of the benzodiazepines?
8. Identify an agent that can reverse the effects of benzodiazepines, such as midazolam and triazolam.
9. Would barbiturates be helpful in managing pain in a ventilated patient?
10. Would meperidine be helpful to prevent or lessen perception of pain?
11. Suggest an analgesic for minor pain for a patient with a bleeding disorder, such as hemophilia, or a patient who is taking an anticoagulant, such as warfarin.
12. Are there any serious side effects to use of a ventilatory stimulant such as doxapram?

CLINICAL SCENARIO

Answers can be found in Appendix A.

A 35-year-old black man was admitted to the hospital with lethargy after being found in his apartment by a friend. An empty bottle of amitriptyline pills was lying next to the man. In the emergency department, the patient became more lethargic to the point of unresponsiveness and developed hypopnea and bradypnea. He was subsequently intubated and mechanically ventilated with a volume-cycled ventilator. The patient had a history of depression but had been in good physical health. He was taking amitriptyline, which was prescribed by his psychiatrist for his depression. In an act of despair, he had taken an overdose of his medication. The man had no allergies, and his past medical history and family history were unremarkable.

Physical examination revealed a mesomorphic man appearing his stated age, markedly sedated, intubated, and mechanically ventilated. His vital signs were as follows: rectal temperature (T) of 39° C, pulse (P) of 140 beats/min, respiratory rate (RR) of 12 breaths/min on an assist/control (A/C) rate of 12 breaths/min, and blood pressure (BP) of 110/60 mm Hg taken in right arm while supine. Head, eyes, ears, nose, and throat (HEENT) were unremarkable except for the oral endotracheal tube (ETT) in place. His chest had normal resonance to percussion, and his lungs had clear breath sounds bilaterally. Cardiovascular examination revealed on palpation the point of maximal impulse was located normally in the fifth intercostal space in the midclavicular line. Auscultation revealed normal S_1 and S_2 without murmurs, gallops, or rubs. He had normal jugular venous pressure, and his pulses were 2+ throughout. His abdomen was mildly distended with absent bowel sounds. No masses or organomegaly were present. His extremities were unremarkable, and his skin was very warm and dry. He was unresponsive to visual, auditory, or tactile stimuli, and his pupils were equally dilated and sluggishly responsive to light. All extremities were flaccid, and his reflexes were 1+ throughout. His plantar reflexes were downgoing.

Laboratory results revealed normal hemogram, electrolytes, blood urea nitrogen (BUN), creatinine, and liver function test results. The tricyclic antidepressant (TCA) level was in the toxic range. His chest radiograph was normal. The ETT was approximately 2 cm above the carina. The electrocardiogram (ECG) showed sinus tachycardia at 140 beats/min, with prolonged P–R and QRS intervals. Arterial blood gas (ABG) results on A/C ventilation at 12 breaths/min, with a tidal volume (VT) of 800 mL and a fraction of inspired oxygen (FIO_2) of 1, were as follows: pH of 7.44, arterial carbon dioxide pressure ($PaCO_2$) of 38 mm Hg, and arterial oxygen pressure (PaO_2) of 550 mm Hg.

TCA overdose was diagnosed, and the patient was admitted to the medical intensive care unit (MICU),

Continued

CLINICAL SCENARIO—cont'd

where he was treated with activated charcoal 30 g via nasogastric tube q6h, along with normal saline hydration intravenously. After the first dose of charcoal, his heart rate dropped to approximately 120 beats/min, and FIO_2 was eventually tapered to 0.35, with the resulting ABG values: pH of 7.43, $PaCO_2$ of 40 mm Hg, and PaO_2 of 175 mm Hg. Several hours after the second charcoal dose, the patient awoke and was able to write notes to the MICU staff, stating that he was anxious to be extubated. The staff wanted to oblige and placed him on a T-piece with 35% O_2 from a large-reservoir nebulizer. About 2 hours later, the patient fell asleep while on the T-piece, and ABG results at that time were pH of 7.36, $PaCO_2$ of 48 mm Hg, and PaO_2 of 165 mm Hg. An astute respiratory therapist noticed the marked change in the ABG parameters and placed the patient back on the ventilator. The patient was eventually able to be extubated uneventfully several hours after the fourth dose of charcoal. He was transferred in stable medical condition to the psychiatry service the day after extubation.

Using the SOAP method, assess this clinical scenario.

REFERENCES

1. Olanow CW, Hauser RA, Gauger L, et al: The effect of deprenyl and levodopa on the progression of Parkinson disease. *Ann Neurol* 38:771, 1995.
2. Lozano AM, Lang AE, Hutchison WD, et al: New developments in understanding the etiology of Parkinson disease and in its treatment. *Curr Opin Neurobiol* 8:783, 1998.
3. Ressler KJ, Nemeroff CB: Role of norepinephrine in the pathophysiology and treatment of mood disorders. *Biol Psychiatry* 46:1219, 1999.
4. Kessler RC, Berglund P, Demler O, et al: The epidemiology of major depressive disorder: results from the National Comorbidity Survey Replication (NCS-R). *JAMA* 289:3095–3105, 2003.
5. Chisholm D, Sanderson K, Ayuso-Mateos JL, et al: Reducing the global burden of depression. *Br J Psychiatry* 184:393–403, 2004.
6. Murray C, Lopez A: Alternative projections of mortality and disability by cause 1990-2020. *Lancet* 349:1498, 1997.
7. American Psychiatric Association: *Diagnostic and statistical manual of mental disorders*, ed 4, Washington, DC, 2000, American Psychiatric Association.
8. American College of Physicians: *ACP Medicine*, section II, New York, 2006, WebMD Professional Publishing.
9. Abramowicz M, editor: Tacrine for Alzheimer's disease. *Med Lett Drugs Ther* 35:87, 1993.
10. Chen AC, Dworkin SF, Haug J, et al: Human pain responsively in a tonic pain model: psychological determinants. *Pain* 37:143, 1989.
11. Carragee EJ, Vittum D, Truong TP, et al: Pain control and cultural norms and expectations after closed femoral shaft fractures. *Am J Orthop* 28:97, 1999.
12. Feine JS, Lavigne GJ, Dao TT, et al: Memories of chronic pain and perceptions of relief. *Pain* 77:137, 1998.
13. Chambers CT, Reid GJ, McGrath PJ, et al: Development and preliminary validation of a postoperative pain measure for parents. *Pain* 68:307, 1996.
14. McGrath PA, Seifert CE, Speechley KN, et al: A new analogue scale for assessing children pain: an initial validation study. *Pain* 64:435, 1996.
15. Colwell C, Clark L, Perkins R: Postoperative use of pediatric pain scales: children self-report versus nurse assessment of pain intensity and affect. *J Pediatr Nurs* 11:375, 1996.
16. Wong DL, Baker CM: Pain in children: comparison of assessment scales. *Pediatr Nurs* 14:9, 1988.
17. Todd KH, Samaroo N, Hoffman JR: Ethnicity as a risk factor for inadequate emergency department analgesia. *JAMA* 269:1537, 1993.
18. Sjostrom B, Haljamae H, Dahlgren LO, et al: Assessment of postoperative pain: impact of clinical experience and professional role. *Acta Anaesthesiol Scand* 41:339, 1997.
19. Beauregard L, Pomp A, Choiniere M: Severity and impact of pain after day-surgery. *Can J Anaesth* 45:304, 1998.
20. Abramowicz M: COX2 alternatives and GI protection. *Med Lett Drugs Ther* 46:91, 2004.
21. Hurwitz ES, Barrett MJ, Bregman D, et al: Public Health Service study of Reye syndrome and medications: report of the main study. *JAMA* 257:1905, 1987.
22. Forsyth BW, Horwitz RI, Acampora D, et al: New epidemiologic evidence confirming that bias does not explain the aspirin/Reye syndrome association. *JAMA* 261:2517, 1989.
23. Manning HL: Dyspnea treatment. *Respir Care* 45:1342, 2000.
24. Ballantyne JC, Carr DB, deFerranti S, et al: The comparative effects of postoperative analgesic therapies on pulmonary outcome: cumulative meta-analyses of randomized, controlled trials. *Anesth Analg* 86:598, 1998.
25. McNeely JK, Farber NE, Rusy LM, et al: Epidural analgesia improves outcome following pediatric fundoplication: a retrospective analysis. *Reg Anesth* 22:16, 1997.
26. Yeager MP, Glass DD, Neff RK, et al: Epidural anesthesia and analgesia in high-risk surgical patients. *Anesthesiology* 66:729, 1987.
27. Pelton JJ, Fish DJ, Keller SM: Epidural narcotic analgesia after thoracotomy. *South Med J* 86:1106, 1993.
28. Ackerman WE, III, Molnar JM, Juneja MM: Beneficial effect of epidural anesthesia on oxygen consumption in a parturient with adult respiratory distress syndrome. *South Med J* 86:361, 1993.
29. Kirsch JR, Diringer MN, Borel CO, et al: Preoperative lumbar epidural morphine improves postoperative analgesia and ventilatory function after transsternal thymectomy in patients with myasthenia gravis. *Crit Care Med* 19:1474, 1991.
30. Hayes C, Malloy AR: Neuropathic pain in the postoperative period. *Int Anesthesiol Clin* 35:67, 1997.
31. American Association for Respiratory Care: Administration of sedative and analgesic medications by respiratory therapists: a position statement, 2007. Retrieved from <http://c.aarc.org/resources/position_statements/documents/sedative.pdf>.
32. Durbin CG, Jr: Respiratory therapists and conscious sedation. *Respir Care* 44:909, 1999.
33. American Society of Anesthesiologists: Practice guidelines for sedations and analgesia by non-anesthesiologists. *Anesthesiology* 96:1004–1017, 2002.
34. Phero JC: Pharmacologic management of pain, anxiety, and behavior: conscious sedation, deep sedation, and general anesthesia. *Pediatr Dent* 15:429, 1993.
35. Rosenberg MB, Campbell RL: Guidelines for intraoperative monitoring of dental patients undergoing conscious sedation, deep sedation, and general anesthesia. *Oral Surg Oral Med Oral Pathol* 71:2, 1991.
36. Matthews RW, Malkawi Z, Griffiths MJ, et al: Pulse oximetry during minor oral surgery with and without intravenous sedation. *Oral Surg Oral Med Oral Pathol* 74:537, 1992.
37. Glassman P, Garrison R: A suggested curriculum for teaching conscious sedation in advanced general practice programs: GPR and AEGD. *Spec Care Dentist* 13:27, 1993.

CHAPTER 21

Vasopressors, Inotropes, and Antiarrhythmic Agents

Henry Cohen

OBJECTIVES

After reading this chapter, the reader will be able to:

1. Define terms that pertain to vasopressors, inotropes, and antiarrhythmic drugs
2. List the various components that make up blood pressure
3. Compare and contrast the mechanism of action of inotropes and vasopressors
4. Describe the various drug interactions that may occur with the use of vasopressors and inotropes
5. Design an algorithm for the management of hypotension
6. Manage extravasation injuries that occur with use of vasopressor therapy
7. Describe the normal conduction of the heart
8. Define nonpharmacologic methods of treating dysrhythmias
9. Compare and contrast the categories of the Vaughan Williams classification system
10. Define the mechanism of action of digoxin
11. List all the dysrhythmias associated with cardiac arrest
12. Design an algorithm that may be used in the management of ventricular fibrillation and pulseless ventricular tachycardia
13. Design an algorithm that may be used in the management of torsades de pointes
14. Describe the proper dosage technique of intravenous magnesium therapy in the management of torsades de pointes
15. List the routes of administering medications during cardiac arrest

KEY TERMS AND DEFINITIONS

Antiarrhythmics Group of cardiac medications that are classified according to mechanism of action; in some instances, they may have multiple mechanisms of action. The most common classification system of antiarrhythmics is the Vaughan Williams classification system, which is divided into four distinct categories and a miscellaneous section.

Arrhythmias/dysrhythmias Irregular (faster or slower) heartbeats; the term *arrhythmia* is used more frequently than *dysrhythmia*.

Continued

KEY TERMS AND DEFINITIONS—cont'd

Atrioventricular (AV) node Link between atrial depolarization and ventricular depolarization.

Bohr effect Presence of carbon dioxide aids in the release and delivery of oxygen from hemoglobin.

Cardiac output (CO) Amount of blood that is pumped out of the heart per unit of time.

Catecholamines Endogenous products that are secreted into the bloodstream and travel to nerve endings to stimulate an excitatory response.

Chronotropic Agent affecting the rate of contraction of the heart.

Diastolic blood pressure (DBP) Lowest pressure reached before ventricular ejection.

Dromotropic An agent that influences the conduction of electrical impulses. A positive dromotropic agent enhances the conduction of electrical impulses to the heart.

Inotropic Agent affecting the strength of muscular contraction.

Mean arterial pressure (MAP) Pressure that drives blood into the tissues averaged over the entire cardiac cycle.

Phosphodiesterase Enzyme responsible for the breakdown of cyclic adenosine 3′,5′-monophosphate (cAMP).

Sudden cardiac death (SCD) Episode of ventricular fibrillation, pulseless ventricular tachycardia, pulseless electrical activity, or asystole leading to loss of life.

Systolic blood pressure (SBP) Peak pressure reached during ventricular ejection.

Tachycardia Overly rapid heartbeat, usually defined as greater than 100 beats/min in adults.

Vasodilator Agent causing dilation of blood vessels.

Vasopressors Agents causing contraction of capillaries and arteries.

Ventricular fibrillation (VF) Cardiac condition in which normal ventricular contractions are replaced by coarse or fine, rapid movements of the ventricular muscle.

OVERVIEW OF CARDIOVASCULAR SYSTEM

The cardiovascular system regulates blood flow to the various regions of the body. Blood flow generally travels via a pressure gradient, shifting from areas of higher pressure to lower pressure. The central nervous system (CNS) relays electrical impulses through sensory receptors found systemically within the vasculature, affecting vascular tone and causing shunting of blood to and from various organ systems within the body. Vascular tone is regulated via the sympathetic nervous system and the circulation of neurotransmitters and hormones, such as epinephrine, vasopressin, and angiotensin. Several factors exert an effect on vascular tone as a response to tissue perfusion and circulatory volume. Hypotension is commonly present in patients with autonomic dysfunction and shock. *Shock* is a life-threatening medical emergency characterized by organ hypoperfusion leading to decreased delivery of oxygen and nutrients to tissues throughout the body. There are six types of shock; their effects on hemodynamic parameters can be seen in Table 21-1.

Factors Affecting Blood Pressure

 KEY POINT

Blood pressure is dependent on cardiac function, vascular tone, and vascular volume.

Typical measurement of blood pressure is relative to a recurring cardiac cycle of atrial and ventricular contractions and relaxations (Figure 21-1). The cycle is divided into the systolic phase and the diastolic phase. The systolic phase is the portion in which ventricular contraction occurs, resulting in ejection of blood through the aorta. Conversely, diastole is the period of ventricular relaxation and blood filling. **Systolic blood pressure (SBP)** is the peak pressure reached during ventricular ejection, and **diastolic blood pressure (DBP)** is the lowest pressure reached right before ventricular ejection. Arterial pressure is typically recorded as SBP/DBP, for example, 120/80 mm Hg. **Mean arterial pressure (MAP)** refers to the pressure that drives blood into the tissues averaged over the entire cardiac cycle. Because the cardiac cycle is pulsatile rather than continuous and because two-thirds of the normal cardiac cycle is spent in

TABLE 21-1	Hemodynamic Changes in Various Shock States			
HEMODYNAMIC PARAMETER	**HYPOVOLEMIC/ HEMORRHAGIC**	**NEUROGENIC**	**CARDIOGENIC**	**SEPTIC/DISTRIBUTIVE**
HR	↑	↔	↔/↑	↑
MAP	↓	↑/↓	↑	↓
CVP (5-12 mm Hg)	↓	↓	↑	↓
PCWP (10-12 mm Hg)	↓	↓	↑	↓
CO (5-7 L/min)	↓	↔/↓	↓	↑
SVR (80-1440 dyn•sec•cm⁻5)	↑	↓	↑	↓

CO, cardiac output; *CVP*, central venous pressure; *HR*, heart rate; *MAP*, mean arterial pressure; *PCWP*, pulmonary capillary wedge pressure; *SVR*, systemic vascular resistance.

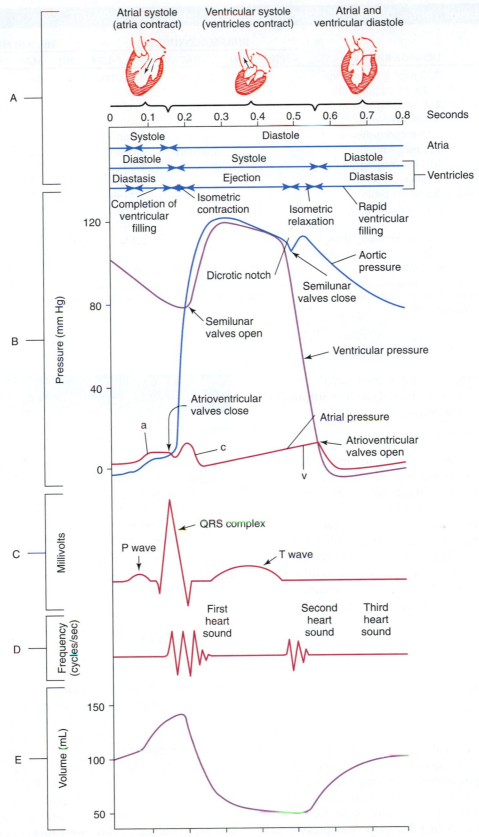

Figure 21-1 The cardiac cycle. *A,* Timing of cardiac events; *B,* simultaneous pressures created in the aorta, left ventricle, and right atrium during the cardiac cycle; *C,* electrical activity during the cardiac cycle; *D,* heart sounds corresponding to the cardiac cycle; *E,* ventricular blood volume during the cardiac cycle. (From Kacmarek RM, Stoller JK, Heuer AJ, et al: *Egan's fundamentals of respiratory care,* ed 10, St. Louis, 2013, Mosby.)

TABLE 21-2   Cardiac Drugs: Dosing, Pharmacokinetics, and Hemodynamic Effects

AGENT	DOSAGE RANGE	PHARMACOKINETICS			HEMODYNAMIC EFFECTS				
		ONSET (MIN)	DURATION	HALF-LIFE	HR	MAP	PCWP	SVR	CO
Amrinone	0.75 mg/kg bolus, then 2.5-15 mcg/kg/min	5-10	0.5-2 hr	4.8-8.3 hr	↓	0-↓	0-↓	0-↓	↓-0-↑
Dobutamine (Dobutrex)	2-20 mcg/kg/min	1-2	10-15 min	2 min	0*	0-↓	↓	↓	↑
Dopamine (Inotropin)	1-5 mcg/kg/min	5	<10 min	2 min	0	0	0	0	0
	5-15 mcg/kg/min	5	<10 min	2 min	↑	0-↓	0-↑	↑	↑
	>15 mcg/kg/min	5	<10 min	2 min	↑	0-↓	0-↑	↑	↑
Epinephrine (Adrenalin)	0.01-0.1 mcg/kg/min	1	3-5 min	3-5 min	↑	↑	0-↓	↓†-↑*	↑
	0.1 mcg/kg/min				↑↑	↑↑	↑	↑↑	↑↑
Norepinephrine (Levophed)	0.5-30 mcg/min	1-3	5-10 min	1-2 min	0-↑	↑↑↑	↑↑	↑↑↑	0-↓
Phenylephrine (Neo-Synephrine)	0.5-5 mcg/kg/min	10-15	1-3 hr	2-3 hr	↓	↑	↑	↑	↓
Milrinone (Primacor)	50 mcg/kg bolus, then 0.375-0.75 mcg/kg/min	90	3-5 hr	2.3 hr	0-↑	↓	↓	↓	↑
Vasopressin (Pitressin)	0.04 U/min	30-60	30-60 min	10-20 min	0	↑	↑	↑	↓†

CO, Cardiac output; *HR*, heart rate; *MAP*, mean arterial pressure; *PCWP*, pulmonary capillary wedge pressure; *SVR*, systemic vascular resistance; ↑, effect increased;
↓, effect decreased; *0*, effect unchanged.
*At high doses.
†At low doses.

diastole, MAP is not the arithmetic mean of the SBP and DBP. MAP is defined as the product of **cardiac output (CO)** and systemic vascular resistance (SVR), as follows:

$$[2(DBP) + SBP]/3 \; or \; MAP = CO \times SVR$$

SVR is used to define the resistance to flow of the vasculature that must be overcome to push blood through the peripheral circulation. CO is the amount of blood that is ejected into the aorta and travels through the systemic circulation per unit of time. CO is dependent on the sum of all local blood flow regulations and is shown in the following equation as the product of heart rate (HR) and stroke volume (SV). *SV* is the amount of blood ejected from the heart during systole. Changes in any of these components may alter the effects of the others.

$$CO = HR \times SV$$

Summing up all components that affect the MAP, the following equation may better illustrate how these components relate to blood pressure:

$$MAP = HR \times SV \times SVR$$

The use of therapies such as fluids, vasopressors, and inotropes to maintain cardiovascular stability is directed toward altering each of these components, as seen in Table 21-2. The various **vasopressors** currently on the market have different affinities for the various receptors located within the body and exert different effects on the hemodynamic parameters, as seen in Table 21-3. Vasopressors and inotropes are not always first-line therapy; on the contrary, fluids are the mainstays for improving hypotensive episodes. Vasopressors and inotropes have considerable side effects, and certain medications interact with various vasopressors and inotropes, leading to alterations in hemodynamic parameters, as seen in Table 21-4.

TABLE 21-3   Inotropes and Vasopressors: Receptor Affinity

DRUG	α	β₁	β₂	DA
Dopamine (Inotropin)	+ to +++*	+++*	+	0/+
Dobutamine (Dobutrex)	0 to +*	0 to +*	+	0
Epinephrine (Adrenalin)	+++*	+++	++*	0
Isoproterenol (Isuprel)	0	+++	+++	0
Norepinephrine (Levophed)	+++	++	++	0
Phenylephrine (Neo-Synephrine)	+++	0	0	0

DA, Dopamine; *0*, no effect; +, slight effect; ++, moderate effect; +++, pronounced effect.
*At higher doses.

In addition to vascular tone, another component that may affect changes in tissue perfusion is vascular volume. Intravascular volume depletion may influence SV and affect MAP as well. This component may be indirectly measured as the pulmonary capillary wedge pressure (PCWP), central venous pressure, or preload. In other words, by using a device called a pulmonary artery catheter to measure the amount of fluid returning to the heart, the PCWP can be estimated. With this measurement, the clinician can evaluate a patient-specific response to fluid therapy and vasoactive therapy. The use of a pulmonary artery catheter is associated with complications such as infection, pneumothorax, bleeding, or thrombus formation.

 KEY POINT

Cardiac drugs are used to influence cardiac function and include agents that increase myocardial contractility, regulate arrhythmias, and treat cardiac arrest.

TABLE 21-4	Drug Interactions

PRECIPITANT DRUG*	EFFECT	OBJECT DRUG*	COMMENTS
Dobutamine, Isoproterenol, Norepinephrine			
Bretylium	↑	Dobutamine, isoproterenol, norepinephrine	Concomitant use may potentiate effects of vasopressors, causing arrhythmias
Halogenated hydrocarbon anesthetics			
Guanethidine			May increase pressor response, causing severe hypertension
Oxytocic drugs			
Tricyclic antidepressants			
Phenylephrine			
Bretylium	↑	Phenylephrine	Concomitant use may potentiate effects of vasopressors
Guanethidine			
Halogenated hydrocarbon anesthetics			
Oxytocic drugs			
Tricyclic antidepressants	↔		Tricyclic antidepressants may increase effects of phenylephrine
Dopamine			
Dopamine	↓	Guanethidine	Antihypertensive effects of guanethidine may be reversed
		Phenytoin	Concomitant use may lead to seizures, severe hypotension, and bradycardia
Tricyclic antidepressants		Dopamine	Tricyclic antidepressants may increase effects of dopamine
Halogenated hydrocarbon anesthetics	↑	Dopamine	May sensitize myocardium to actions of vasopressors, causing arrhythmia
MAOIs			Dopamine is metabolized by MAOIs. MAOIs increase pressor response to dopamine by sixfold to twentyfold
Oxytocic drugs			Concomitant use may cause severe hypertension
Epinephrine			
Cardiac glycosides	↑	Epinephrine	May sensitize myocardium to actions of vasopressors, causing arrhythmia
Halogenated hydrocarbon anesthetics			
Levothyroxine antihistamines (chlorpheniramine, diphenhydramine)			
MAOIs			Concomitant use may cause severe hypertension
Methyldopa			
Oxytocic drugs			
Reserpine			
Sympathomimetics			
Tricyclic antidepressants			
β Blockers			
α Blockers	↓	Epinephrine	Vasoconstricting and hypertensive effects of pressor may be reversed
Chlorpromazine			
Diuretics			
Epinephrine		Guanethidine	Epinephrine may antagonize effects of guanethidine, resulting in decreased antihypertensive effects
Digoxin			
Amiodarone	↑	Digoxin	Amiodarone may increase digoxin blood level; reduce digoxin dose by 50%
β Blockers			Combination may cause advanced or complete heart block
Calcium channel blockers			
Calcium			Rapid administration of intravenous calcium may result in fatal arrhythmias
Succinylcholine			Succinylcholine may cause sudden extrusion of K$^+$ from muscle cells, leading to arrhythmias
Sympathomimetics			Combination may cause increased risk of cardiac arrhythmias
Thiazide and loop diuretics			Diuretic-induced electrolyte disturbances may predispose to digitalis toxicity
Thyroid hormones	↓	Digoxin	Thyroid hormones may reduce digoxin blood levels; hypothyroid patients may require higher dose of digoxin

MAOIs, Monoamine oxidase inhibitors.
*Precipitant drug refers to the drug that causes the interaction; object drug refers to the drug affected by the interaction. ↑, Object drug increased; ↓, object drug decreased; ↔, object drug unaffected.

AGENTS USED IN THE MANAGEMENT OF SHOCK

 KEY POINT

Cardiotonic agents stimulate the myocardium and produce a positive effect. These agents include cardiac glycosides (digitalis family), β-adrenergic stimulants, dobutamine, dopamine (DA), isoproterenol, epinephrine, and phosphodiesterase inhibitors.

Catecholamines

Norepinephrine (Levophed) and Epinephrine (Adrenalin Chloride)

Norepinephrine (Levophed) and epinephrine (Adrenalin Chloride) are endogenous **catecholamines** that are secreted by the adrenal medulla. Epinephrine is ultimately synthesized by the catalytic actions of tyrosine hydroxylase, which converts the amino acid tyrosine to levodopa and subsequently to dopamine (DA), norepinephrine, and epinephrine.[1,2] These neurotransmitters travel to sympathetic nerve endings where they are released to stimulate other nerve fibers and to stimulate an excitatory response. Norepinephrine and epinephrine stimulate α receptors (on the vasculature) and β receptors within the vasculature and in the myocardium. α Receptors within the vasculature cause vasoconstriction, whereas β receptors cause vasodilation. Most vascular beds within the body contain β receptors; however, they are outnumbered by α receptors, so any epinephrine and norepinephrine stimulation of β receptors is negligible or of no effect, yielding a net response of vasoconstriction. In addition, β receptors more densely populate the myocardium compared with α receptors, leading to a net effect of **tachycardia**.[3,4]

Isoproterenol (Isuprel)

Isoproterenol (Isuprel) is a synthetic catecholamine used for the treatment of symptomatic bradycardia or torsades de pointes. Isoproterenol works solely as an agonist of β receptors. By stimulating β_1-adrenergic receptors, it exerts pronounced **inotropic** and **chronotropic** effects. By stimulating β_2-adrenergic receptors, it leads to smooth muscle relaxation of the bronchi, skeletal muscle, vasculature, and gastrointestinal tract. Venous return to the heart is also increased by vasodilation of the venous bed. The use of isoproterenol is limited because of its pronounced stimulatory effect on the HR.[4]

Dopamine

DA is an endogenous catecholamine that is a precursor to norepinephrine. The usual vasopressor dose of DA is 5 to 20 mcg/kg/min; DA directly stimulates β receptors, producing chronotropic and inotropic effects and leading to increased CO, and stimulates peripheral α receptors, causing increased SVR.

Previously, low-dose DA (1 to 5 mcg/kg/min) was thought to stimulate selectively the DA_1 and DA_2 receptors in the splanchnic and renal artery beds, causing vasodilation and increased blood flow. This belief has been nullified, and use of low-dose DA is considered an antiquated form of practice. It has been suggested that improvement of renal and splanchnic blood flow as a result of DA stems from its benefits on CO, which enhances perfusion to all major organs, including blood flow to the kidney.

There is a higher likelihood of adverse effects occurring with higher doses of DA when used in patients with cardiac failure because of the increase in afterload and myocardial oxygen demand. Adverse effects include tachyarrhythmias, ectopic beat, palpitations, and decreased perfusion.

At doses that are often required for patients with septic shock (e.g., "high-dose DA"), there is an increased risk of tachyarrhythmias compared with the risk with other vasopressors. This is an artifact of the higher affinity of DA for β_1 receptors. Consequently, the updated 2012 Surviving Sepsis Guidelines[5] recommend the use of DA be limited to highly selected patients (i.e., those with low risk of tachyarrhythmia or profound bradycardia). Overall, norepinephrine is considered a more potent vasopressor than DA and should be used as an initial therapy over DA in the setting of septic shock.[5]

Phenylephrine

In contrast to epinephrine, phenylephrine is purely an α agonist, yet it differs from epinephrine only in that it lacks a hydroxyl group (−OH) on the benzene ring. Phenylephrine induces vasoconstriction in most vascular beds, elevating SBP and DBP. Phenylephrine exerts an effect on systemic blood pressure by elevating total peripheral resistance.

Because of the unopposed α_1 stimulation in the vasculature causing increased SVR, patients on phenylephrine infusions develop a reflex bradycardia. This effect may be useful in patients who develop tachyarrhythmia while taking norepinephrine infusions. Initial phenylephrine infusions are usually started at 5 mcg/kg/min (or alternatively 100 to 180 mcg/min) and similarly to other vasopressors, rates can be titrated higher as needed to maintain the targeted blood pressure.[6]

Vasopressin (Pitressin)

Aside from the pressor effects of vasopressin (which are discussed subsequently in the section on advanced cardiac life support), vasopressin may be used in the setting of septic shock, not only because of its pressor effect, but also because of its water-retentive effects. Vasopressin is a naturally occurring hormone also known as antidiuretic hormone. Vasopressin shows affinity for V_1 and V_2 (vasopressin-1 and vasopressin-2) receptors located in the collecting ducts in the kidneys, which contribute to water conservation and concentration of urine. The use of vasopressin may be especially beneficial in the setting of sepsis because vasopressin is deficient in septic patients.

The dose of vasopressin in septic shock is generally 0.01 to 0.04 U/min. Although higher doses of vasopressin may be used, the Surviving Sepsis Guidelines recommend avoiding use of higher vasopressin doses because of its propensity to cause adverse cardiovascular events such as myocardial ischemia. Higher doses of vasopressin should be limited to refractory septic shock when adequate MAP is unable to be achieved with other vasopressors.[5] Doses of up to 0.8 U/min have been employed for patients with variceal hemorrhage, but it is often combined with nitroglycerin infusion to limit the development of myocardial ischemia. Vasopressin can be titrated down by 0.01 U/min increments when therapy is no longer required for maintenance of MAP.

Vasopressin should not be utilized as a sole agent for management of hypotension in the setting of septic shock.[5] Precaution stems from the fact that vasopressin infusion may decrease splanchnic blood flow. When vasopressin is used, it should be used when other vasopressors are insufficient and should be used as add-on therapy in combination with one or two additional cathecholamines or to reduce the doses required of other vasopressors.

Other settings in which vasopressin may be used include diabetes insipidus at doses of 5 to 10 U given intramuscularly or subcutaneously and repeated two or three times per day or given as a continuous infusion.[7] Vasopressin has also been used to treat variceal bleeding at high doses (i.e., up to 2 U/min). Caution is needed when treating conditions with vasopressin other than shock; myocardial ischemia may ensue as a result of the potent vasoconstrictive properties at higher doses.[8]

Midodrine (Proamatine)

Midodrine hydrochloride is an oral inactive prodrug that converts to the active species, desglymidodrine, via deglycination. Desglymidodrine is an α_1 agonist. Midodrine is indicated for the management of orthostatic hypotension. However, because midodrine can cause significant hypertension and reflex bradycardia, it should only be used in refractory patients with orthostatic hypotension that is severe enough to impair daily living—this is also noted as a U.S. Food and Drug Administration (FDA) boxed warning (so called for the box surrounding the warning located in the manufacturer information sheet or the package insert) in the product labeling.[9] Although not labeled for use in shock, midodrine has been used to wean patients from intravenous (IV) vasopressors and transition them from the intensive care unit to general medical floors.[10]

Vasopressor-Induced Extravasation and Management

All IV vasopressors can cause immense vasoconstriction in the vessels that supply subcutaneous tissue, and when extravasation occurs it can lead to necrosis and gangrene. Initial signs and symptoms of extravasation include pain, swelling, erythema, blistering, blanching, and/or mottling of the skin. As a general rule, the risk of vasopressor extravasation increases with more concentrated IV solutions. The two vasopressors most frequently implicated to cause severe extravasation are norepinephrine and epinephrine.

To minimize the risk of extravasation, vasopressors should be preferentially administered via a central line

rather than a peripheral line because of the large vein size and increased blood flow, such as from the vena cava. Administration of vasopressors through a peripheral line leads to high vasopressor concentrations in the area of the peripheral line, which increases the risk of extravasation injury. Management of extravasation includes discontinuing the infusion or switching administration to a different access site and administering an α-antagonist, such as phentolamine. The phentolamine dose for extravasation is 5 to 10 mg mixed with 10 mL of normal saline injected into the area of extravasation. Phentolamine is also indicated for the prevention of dermal necrosis caused by norepinephrine extravasation by adding 10 mg of phentolamine to each liter of solution containing norepinephrine.

Inotropic Agents

Dobutamine

Dobutamine is indicated for the short-term treatment of decompensated heart failure secondary to depressed contractility. Dobutamine is a synthetic catecholamine that is chemically related to DA; however, in contrast to DA, it is not metabolized to norepinephrine, and it does not stimulate DA receptors.[4] Its pharmacologic actions are due to the effects of its racemic components. The (R)-isomer is responsible for its activity on the β_1 and β_2 receptors, causing predominant positive inotropic and chronotropic effects and vasodilatory effects, respectively. This combination of effects enhances CO and SV. The (S)-isomer is responsible for its activity on the α_1 receptors, causing vasoconstriction.[1,6] The vasodilatory β_2-adrenergic effects counterbalance the vasoconstrictive α_1 effects, leading to minor changes in SVR usually seen at lower doses. With increasing doses, the β_2-vasodilatory actions predominate over the α_1-vasoconstrictive effect, causing a decrease in systemic and pulmonary vascular resistance. The decline in systemic and pulmonary vascular resistance may also be secondary to enhanced CO.

As an inotropic agent, dobutamine has adverse cardiac effects, which include **arrhythmias/dysrhythmias**, increase in myocardial oxygen consumption and demand, tachycardia, and hypotension. A limiting factor when dobutamine is used for more than 72 hours is tachyphylaxis; this may be due to a downregulation of β_1 receptors and may be overcome by increasing the dose. In patients with sulfite sensitivity, allergic reactions such as anaphylaxis or life-threatening asthmatic episodes may occur because dobutamine formulations contain sulfites.[4]

Phosphodiesterase Inhibitors: Inamrinone and Milrinone

Phosphodiesterase inhibitors (also known as inodilators), such as inamrinone (formerly known as amrinone) and milrinone, are both inotropic and **vasodilator** agents because they increase myocardial contractility and induce vascular smooth muscle relaxation. These effects are mitigated by inhibition of intracellular phosphodiesterase (subclass III). **Phosphodiesterase** is an enzyme responsible for the breakdown of cyclic adenosine 3′,5′-monophosphate (cAMP). An increase in cAMP concentration mediates an increase in intracellular ionized calcium, which is responsible for its inotropic effect, and cAMP-dependent protein phosphorylation, causing relaxation of vascular muscle. Hemodynamically, phosphodiesterase inhibitors cause a decrease in SVR and PCWP and an increase in CO without increasing HR or myocardial oxygen demand. These hemodynamic changes are related to plasma concentration.

Milrinone is the phosphodiesterase inhibitor most commonly used in practice today because it has a shorter half-life than inamrinone and is less likely to cause thrombocytopenia. It undergoes renal elimination with an elimination half-life of 1 to 3 hours in patients with normal renal function; steady-state concentrations are reached in 4 to 6 hours if initiated without a loading dose. The risk of hypotension occurring is higher when a loading dose is given. Milrinone may be given as an initial IV bolus dose of 50 mcg/kg administered slowly over 10 minutes followed by continuous infusion at a rate of 0.375 to 0.75 mcg/kg/min and titrated to effect. Dosage adjustment should be made in patients with severe cardiac failure or renal impairment because of the considerable reduction in clearance.[1,4,6]

Cardiac Glycosides: Digoxin (Lanoxin)

The cardiac glycoside class consists of one medication, digoxin (Lanoxin), which is used in the management of congestive heart failure (CHF). The implementation of digoxin in the treatment of CHF stems from its capacity to exert an inotropic effect on the myocardium. Cardiac glycosides reversibly inhibit the sodium-potassium pump (Na^+, K^+-ATPase pump) located in the cardiac heart muscle, leading to a net loss of potassium (K^+) and a net gain in intracellular sodium (Na^+) concentration. As a result, the sodium-calcium active transport system, which pumps sodium out of the cell and calcium into the cell, is activated. Elevated intracellular calcium (Ca^{++}) concentrations result in further calcium secretion from the endoplasmic reticulum, ultimately stimulating the actin-myosin light chain reaction, resulting in myocardial contraction. Digoxin also has an inhibitory effect on the vagus nerve, leading to decreased HR and **atrioventricular (AV) node** prolongation. In contrast to other inotropic agents such as dobutamine and milrinone, digoxin generally does not exert hypotensive effects, unless directly caused by bradycardia.

Digoxin undergoes renal elimination. In the presence of renal insufficiency, accumulation of digoxin may occur. Generally, digitalis intoxication is diagnosed when the mean serum digoxin concentration exceeds 2 ng/mL; however, the clinical significance of this value depends on the time of ingestion and the time of serum sampling. Digoxin has a long distribution phase. It may take 4 hours after IV administration and 6 hours after oral administration for digoxin to distribute fully out of the circulatory compartment and into other regions of the body. Serum sampling of digoxin before the distribution phase may give

the impression that the serum concentration is greater than it actually is. Digoxin displays a very narrow therapeutic range (0.5 to 2 ng/mL), particularly in the setting of hypokalemia. Hypokalemia may potentiate the adverse effects of digoxin and render the risk of arrhythmias and death more imminent. Adequate potassium supplementation should be used to maintain the serum potassium level within a normal range.

In contrast, digitalis toxicity may cause hyperkalemia by its inhibitory actions on the Na^+,K^+-ATPase pump. Digoxin toxicity may manifest as serious life-threatening ventricular arrhythmias (VAs), including premature ventricular contractions, AV junctional rhythm, bigeminal rhythm, and second-degree AV blockade. Bradycardia may also occur early on in the setting of digoxin toxicity. The initial symptoms of digitalis toxicity are nausea, vomiting, anorexia, and abdominal pain. These symptoms may be due to a direct effect on the gastrointestinal tract or result from CNS stimulation of the chemoreceptor trigger zone. Other rare but possible neuropsychiatric effects may manifest as disorientation and hallucination, especially in elderly patients, and visual disturbances, such as yellow-green halos. Digoxin immune Fab is the antidote used to facilitate the speedy elimination of digoxin from the body. Digoxin immune Fab is indicated in the setting of life-threatening toxicity such as VAs, bradyrhythmias, ingestion of greater than 10 mg in adults or 4 mg in children, a steady-state level greater than 10 ng/mL, progressive elevation of potassium, or a potassium level greater than 5 mEq/L.[11]

ELECTROPHYSIOLOGY OF MYOCARDIUM

Electrical activity is initiated by an innate pacemaker located at the sinoatrial (SA) node. Electrical potential exists across the cell membrane, and it changes in response to transmembrane movement of Na^+, K^+, Ca^{++}, and Cl^- ions. These ions mediate the process of myocardial contraction and relaxation. When an electrical stimulus is evoked from the SA node, it generates an action potential (AP). Once generated, the AP produces a local current, which evokes further APs along the myocardium. An AP elicits myocardial depolarization or contraction. The link between atrial depolarization and ventricular depolarization is a portion of the conduction system called the AV node. The AV node slows down the electrical impulse to ensure that atrial excitation is completed before ventricular excitation. After leaving the AV node, the impulse travels to the wall between the two ventricles via the conducting system fibers known as the bundle of His. From the bundle of His, the cardiac conduction system bifurcates into three main bundle branches: the right bundle and two left bundles. These bundle branches form a conduction network, referred to as Purkinje fibers (Figure 21-2). The conduction system innervates the myocardium and causes changes in membrane polarization of the muscle fiber.[8]

An AP (Figure 21-3) can be divided into the following five different phases:

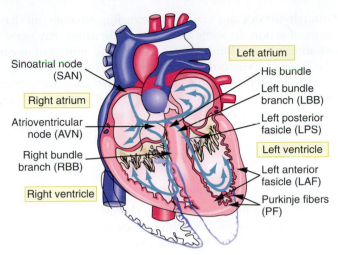

Figure 21-2 Cardiac conduction system.

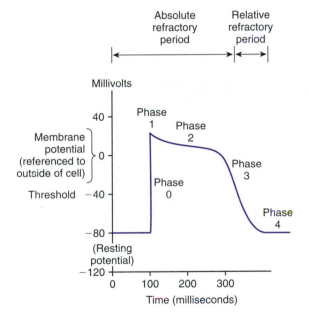

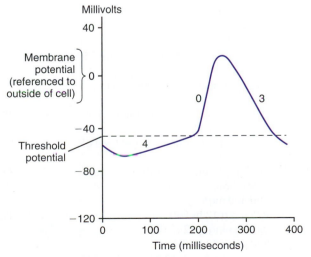

Figure 21-3 Action potential diagram. (From Cairo JM, Pilbeam SP: *Mosby's respiratory care equipment*, ed 8, St. Louis, 2010, Mosby.)

Phase 0: Initial rapid depolarization of myocardial tissues secondary to an abrupt transmembrane influx of sodium through "fast" sodium channels

Phase 1: Fast sodium channels are inactivated; this, coupled with the movement of K^+ and Cl^- ions, leads to a transient net outward current and the beginning of repolarization

Phase 2: "Plateau" phase, maintained by a balance between calcium influx and potassium efflux

Phase 3: Calcium channels close, but membrane remains permeable to potassium, resulting in cellular repolarization

Phase 4: Cell returns to its "resting" state; the resting membrane potential is reached through gradual depolarization related to a constant sodium influx balanced by a decreasing efflux of potassium

During the AP, a second stimulus would not evoke a second AP; at this point, the membrane is said to be in the *absolute refractory period*. The absolute refractory period does not allow the heart to undergo premature contractions or to maintain a tetanic state. Arrhythmias are associated with abnormal impulse generation or conduction. Certain conditions that can precipitate arrhythmias are myocardial ischemia, CHF, oversensitivity to catecholamines, and electrolyte abnormalities.

Ablation With Radiofrequency Current

Catheter ablation is very effective when atrial fibrillation (AF) is due to a single primary circuit. The procedure involves inserting a catheter into a blood vessel in the groin or the neck and guiding it toward the heart. When the tip of the catheter is placed against the part of the heart causing the arrhythmia, radiofrequency electrical current is applied through the catheter to produce a small burn about 6 to 8 mm in diameter. Patients should be adequately anticoagulated at least 1 month before the ablation procedure to prevent the formation of thrombi in the atria. The procedure carries a success rate in maintaining sinus rhythm over the next year of 30% to 90%.[12]

Implantable Cardioverter-Defibrillators

Implantable cardioverter-defibrillators (ICDs) have been used since the 1980s to cardiovert, to terminate ventricular tachycardia (VT), and to provide backup pacing for bradycardia. ICDs are indicated for the following conditions:

- Cardiac arrest caused by pulseless VT or **ventricular fibrillation (VF)** not caused by a transient or reversible cause
- Spontaneous sustained VT
- Syncope of undetermined origin with clinically relevant, electrophysiologically inducible sustained VT or VF when drug therapy is ineffective, not tolerated, or not preferred

- Nonsustained VT in patients with coronary artery disease, before myocardial infarction, left ventricular dysfunction, and electrophysiologically inducible VT or VF not suppressed by class I antiarrhythmics

Of patients with ICDs, 40% to 70% require antiarrhythmic drug therapy, which puts them at risk for drug-ICD interactions.[13,14]

PHARMACOLOGY OF ANTIARRHYTHMICS

 KEY POINT

Antiarrhythmic agents are classified into groups on the basis of their electrophysiologic action. Class I agents depress the inward sodium current and are subdivided further as IA, IB, and IC. Class II agents are β-blocking agents. Class III agents have complex effects that can prolong the action potential (AP) and in some cases exert β-blocking action. Class IV agents are calcium channel blockers. Other antiarrhythmic agents include adenosine, which is used to convert supraventricular tachycardia (SVT) into sinus rhythm.

Antiarrhythmics are classified according to their mechanisms of action. In some instances, these drugs may manifest multiple mechanisms of action. The most common classification system of antiarrhythmics is the Vaughan Williams classification system, which divides antiarrhythmics into classes: I (IA, IB, IC), II, III, IV, and a miscellaneous class. Table 21-5 describes the detailed pharmacology of antiarrhythmics, and Table 21-6 lists their pharmacokinetic parameters.

Class IA

Class IA agents block fast sodium channels in the myocardium, specifically in the atrium. They also block repolarizing potassium currents and may prolong the AP. As a result, class IA agents have been associated with significant proarrhythmic properties, such as Q–T interval prolongation.

Quinidine

Quinidine, although less commonly used, is efficacious in the treatment of atrial fibrillation/flutter (AF/AFL)

TABLE 21-5 Pharmacology of Antiarrhythmics

CLASS/MOA	ION BLOCK	DRUG	QRS	Q–T$_c$	INDICATIONS	DOSAGES	ROUTE
IA/↓ phase 0, ↑ AP	Sodium (intermediate)	Moricizine*	↑	0	VA	600-900 mg/day in three divided doses	PO
		Quinidine	↑	↑	AF/AFL/VA	Quinidine sulfate, 200-600 mg q 4-12 hr; quinidine gluconate, AF/AFL cardioversion and VA, 324-648 mg q 8-12 hr	PO
						Quinidine gluconate, AF/AFL cardioversion and VA, 10 mg/min infusion up to 400 mg	IV
		Procainamide	↑	↑	VA	40-50 kg, 2 g/day; 60-70 kg, 3 g/day; 80-90 kg, 4 g/day; >100 kg, 5 g/day	IV
		Disopyramide	↑	↑	VA	400-800 mg/day in divided doses, IR divided q 6 hr, CR divided q 12 hr	PO
IB/↓ phase 0 slightly; shorten AP	Sodium (fast on/off)	Lidocaine	0	0-↓	VA	50-100 mg (may repeat in 5 min) up to 300 mg in any 1-hr period; maintenance 1-4 mg/min	IV
					VT	1-1.5 mg/kg; may repeat at 0.5-0.75 mg/kg q 5-10 min (maximum 3 mg/kg)	
		Mexiletine	0	0	VA	200-400 mg q 8 hr	PO
						150-250 mg over 10 min, then 250 mg over 30-60 min, then 250 mg over 2.5 hr, then 500 mg over 8 hr; maintenance 250-500 mg q 12 hr	IV
		Tocainide	0	0-↓	VA	400 mg q 8 hr, then 1200-1800 mg/day divided q 8 hr (maximum 2400 mg/day)	PO
		Phenytoin	0	↓	VA	4 mg/kg q 6 hr for 1 day, then 5-6 mg/kg/day divided q 12 hr	PO
						15 mg/kg over 1 hr (or target level of 15-20 mcg/mL)	IV
IC/Marked ↓ of phase 0; affect repolarization	Sodium (slow on/off)	Flecainide	↑↑	0-↑	AF/AFL/PSVT	50 mg q 12 hr; ↑ by 100 mg q 4 days (maximum 300 mg/day)	PO
					VA/VT	200-400 mg/day	
		Propafenone	↑	0-↑	AF	225 mg q 12 hr (SR)	PO
					AFL	325-425 mg q 12 hr (IR)	
					PSVT	150 mg q 12 hr (IR)	
					AF/AFL/ PSVT/VA	AF, 225 mg (SR) q 12 hr, ↑ to 325-425 mg q 12 hr; AFL/PSVT/VA, 150-300 mg (IR) q 8 hr	

TABLE 21-5 Pharmacology of Antiarrhythmics—cont'd

CLASS/MOA	ION BLOCK	DRUG	QRS	Q–T$_c$	INDICATIONS	DOSAGES	ROUTE
II/↓ phase 4 (depolarization)	Calcium (indirect)	Propranolol	0	0-↓	AF/AFL/ PSVT/PVC	Loading dose, 0.5-1 mg q 2 min (up to 0.1-0.15 mg/kg); maintenance dose, 0.04 mg/kg/min	IV
						Maintenance dose, 10-120 mg three times daily	PO
		Esmolol	0	0-↓		Loading dose, 0.5 mg/kg over 1 min; maintenance dose, 50-300 mcg/kg/min (bolus between dose increases)	IV
		Acebutolol	0	0-↓		Initial, 200 mg twice a day; maintenance, 600-1200 mg/day (in two or three divided doses)	PO
		Metoprolol	0	0-↓		Initial, 2.5-5 mg q 2-5 min (up to 15 mg over 10-15 min)	IV
						Maintenance dose, 25-100 mg twice a day	PO
		Atenolol	0	0-↓		0.5 mg/min in aliquots of 2.5 mg with 10-min interval between aliquots (maximum single dose 10 mg)	IV
						Initial, 50-100 mg daily	PO
		Nadolol	0	0-↓		0.01-0.05 mg/kg at 1 mg/min (maximum cumulative dose 10 mg)	IV
						60-160 mg/day in single or divided doses	PO
III/↑ phase 3 (repolarization)	Potassium	Amiodarone	↑	↑↑	VA	800-1600 mg for 1-3 wk, then 600-800 mg for 1 mo, then 400-600 mg daily	PO
						150-300 mg bolus, then 1 mg/min for 6 hr, then 0.5 mg/min for 18 hr	IV
		Dronedarone	↑	↑↑	AF/AFL	400 mg twice a day with meals	PO
		Bretylium	0	0	VA	Loading dose, 5-10 mg/kg bolus, may repeat to a maximum of 30 mg/kg, then 1-2 mg/min or 5-10 mg/kg over 8 min q 6 hr	IV
		Dofetilide			AF/AFL	Q–T$_c$ ≤ 440 msec, 500 mcg twice a day 2-3 hr after first dose if Q–T$_c$ increases >15% or >500 msec, ↓ dose to 250 mcg twice a day	PO
		Sotalol	0	↑↑	AF/AFL	CrCl > 60 mL/min, 160 mg/day; CrCl 40-60 mL/min, 80 mg/day; titrate to Q–T$_c$ <520 msec (maximum 320 mg/day)	PO
					VA	80 mg twice a day, ↑ at 40-80 mg q 2-3 days (maximum 480-640 mg/day)	
		Ibutilide	0	↑↑	AF/AFL	≥60 kg, 1 mg; <60 kg, 0.1 mg/kg over 10 min (may repeat once)	IV
IV/↓ phase 4, ↑ phases 1 and 2	Calcium	Verapamil	0	0	SVT	IR, 240-320 mg/day in three or four divided doses; up to 480 mg/day in three or four divided doses for patients not on digoxin therapy	PO
						0.075-0.15 mg/kg over 2 min; may give 10 mg after 30 min if no response	IV
		Diltiazem	0	↓	PSVT	0.25 mg/kg over 2 min; if no response, may give 0.35 mg/kg after 15 min; maintenance, 5-10 mg/hr; ↑ in 5-mg/hr increments up to 15 mg/hr for up to 24 hr	IV
↑ phase 4 ↓ AP	Na$^+$,K$^+$ pump	Digoxin	0	↓	SVT	8-12 mcg/kg	IV
↓ conduction time; interrupts reentry through AV node	Adenosine receptor	Adenosine	0	0	SVT	6 mg over 1-2 sec; ↑ to 12 mg q 1-2 min as needed for two doses (maximal single dose 12 mg)	IV

AF, Atrial fibrillation; *AFL*, atrial fibrillation/flutter; *AP*, action potential; *AV*, atrioventricular; *CrCl*, creatinine clearance; *CR*, controlled release; *ER*, extended release; *IR*, immediate release; *IV*, intravenous; *MOA*, mode of action; *PO*, per os (orally administered); *PSVT*, paroxysmal supraventricular tachycardia; *PVC*, premature ventricular contraction; *QRS*, QRS interval, time for ventricular depolarization; *Q–T$_c$*, Q–T interval (duration of ventricular electrical activity), corrected for heart rate; *SR*, sustained release; *VA*, ventricular arrhythmia; *VT*, ventricular tachycardia; ↑↑, high increase; ↑, increase; ↓, decrease; 0, no change.

*Moricizine does not belong to any subclass (IA, IB, or IC) of antiarrhythmic but does have some properties of each.

TABLE 21-6 Antiarrhythmics: Pharmacokinetics and Adverse Reactions

DRUG	ONSET (PO) (hr)	DURATION (hr)	HALF-LIFE (hr)	THERAPEUTIC RANGE (mcg/mL)	TOXIC LEVEL (mcg/mL)	ADVERSE REACTIONS
	PHARMACOKINETICS					
Moricizine (Ethmozine)	2	10-24	1.5-3.5	NA	NA	*All class I agents:* Negative inotropic effect, infranodal conduction block
Quinidine (Quinaglute)	0.5	6-8	6-7	2-6	>8	*Class IA:* Torsades de pointes *Quinidine:* N/V/D, cinchonism (tinnitus, blurred vision, dizziness, tremor)
Procainamide (Pronestyl)	0.5	≥3	2.5-4.5	4-8	>16	*Procainamide:* N/V/D (30%), bitter taste, rash, hepatitis, mental depression, psychosis
Disopyramide (Norpace)	0.5	6-7	4-10	40-60	>80	*Disopyramide:* Anticholinergic effects (dry mouth, blurred vision, urinary retention), hypoglycemia, cholestatic jaundice, agranulocytosis
Lidocaine (Xylocaine)	—	0.25	1-2	1.5-6	>7	
Mexiletine (Mexitil)	—	—	10-12	0.5-2	>2	*Class IB:* Muscle twitch, seizures, proarrhythmia, dyspnea
Tocainide (Tonocard)	—	—	11-15	4-10	>10	*Phenytoin:* Hypotension, gingival hyperplasia, antiepileptic hypersensitivity syndrome
Phenytoin (Dilantin)	0.5-1	≥24	22-36	10-20	>20	*Class IC:* Ventricular proarrhythmia *Propafenone:* Dyspnea (2%), worsening of asthma, metallic taste
Flecainide (Tambocor)	—	—	12-27	0.2-1	>1	
Propafenone (Rythmol)	—	—	2-10*	0.6-1	—	
Propranolol (Inderal)	0.5	3-5	2-3	0.05-0.1	—	Sinus bradycardia, AV block, depression of LV function (adrenergic-dependent), masked symptoms of hypoglycemia in diabetics
Esmolol (Brevibloc)	<5 minutes	Minutes	0.15	—	—	
Acebutolol (Sectral)	—	24-30	3-4	—	—	Sudden discontinuation of β blockers may cause rebound hypertension
Amiodarone (Cordarone)	1-3 weeks	Months	26-107 days	0.5-2.5	>2.5	*All:* Sinus bradycardia; torsades de pointes, heart failure exacerbation
Dronedarone (Multaq)	3-6	—	13-19	—	—	*Amiodarone:* GI (25%), ocular (10%), CNS, hepatic (40%-55%), dermatologic (15%), hypothyroidism/hyperthyroidism (4%)
Bretylium (Bretylol)	—	6-8	5-10	0.5-1.5	—	
Dofetilide (Tikosyn)	—	—	10	—	—	*Dronedarone:* N/V/D, asthenia, elevated serum creatinine (51%)
Sotalol (Betapace, Betapace AF)	—	—	12	—	—	*Dofetilide:* Headache (11%), chest pain (10%), dizziness (8%), dyspnea (6%)
Ibutilide (Corvert)	—	—	2-12	—	—	*Ibutilide:* Proarrhythmia, nausea, headaches
Verapamil (Isoptin)	0.5	6	3-7	0.08-0.3	—	Sinus bradycardia, AV block, negative inotropic effect
Diltiazem (Cardizem)	2-4	4-6	3-6	—	—	
Digoxin (Lanoxin)	0.5-2	≥24	30-40	0.5-2 ng/mL	>2.5 ng/mL	VF/VT, N/V as first sign of toxicity
Adenosine (Adenocard)	34 seconds (IV)	1-2 minutes	<10 seconds	NA	—	Dyspnea (12%), cough (6%), respiratory failure, bronchospasms (28%), chest pressure (7%), facial flushing (18%)

TABLE 21-6   Antiarrhythmics: Pharmacokinetics and Adverse Reactions—cont'd

DRUG	PHARMACOKINETICS					ADVERSE REACTIONS
	ONSET (PO) (hr)	DURATION (hr)	HALF-LIFE (hr)	THERAPEUTIC RANGE (mcg/mL)	TOXIC LEVEL (mcg/mL)	
Moricizine (Ethmozine)	2	10-24	1.5-3.5	NA	NA	*All class I agents:* Negative inotropic effect, infranodal conduction block
Lidocaine (Xylocaine)	—	0.25	1-2	1.5-6	>7	*Class IA:* Torsades de pointes
Mexiletine (Mexitil)	—	—	10-12	0.5-2	>2	*Class IB:* Muscle twitch, seizures, proarrhythmia, dyspnea
Tocainide (Tonocard)	—	—	11-15	4-10	>10	*Class IC:* Ventricular proarrhythmia
Flecainide (Tambocor)	—	—	12-27	0.2-1	>1	
Quinidine (Quinaglute)	0.5	6-8	6-7	2-6	>8	*Quinidine:* N/V/D, cinchonism (tinnitus, blurred vision, dizziness, tremor)
Procainamide (Pronestyl)	0.5	≥3	2.5-4.5	4-8	>16	*Procainamide:* N/V/D (30%), bitter taste, rash, hepatitis, mental depression, psychosis
Disopyramide (Norpace)	0.5	6-7	4-10	40-60	>80	*Disopyramide:* Anticholinergic effects (dry mouth, blurred vision, urinary retention), hypoglycemia, cholestatic jaundice, agranulocytosis
Phenytoin (Dilantin)	0.5-1	≥24	22-36	10-20	>20	*Phenytoin:* Hypotension, gingival hyperplasia, antiepileptic hypersensitivity syndrome
Propafenone (Rythmol)	—	—	2-10*	0.6-1	—	*Propafenone:* Dyspnea (2%), worsening of asthma, metallic taste
Propranolol (Inderal)	0.5	3-5	2-3	0.05-0.1	—	Sinus bradycardia, AV block, depression of LV function (adrenergic-dependent), masked symptoms of hypoglycemia in diabetics
Esmolol (Brevibloc)	<5 minutes	Minutes	0.15	—	—	
Acebutolol (Sectral)	—	24-30	3-4	—	—	Sudden discontinuation of β blockers may cause rebound hypertension
Bretylium (Bretylol)	—	6-8	5-10	0.5-1.5	—	*All:* Sinus bradycardia; torsades de pointes, heart failure exacerbation
Sotalol (Betapace, Betapace AF)	—	—	12	—	—	
Amiodarone (Cordarone)	1-3 weeks	Months	26-107 days	0.5-2.5	>2.5	*Amiodarone:* GI (25%), ocular (10%), CNS, hepatic (40%-55%), dermatologic (15%), hypothyroidism/hyperthyroidism (4%)
Dronedarone (Multaq)	3-6	—	13-19	—	—	*Dronedarone:* N/V/D, asthenia, elevated serum creatinine (51%)
Dofetilide (Tikosyn)	—	—	10	—	—	*Dofetilide:* Headache (11%), chest pain (10%), dizziness (8%), dyspnea (6%)
Ibutilide (Corvert)	—	—	2-12	—	—	*Ibutilide:* Proarrhythmia, nausea, headaches
Verapamil (Isoptin)	0.5	6	3-7	0.08-0.3	—	Sinus bradycardia, AV block, negative inotropic effect
Diltiazem (Cardizem)	2-4	4-6	3-6	—	—	
Digoxin (Lanoxin)	0.5-2	≥24	30-40	0.5-2 ng/mL	>2.5 ng/mL	VF/VT, N/V as first sign of toxicity
Adenosine (Adenocard)	34 sec (IV)	1-2 min	<10 sec	NA	—	Dyspnea (12%), cough (6%), respiratory failure, bronchospasms (28%), chest pressure (7%), facial flushing (18%)

AV, Atrioventricular; *GI,* gastrointestinal; *LV,* left ventricular; *NA,* not applicable; *N/V/D,* nausea/vomiting/diarrhea; *VF/VT,* ventricular fibrillation/ventricular tachycardia; —, none.

*Half-life is 6 to 36 hours in patients who are poor metabolizers of propafenone (i.e., patients with low-activity CYP2D6 isozyme).

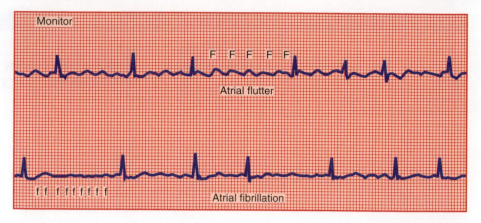

Figure 21-4 Atrial flutter and fibrillation. Notice the "sawtooth" waves (F waves) with atrial flutter and the irregular fibrillatory. (From Miller RD, Eriksson LA, Wiener-Kronish JP, et al: *Miller's anesthesia*, ed 7, Philadelphia, 2010, Churchill Livingstone.)

(Figure 21-4). The effects of quinidine on the AV node are bimodal. At lower concentrations, quinidine has antivagal properties, enhancing AV nodal conduction. At higher concentrations, the AV nodal conduction is slowed down. Because of difficulty in predicting response to quinidine, it is important to initiate a rate-controlling agent first. Quinidine should be used with caution in patients with preexisting asthma, muscle weakness, or infection with fever because hypersensitivity reactions to this medication may be masked by these conditions. Overdosage of quinidine has produced respiratory depression or distress, apnea, diarrhea, vomiting, seizures, hypotension, syncope, and electrocardiogram (ECG) changes.[15]

Procainamide

Procainamide is available only as an IV formulation in the United States and is indicated for the treatment of VT (Figure 21-5) that is life-threatening; because of its proarrhythmic effects, including torsades de pointes (Figure 21-6), the use of this agent for lesser arrhythmias is not recommended. In addition, procainamide has the potential to produce serious hematologic disorders, particularly leukopenia and agranulocytosis; it is used only when benefits outweigh the risks. Procainamide has also been used to convert AF/AFL to sinus rhythm. It is necessary to monitor levels of both procainamide and its active metabolite *N*-acetyl procainamide (NAPA) for efficacy and toxicity. An adverse effect unique to procainamide is the development of lupus erythematosus–like syndrome, which can manifest with pleural or abdominal pain, myalgias, arthralgias, pleural effusion, pericarditis, fever, chills, and skin lesions. Lupus erythematosus–like syndrome occurs in 30% of patients after prolonged administration of procainamide, especially in slow acetylators, who are at risk of accumulating the hydroxylamine metabolite responsible for the pathogenesis of this syndrome. If the lupoid syndrome does not resolve with discontinuation of procainamide, treatment with corticosteroids may be warranted.[4]

Disopyramide

Disopyramide is indicated for the treatment of life-threatening VT; it is also used for the treatment of paroxysmal supraventricular tachycardia (PSVT). Treatment with

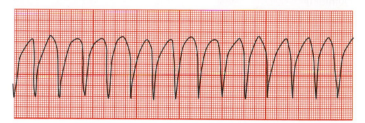

Figure 21-5 Ventricular tachycardia. (From DesJardins T, Burton G: *Clinical manifestations and assessment of respiratory care*, ed 6, St Louis, 2011, Mosby.)

disopyramide should be initiated in the hospital. Patients with AF/AFL must receive digoxin therapy to achieve an adequate serum digoxin level before administration of disopyramide to ensure there is no further elevation of ventricular rate. Potassium should be corrected before initiation of therapy because the drug may be ineffective in patients with hypokalemia, and its toxic effects may be enhanced in hyperkalemia. Disopyramide may cause or aggravate CHF or episodes of hypotension because of its negative inotropic properties. Overdose with disopyramide may be followed by apnea, loss of consciousness, cardiac arrhythmias, and loss of spontaneous respirations requiring mechanical ventilation or other vigorous treatment modalities. This agent has limited use because of its anticholinergic side effects, including dry mouth, difficulty in urination, dizziness, tachycardia, hyperthermia, and blurred vision.[4]

Class IB

Class IB agents are often used and have less proarrhythmic potential compared with class IA agents. The actions of class IB agents are limited to VAs.

Lidocaine

Lidocaine is used frequently to treat VA occurring during cardiac surgery or after an acute myocardial infarction. After administering IV bolus doses (owing to its short half-life of approximately 1.5 to 2 hours), continuous infusion is necessary to maintain sinus rhythm. Lidocaine is metabolized extensively in the liver to two toxic metabolites, monoethylglycinexylidide and glycinexylidide; these metabolites

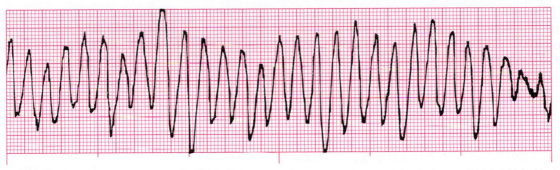

Figure 21-6 Torsades de pointes arrhythmia. (From Aehlert B: *ECGs made easy*, ed 4, St Louis, 2010, Mosby.)

display antiarrhythmogenic properties but are also highly prone to seizure activity. Patients need to be monitored vigilantly for signs of seizure, such as tremors.[15] Other CNS side effects associated with lidocaine are insomnia, drowsiness, ataxia, agitation, and dysarthria. Caution should also be exercised in patients with hepatic failure or CHF because the rate of drug clearance is significantly reduced in either condition. Lidocaine infusions lasting longer than 24 hours may prolong the half-life of lidocaine to approximately 3 hours, leading to a greater risk of lidocaine accumulation and toxicity. In the setting of lidocaine infusion longer than 24 hours, the infusion rate should be reduced by approximately 50%. Lidocaine has also been implicated in causing respiratory depression and arrest.[4]

Mexiletine

Mexiletine has a mechanism of action similar to lidocaine and is available as an oral formulation. It is indicated for the treatment of life-threatening VAs. Because of its anesthetic properties, it is also used at lower doses to reduce neuropathic pain associated with diabetic neuropathy. In controlled trials, the most frequent adverse events were gastrointestinal disturbances (41%), tremor (12%), and lightheadedness and difficulty in coordination (more than 10%). Dyspnea and respiratory problems occurred in 5.7% of patients. Coma and respiratory arrest may occur with massive overdoses.[15]

Tocainide

Tocainide is the oral congener of lidocaine and is used to treat VAs and may also be used to treat myotonic dystrophy and trigeminal neuralgia. Tocainide carries an FDA boxed warning for causing pulmonary disorders, including pulmonary edema, fibrosing alveolitis, pneumonitis, and respiratory arrest (0.11%). These pulmonary manifestations are detectable on radiographic studies within 3 to 18 weeks of therapy. Another boxed warning is for blood dyscrasias, which is not that prevalent (0.18%) but is associated with a fatality rate of up to 25%.[4]

Class IC

Class IC agents are generally not used mainly because of their relatively higher proarrhythmic potential. Other agents from this class have been withdrawn from the market (i.e.,

encainide and moricizine) because of their substantial proarrhythmic potential as shown in two landmark trials: Cardiac Arrhythmia Suppression Trial I (CAST I)[16] and CAST II.[17] Class IC agents are commonly used in the management of supraventricular arrhythmias, but they have activity against VAs as well.

Flecainide (Tambocor)

Flecainide (Tambocor) is indicated for the prevention of paroxysmal AF/AFL associated with disabling symptoms and PSVT, including AV nodal reentrant tachycardia, AV tachycardia, other supraventricular tachycardia (SVT) in patients without structural heart disease, and sustained VT. It is efficacious in suppressing AF in 61% to 92% of patients treated. Flecainide has a long half-life, and the dose should not be increased more often than every 4 days. Flecainide was one of the antiarrhythmics studied in CAST in patients with asymptomatic non–life-threatening arrhythmias occurring 6 days to 2 years after documented myocardial infarction. Flecainide contributed to an excessive mortality or nonfatal cardiac arrest rate of 5.1% versus 2.3% for its matched placebo. Long-term oral prophylaxis with an antiarrhythmic agent poses a great risk of adverse events, and relapse rates are high. Also, flecainide elimination is affected by urinary pH, leading to either toxic or subtherapeutic levels. Alkaline pH decreases and acidic pH increases renal excretion of flecainide.[4]

The "pill-in-the-pocket" approach is the alternative treatment of recurrent arrhythmias, in which a pill is taken by the patient at the time of onset of palpitations. One study assessed this approach in the conversion of AF to sinus rhythm with class IC agents, using either flecainide or propafenone as a single oral dose to convert patients to sinus rhythm out of hospital. Flecainide was shown to be equally effective for pill-in-the-pocket treatment of recurrent AF, with a 94% efficacy rate.[18]

Propafenone (Rythmol)

Propafenone (Rythmol) seems to be comparable to other antiarrhythmics in preventing PSVT and maintaining sinus rhythm after successful cardioversion. It is considered a first-line agent for conversion of recent-onset (less than 48 hours) AF, with efficacy rates of 60% to 90%. Therapy is 15% to 30% less effective in patients manifesting symptoms of AF for more than 48 hours. Propafenone displays nonselective β-blocking activity, and it generally should not be used to treat patients with asthma or bronchospastic disease because β-blocking properties may inhibit bronchodilation. The highest concentrations of the drug are found in the lungs (10-fold higher than in the heart muscles or liver and 24-fold higher than in the kidneys).[19]

Class II

Class II agents consist mainly of β-blocking agents. These agents are used in the management of hypertension and post–myocardial infarction; metoprolol is the only agent in this class that may be used in the setting of CHF.

β Blockers

Propranolol (Inderal), metoprolol (Lopressor), atenolol (Tenormin), and nadolol (Corgard) are available as IV and oral formulations; esmolol (Brevibloc) is available only in the intravenous form. These agents have negative **dromotropic** activity but are more commonly used for negative chronotropic properties in AF/AFL and to prevent or convert SVT to normal sinus rhythm. β Blockers should not be used in settings of acute decompensated heart failure because they can exacerbate symptoms of heart failure. However, after the symptoms of heart failure are stabilized, β blockers may be initiated at lower doses. In settings in which patients with airway disease are overly sensitive to the bronchoconstrictive effects of β blockers, esmolol may be a convenient selection because of its β1-selective property. Because of the short half-life of esmolol (approximately 10 minutes), one may titrate the dose to meet the patient's therapeutic and safety goals.

Class III

Class III agents are used to treat SVAs and VAs. Bretylium, which is considered a member of this class, is no longer manufactured in the United States because of a lack of substantial efficacy data.

Amiodarone (Cordarone)

Amiodarone (Cordarone) is effective in the management of VAs and SVAs. In the past, the life-threatening adverse effects of amiodarone prevented it from being used as a first-line agent; it was reserved for patients with life-threatening VAs. Amiodarone seems to exhibit greater efficacy and a lower incidence of proarrhythmic effects than class I or III antiarrhythmics. Today, amiodarone has become a mainstay in the management of AF, VF, and VT.

Amiodarone-induced pulmonary toxicity warrants substantial concern when treating patients with arrhythmias. The main caveat associated with amiodarone is its distinctive side effect profile.[5] Baseline parameters that must be obtained before starting therapy, along with incidences of various side effects, are presented in Table 21-7. Pulmonary toxicity is quite common, as evidenced by cough and by local or diffuse infiltrates on chest radiographs, and occurs at a rate of up to 20%. Amiodarone-induced pulmonary

TABLE 21-7	Routine Laboratory Testing in Patients Receiving Amiodarone
TYPE OF TEST	**TIME WHEN TEST IS PERFORMED**
Liver enzyme tests	Baseline and then every 6 months
Thyroid function (T$_4$ and TSH)	Baseline and then every 6 months
Serum creatinine and electrolytes	Baseline and then every 6 months
Chest radiograph	Baseline and then yearly
Ophthalmic evaluation	Baseline and for visual impairment or symptoms, and then every 6 months
Pulmonary function tests	Baseline and for unexplained dyspnea, especially in patients with underlying lung disease, and if there are suggestive abnormalities on chest radiograph
ECG	Baseline and then yearly

ECG, Electrocardiogram; *T$_4$*, thyroxine; *TSH*, thyroid-stimulating hormone.

toxicity is managed best by discontinuation or by corticosteroid therapy; in some cases, fatalities of approximately 10% have been reported.[15] In addition, amiodarone is regarded as one of the most potent inhibitors of the cytochrome (CY) P450 3A4 isoenzyme system, and it inhibits CYP2C9 and CYP2C19 (hepatic drug-metabolizing enzymes); concomitant prescription medications, herbals, and over-the-counter (OTC) products must be evaluated for detection of severe, often life-threatening interactions.

Dronedarone (Multaq)

Although similar in chemical structure to amiodarone, dronedarone (Multaq) differs from amiodarone by the removal of the iodine moiety and addition of a methylsulfonamide group (Figure 21-7). These structural changes result in decreased accumulation of the drug inside various tissues, leading to reduced toxicities of the thyroid gland and other organs associated with amiodarone toxicity (Table 21-8 provides monitoring parameters specifically for dronedarone). In addition, the modifications allow dronedarone to achieve steady-state faster than amiodarone because a shorter half-life of approximately 1 day versus more than 50 days. Similar to amiodarone, dronedarone is primarily a class III antiarrhythmic, but it shows properties of all four Vaughan Williams classes. It is indicated to reduce risk for hospitalization in patients with paroxysmal or persistent AF/AFL who are currently in sinus rhythm or pending cardioversion to sinus rhythm.[20] It is available only by the oral route.

Also, similar to amiodarone, Q–T interval prolongation is rare at an incidence of less than 1%. The same precautions taken with amiodarone for risks of Q–T interval prolongation should also be taken with dronedarone therapy based on the ATHENA trial,[21] in which dronedarone exhibited a 40% risk of Q–T interval prolongation compared

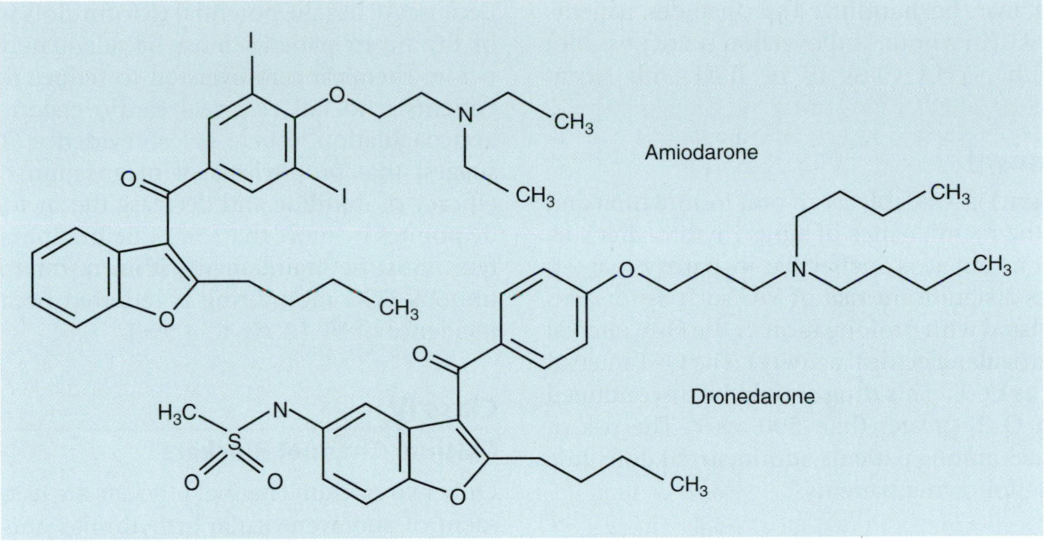

Figure 21-7 Structural difference between amiodarone and dronedarone. (From Zimetbaum PJ: Dronedarone for atrial fibrillation—an odyssey, *N Engl J Med* 360:1811-1813, 2009.)

TABLE 21-8	Laboratory Tests in Patients Receiving Dronedarone
TYPE OF TEST	**TIME WHEN TEST IS PERFORMED**
Liver enzyme tests	Baseline and then periodically during the first 6 months of treatment; then every 6 months
Serum creatinine	Baseline and then 7 days after initiation; then every 6 months
Electrolytes	Baseline and then every 6 months
ECG	Baseline and then every 3 months
Pulmonary function tests	Not necessary unless there is an unexplained dyspnea or nonproductive cough

with placebo. Q–T interval prolongation can be monitored by obtaining a 12-lead ECG and measuring the *corrected Q–T interval (Q–T$_c$)*. The Q–T$_c$ takes into account the measurements of all Q–T intervals on the 12-lead ECG. Generally, strong precautions should be taken when the Q–T$_c$ interval exceeds 450 msec; however, therapy should be withheld and alternatives should be considered when Q–T$_c$ exceeds 500 msec.

Similar to amiodarone, this medication is a CYP450 3A4 substrate and a moderator inhibitor for both CYP3A4 and CYP2D6 isoenzymes. It is contraindicated for use with potent CYP3A4 inhibitors (e.g., clarithromycin, telithromycin, cyclosporine, itraconazole, voriconazole) and inducers (e.g., carbamazepine, phenobarbital, phenytoin, rifampin). If used concurrently with nondihydropyridine calcium channel blockers (e.g., diltiazem or verapamil) or β blockers, these medications should be initiated at a lower dose

to minimize risk for bradycardia or heart block. Dronedarone is also an inhibitor of P-glycoprotein, and digoxin should be avoided; however, if use of digoxin is necessary, the dose should be empirically reduced by 50% with increased monitoring for clinical response and potential adverse effects.[20] A greater than twofold increased risk in mortality was found in patients with New York Heart Association (NYHA) class III and IV CHF who were treated with dronedarone compared with a placebo in the Antiarrhythmic Trial with Dronedarone in Moderate Severe CHF Evaluating Morbidity Decrease (ANDROMEDA)[22] study. Therefore the drug is contraindicated in any patients with NYHA class IV CHF and NYHA class II-III CHF with recent decompensation requiring hospital admission or referral to a specialized CHF clinic. Other contraindications include Q–T$_c$ greater than 500 msec, HR less than 50 beats/min, concomitant use of Q–T interval-prolonging medications or herbals owing to risk for torsades de pointes, sick sinus syndrome, or second- or third-degree AV block unless a functional pacemaker is present.

Amiodarone and dronedarone are the only two agents in this class of antiarrhythmics. Amiodarone is considered more effective than dronedarone in the management of chronic AF. If a patient is tolerating amiodarone, has not developed any adverse effects, and is able to maintain a favorable rhythm, current evidence suggests that it would be prudent to continue amiodarone therapy. However, the clinician must weigh the risks versus benefits against the fact that dronedarone is associated with fewer systemic adverse events that lead to discontinuation. In addition, dronedarone may have the same risks of Q–T interval prolongation or even greater risks. The decision to choose one agent over another is based on multiple patient-specific factors.

Providers prescribing dronedarone must enroll in the $_m$PACT REMS[20] program. This REMS program was developed to halt prescribing of dronedarone to patients in whom the drug may be harmful. This includes patients with permanent AF (in whom cardioversion is not possible) and patients with NYHA Class IV or II-III with recent decompensation.

Dofetilide (Tikosyn)

Dofetilide (Tikosyn) is available as an oral formulation and is indicated for the maintenance of sinus rhythm after successful conversion, but it is ineffective in paroxysmal AF. Dofetilide carries a significant risk of VAs such as torsades de pointes associated with prolongation of the Q–T interval (duration of ventricular electrical activity). The Q–T interval can be reported as $Q-T_c$. This drug should be discontinued in patients with $Q-T_c$ greater than 500 msec. The risk of torsades de pointes among patients administered dofetilide is greatest for the following patients:[4]

- Women
- Patients with congenital heart disease or ischemic heart disease
- Patients with diminished renal function
- Patients receiving dofetilide doses exceeding 500 mg twice daily

This medication must be adjusted to avoid renal accumulation. Drug interactions with dofetilide pose a significant problem. Agents such as cimetidine, azole antifungals, prochlorperazine, metformin, and the trimethoprim component of trimethoprim-sulfamethoxazole (Bactrim) may inhibit active tubular secretion of dofetilide and increase the plasma concentration. Therapy with dofetilide must be initiated in a facility that can provide continuous ECG monitoring and the presence of personnel trained to manage severe VAs for at least 3 days. Both the prescriber and the pharmacy must be participants in a program known as the Tikosyn in Pharmacy System (TIPS) before prescribing and dispensing dofetilide.[23]

Sotalol (Betapace and Betapace AF)

Sotalol (Betapace and Betapace AF) is available only by the oral route and works by prolonging the AP duration and the relative refractory period. Sotalol can be used for SVAs and VAs. When initiating sotalol, the patient should be kept in a facility that can provide continuous ECG monitoring and the presence of personnel trained to manage severe VAs for at least 3 days.[4] As with any β-blocking agent, caution must be exercised when treating patients with restrictive airway disease.

Ibutilide (Corvert)

Ibutilide (Corvert) is available as an IV formulation and is an alternative to electrical cardioversion. Ibutilide is the first antiarrhythmic agent indicated for rapid conversion of AF/ AFL of recent onset by the FDA. In clinical trials, ibutilide was more effective for the treatment of AFL than AF (more than 50% versus less than 40%). Class I antiarrhythmics and other class III antiarrhythmics should not be given with this medication or within 4 hours of an ibutilide infusion because of the potential for prolonged refractoriness.[24]

Because AF has the potential to form clots within the atrium of the heart, patients must be adequately anticoagulated before chemical cardioversion to reduce the risk of stroke. Patients who fail electrical cardioversion require lifelong anticoagulation.[4] There is also evidence (TIME study)[25] to suggest that prophylaxis of magnesium can enhance the efficacy of ibutilide and decrease the incidence of torsades de pointes by more than 30%. Before initiation, all electrolytes must be maintained within normal limits, and continuous ECG monitoring is required because of the high incidence of VF (2.7% to 4.9%).[24]

Class IV
Calcium Channel Blockers

Only two calcium channel blockers are used in the management of supraventricular arrhythmias and ventricular rate control for AF: verapamil (Isoptin) and diltiazem (Cardizem). These agents exert their effects by blocking calcium channels in the AV node and slowing AV nodal conduction. In contrast to β blockers, verapamil and diltiazem are not favorable agents for use in the setting of CHF; however, they are good alternatives to β blockers in the setting of airway disease.

Miscellaneous
Digoxin (Lanoxin)

Digoxin (Lanoxin) has direct AV-blocking effects and vagotonic properties that aid in reducing the HR. Although digoxin prolongs the relative refractory period of the AV node and reduces the number of impulses through the AV node, it is not regarded as a first-line agent for AF.[4,15] Digoxin does not have a rapid onset of effect, especially for the management of an acute condition such as AF; it requires approximately 2 hours to achieve maximal effect. Additionally, digoxin has the potential to shorten the refractory period of atrial muscles, allowing electrical impulses to be conducted throughout the myocardium and ultimately potentiating episodes of AF. It is less effective than β blockers and calcium channel blockers during states of increased sympathetic tone, such as in exercise and stress. Digoxin is not regarded as a first-line agent for the control of ventricular rate in AF except in patients with impaired left ventricular function or heart failure.[15]

Adenosine (Adenocard)

Rapid administration of adenosine (Adenocard) is implemented to terminate SVTs only. Adenosine has a half-life of approximately 12 seconds, and because of its ultrashort half-life, adenosine is best administered through a central line for rapid arrival at the site of action, or if given through a brachial line, the arm should be held in the upright position followed almost instantly by a saline flush. Dyspnea, hyperpnea, and cough have been reported after administration of IV adenosine in patients with asthma and chronic obstructive pulmonary disease; these symptoms are generally benign and short-lasting.[26,27]

KEY POINT

Drugs used in advanced cardiac life support included antiarrhythmics, vasopressors such as epinephrine and vasopressin, the electrolyte magnesium, and atropine for bradycardia or asystole.

MANAGEMENT AND PHARMACOTHERAPY OF ADVANCED CARDIAC LIFE SUPPORT

Sudden Cardiac Death

Death from heart disease is the leading cause of death in the United States. Of deaths caused by heart disease, nearly three quarters of these are due to **sudden cardiac death (SCD)**.[28] SCD can be defined as an episode of VF, pulseless VT, pulseless electrical activity (PEA), or asystole, all of which are life-threatening arrhythmias.[29] Although the fatalities associated with episodes of SCD are unacceptably high, an individual may be resuscitated, and it is common to encounter patients having a "history" of SCD. The goal in treating SCD is to restore sinus rhythm, to prevent further episodes of SCD, and to prevent impairment of neurologic function. Several studies have shown benefits in mortality reduction by minimizing time to defibrillation and by delivery of cardiopulmonary resuscitation (CPR).[29]

In a patient with VF, survival decreases by 7% to 10% for every minute that passes from the time of symptom onset to defibrillation.[29] When CPR is initiated, the decline in survival occurs at a more gradual rate of approximately 3% to 4% for every minute between onset of symptoms and time to defibrillation.[29] Needless to say, efficient and timely delivery of defibrillation and CPR is imperative for successful management of SCD.

After beginning CPR and attempting defibrillation, health care workers may begin establishing other therapeutic modalities such as IV access; medication therapy and the insertion of an advanced airway should be considered. VF and pulseless VT are managed primarily by defibrillation and CPR and secondarily by pharmacotherapy; conversely, asystole and PEA are not managed by defibrillation and are managed first by CPR only and second by pharmacotherapy as depicted in the algorithms in Figures 21-8, 21-9, and 21-10. It may be prudent to review the national consensus guidelines for further details of advanced cardiac life support algorithms.

Epinephrine

Epinephrine, an endogenous neurotransmitter, is administered in 1-mg doses as a 10-mL solution. Epinephrine stimulates β_1-adrenergic and β_2-adrenergic receptors, which are

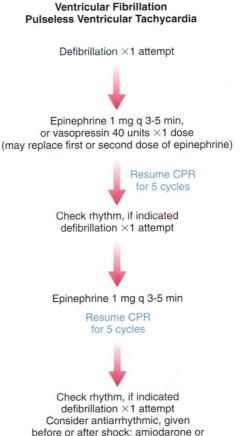

Figure 21-8 *Left,* Ventricular fibrillation pattern and ventricular tachycardia pattern. *Right,* Algorithm for treatment of ventricular fibrillation and pulseless ventricular tachycardia.

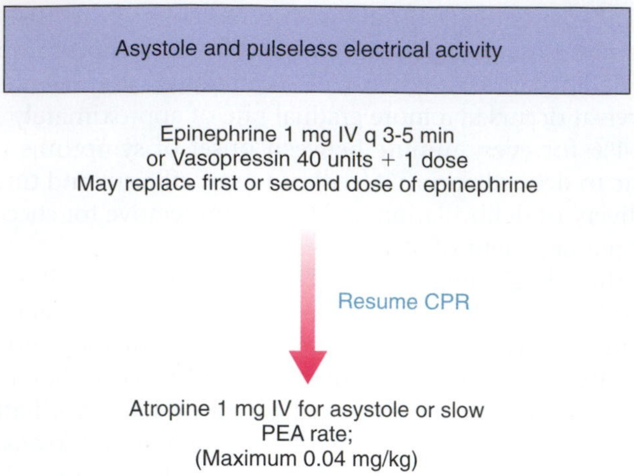

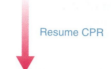

Asystole and pulseless electrical activity

Epinephrine 1 mg IV q 3-5 min
or Vasopressin 40 units + 1 dose
May replace first or second dose of epinephrine

Resume CPR

Atropine 1 mg IV for asystole or slow
PEA rate;
(Maximum 0.04 mg/kg)

Figure 21-9 Algorithm for treatment of asystole and pulseless electrical activity (PEA).

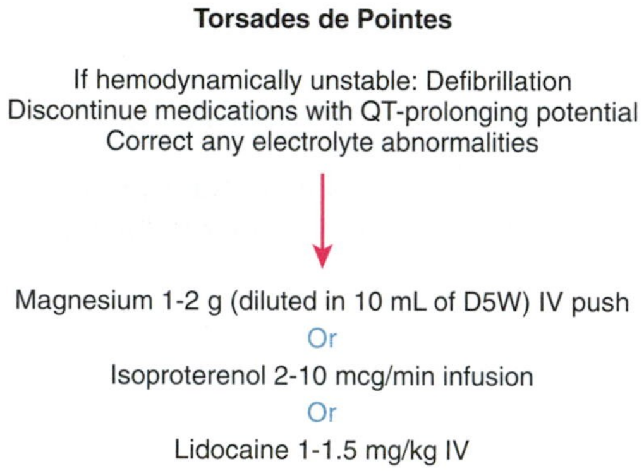

Torsades de Pointes

If hemodynamically unstable: Defibrillation
Discontinue medications with QT-prolonging potential
Correct any electrolyte abnormalities

Magnesium 1-2 g (diluted in 10 mL of D5W) IV push

Or
Isoproterenol 2-10 mcg/min infusion

Or
Lidocaine 1-1.5 mg/kg IV

Figure 21-10 Algorithm for treatment of torsades de pointes. *D5W*, 5% dextrose in water.

found in dense proportions in the heart and lungs. The effect of epinephrine on α_1 receptors, located within the coronary and cerebral vasculature, is more closely correlated with efficacy. Stimulation of α_1 receptors causes vasoconstriction of the coronary and cerebral vasculature, increasing blood flow to the heart's myocardium and the CNS. In contrast, stimulation of β_1 receptors increases cardiac HR, resulting in increased oxygen demand on the heart and impairing oxygen delivery to the myocardium and the CNS.

One main caveat associated with epinephrine use is the occurrence of decreased receptor affinity in the setting of metabolic acidosis. Metabolic acidosis may readily ensue during SCD, owing to hypoxic conditions leading to a shift in anaerobic respiration. At the present time, there is no recommended maximal dose of epinephrine in the management of SCD. Postresuscitation side effects include hypertension and tachycardia.

Vasopressin

Vasopressin, also known as antidiuretic hormone, is an endogenous hormone that acts as a potent vasoconstrictor.

Vasopressin is administered as a one-time IV dose of 40 U. Because the effects of vasopressin have not been shown to be exceedingly different from the effects of epinephrine, this dose may be administered in lieu of the first or second dose of epinephrine when treating any form of SCD.[29] In contrast to epinephrine, vasopressin is a nonadrenergic vasoconstrictor; its vasoconstricting properties are manifested by activation of V_1 receptors, which are found in the vasculature. Once stimulated, V_1 receptors release calcium from the sarcoplasmic reticulum in vascular smooth muscle, leading to vasoconstriction and increasing SVR and coronary and cerebral blood flow. In contrast to epinephrine, vasopressin receptor affinity is not compromised in the setting of metabolic acidosis. In the setting of long-term continuous infusion therapy, vasopressin may cause gastrointestinal and skin ischemia; however, in the setting of SCD, these adverse events would be unlikely.

Atropine (AtroPen)

Atropine (AtroPen) is indicated for certain forms of SCD, such as asystole or PEA, usually given at a dose of 1 mg as IV push, along with epinephrine or vasopressin. Atropine acts by blocking the actions of acetylcholine, an endogenous cholinergic agent. The cholinergic system is typically involved with HR reduction, and by blocking this effect, atropine exerts a pronounced (albeit short-lived) chronotropic effect on the heart. The recommended maximal dose of atropine used during resuscitation is 0.04 mg/kg. Because atropine affects acetylcholine globally within the body, noticeable adverse effects include meiosis, dry mouth, urinary retention, and constipation.

Sodium Bicarbonate

Sodium bicarbonate ($NaHCO_3$) is routinely and frequently used for the management of metabolic acidosis. It is indicated in a variety of settings that may induce acidemia, including metabolic acidosis from severe renal disease, shock, cardiac arrest, uncontrolled diabetes, extracorporeal circulation of blood, severe diarrhea, or certain drug intoxications such as tricyclic antidepressants, barbiturates, and salicylates.[30] The current Surviving Sepsis Guidelines[5] do not endorse sodium bicarbonate infusions for hypoperfusion-induced lactic acidosis unless acidosis is severe (i.e., pH <7.15) because of a lack of evidence supporting its benefit.[31] Furthermore, several studies in patients with diabetic ketoacidosis (DKA) have shown no decrease in time to resolution of acidemia with administration of sodium bicarbonate.[32] On the other hand, adverse effects of sodium bicarbonate infusions include fluid overload due to the sodium content (1 mL of 4.2% $NaHCO_3$ contains 11.5 mg of Na^+; 1 mL of 8.4% $NaHCO_3$ contains 22.9 mg of Na^+), a decrease in serum ionized calcium, and elevations in CO_2 caused by the conversion of sodium bicarbonate to CO_2.[30] Because of the increase in CO_2 that occurs with bicarbonate infusions, patients must be on adequate ventilatory support.

Despite these concerns, critical care practitioners frequently utilize sodium bicarbonate infusions for management of severe acidosis.

Treatment of metabolic acidosis should first and foremost involve correction of the underlying cause of acidosis. When administering bicarbonate infusions, the goal of therapy should be to normalize serum bicarbonate levels. Symptoms of acidemia and serum pH (goal pH of 7.2) should be considered in determining whether a bicarbonate infusion is necessary. The package insert lists a standard dose of sodium bicarbonate at 2 to 5 mEq/kg. Most drug references recommend replacement of 50% of total bicarbonate dose over 3 to 4 hours followed by the remainder of the dose over 8 to 24 hours.[1,4,15] To avoid the overcorrection of acidemia, the initial goal of bicarbonate administration should be to lower the serum bicarbonate by 10 to 12 mEq/L, rather than to normalize the serum bicarbonate level. Full correction of CO_2 may cause rebound acidosis because there is a delay in ventilation readjustment to CO_2 levels. Although bicarbonate infusions can be prepared in several diluents, including 5% dextrose in water (D5W) or normal saline, preparation in normal saline increases risk of developing hypernatremia. In patients with cardiac arrest and acidosis, undiluted bicarbonate can be given as an intravenous push at a dose of 0.5 to 1 mEq/kg of body weight.[30]

The presence of carbon dioxide helps the release and delivery of oxygen from hemoglobin, also known as the **Bohr effect**. When comparing the oxygen dissociation curves of a serum sample with carbon dioxide and another with no carbon dioxide, oxygen is able to dissociate more readily in the former state, as depicted in Figure 21-11.

In addition, sodium bicarbonate decreases hydrogen ion concentration in the serum by reacting with it, yielding carbon dioxide and water. For this reaction to continue, the product (carbon dioxide) must be removed. Sodium bicarbonate therapy aids in increasing extracellular pH only if ventilation is sufficient to remove the carbon dioxide. If *hypercapnia* (excess carbon dioxide in the blood) ensues, as carbon dioxide accumulates in the serum it eventually crosses cellular membranes readily; intracellular pH may continue to decline, and further deterioration of cellular function occurs.

Magnesium Sulfate

Magnesium is often implemented in the management of torsades de pointes. Although its mechanism has not been fully elucidated, magnesium may exert its pharmacologic effect by prolonging conduction time; however, its role has been clearly delineated. Intravenous magnesium may be effective whether or not a patient is *eumagnesemic* (having a normal serum magnesium level). The typical dose consists of 1 to 2 g and may be repeated, separated by several minutes. No maximal dose of magnesium has been determined as yet; however, patients with normal renal function are reported to tolerate up to 16 g in a 24-hour period. A continuous infusion regimen may be initiated at a rate of 0.5 to 1 g/hr. Caution is warranted when treating patients with renal insufficiency. Signs and symptoms of magnesium intoxication include the following:

- Sweating
- Hypotension
- Hypothermia
- Depression of reflexes
- CNS depression

Severe hypermagnesemia may result in respiratory depression or fatal respiratory paralysis, circulatory collapse, and flaccid paralysis. Absence of patellar reflex is a clinical sign of magnesium intoxication.

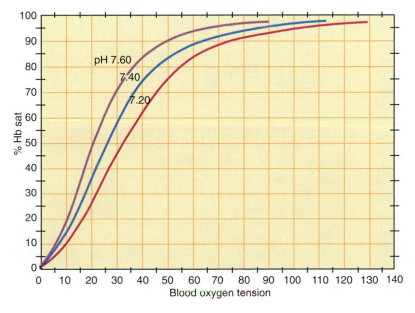

Figure 21-11 Bohr effect. (Kacmarek RM, Wilkins RL, Stoller JK, et al: Egan's fundamentals of respiratory care, ed 10, St. Louis, 2013, Mosby.)

ALTERNATIVE ROUTES OF MEDICATION ADMINISTRATION

Intraosseous Route

In the face of life-threatening medical emergencies in which there is a dire need for medication and fluid delivery, it is incumbent on the health care worker to provide vascular access in the most efficient and safest way possible. Often, IV access is difficult if not impossible in infants and young children, elderly patients with circulatory collapse, and IV drug abusers. In such situations, an intraosseous (IO) needle may be inserted with relative ease, even in the most poorly perfused patients. The 2010 American Heart Association guidelines[29] for CPR and emergency cardiovascular care recommend IO therapy as an alternative to direct IV therapy.

The marrow of IO bone provides a rich network of vessels that ultimately drains into the central circulation, allowing medications and fluids to gain almost instant access to the central circulation. IO access is recommended for use in children and adults. IO access may be problematic when implemented in elderly patients owing to the presence of a thicker cortex of bone and smaller marrow cavity; inability to enter the marrow may increase the risk of bone fracture. Typically, an IO needle should not remain at the site of insertion for more than 3 to 4 hours.

Endotracheal Route

In the event that the IV route is inaccessible, a few agents are amenable to endotracheal delivery; these agents have come to be known by the acronym *NAVEL*:

*N*aloxone
*A*tropine
*V*asopressin
*E*pinephrine
*L*idocaine

The following should be done when administering the previously listed agents by the endotracheal route:

- The patient should be positioned horizontally, as opposed to being in the Trendelenburg position, and chest compressions should cease.
- A catheter should be inserted into the endotracheal tube and allowed to pass the tip of the tube. The medication solution should be sprayed down the tube, followed by 5 to 10 rapid ventilations with a respirator bag.
- Medications should be diluted with approximately 10 mL of distilled water or normal saline. Endotracheal absorption is greater with distilled water, but distilled water has a negative effect on the partial pressure of oxygen. Generally, the systemic absorption of these medications is reduced via the endotracheal route, and the dose administered should always be 2 to 2.5 times the usual IV dose, except for vasopressin; the vasopressin IV dose of 40 U may be given via the endotracheal route.

 SELF-ASSESSMENT QUESTIONS

Answers can be found in Appendix A.

1. In which phase of the cardiac cycle does ventricular contraction occur?
2. Identify three functions that regulate mean arterial pressure.
3. Which measurements, taken by a pulmonary artery catheter, are estimates of intravascular volume?
4. Hypotension is first managed by what mode of therapy?
5. What vasopressor acts only on the α receptors within the vasculature?
6. Which agents exert an inotropic effect on the heart?
7. What electrolyte abnormality may potentiate the adverse effects of digoxin?
8. What drug should be given for the management of extravasation caused by vasopressors?
9. What Vaughan Williams class of antiarrhythmics acts on the fast sodium channels in the myocardium?
10. What antiarrhythmic agent is structurally similar to amiodarone but has an improved side effect profile?
11. In patients taking dofetilide, at what $Q-T_c$ interval should the drug be discontinued because the risk for torsades de pointes becomes too great?
12. Which antiarrhythmic agent is highly associated with the development of lupus erythematosus?
13. Identify the four categories of sudden cardiac death.
14. What medication is indicated for treatment of asystole and pulseless electrical activity but not ventricular fibrillation or pulseless ventricular tachycardia during cardiac arrest?
15. What are the two alternative routes of medication administration during cardiac arrest when an intravenous route is not available?
16. In a patient with septic shock, what is the pH in which the Surviving Sepsis Guidelines recommend utilizing sodium bicarbonate therapy?
17. When medications are administered via the endotracheal route during cardiac arrest, the dose should be increased by how many times the usual intravenous dose?

 CLINICAL SCENARIO 1

Answers can be found in Appendix A.

A.M. is a 28-year-old female who was rushed to the emergency department of a local hospital by paramedic staff after she collapsed suddenly at work. When she collapsed, the staff in her office called for an ambulance although basic life support was not started. It was reported that she was in ventricular fibrillation when the paramedic staff arrived at the scene. The paramedics promptly administered two shocks with a defibrillator,

CLINICAL SCENARIO 1—cont'd

and after the second shock a pulse could be felt. On arrival to the hospital, the patient's blood pressure dropped to 85/42 and the cardiac monitor showed a supraventricular tachycardia of 170 beats/minute. The patient was admitted to the intensive care unit for management of hypotension.

Using the SOAP method, assess this clinical scenario.

CLINICAL SCENARIO 2

Answers can be found in Appendix A.

R.W., a 49-year-old man, is visiting his mother, who was admitted to a nursing home for long-term rehabilitation because of a spinal cord injury. He goes to the bathroom, and a few minutes later his mother hears a loud thud; she calls out to him, but there is no response. After an additional 3 minutes, the head nurse and the clinical pharmacist initiate CPR and obtain the code cart. The initial ECG reading reveals pulseless electrical activity, and they administer one dose of epinephrine and atropine given as a rapid IV push followed by a saline flush. The code team arrives to continue CPR, and a subsequent ECG reading reveals ventricular fibrillation. One shock is delivered, and a dose of amiodarone 300 mg IVPB (intravenous piggyback) over 10 minutes is administered. The patient regains consciousness and becomes hemodynamically stable.

Using the SOAP method, assess this clinical scenario.

REFERENCES

1. Barnes AD, Lee SH: Shock. In Koda-Kimble MA, Young Yee L, Kradjan WA, et al, editors: *Applied therapeutics*, ed 10, Baltimore, 2012, Lippincott Williams & Wilkins.
2. Guyton AC, Hall JE: *Textbook of medical physiology*, Philadelphia, 2006, Saunders.
3. Widmaier E, Raff H, Strang K: *Vander's human physiology: the mechanisms of body functions*, ed 13, New York, 2013, McGraw-Hill.
4. *Drug facts and comparisons*, St Louis, 2013, Facts & Comparisons, Lippincott Williams & Wilkin.
5. Dellinger RP, Levy MM, Rhodes A, et al: Surviving Sepsis Campaign: International guidelines for management of severe sepsis and septic shock: 2012. *Crit Care Med* 41:580–637, 2013.
6. Phenylephrine hydrochloride [Package Insert]. Baxter Healthcare, Deerfield, IL: 2010.
7. Pitressin (vasopressin) [Package Insert]. JHP Pharmaceuticals LLC. Rochester, MI: 2013.
8. Garcia-Tsao G, Sanyal AJ, Grace ND, et al: Prevention and management of gastroesophageal varices and variceal hemorrhage in cirrhosis. *Hepatology* 46:922, 2007.
9. Midodrine [Package Insert]. Shire Manufacturing, Wayne PA: 2005.
10. Van de Wal RM, Swaans MJ, Deneer VH, et al: Midodrine for ICU patients suffering from refractory hypotension. *Neth J Crit Care* 14(1):36–38, 2010.
11. Hack JB, Lewin NA: Cardioactive steroids. In Flomenbaum NE, Goldfrank LR, Hoffman RS, et al, editors: *Goldfrank's toxicologic emergencies*, ed 8, New York, 2006, McGraw-Hill.

12. White MC, Song SC, Chow MS: Cardiac arrhythmias. In Koda-Kimble MA, Young Yee L, Kradjan WA, et al, *editors: Applied therapeutics*, ed 8, Baltimore, 2005, Lippincott Williams & Wilkins.
13. Nattel S, Opie LH: Controversies in atrial fibrillation. *Lancet* 367:262, 2006.
14. Link MS, Atkins AL, Rod S, et al: ACC/AHA/NASPE 2010 guideline update for Electrical Therapies: Automated External Defibrillators, Defibrillation, Cardioversion, and Pacing 2010 American Heart Association Guidelines for Cardiopulmonary Resuscitation and Emergency Cardiovascular Care: a report of the American College of Cardiology/American Heart Association Task Force on Practice Guidelines (ACC/AHA/NASPE Committee on Pacemaker Implantation). Retrieved from <http://circ.ahajournals.org/content/122/18_suppl_3.toc>, 2010
15. *AHFS Drug Information*, Bethesda, MD, 2014, American Society of Health-System Pharmacists.
16. Echt DS, Liebson PR, Mitchell LB, et al: Mortality and morbidity in patients receiving encainide, flecainide, or placebo. The Cardiac Arrhythmia Suppression Trial. *N Engl J Med* 324:781–788, 1989.
17. The Cardiac Arrhythmia Suppression Trial-II Investigators: Effect of antiarrhythmic agent moricizine on survival after myocardial infarction: the Cardiac Arrhythmia Suppression Trial-II. *N Engl J Med* 327:227–233, 1992.
18. Alboni P, Botto GL, Baldi N, et al: Outpatient treatment of recent-onset atrial fibrillation with the "pill-in-the-pocket" approach. *N Engl J Med* 351:2384, 2004.
19. Rhytmol [Package Insert], Smith-Kline Beecham Co, Research Triangle Park, 2009.
20. Multaq Product Information, Sanofi-Aventis U.S. LLC. Retrieved from <http://products.sanofi-aventis.us/Multaq/Multaq.pdf>, 2009.
21. Hohnloser SH, Crijns HJGM, van Eickels M, et al: for the ATHENA Investigators. Effect of dronedarone on cardiovascular events in atrial fibrillation. *N Engl J Med* 360:668–678, 2009.
22. Kober L, Torp-Pedersen C, McMurray JJ, et al: Increased mortality after Dronedarone therapy for severe heart failure. *N Engl J Med* 358:2678–2687, 2008.
23. Tikosyn Product Information, Pfizer. Retrieved from <http://www.pfizer.com/files/products/uspi_tikosyn.pdf>, 2006.
24. Corvert Product Information, Pfizer. Retrieved from <http://www.pfizer.com/pfizer/download/uspi_corvert.pdf>, 2006.
25. Kalus JS, Spencer AP, Tsikouris JP, et al: Impact of prophylactic i.v. magnesium on the efficacy of ibutilide for conversion of atrial fibrillation or flutter. *Am J Health Syst Pharm* 60:2308–2312, 2003.
26. Fan MS, Mustafa J: Role of adenosine in airway inflammation in an allergic mouse model of asthma. *Int Immunopharmacol* 6:36, 2006.
27. Burki NK, Alam M, Lee L: The pulmonary effects of intravenous adenosine in asthmatic subjects. *Respir Res* 7:139, 2006.
28. Zheng ZJ, Croft JB, Giles WH, Mensah GA: Sudden cardiac death in the United States, 1989 to 1998. *Circulation* 104(18):2158–2163, 2001.
29. American Heart Association: The American Heart Association 2010 guidelines for cardiopulmonary resuscitation and emergency cardiovascular care. *Circulation* 122:S729–S767, 2010.
30. Sodium Bicarbonate [Package Insert]. Hospira, Inc.; 2006: Lake Forest, IL.
31. Viallon A, Zeni F, Lafond P, et al: Does bicarbonate therapy improve the management of severe diabetic ketoacidosis? *Crit Care Med* 27(12):2690–2693, 1999.
32. Duhon B, Attridge RL, Franco-Martinez AC, et al: Intravenous sodium bicarbonate therapy in severely acidotic diabetic ketoacidosis. *Ann Pharmacother* 47(7–8):970–975, 2013. doi: 10.1345/aph.1S014. [Epub 2013 Jun 4].

CHAPTER **22**

Drugs Affecting Circulation: Antihypertensives, Antianginals, Antithrombotics

Henry Cohen

CHAPTER OUTLINE

OBJECTIVES

After reading this chapter, the reader will be able to:

1. Define terms that pertain to drugs affecting circulation: antihypertensives, antianginals, and antithrombotics
2. Categorize the stages of normal to high blood pressure
3. Define a hypertensive crisis, and differentiate between hypertensive emergency and hypertensive urgency
4. Design an algorithm for the pharmacotherapy of hypertension
5. Compare and contrast the clinical pharmacology of the agents used for hypertensive pharmacotherapy
6. Describe the chronotherapeutic effect of blood pressure, and design a pharmacotherapy regimen based on this principle
7. Describe the mechanism of action of angiotensin-converting enzyme inhibitors, calcium channel blockers, and β blockers
8. Compare and contrast the clinical pharmacology of spironolactone and eplerenone

9. List drug-drug interactions relevant to antihypertensives and plausible mechanisms
10. Describe the formation and elimination of an acute coronary thrombus
11. Describe the pathophysiology of angina and the drugs used to treat angina
12. List the agents in each of the following antithrombotic classes: anticoagulants, antiplatelets, and thrombolytics
13. Describe the mechanism of action of heparin
14. Compare and contrast the clinical pharmacology of heparin and low-molecular-weight heparin (LMWH)
15. List the laboratory parameters that may be used to monitor for the effect of heparin, LMWH, and direct thrombin inhibitors
16. Describe the mechanism of heparin-induced and warfarin-induced paradoxical thrombosis

OBJECTIVES—cont'd

17. Compare and contrast the clinical pharmacology of aspirin, clopidogrel, ticlopidine, and dipyridamole
18. Describe the role of genetic polymorphism in the antiplatelet activity of clopidogrel and anticoagulant effect of warfarin
19. Describe the indication and mechanism of action of glycoprotein IIb/IIIa inhibitors
20. List the indications and contraindication of thrombolytic agents

KEY TERMS AND DEFINITIONS

Antithrombotics Drugs that prevent or break up blood clots in conditions such as thrombosis or embolism; antithrombotics include anticoagulants, antiplatelets, and thrombolytics.

Arterial blood pressure (blood pressure) Defined hemodynamically as the product of systemic vascular resistance and cardiac output (heart rate × stroke volume).

Cardiovascular disease (CVD) Damage to the heart and the blood vessels or circulation, including to the brain, kidney, and the eyes.

Chronotropic Influencing the rate of rhythmic movements (heartbeat).

Circadian rhythm Human biologic variations of rhythm within a 24-hour cycle.

Creatinine clearance (CrCl) Measurement of the renal clearance of endogenous creatinine per unit of time; approximates glomerular filtration rate (GFR) but overestimates GFR by 10% to 15%; used for drug dosage guidelines.

D-dimers Covalently cross-linked degradation fragments of the cross-linked fibrin polymer during plasmin-mediated fibrinolysis; level increases after the onset of fibrinolysis and allows for identification of the presence of fibrinolysis.

Dose-ceiling effect Maximum dose of a drug, beyond which it no longer exerts a therapeutic effect; however, its toxic effect increases.

Fibrin split or fibrinogen degradation products (FDPs) Small peptides that result after the action of plasmin on fibrinogen and fibrin in the fibrinolytic process. FDPs are anticoagulant substances that can cause bleeding if fibrinolysis becomes uncontrolled and excessive.

Glomerular filtration rate (GFR) Volume of water filtered from the plasma by the kidney via the glomerular capillary walls into Bowman capsules per unit time; considered to be 90% of creatinine clearance and equivalent to insulin clearance.

Hypertensive emergency Blood pressure greater than 180/120 mm Hg, with the elevation of blood pressure accompanied by acute, progressing target organ injury.

Hypertensive urgency Blood pressure greater than 180/120 mm Hg without signs or symptoms of acute target organ complications.

Inotropes Drugs influencing the contractility of a muscle (heart).

Intrinsic sympathomimetic activity (ISA) Having the ability to activate and block adrenergic receptors, producing a net stimulatory effect on the sympathetic nervous system.

Renin Enzyme, also known as angiotensinogenase, released by the kidney in response to a lack of renal blood flow and responsible for converting angiotensinogen into angiotensin I.

Substitute neurotransmitters Neurotransmitter or hormone replacements that may be weaker or inert.

The circulatory system comprises an integral functional part of the cardiopulmonary system. Drug therapy affecting the circulation is seen in the acute critical care, outpatient care, and home care environments. This chapter presents three classes of drug therapy targeted at the circulatory system. After a brief review of the epidemiology, etiology, and pathophysiology of hypertension, the multiple drug groups used as antihypertensives are described. Drugs used to treat angina pectoris are the second group of drugs described. The third group of agents affecting circulation, antithrombotics, comprises several classes of drugs used to regulate clotting mechanisms.

HYPERTENSION

KEY POINT

Normal blood pressure is defined as blood pressure of less than 120/80 mm Hg. The diagnosis of hypertension and goal blood pressure are based on individual risk factors.

Epidemiology and Etiology

More than 1 billion people worldwide and 1 in every 4 Americans has high blood pressure (≥140/90 mm Hg). High blood pressure (≥140/90 mm Hg) is present in 78 million American adults or 33% of Americans 20 years of age and older. Among those with hypertension, approximately 18% are unaware of their condition and only about half have achieved their target blood pressure.[1-2] Hypertension adversely affects numerous body organs, including the heart, brain, kidney, and eyes. Damage to these organ systems resulting from hypertension is termed **cardiovascular disease (CVD)**. Uncontrolled hypertension increases CVD morbidity and mortality by increasing the risk of developing left ventricular hypertrophy, angina, myocardial infarction (MI), heart failure, stroke, peripheral arterial disease, retinopathy, and kidney disease. One of eight deaths can be attributed to hypertension, and the World Health Organization reports that suboptimal blood pressure (systolic blood pressure [SBP] above 115 mm Hg) is responsible for 62% of cerebrovascular disease and 49% of ischemic heart disease. Blood pressure increases with age, and hypertension is more prevalent in adults older than 65 years. This fact is of great concern because it is estimated that by 2040, 25% of the American population will be older than 65. Hypertension occurs more frequently in men than in women and occurs in more blacks than whites. Evidence suggests that individuals who are normotensive have a greater than 90% lifetime risk for developing hypertension by age 55.[3]

2014 Antihypertension Guidelines Update

The 2014 Evidenced-Based Guideline for the Management of High Blood Pressure in Adults Report From the Panel Members Appointed to the Eighth Joint National Committee (JNC 8) is the most up-to-date guideline for the management of hypertension.[4] This guideline addresses thresholds for pharmacologic treatment, agents of choice for hypertension management, and treatment goals for various hypertensive populations. It defines hypertension as blood pressure ≥140/90 mm Hg but does not categorize blood pressure classification into stages.

Blood pressure targets vary by age and presence of diabetes mellitus or chronic kidney disease (CKD). The guideline recommends that for the general population age ≥60 years, pharmacologic treatment should be initiated when SBP is ≥150 mm Hg or diastolic blood pressure (DBP) is ≥90 mm Hg to target a goal SBP <150 mm Hg and DBP <90 mm Hg. In cases where pharmacologic treatment results in a lower SBP, such as SBP <140 mm Hg, treatment need not be adjusted provided the patient tolerates therapy without experiencing adverse effects on health and quality of life.

In the general population under 60 years of age pharmacologic treatment should be initiated when SBP is ≥140 mm Hg and DBP is ≥90 mm Hg to target a goal SBP <140 mm Hg and DBP <90 mm Hg. In patients with CKD or diabetes, pharmacologic therapy should be initiated for all patients age 18 years or older at SBP ≥140 mm Hg or DBP ≥90 mm Hg to achieve a goal SBP <140 mm Hg and DBP <90 mm Hg (Table 22-1).

Preferred agents for initial management of hypertension in nonblack patients without CKD include thiazide-type diuretics, calcium channel blockers (CCBs),

angiotensin-converting enzyme inhibitors (ACEIs), and angiotensin II receptor blockers (ARBs). In black patients without CKD, thiazide-type diuretics and CCBs are preferred because of evidence of improved outcomes compared with ACEIs and insufficient evidence comparing these agents to other drug classes. In adult patients with CKD and hypertension, evidence shows improved kidney outcomes with use of an ACEI or ARB; therefore all hypertensive CKD patients, regardless of race or diabetes status, should be on an ACEI or ARB as first-line therapy. β Blockers are no longer considered first-line antihypertensive agents for any of the described hypertensive populations because of a study that showed a higher composite rate of cardiovascular death, MI, or stroke with β blockers compared with ARBs. Studies comparing β blockers to the other first-line antihypertensive agents (ACEIs, CCBs, thiazide-type diuretics) showed similar efficacy among agents or had insufficient evidence to determine a difference between agents.

Blood pressure medication doses and agents should be adjusted to achieve target blood pressure (Table 22-2). If

TABLE 22-2	Titration of Antihypertensive Agents to Achieve Target Blood Pressure
Strategy A	• Start with <u>one</u> antihypertensive medication • If goal BP is not achieved: titrate dose of initial agent to maximum recommended dose as necessary to achieve target BP • If goal BP is still not achieved: add additional agent and titrate dose to maximum recommended dose as necessary to achieve target BP • If goal BP is still not achieved: add a third antihypertensive agent and titrate dose to maximum recommended dose as necessary to achieve target BP
Strategy B	• Start with <u>one</u> antihypertensive medication • If goal BP is not achieved: add a second medication • If goal BP is still not achieved: titrate doses of both medications to maximum recommended dosages as necessary to achieve target BP • If goal BP is still not achieved: add a third drug and titrate to maximum recommended dose as necessary to achieve target BP
Strategy C	• Start with <u>two</u> antihypertensive medications • If goal BP is not achieved: titrate doses of both medications as necessary • If goal BP is still not achieved: add a third agent and titrate dose to maximum as necessary to achieve target BP • Strategy C may be preferred if SBP >160 mm Hg and/or DBP >100 mm Hg and/or SBP >20 mm Hg above goal and/or DBP >10 mm Hg above goal

TABLE 22-1	Target Blood Pressure by Age and Comorbidities

PATIENT POPULATION	TARGET BLOOD PRESSURE
• Age ≥60 years	SBP <150 mm Hg
• No diabetes or CKD	DBP < 90 mm Hg
• Age <60 years	SBP <140 mm Hg
• No diabetes or CKD	DBP <90 mm Hg
• Age ≥18 years	SBP < 140 mm Hg
• Diabetes or CKD present	DBP <90 mm Hg

CKD, Chronic kidney disease; *DBP,* diastolic blood pressure; *SBP,* systolic blood pressure.

BP, Blood pressure; *DBP,* diastolic blood pressure; *SBP,* systolic blood pressure.

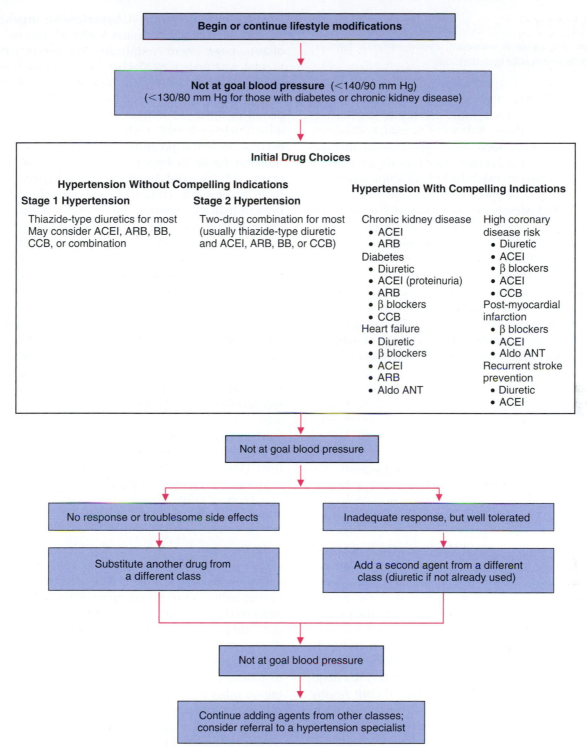

Begin or continue lifestyle modifications

Not at goal blood pressure (<140/90 mm Hg)
(<130/80 mm Hg for those with diabetes or chronic kidney disease)

Initial Drug Choices

Hypertension Without Compelling Indications

Stage 1 Hypertension

Thiazide-type diuretics for most
May consider ACEI, ARB, BB,
CCB, or combination

Stage 2 Hypertension

Two-drug combination for most
(usually thiazide-type diuretic
and ACEI, ARB, BB, or CCB)

Hypertension With Compelling Indications

Chronic kidney disease
- ACEI
- ARB

Diabetes
- Diuretic
- ACEI (proteinuria)
- ARB
- β blockers
- CCB

Heart failure
- Diuretic
- β blockers
- ACEI
- ARB
- Aldo ANT

High coronary
disease risk
- Diuretic
- ACEI
- β blockers
- ACEI
- CCB

Post-myocardial
infarction
- β blockers
- ACEI
- Aldo ANT

Recurrent stroke
prevention
- Diuretic
- ACEI

Not at goal blood pressure

No response or troublesome side effects

Inadequate response, but well tolerated

Substitute another drug from
a different class

Add a second agent from a different
class (diuretic if not already used)

Not at goal blood pressure

Continue adding agents from other classes;
consider referral to a hypertension specialist

Figure 22-1 An algorithm for the management of hypertension. *ACEI,* Angiotensin-converting enzyme inhibitor; *aldo ANT,* aldosterone antagonists; *ARBs,* angiotensin II receptor blockers; *BB,* beta blocker; *CCB,* calcium channel blockers.

goal blood pressure is not achieved within a month of initiation of drug therapy, increase the dose of the initial antihypertensive or add on a second agent from the four preferred drug classes (ACEIs, ARBs, CCBs, and thiazide-type diuretics). If goal blood pressure is still not achieved, titrate up medication dosages and add a third antihypertensive agent. Antihypertensives from nonpreferred medication classes can be used if target blood pressure cannot be achieved despite use of three antihypertensives or in the presence of contraindications to preferred medication classes. In complicated patients or those in whom target blood pressure cannot be achieved, consider referral to a hypertension specialist.[4] An algorithm for the management of hypertension is depicted on Figure 22-1.

KEY POINT

When the cause is unknown, hypertension is termed *primary* or *essential* hypertension.

In almost all cases, the etiology of hypertension is unknown, and it is termed either *primary hypertension* or *essential hypertension*. The prevalence of secondary hypertension is less than 10%; secondary hypertension includes many disease-induced and drug-induced etiologies. Disease-induced causes of hypertension include Cushing syndrome, hyperparathyroidism, hyperthyroidism, pheochromocytoma, primary aldosteronism, and kidney disease. Drug-induced causes of hypertension include amphetamines, corticosteroids, cyclosporine, erythropoietin, estrogens, nonsteroidal antiinflammatory drugs (NSAIDs) including cyclooxygenase-1 inhibitors (e.g., ibuprofen and naproxen) and cyclooxygenase-2 inhibitors (e.g., celecoxib), pseudoephedrine, sibutramine, tacrolimus, venlafaxine, high sodium–containing over-the-counter (OTC) products (e.g., Alka-Seltzer effervescent antacid tablets), OTC weight loss products (e.g., ephedrine-containing diet pills), and chronic alcohol ingestion.[5,6]

Pathophysiology

KEY POINT

Arterial blood pressure is a product of systemic vascular resistance and cardiac output ([heart rate] × [stroke volume]).

Arterial blood pressure, termed *blood pressure*, is generated by the interplay between blood flow and the resistance to blood flow. Arterial blood pressure reaches a peak during cardiac systole and a nadir at the end of diastole. Arterial blood pressure is defined hemodynamically as the product of cardiac output (heart rate × stroke volume) and total peripheral resistance. Venous capacitance, which affects the volume of blood *(preload)*, is a major determinant of cardiac output and SBP. Arteriolar capacitance *(afterload)* is a major determinant of total peripheral resistance and DBP. Antihypertensives elicit actions on some or all of the hemodynamic parameters that define arterial blood pressure.

Hypertensive Crisis

KEY POINT

Hypertensive crisis is defined as systolic blood pressure (SBP) 180 mm Hg or greater and diastolic blood pressure (DBP) 120 mm Hg or greater, encompassing both hypertensive emergency and urgency.

A patient with blood pressure greater than 180/120 mm Hg is considered to be in a hypertensive crisis. A hypertensive crisis represents either a hypertensive urgency or a hypertensive emergency. A **hypertensive urgency** usually signifies high blood pressures without signs or symptoms of acute target organ complications; however, patients may present with severe headaches, shortness of breath, nosebleeds, or severe anxiety. In these situations, improvement in blood pressure control can be accomplished over a period of 24 to 48 hours.[7] Overaggressive use of intravenous drugs and oral medications can cause too rapid a decrease in blood pressure. Rapid decrease in blood pressure can result in hypoperfusion of organs such as the brain, kidneys, and heart. Oral antihypertensive agents such as captopril, clonidine, and labetalol are routinely used to manage hypertensive urgencies, followed by close observation for several hours. Patients can benefit from antihypertensive medication adjustments if they are found to be noncompliant with taking their medications.

A **hypertensive emergency** exists when the elevation of blood pressure is accompanied by acute progressing target organ injury. Examples of acute target organ injury include encephalopathy, intracranial hemorrhage, severe retinopathy, renal failure, unstable angina, acute left ventricular failure with pulmonary edema, dissecting aortic aneurysm, and eclampsia. Hypertensive emergencies require admission to an intensive care unit, invasive arterial blood pressure monitoring, and immediate but gradual blood pressure reduction over minutes to several hours with intravenous antihypertensives. The initial goal as outlined in JNC-VII is to reduce the mean arterial pressure (MAP) by no more than 25% within minutes to 1 hour after starting therapy. MAP can be calculated by adding one-third of the SBP to two-thirds of DBP:

$$([\tfrac{1}{3}\,SBP] + [\tfrac{2}{3}\,DBP]) = MAP$$

In the next 2 to 6 hours, the blood pressure must be gradually decreased to 160/100 to 160/110 mm Hg. If the decreased blood pressure is well tolerated by the patient, further reduction of blood pressure toward normal can be attempted over the next 24 to 48 hours. Recommendations differ for patients with ischemic stroke, patients with aortic dissection, and patients awaiting antithrombolytic therapies. Intravenous labetalol and nitroprusside can be used to manage most types of hypertensive emergencies. Depending on other comorbid conditions, alternative intravenous medications can be employed (e.g., nicardipine, esmolol, nitroglycerin, ACEI, and hydralazine). Nitroprusside at high doses or when used for long durations can cause methemoglobinemia. Classic methemoglobin blood is chocolate brown and is without color change despite exposure to air.

HYPERTENSION PHARMACOTHERAPY

KEY POINT

First-line drug groups used to treat hypertension include thiazide-type diuretics, angiotensin-converting enzyme inhibitors (ACEIs), angiotensin II receptor blockers (ARBs), and calcium channel blockers (CCBs).[4]

Angiotensin-Converting Enzyme Inhibitors

ACEIs act primarily through suppression of the renin-angiotensin-aldosterone system (RAAS). Because of a lack of renal blood flow, **renin** is released into the circulation, where it acts on angiotensinogen to produce angiotensin I. In the pulmonary vasculature, angiotensin I is converted by angiotensin-converting enzyme (ACE) to angiotensin II. Angiotensin II is a highly potent endogenous vasoconstrictor that also stimulates aldosterone secretion from the zona glomerulosa cells of the adrenal cortex, contributing to sodium and water retention.[8] Angiotensin II also stimulates the release of catecholamines from the adrenergic nerve endings and mediates the release of central sympathetic outflow. ACE is abundant in the endothelial cells of blood vessels and to a lesser extent in the kidneys.

ACEIs block the conversion of angiotensin I to angiotensin II by competing with the physiologic substrate angiotensin I for the active site of ACE (Figure 22-2). The affinity of ACEIs for ACE is approximately 30,000 times greater than for angiotensin I. ACEIs also inhibit kininase which is responsible for the degradation of bradykinin and other vasodilating substances, including prostaglandin E_2 (PGE_2) and prostacyclin (PGI_2), which enhances the antihypertensive effects of these drugs. Because ACEIs are potent antihypertensives in patients with low-renin hypertension, the effects on bradykinin may have an integral role in the mechanism of action of these agents. The hemodynamic effects of ACEIs are a reduction of peripheral arterial resistance, an increase in cardiac output, little or no change in heart rate, an increase in renal blood flow, and unchanged **glomerular filtration rate (GFR)**. ACEIs have mild antihyperlipidemic effects.

Ten ACEIs are available in the United States. ACEIs and ARBs are the preferred antihypertensives in the setting of CKD. ACEIs generally decrease SBP and DBP by 15% to 25%. ACEIs are most effective in normal-renin or high-renin hypertension; however, they are also effective in low-renin hypertension, especially when used at maximal doses. ACEIs are effective alone and in combination with other antihypertensive agents, especially thiazide-type diuretics.

ACEIs are homogeneous, which means there is very little variability among ACEIs in terms of efficacy and toxicity. In contrast to β blockers and thiazide diuretics, ACEIs do not induce glucose intolerance, hyperlipidemia, or hyperuricemia. With the exception of captopril, all ACEIs are generally administered once or twice daily. Enalaprilat is the only available parenteral ACEI. Table 22-3 presents the pharmacokinetics and dosage guidelines for ACEIs.[5]

The most common adverse effect associated with ACEIs is a persistent nonproductive dry cough (20% to 30%). The cough may be due to ACEI-induced accumulation of kinins, prostaglandins, or substance P in the respiratory tract. The cough may develop within days to 1 year after the start of therapy. Antitussives are ineffective in relieving ACEI-induced cough. Cross-reactivity among the ACEIs is absolute; however, ARBs rarely cause cough and may be considered an alternative. ACEI-induced rash is also

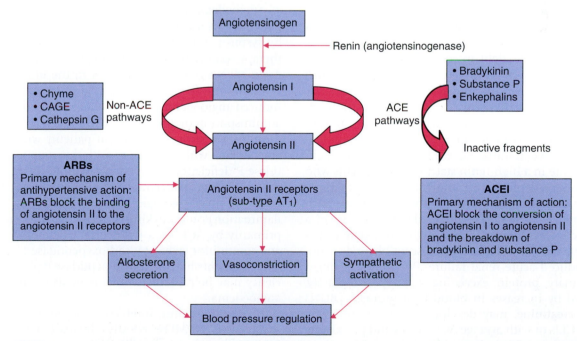

Figure 22-2 Angiotensin II formation and actions. *ACE*, Angiotensin-converting enzyme; *ACEI*, angiotensin-converting enzyme inhibitor; *ARBs*, angiotensin II receptor blockers; *AT₁*, angiotensin II type 1; *CAGE*, chymostatin-sensitive angiotensin II–generating enzyme.

TABLE 22-3   Pharmacokinetics and Dosage Guidelines for Angiotensin-Converting Enzyme Inhibitors

ACEI GENERIC NAME (BRAND NAME)	ACTIVE METABOLITE	ELIMINATION TOTAL	HALF-LIFE OF PARENT DRUG (hr)*	DURATION OF ACTION (hr)	DOSAGE RANGE (mg/day)	DAILY FREQUENCY	EFFECT OF FOOD ON ABSORPTION
Benazepril (Lotensin)	Benazeprilat	11%-12% bile	22	24+	5-80	1	Slightly reduced
Captopril (Capoten)	None	95% urine	2	6-10	12.5-450	2-4	Reduced by 30%-40%
Enalapril (Vasotec)	Enalaprilat	94% urine and feces	11	24	2.5-40	1-2	None
Enalaprilat (Vasotec IV)	None	No data	35		1.25-5	Every 6 hr	NA
Fosinopril (Monopril)	Fosinoprilat	50% urine, 50% feces	12-15	24	10-80	1	Slightly reduced
Lisinopril (Prinivil; Zestril)	None	29% urine, 69% feces, 2% unchanged	13	24	10-40	1	None
Moexipril (Univasc)	Moexiprilat	13% urine, 53% feces	2-9	24	7.5-30	1-2	Markedly reduced
Quinapril (Accupril)	Quinaprilat	60% urine, 37% feces	2-3	24+	20-80	1-2	Reduced
Perindopril (Aceon)	Perindoprilat	96%-78% bile, 4%-12% urine	0.8-1	24	4-16	1	Reduced
Ramipril (Altace)	Ramiprilat	60% urine, 40% feces	11-17	24+	2.5-20	1-2	Slightly reduced
Trandolapril (Mavik)	Trandolaprilat	33% urine, 56% feces	24	24+	1-4	1	Reduced

NA, Not applicable.

*Assuming normal renal function.

common; the incidence is 10%, and the reaction is usually transient. The rash often occurs in the upper extremities and is often accompanied by pruritus and erythema. A higher incidence of rash with captopril relative to other ACEIs may be due to the sulfhydryl-containing structure of captopril. All other ACEIs, with the exception of fosinopril (phosphorus-containing), possess a dicarbocyl group. ACEIs are known to cause dysgeusia (6%), manifesting as a metallic or salty taste or loss of taste perception.

ACEIs may cause a slight increase in potassium that is generally inconsequential. The risk of hyperkalemia may be increased with concomitant use of β blockers, heparin, low-molecular-weight heparin (LMWH), trimethoprim, amiloride, spironolactone, and salt substitutes, and in patients with diabetes or renal failure. Orthostatic hypotension is common when initiating ACEI therapy, especially in patients who are in a high-renin state, such as patients who are salt or volume depleted (e.g., patients with heart failure, cirrhosis, or diabetes, or receiving diuretics). Patients with bilateral renal artery stenosis, with unilateral stenosis of a solitary functioning kidney, or in a high-renin state (especially patients with heart failure) are susceptible to developing ACEI-induced acute renal failure. Proteinuria, defined as total urinary protein exceeding 1 g/day and, rarely, accompanied by increases in blood urea nitrogen (BUN) and serum creatinine, may develop in patients receiving high-dose ACEIs or with average ACEI doses and preexisting renal dysfunction. ACEI-induced blood dyscrasias such as neutropenia and agranulocytopenia occur with an incidence of less than 1% and are more common in patients

with connective tissue diseases (e.g., systemic lupus erythematosus). ACEIs should be avoided in women of childbearing age because of the potential for fetal and neonatal morbidity and mortality in the second and third trimesters of pregnancy manifesting as skull hypoplasia, hypotension, anuria, and death (pregnancy category D).

Angioedema is rare, occurring in about 1 to 5 of 1000 patients, but it can be life-threatening when accompanied by dyspnea. Angioedema can occur at any time during ACEI therapy, especially when starting and stopping regimens. Angioedema generally manifests in the upper extremities, primarily the face, lips, tongue, glottis, and larynx. ACEI-induced angioedema is an absolute contraindication for the administration of alternative ACEIs and a relative contraindication for ARBs, especially in patients with a history of angioedema with dyspnea or with documented aminopeptidase P deficiency. Angioedema symptoms may be associated with high concentrations of bradykinin. Bradykinin exerts its pharmacologic effects (vasodilation and proinflammation) on bradykinin-2 receptors and is metabolized primarily by ACE, to a lesser extent by aminopeptidase P, and to a minor extent by carboxypeptidase N. Delineating which patients have an aminopeptidase P plasma level deficiency may help predict which patients are predisposed to angioedema.

A significant drug interaction occurs when combining ACEIs with NSAIDs. NSAIDs increase renin release by inhibiting renal vasodilating prostaglandins (PGE$_2$ and PGI$_2$), therefore blunting or negating the antihypertensive effects of ACEIs. NSAIDs less likely to reduce renal prostaglandins and to minimize or circumvent the interaction with ACEIs are sulindac (Clinoril), nabumetone (Relafen), etodolac (Lodine), salsalate (Disalcid), and choline magnesium trisalicylate (Trilisate). ACEIs may increase lithium concentrations and have been associated with life-threatening lithium toxicity. ACEI-induced renal sodium depletion may increase lithium renal tubule reabsorption. Patients receiving this combination should be monitored for symptoms of lithium toxicity such as nausea, vomiting, diarrhea, tremor, and mental status changes. Lithium levels should be monitored before and after initiating the ACEI. A quinapril tablet, in contrast to other ACEIs, contains magnesium carbonate at sufficient concentration to reduce tetracycline absorption by 40%. The mechanism of this interaction may be chelation and plausibly may occur with quinolones. To circumvent this interaction, quinapril administration should be spaced 2 to 6 hours apart from tetracycline and quinolone antimicrobials.

Angiotensin II Receptor Blockers

Several nonrenin and nonACE pathways are used for the production of angiotensin II (see Figure 22-2). Nonrenin pathways generate angiotensin II from angiotensinogen via tissue plasminogen activator, cathepsin G, and tonin. NonACE enzymes that generate angiotensin II from angiotensin I are cathepsin G, chymostatin-sensitive angiotensin II–generating enzyme, and chymase. ACEIs incompletely block the synthesis of angiotensin II. ARBs are angiotensin II type 1 (AT_1) receptor antagonists. AT_1 receptors are found in many tissues, such as adrenal glands (cortex and medulla); vascular smooth muscle; and brain, kidney, liver, uterus, and myocardial tissue. Many tissues also have an angiotensin II type 2 (AT_2) receptor; however, it is not known to have effects on myocardial hemostasis. ARBs have 1000-fold greater affinity for AT_1 receptors than AT_2 receptors and generally do not block the AT_2 receptor. Because ARBs do not inhibit ACE, they do not interfere with the concentrations of bradykinins and substance

P. This kinin-sparing effect may explain why ARBs have a low incidence of inducing cough or angioedema. However, the beneficial effects of kinins, including blood pressure–lowering potency, may be sacrificed.

Eight ARBs are available in the United States. ARBs are indicated for hypertension and can be used to treat heart failure. ARBs have been shown to reduce morbidity, such as target organ damage (e.g., nephropathy) in patients with hypertension, cardiovascular events in patients with systolic heart failure, and progression of nephropathy in patients with type 2 diabetes. In black patients, ARBs and ACEIs may be less potent antihypertensives; however, this can be circumvented by administering maximal doses.

Compared with ACEIs, ARBs are considered as potent or slightly weaker antihypertensive agents. The inhibition of bradykinin by ACEIs may account for its augmented antihypertensive effect. Angiotensin II receptor blockers arguably are considered second-line agents to ACEIs for hypertension and heart failure and are indicated when ACEI-induced cough or other adverse effects are intolerable. Both ACEIs and ARBs are considered first-line agents for hypertension in nonblack patients and in patients with CKD, regardless of race (JNC8).[4] However, ARBs may be considered superior to ACEIs in patients with type 2 diabetic nephropathy. ARBs are administered once or twice daily. Using the combination of an ACEI and an ARB has not been well studied; however, its beneficial effects have been observed in patients with heart failure and nephrotic syndrome. Table 22-4 presents the pharmacokinetics and dosage guidelines for ARBs.[5,6,8]

The side effect profile of ARBs seems to be similar to that of ACEIs. ARBs may cause orthostatic hypotension, hyperkalemia, neutropenia, nephrotoxicity, and fetotoxicity. Similar warnings and precautions exhibited with ACEIs should be undertaken for ARBs. ARBs can cause cough; however, the incidence is significantly less than with ACEIs. ARBs cause significantly less angioedema than ACEIs; cross-reactivity has been reported. ARBs are not absolutely contraindicated in ACEI-induced angioedema; however, their

TABLE 22-4	Pharmacokinetics and Dosage Guidelines for Angiotensin II Receptor Blockers				
ARB GENERIC NAME (BRAND NAME)	**ELIMINATION**	**TERMINAL HALF-LIFE (hr)**	**DOSAGE RANGE (mg/day)**	**DAILY FREQUENCY**	**EFFECT OF FOOD ON ABSORPTION**
Azilsartan (Edarbi)	55% in feces and 42% in urine	11	40-80	1	No effect
Candesartan (Atacand)	Ester hydrolysis/ O-deethylation	9	8-32	1-2	No effect
Eprosartan (Teveten)	80% unchanged, 20% acyl glucuronide	5-9	400-800	1-2	No effect
Irbesartan (Avapro)	CYP2C9, CYP3A4	11-15	150-300	1	No effect
Losartan (Cozaar)	CYP2C9, CYP3A4	2	25-100	1-2	Slightly reduced
Olmesartan (Benicar)	35%-50% in urine and remainder in feces	13	20-40	1	No effect
Telmisartan (Micardis)	Conjugation to acyl glucuronide	24	20-80	1	Slightly reduced
Valsartan (Diovan)	Biliary metabolism	6	80-320	1	Markedly reduced

CYP, Cytochrome P450.

use in this setting can be dangerous and should be avoided. Rash and dysgeusia are rarely reported with ARBs.

Losartan is extensively metabolized by the hepatic cytochrome P450 (CYP) 3A4 and CYP2C9 isoenzymes to an active carboxylic acid metabolite that is predominantly responsible for the AT_1 blockade and antihypertensive effects of losartan. Drugs that induce these enzyme systems (e.g., phenytoin, phenobarbital, carbamazepine, oxcarbazepine, rifampin, and rifabutin) may increase the antihypertensive effects of losartan by increasing the concentration of the active metabolite. Phenobarbital has been shown to decrease the levels of losartan and its metabolite by 20%. Conversely, drugs that inhibit CYP3A4 (e.g., ketoconazole, fluconazole, erythromycin, clarithromycin, fluoxetine, and amiodarone) or CYP2C9 (e.g., amiodarone, cimetidine, and fluoxetine) or CYP3A4 and CYP2C9 simultaneously (e.g., fluoxetine, amiodarone) may decrease the antihypertensive effects of losartan by decreasing the concentration of the active metabolite. However, a study evaluating the effects of cimetidine (CYP3A4 and CYP2C9 inhibitor) on losartan did not yield any changes in the disposition of losartan's carboxylic acid metabolite.

Telmisartan has been shown to increase digoxin peak plasma concentrations by 50%. Digoxin serum concentrations should be monitored before and after the addition of telmisartan. Several mechanistically similar drug-drug interactions that occur with ACEIs are likely to occur with ARBs, such as with NSAIDs and lithium.

Direct Renin Inhibitors

DRIs act by inhibiting renin, the enzyme that is the first step of the RAAS (see Figure 22-2). Renin is responsible for the conversion of angiotensinogen to angiotensin I, which is the rate-limiting step in RAAS. Renin inhibition also leads to decreased formation of angiotensin II and aldosterone. However, all agents that inhibit the RAAS, such as ACEIs, have the potential to inhibit feedback inhibition of renin, leading to increases in renin and its activity. This effect can be blocked with the use of a renin inhibitor. DRIs can be used alone or in combination with other antihypertensive agents.

Aliskiren (Tekturna) is currently the only DRI available on the market. It is indicated only for the treatment of hypertension. Similar to ACEIs and ARBs, aliskiren is considered a poor antihypertensive agent for black patients. In addition, no studies show that aliskiren is effective in reducing cardiovascular risk. It can be used in combination with any other antihypertensive agents, but it has been studied most comprehensively in combination with ARBs and diuretics.

The most common side effects observed with aliskiren include diarrhea, headache, dizziness, fatigue, upper respiratory tract infection, nasopharyngitis, and back pain. Aliskiren can also cause dry cough, but its incidence is much less than that reported with ACEIs. Similar to other agents that affect the RAAS, aliskiren has been associated with angioedema, and has occurred in patients with and without a history of angioedema with ACEI or ARB therapy. Aliskiren possibly may be fetotoxic and is not recommended for use in pregnant patients (pregnancy category D). Rare side effects include increased uric acid levels, renal stones, anemia, rash, renal impairment, myositis, and rhabdomyolysis. Aliskiren monotherapy has a low incidence of hyperkalemia; however, hyperkalemia occurs more frequently when aliskiren is used in combination with ACEIs. It should be used cautiously in combination with other agents that cause hyperkalemia, such as potassium-sparing diuretics and sulfamethoxazole-trimethoprim (Bactrim). Aliskiren is contraindicated in diabetic patients using an ACEI or ARB.

Aliskiren is administered once daily at a dose of 150 to 300 mg. It has very poor oral bioavailability; only about 2.5% is absorbed. Absorption of aliskiren is substantially decreased by high fatty meals; patients should always take it the same way: either with or without food. It undergoes minimal hepatic metabolism by CYP3A4. Cyclosporine and itraconazole, which are potent inhibitors of CYP3A4, were shown to increase aliskiren levels significantly and should not be used concomitantly. Other CYP3A4 inhibitors were also shown to increase aliskiren levels, but the clinical significance of their interaction is unknown. Aliskiren has also been shown to reduce the effectiveness of furosemide by 30% to 50%. The effectiveness of furosemide should be monitored when these two agents are used concomitantly. Approximately 25% of the absorbed dose is excreted unchanged in the urine. Most of the unabsorbed drug is excreted in the feces. No dosage adjustments are recommended at this time in patients with renal or hepatic impairment.[9,10]

Calcium Channel Blockers

Vascular smooth muscle and cardiac cell contraction depends on free intracellular calcium ion concentration. Calcium enters vascular smooth muscle cells, myocardial cells, and pacemaker cells through voltage-gated L-type and T-type calcium channels. L-channel blockade mediates coronary and peripheral vasodilation and may cause reflex sympathetic activation or a negative inotropic effect. T-channel blockade also mediates coronary and peripheral vasodilation but is devoid of a reflex sympathetic activation. The influx of calcium from extracellular fluid into cells triggers a second messenger, *inositol triphosphate,* to release stored intracellular calcium from the sarcoplasmic reticulum. This increase in cytosolic calcium results in enhanced binding to the protein *calmodulin.* A calcium-calmodulin complex activates myosin kinase, promoting the interaction between actin and myosin, culminating in cellular contraction. Conventional CCBs inhibit only L-channels. The pharmacodynamic effects of the calcium antagonists on smooth muscle, myocardium, or specialized conduction and pacemaker tissues differ among the agents because of different receptor distribution and densities and the drug's inherent receptor selectivity and affinity.

Nondihydropyridine CCBs include verapamil and diltiazem. Verapamil and to a lesser extent diltiazem possess negative **chronotropic** effects by lowering sinoatrial (SA) node automaticity and decreasing atrioventricular (AV) node conduction; these agents are indicated for the treatment of angina and arrhythmias in addition to hypertension. Verapamil and to a lesser extent diltiazem are also potent negative **inotropes** and may exacerbate heart failure, and should be avoided in patients with severe left ventricular dysfunction.

Dihydropyridine CCBs are potent vasodilators; these agents include amlodipine, felodipine, isradipine, nicardipine, nifedipine, and nisoldipine. With the exception of nifedipine, dihydropyridine CCBs have negligible chronotropic effects. Immediate-release nifedipine, especially when administered as a liquid, causes a potent reflex tachycardia that increases coronary oxygen demand and has been implicated with an increased risk of MI and stroke. Only sustained-release dosage forms of nifedipine are indicated for hypertension.[11] Amlodipine and plausibly felodipine may be used in patients with heart failure because these agents do not decrease cardiac contractility. CCBs are very effective antihypertensive agents in both elderly and black patients. Table 22-5 presents the pharmacokinetics and dose guidelines for calcium antagonists.[4,5,6]

Verapamil (e.g., Covera-HS, Verelan PM) and diltiazem (Cardizem LA) have long-acting formulations that are specifically designed to target the **circadian rhythm** of blood pressure throughout the day. Many hypertensive patients have a catecholamine surge with a blood pressure peak in the morning between 6 AM and 12 PM, followed by sustained high (but lower than the peak) blood pressures throughout the day and a nadir at night. Most MIs, strokes, dysrhythmias, and venous thromboembolic events occur in the morning hours, in concert with the circadian blood pressure peaks. CCB formulations are generally designed to be administered at bedtime and begin to release medication in the early morning to achieve a peak effect in the morning hours and a sustained effect during the day.

These novel circadian dosage forms may have limited utility in hypertensive patients who do not have a nadir in blood pressure in the nighttime, or "nondippers." These formulations leave patients unprotected with a high risk of a coronary event and have not been shown to have better effects on morbidity compared with thiazides and β blockers. Typical hypertensive nondippers (no nighttime nadir) are elderly patients, patients with renal insufficiency, and patients with secondary hypertension. Both verapamil and diltiazem are available in several immediate, extended, and sustained release products. The different dosage

TABLE 22-5   Pharmacokinetics and Dosage Guidelines for Calcium Channel Blockers

CALCIUM ANTAGONIST GENERIC NAME (BRAND NAME)	ONSET OF ACTION OF ORAL DOSE FORMS (hr)	HALF-LIFE (hr)	DOSAGE RANGE (mg/day)	DAILY FREQUENCY
Nondihydropyridines				
Verapamil (Calan, Isoptin)	0.5	3-7	180-480	3-4
Verapamil SR (Calan SR, Isoptin SR)	0.5	3-7	120-480	1-2
Verapamil ER (Covera-HS)	4-5	2.8-7.4	180-420	Once at bedtime
Verapamil chronotherapeutic oral drug absorption (Verelan PM)	4-5	3-7	100-400	Once at bedtime
Diltiazem (Cardizem)	0.5	3.5	90-360	3-4
Diltiazem ER capsules (Cardizem CD, Cartia XT, Dilacor XR, Diltia XT, Tiazac, Taztia XT)	1	5	90-540	1-2
Diltiazem ER tablets (Cardizem LA)	3-4	6-9	120-540	Once daily (morning or evening)
Dihydropyridines				
Amlodipine (Norvasc)	6-12	30-50	2.5-10	1
Felodipine (Plendil)	2-5	11-16	5-20	1
Isradipine (DynaCirc)	2	8	2.5-10	2
Isradipine CR (DynaCirc CR)	2	8	2.5-10	1
Nicardipine (Cardene)	20 min	2-4	60-120	3
Nicardipine SR (Cardene SR)	20 min	2-4	60-120	2
Nifedipine (Adalat, Procardia)*	20 min	2-5	30-120	3-4
Nifedipine LA (Adalat CC, Procardia XL)	20 min	7	30-120	1
Nimodipine (Nimotop)†	ND	1-2	360	Every 4 hr for 21 days
Nisoldipine (Sular)	ND	7-12	20-60	1

CC, Coat core; *CD,* controlled delivery; *CR,* controlled release; *ER,* extended release; *HS,* half strength; *LA,* long acting; *SR,* sustained release; *XL, XR,* extended release; *XT,* extended technology.
*Nifedipine (prompt release) is not indicated for hypertension.
†Indicated for subarachnoid hemorrhage, not hypertension.

formulations of the same drug, with or without circadian effects, are usually not interchangeable and should not be switched on a milligram-to-milligram basis.

The incidence of verapamil-induced and to a lesser extent diltiazem-induced constipation is high and often necessitates the use of a stimulant laxative such as bisacodyl or sennosides. Dihydropyridines have potent peripheral vasodilating effects, and they have a high incidence of palpitations, orthostatic hypotension, flushing, headaches, lightheadedness, and syncope. These adverse effects are minimized with long-acting agents. All CCBs may cause peripheral edema, gingival hyperplasia, and gastroesophageal reflux (except diltiazem). CCB-induced peripheral edema does not respond to diuretic therapy and requires discontinuation of the offending agent.

Diltiazem and verapamil inhibit CYP3A4 metabolism and plausibly the P-glycoprotein (P-gp) transport of alfentanil, buspirone, carbamazepine, cyclosporine, digoxin, lovastatin, methylprednisolone, quinidine, simvastatin, and tacrolimus, resulting in higher serum levels and potential toxicity. Verapamil and diltiazem inhibit the hepatic metabolism of theophylline. Although dihydropyridine CCBs are not inhibitors of CYP3A4, they are major substrates of CYP3A4 and may result in significant drug and food interactions through competitive inhibition. Grapefruit juice inhibits the CYP3A4 in the gut and may increase significantly the levels of felodipine, nifedipine, and nisoldipine. Because many CCBs are significantly metabolized by the CYP system, CYP enzyme inducers, such as carbamazepine, oxcarbazepine, phenobarbital, phenytoin, and rifampin, may lower the serum concentrations of CCBs and compromise efficacy.

β Blockers

The antihypertensive effects of β blockers have multiple mechanisms of action and are as follows:

- Blockade of the β receptors on the renal juxtaglomerular cells, leading to renin blockade and decreased angiotensin II concentrations
- Blockade of myocardial β receptors, leading to decreased cardiac contractility and heart rate, diminishing cardiac output
- Blockade of central nervous system (CNS) β receptors, leading to decreased sympathetic output from the CNS and plausibly blockade of peripheral β receptors, decreasing norepinephrine concentrations

β Blockers cannot be used interchangeably with each other. Instead, disease state guidelines dictate which β blockers to use for each comorbidity. β Blockers with **intrinsic sympathomimetic activity (ISA)**, including acebutolol, carteolol, penbutolol, and pindolol, cause less reduction of resting heart rate, cardiac output, and peripheral blood flow. ISA may be beneficial in patients with stable angina, bradyarrhythmias, compromised pulmonary function, and peripheral vascular (arterial) disease. Labetalol is an α and β blocker with weak β₂ ISA; nevertheless, it is relatively

contraindicated in patients with asthma and chronic obstructive pulmonary disease. Labetalol is indicated for hypertension and is often used to manage hypertensive urgencies (oral formulation) and hypertensive emergencies (parenteral formulation). The α and β blocker carvedilol is indicated for patients with hypertension and for patients with mild to moderate heart failure.

Nebivolol (Bystolic), is a highly cardioselective third-generation β_1 blocker that also exhibits vasodilatory properties mediated through nitric oxide, resulting in decreased peripheral vascular resistance, increased stroke volume, and preserved cardiac output. It is approximately three times more β_1-selective than bisoprolol. It is indicated for the treatment of hypertension and has similar blood pressure reduction effects as atenolol, bisoprolol, ACEIs, ARBs, and CCBs.

β Blockers are indicated for hypertension, angina pectoris, cardiac dysrhythmias, secondary prevention of MI, chronic heart failure, and pheochromocytoma. β Blockers are no longer considered first-line agents in treatment of essential hypertension but should be reserved as add-on therapy to other antihypertensive agents. β Blockers are also used for migraine prophylaxis, hypertrophic subaortic stenosis, tremors, alcohol withdrawal syndrome, prophylaxis of esophageal variceal rebleeding, anxiety, symptoms of thyrotoxicosis, and in combination with α blockers for pheochromocytoma. Table 22-6 presents the pharmacokinetics and dose guidelines for β blockers.[4,7,6,9]

β Blockers increase triglycerides and decrease high-density lipoproteins; however, this deleterious effect may diminish after prolonged therapy (1 year). β Blockers may cause hyperglycemia and glucose intolerance. These agents can be especially dangerous in diabetics because they mask some of the common symptoms of hypoglycemia, such as palpitations, tremors, and hunger. The use of β blockers in patients with hyperlipidemia or diabetes is acceptable if the lipid and glucose profiles are closely monitored. α and β Blockers and agents with ISA are less likely to affect the lipid and glucose profiles adversely.

β Blocker–induced pulmonary dysfunction may manifest as bronchospasm, bronchial obstruction, wheezing, dyspnea, cough, and exacerbation of previously stable asthma or chronic airway obstruction. Agents with β_1 selectivity, such as atenolol and metoprolol, are less likely to cause pulmonary dysfunction; however, they lose their selectivity with increasing doses. β-Blocking agents may exacerbate intermittent claudication and Raynaud phenomenon, and they may cause CNS disturbances, such as vertigo, tiredness, fatigue, somnolence, mental depression, and nightmares. A correlation between the individual lipid solubility of a β blocker and its ability to penetrate the blood-brain barrier and cause CNS adverse effects may exist. Consequently, agents with high lipophilicity, such as propranolol and penbutolol, have a high incidence of CNS adverse effects. β Blockers should not be discontinued abruptly because this causes a rebound (pretreatment blood pressure) or overshoot (blood pressure higher than pretreatment) hypertension; the drug should be

TABLE 22-6   Pharmacokinetics and Dosage Guidelines for β Blockers

β BLOCKER GENERIC NAME (BRAND NAME)	α BLOCKADE	β₁ SELECTIVITY	ISA	LIPID SOLUBILITY	HALF-LIFE (hr)	DOSAGE RANGE (mg)	DAILY FREQUENCY
Acebutolol (Sectral)	0	+	+	Low	3-4	200-200	2
Atenolol (Tenormin)	0	+	0	Low	6-9	25-100	1
Betaxolol (Kerlone)	0	+	0	Low	14-24	5-20	1
Bisoprolol (Zebeta)	0	++	+	Low	9-12	25-200	1
Carteolol (Cartrol)	0	0	+	Low	6	2.5-10	1
Carvedilol (Coreg)	+	0	0	High	7-10	6.25-50	2
Labetalol (Trandate, Normodyne)	+	0	0	Moderate	3-5	100-2400	2
Metoprolol (Lopressor)	0	+	0	Moderate	3-5	50-200	1-2
Metoprolol ER (Toprol-XL)	0	+	0	Moderate	3-7	25-200	1
Nadolol (Corgard)	0	0	0	Low	14-24	20-240	1
Nebivolol (Bystolic)	0	+++	?	Low	11-30	5-40	1
Penbutolol (Levatol)	0	0	+	High	5	20-80	1
Pindolol (Visken)	0	0	+++	Moderate	3-4	10-60	2
Propranolol (Inderal)	0	0	0	High	4-6	40-240	2
Propranolol LA (Inderal, InnoPran XL)	0	0	0	High	8-10	80-640	1
Timolol (Blocadren)	0	0	0	Low	3-4	20-40	2

ER, Extended release; *ISA*, intrinsic sympathomimetic activity; *LA*, long acting; *XL*, extended release; *0*, none; +, ++, +++, equals higher degree.

tapered slowly over 1 to 2 weeks before discontinuing entirely.

Several β blockers, including carvedilol, metoprolol, nebivolol, propranolol, and timolol, are CYP2D6 substrates. Fluoxetine, paroxetine, and sertraline are potent CYP2D6 inhibitors and may significantly increase the effect of the substrate β blocker. Because almost all β blockers are significantly metabolized by the CYP system, CYP enzyme inducers, such as cigarettes and marijuana, carbamazepine, oxcarbazepine, phenobarbital, phenytoin, and rifampin, may lower serum concentrations of β blockers and compromise efficacy. Atenolol is almost entirely renally eliminated and may be used as an alternative to β blockers that interact via hepatic mechanisms or in patients with liver disease.

Diuretics

Diuretics are divided into the following five classes:

1. Thiazides and thiazide-like agents
2. Loop diuretics
3. Potassium-sparing agents
4. Carbonic anhydrase inhibitors (CAIs) (e.g., acetazolamide [Diamox])
5. Osmotics (e.g., mannitol)

Thiazides are used primarily as a first line for the management of hypertension in nonblack patients without comorbidities.[4] Thiazides, loop diuretics (except ethacrynic acid), and CAIs are sulfonamide-containing agents and may cross-react in patients who have a history of sulfonamide allergy. Sulfonamide-containing agents include sulfonylurea antidiabetics, silver sulfadiazine, tamsulosin, celecoxib, and probenecid. A significant drug-drug interaction occurs when combining diuretics with NSAIDs and combining sodium-depleting diuretics with lithium. The mechanisms of these interactions are similar to the mechanisms of ACEIs and have been discussed previously in this chapter.

Potassium-Sparing Diuretics

Potassium-sparing agents are weak hypotensive agents when used alone, but they provide an additive hypotensive effect when used in combination with thiazide diuretics. The two agents used clinically are amiloride (Midamor) and triamterene (Dyrenium). These agents are employed primarily for their antikaliuretic effects, which offset the potassium excretion effects of other diuretics. These agents work by blocking sodium channels in the luminal membrane of cells in the distal tubule and collecting duct, attenuating the excretion of potassium, calcium, and magnesium. Both hypokalemia and hypomagnesemia have been implicated as a cause of cardiac arrhythmias; there is an advantage to adding these agents to diuretic antihypertensive therapy. The magnesium-sparing effects of potassium-sparing diuretics may be an added benefit compared with a diuretic plus a potassium supplement.

Both potassium-sparing diuretics can cause gastrointestinal side effects, such as dyspepsia, abdominal cramps, nausea, and diarrhea; CNS side effects, such as mental confusion, lethargy, headache, and dizziness; and hematologic, dermatologic, and musculoskeletal (leg cramps) adverse effects. Triamterene has been associated with interstitial nephritis and nephrolithiases; the incidence may be 1 in 200. Triamterene is photosensitizing, which may be additive when combined with phototoxic sulfonamide-containing thiazide diuretics. Triamterene may cause hyperuricemia and hyperglycemia.

Thiazide and Thiazide-Like Diuretics

Thiazide diuretics increase sodium and chloride excretion by interfering with their reabsorption in the distal tubule; a mild diuresis of slightly concentrated urine results. Excretion of potassium, bicarbonate, magnesium, phosphate, and iodide is also increased, whereas calcium excretion is decreased. Although thiazides decrease extracellular fluid volume, antihypertensive activity is caused primarily by direct vasodilation. Thiazides are indicated for hypertension, chronic edema, chronic heart failure, and ascites. Thiazides generally take 2 to 4 weeks to elicit their full pharmacologic effect. Thiazides have a **dose-ceiling effect**, at which point the antihypertensive effects do not increase despite dose increases; however, the toxic effects do *not* have a dose-ceiling effect.

Because thiazides cause hypercalcemia, they may be a useful adjunct in the management and prevention of osteoporosis. Although chlorthalidone, indapamide, and metolazone do not possess the benzothiadiazine structure, pharmacologically they act like thiazide diuretics—they are thiazide-like in structure and activity. Thiazide diuretics lose their antihypertensive potency in patients with a **creatinine clearance (CrCl)** less than 30 mL/min. Indapamide retains its potency, however, in patients with a CrCl greater than 15 mL/min. Metolazone is the only thiazide-like diuretic that retains potency in patients with a CrCl less than 15 mL/min. Despite the thiazide-like structure of metolazone, its pharmacologic effects are similar to those of loop diuretics. Metolazone is often added to a loop diuretic in patients with diuretic resistance, achieving a synergistic diuretic effect. Mykrox tablets are a formulation of metolazone with a higher bioavailability than conventional metolazone, resulting in a more rapid diuretic effect; Mykrox is not therapeutically equivalent to Zaroxolyn. Table 22-7 presents the pharmacokinetics and dose guidelines for thiazide and thiazidelike diuretics.[4,5,6]

Common side effects observed with thiazide and thiazide-like diuretics include hypokalemia, hypomagnesemia, hypercalcemia, hyperuricemia, hyperglycemia, hyperlipidemia, and sexual dysfunction. These abnormalities are dose-related and may be minimized by using low-dose agents such as chlorthalidone, 12.5 to 25 mg daily, or hydrochlorothiazide, 12.5 mg twice daily. Less common thiazide-induced adverse effects include dyspepsia, rashes, photosensitivity, thrombocytopenia, and pancreatitis.

Loop Diuretics

Loop diuretics, often referred to as *high-ceiling diuretics*, act principally at the thick ascending limb of the loop of Henle, where they decrease sodium reabsorption by competing for the chloride site on the Na^+-K^+-$2Cl^-$ symporter (a transport molecule). Excretion of sodium, chloride, potassium, hydrogen ion, calcium, magnesium, ammonium, bicarbonate, and possibly phosphate is enhanced. Diuretics such as thiazides have a limited diuretic potency with a plateau effect because they act primarily at sites past the ascending limb; only a small percentage of the filtered load reaches these more distal sites. Because more than 25% of the filtered load is reabsorbed in the ascending limb, loop diuretics are highly efficacious with increasing doses, and this is why they are termed high-ceiling diuretics.

Loop diuretics are indicated for chronic heart failure, ascites with or without hepatic cirrhosis, renal failure, pulmonary edema, hypercalcemia, hypermagnesemia, and syndrome of inappropriate antidiuretic hormone. Loop diuretics are second-line diuretics in the management of hypertension; however, they are superior to thiazide diuretics in diuresis and decreasing blood pressure for patients with renal insufficiency. Table 22-8 presents the pharmacokinetics and dose guidelines for oral loop diuretics.[4,5,6]

Loop diuretics are very potent and consequently may cause severe dehydration, hypotension, hypochloremic alkalosis, and hypokalemia. Loop diuretics should not be administered at bedtime because the patient will have to urinate frequently, causing sleep disturbances. Loop diuretics may cause hyperglycemia (not reported with bumetanide), hyperuricemia, dyspepsia, photosensitivity, and ototoxicity. Ethacrynic acid is the most auditory ototoxic loop diuretic and should be considered only for patients refractory to other loop diuretics or when there is a history of a life-threatening sulfonamide allergy.

TABLE 22-7   Pharmacokinetics and Dosage Guidelines for Thiazides and Thiazide-Like Diuretics

THIAZIDE/THIAZIDE-LIKE DIURETIC GENERIC NAME (BRAND NAME)	BIOAVAILABILITY	PEAK EFFECT (hr)	DURATION OF DIURESIS (hr)	HALF-LIFE (hr)	DOSAGE RANGE (mg/day)	DAILY FREQUENCY
Chlorothiazide (Diuril)	10-20	2 (PO), 0.5 (IV)	6-12 (PO), 2 (IV)	1-2	500-2000	1-2
Chlorthalidone (Hygroton)	65	2	24-72	35-55	15-200	1
Hydrochlorothiazide (Esidrix, HydroDIURIL, Oretic, Microzide)	65-75	4-6	6-12	2.5-4.5	25-100	1-3
Indapamide (Lozol)	95	2	24-36	14-18	1.25-5	1
Metolazone (Zaroxolyn)	65	2	12-24	6-20	5-20	1
Metolazone (Mykrox)		2-4	12-24	14	0.5-1	1

IV, Administered intravenously; *PO*, administered orally.

TABLE 22-8   Pharmacokinetics and Dosage Guidelines for Oral Loop Diuretics

LOOP DIURETIC GENERIC NAME (BRAND NAME)	BIOAVAILABILITY (%)	ONSET (hr)	DURATION (hr)	HALF-LIFE (hr)	DOSAGE RANGE (mg/day)	DAILY FREQUENCY
Bumetanide (Bumex)	70-95	0.5-1	5-6	0.8 ±0.2	0.5-10	1
Ethacrynic acid (Edecrin)	100	0.5	6-8	2-4	50-200	1-2
Furosemide (Lasix)	60	0.5-1	6-8	0.5-1.1	40-240	1-2
Torsemide (Demadex)	80	0.5-1	1	2-4	5-200	1

TABLE 22-9   Pharmacokinetics and Dosage Guidelines for Aldosterone Antagonists

ALDOSTERONE ANTAGONIST GENERIC NAME (BRAND NAME)	ACTIVE METABO-LITE	ELIMINA-TION TOTAL	ONSET OF ACTION (hr)	PEAK RESPONSE	DURATION OF ACTION (hr)	HALF-LIFE OF PARENT DRUG (hr)	DOSAGE RANGE (mg/day)	DAILY FRE-QUENCY	EFFECT OF FOOD ON ABSORP-TION
Spironolactone (Aldactone)	Canrenone	47%-57% renal, 35%-41% fecal	2-4	6-8 hours	16-24	1.4	25-400	1-2	Increased
Eplerenone (Inspra)	None	67% renal, 32% fecal	1-2	4 weeks	24	3.5-6	50-100	1-2	No effect

Aldosterone Antagonists

Spironolactone (Aldactone) and eplerenone (Inspra) are aldosterone antagonists that exert their effect on the late distal tubule and collecting duct. Spironolactone, a weak diuretic, is used primarily for its aldosterone antagonist effects. Spironolactone is indicated for hypertension, management of hepatic cirrhosis (diuretic of choice), primary hyperaldosteronism, hypokalemia, and heart failure. For hypertension, spironolactone is used in combination with other antihypertensives or to spare potassium when administered with diuretics. The chemical structure of spironolactone resembles the structure of the corticosteroids and may explain its sexual adverse effects, such as impotence, decreased libido, gynecomastia, deepening of the voice, menstrual irregularities, and hirsutism. Other spironolactone-induced adverse effects include diarrhea, gastritis, skin rashes, drowsiness, lethargy, ataxia, headaches, and confusion. Similar to the other potassium-sparing diuretics, spironolactone may cause hyperkalemia. Table 22-9 presents the pharmacokinetics and dosage guidelines for the aldosterone antagonists.[4,5,6]

Eplerenone is indicated for heart failure after MI and hypertension. Similar to spironolactone, eplerenone blocks the mineralocorticoid receptor, but, in contrast to spironolactone, it does not block the progesterone or androgen receptor, minimizing the sexual adverse effects such as gynecomastia, breast pain, impotence, and menstrual irregularities. Eplerenone has a higher incidence of severe hyperkalemia, especially in patients with reduced renal function.

Because of the risk of severe hyperkalemia, eplerenone is contraindicated in all patients with potassium values greater than 5.5 mEq/L or CrCl less than 30 mL/min and in hypertensive patients with type 2 diabetes and microalbuminemia, concomitant use of potassium supplements or potassium-sparing diuretics, or serum creatinine greater than 2 mg/dL in men and greater than 1.8 mg/dL in women or a CrCl less than 50 mL/min. Vigilant monitoring of serum potassium levels is necessary when eplerenone is administered with ACEIs, ARBs, or β blockers. Eplerenone is a CYP3A4 substrate; CYP3A4 inhibitors such as verapamil, diltiazem, erythromycin, fluconazole, and saquinavir may increase eplerenone levels by 50%. Grapefruit juice may also increase levels of eplerenone but to a lesser extent (approximately 25%). It is recommended to initiate eplerenone at a lower dose of 25 mg/day in patients who are taking CYP3A4 inhibitors.

Centrally Acting Adrenergic Agents

The centrally acting adrenergic agents, or α_2 agonists, decrease blood pressure by affecting cardiac output and peripheral resistance; they are negative inotropes and chronotropes. α_2 Agonists stimulate brainstem α_2 receptors, resulting in a decrease in sympathetic outflow from the CNS. α_2 Agonists are very effective antihypertensives; however, they are not considered first-line therapy because of their side effect profile. They have a high incidence of anticholinergic-like side effects, such as sedation, blurred vision, dry mouth, constipation, and urinary retention, and

CNS side effects, such as drowsiness, fatigue, headaches, depression, psychosis, and nightmares. Long-term use of these agents results in sodium and fluid retention and almost always necessitates the use of concomitant diuretics; this is especially seen with methyldopa. α_2 Agonists are not recommended for noncompliant patients and should never be withdrawn abruptly because of the risk of either rebound hypertension or overshoot hypertension.

The most effective and least toxic α_2 agonist is the clonidine transdermal therapeutic system (Catapres-TTS), which achieves sustained levels of clonidine for 7 days. The sustained clonidine levels avoid the peaks and troughs associated with the prompt release dosage form, and treatment is relatively devoid of the troublesome anticholinergic and CNS side effects. The clonidine patch is applied to a hairless area of intact skin on the upper torso. On the initial application, the clonidine patch takes 2 to 3 days to achieve target blood levels and a therapeutic effect. It is recommended to coadminister clonidine oral tablets along with the patch for the first 2 to 3 days of therapy. The most common adverse effects of the patch are local skin rashes and irritation. Table 22-10 presents the pharmacokinetics and dosage guidelines for α_2 agonists.[4,5,6]

α_1-Adrenergic Antagonists

α_1-Adrenergic receptor antagonists selectively block postsynaptic α_1 receptors. Total peripheral resistance is reduced through arterial and venous dilation; these agents decrease both preload and afterload and cause a potent first-dose sympathetic reflex increase in heart rate and renin activity.[12] α_1-Adrenergic antagonists cause a first-dose phenomenon that manifests with orthostatic hypotension, tachycardia, palpitations, dizziness, headaches, and syncope. After several doses, despite persistent vasodilation, tolerance to the first-dose phenomenon develops, and heart rate, renin, and cardiac output return to normal. To minimize the first-dose phenomenon, initial doses of α_1-adrenergic antagonists should be low and administered at bedtime.

α_1-Adrenergic antagonists are indicated for hypertension, benign prostatic hyperplasia (BPH), heart failure, and Raynaud vasospasm; an exception is uroselective α_1-adrenergic antagonists (tamsulosin and alfuzosin), which are indicated only for BPH. In contrast to other antihypertensives, α_1-adrenergic antagonists have favorable effects on the lipoprotein profile and may decrease triglycerides and low-density lipoproteins and increase high-density lipoproteins by 5% to 10%, making them an ideal drug of choice. However, the ALLHAT (Antihypertensive and Lipid-Lowering Treatment to Prevent Heart Attack Trial) study compared doxazosin with other antihypertensives (chlorthalidone) and revealed a 25% higher incidence of combined cardiovascular morbidity in patients receiving doxazosin.[13] A higher incidence of doxazosin-induced stroke, heart failure, angina, and coronary revascularization was reported. On the basis of the results of this study, α_1-adrenergic antagonists are considered second-line antihypertensive therapy. Table 22-11 presents the pharmacokinetics and dosage guidelines for α_1-adrenergic antagonists.[4,5,6]

TABLE 22-10 Pharmacokinetics and Dosage Guidelines for Centrally Acting Adrenergic Agents (α_2 Agonists)

α_2 AGONIST GENERIC NAME (BRAND NAME)	ONSET OF ACTION (hr)	PEAK EFFECT (hr)	DURATION OF ACTION (hr)	HALF-LIFE (hr)	ELIMINATION	DOSAGE RANGE (mg/day)	DAILY FREQUENCY
Methyldopa (Aldomet)	4-6	6-9	24-48	1.25	Renal (biphasic)	500-2000	2-3
Clonidine (Catapres)	0.5-1	3-5	24	6-20	Renal (40%-60%)	0.1-2.4	2-4
Guanfacine (Tenex)	2.5	6	24	17	Renal (50%)	1-3	Once at bedtime
Guanabenz (Wytensin)	1	2-5	6-8	7-10	Renal (70%-80%)	4-32	2

TABLE 22-11 Pharmacokinetics and Dosage Guidelines for α_1-Adrenergic Receptor Antagonists

α_1 ANTAGONIST GENERIC NAME (BRAND NAME)	ELIMINATION ROUTES	PEAK EFFECT (hr)	DURATION OF ACTION (hr)	HALF-LIFE (hr)	DOSAGE RANGE (mg/day)	DAILY FREQUENCY
Doxazosin (Cardura)	63% feces, 9% urine	6	18-36	11	1-16	1
Prazosin (Minipress)	90% feces, 10% urine	1.5	8-10	2	3-40	2-3
Terazosin (Hytrin)	60% feces, 40% urine	2	24	14	120	1-2

Antiadrenergic Agents

Reserpine, guanethidine (Ismelin), and guanadrel (Hylorel) are antiadrenergic antihypertensive agents. All three of these agents are second-line antihypertensives. Reserpine works by binding to storage vesicles of peripheral and central postganglionic adrenergic neurons and depleting norepinephrine. Subsequently, reserpine renders the neuronal storage vesicles dysfunctional. Reserpine may cause sedation, depression, suicidal ideation, psychosis, peptic ulcer disease, and nasal stuffiness. The side effects of reserpine can be minimized with low yet effective antihypertensive doses (0.25 mg or less). Guanethidine and guanadrel are postganglionic sympathetic inhibitors that produce a selective block of efferent peripheral sympathetic pathways. Guanethidine and guanadrel act as **substitute neurotransmitters** by replacing norepinephrine in the neuronal storage vesicle. Guanethidine and guanadrel cause similar adverse effects, such as orthostatic hypotension, sexual dysfunction, and diarrhea that can be occasionally explosive. The antihypertensive effects of these agents may be diminished when combined with tricyclic antidepressants, amphetamines, and ephedrine.

Vasodilators

The two common vasodilators used in the management of hypertension are hydralazine (Apresoline) and minoxidil (Loniten). Because of their side effect profile, the vasodilators are second-line antihypertensive agents. Hydralazine has also been used for angina and is indicated for heart failure in combination with isosorbide dinitrate. Hydralazine and isosorbide dinitrate are recommended to reduce morbidity and mortality in black patients with New York Heart Association (NYHA) class III to IV heart failure with reduced ejection fraction receiving optimal therapy with ACEIs and β blockers and in patients with current or prior symptomatic heart failure with reduced ejection fraction who have a contraindication to ACEI or ARB use.[14,15,16]

Hydralazine and minoxidil reduce total peripheral resistance by a direct action on vascular smooth muscle, increasing intracellular concentrations of cyclic guanosine 3′,5′-monophosphate (cGMP). These vasodilators are so potent that they cause a profound activation of baroreceptors, leading to reflex tachycardia, renin release, and an increase in cardiac output. To minimize tachycardia and fluid retention, these agents are often administered concomitantly with a β blocker and a loop diuretic,

respectively. Hydralazine has been associated with peripheral neuropathy and drug-induced systemic lupus erythematosus–like syndrome. When hydralazine is administered with food, its bioavailability may double and may cause cardiac toxicity. Hydralazine should be administered consistently with or without food. Minoxidil-induced adverse effects include hirsutism, nausea and vomiting, and pericardial effusions. Table 22-12 shows the pharmacokinetics and dosage guidelines for the oral vasodilators.

ANGINA

Epidemiology, Etiology, and Pathophysiology

 KEY POINT

Angina pectoris is a marker for myocardial ischemia.

Ischemic heart disease can manifest as many clinical variants such as stable exertional angina; unstable (rest, preinfarction, crescendo) angina; coronary vasomotion; vasospasm associated with atypical, variant, or Prinzmetal angina; silent myocardial ischemia; or MI. Angina pectoris (chest pain) is a symptom or marker of myocardial ischemia. Ischemia is defined as a lack of oxygen and decreased or no blood flow to the myocardium. From 2002 to 2006, more than 10 million Americans older than 20 years were diagnosed with angina pectoris.[17] Women often initially present with angina, whereas men present with MI. Coronary artery disease (CAD), when present, tends to be less severe in women than men.

Angina pectoris can manifest with a heavy weight or pressure on the chest, a burning sensation, or shortness of breath. The chest tightness or pressure can occur over the sternum, left shoulder, and lower jaw. Chest pain can be precipitated by physical exercise, a cold environment, or emotional stress (anger). The duration of pain intensity may range from a few minutes to half an hour. During angina, an imbalance of myocardial oxygen supply and myocardial oxygen demand occurs. Factors that increase myocardial oxygen demand include increased heart rate, increased systolic wall force or tension, or increased contractility. Factors that decrease myocardial oxygen supply include a decrease in the concentration of oxygen (e.g., anemia), a decrease in coronary blood flow (e.g., thrombus), or inability of the myocardium to extract oxygen from the blood.

TABLE 22-12	Pharmacokinetics and Dosage Guidelines for Oral Vasodilators				
VASODILATORS GENERIC NAME (BRAND NAME)	**BIOAVAILABILITY (%)**	**ONSET OF ACTION (min)**	**TERMINAL HALF-LIFE (hr)**	**DOSE RANGE (mg/day)**	**DAILY FREQUENCY**
Hydralazine (Apresoline)	30-5	20-30	2-8 ESRD: 7-16	40-300	3-4
Minoxidil (Loniten)	90	30	3.5-4.2	5-100	1

ESRD, End stage renal disease.

Pharmacotherapy

> **KEY POINT**
>
> Pharmacotherapy for angina includes nitrates (e.g., nitroglycerin), β blockers, and calcium antagonists.

Pharmacotherapy for angina pectoris includes nitrates, β blockers, CCBs, and ranolazine (Ranexa). Ranolazine was approved by the U.S. Food and Drug Administration (FDA) in 2006 for the treatment of chronic stable angina in combination with amlodipine, β blockers, or nitrates.[18] For the management of vasospastic and chronic stable angina, diltiazem, verapamil, amlodipine, and nifedipine are indicated. For the management of angina, β blockers are usually dosed to achieve a resting heart rate of 50 to 60 beats/min and a maximal exercise heart rate of 100 beats/min. The new 2014 antihypertension guidelines (JNC8) do not make a specific goal blood pressure for patients with documented CAD (i.e., chronic stable angina, unstable angina, non–ST segment elevation MI, ST segment elevation MI). The target blood pressure for the general population ≥60 years is SBP of less than 150 mm Hg and DBP of less than 90 mm Hg, and for the general population ≤60 years, target SBP is less than 140 mm Hg and DBP less than 90 mm Hg.[4] All patients with angina should receive daily aspirin (75 to 100 mg/day) to prevent MI.[19-21]

Nitrates

Nitroglycerin reduces myocardial oxygen demand by causing venodilation of coronary arteries and collaterals, resulting in decreased end-diastolic pressures. Venous effects predominate; however, nitroglycerin can affect arteries at high doses. The cellular mechanism of action of nitrates is depicted in Figure 22-3. Nitrates are indicated for acute treatment or prophylaxis of angina, acute MI, acute heart failure, low-output syndromes, and hypertension (intravenous). Nitrates may be administered by various routes and are readily available in multiple preparations, including oral, intravenous, ointment, transdermal, translingual, and sublingual tablets. Sublingual nitroglycerin is indicated for acute anginal relief. Sublingual nitroglycerin has an onset of action of minutes and duration of action of 30 minutes. Sublingual nitroglycerin should be administered every 5 minutes until relief is obtained. If pain relief is not achieved after three doses in 15 minutes, emergency care should be sought. This algorithm is recommended for patients who were previously prescribed nitroglycerin. For patients who were never prescribed nitroglycerin, it is recommended that patients should seek emergency care if symptoms worsen or persist 5 minutes after taking the first sublingual nitroglycerin.[21] Sublingual tablets must always be stored in their original glass container, and any unused tablets should be discarded 6 months after the original container is opened because of loss of potency. Other forms of nitroglycerin are isosorbide dinitrate (Isordil) and isosorbide mononitrate (Imdur, Ismo, and Monoket). Table 22-13 presents the pharmacokinetics and dosage guidelines of nitrates.

Serious adverse reactions to nitrates are uncommon and involve mainly the cardiovascular system. The most frequent adverse effects include tachycardia, palpitations, postural hypotension, dizziness, flushing, and headache. Case reports of clinically significant methemoglobinemia are rare at conventional doses. Methemoglobinemia formation is dose-related and occurs by the nitrite ion reacting with the ferrous hemoglobin. Tolerance to the vascular and antianginal effects may occur after 24 hours of continuous therapy with any formulation. Because most evidence supports the central role of cGMP stimulation in nitrate-induced vasodilation, it has been suggested that the tolerance results from sulfhydryl depletion at the nitrate receptor. Sulfhydryl depletion leads to reduced S-nitrosothiol production and a decreased production of cGMP. Theoretically, administration of a sulfhydryl donor, such as N-acetyl cysteine or captopril, may restore vascular response to nitrates. Increasing doses of nitroglycerin overcome tolerance, but this is short-lived. To circumvent nitrate tolerance, a nitrate-free interval of 10 to 14 hours is suggested. Nitrates are contraindicated in patients concomitantly taking phosphodiesterase type 5 inhibitors for erectile dysfunction, such as sildenafil (Viagra), vardenafil (Levitra), and tadalafil (Cialis), because of pronounced potentiation of nitric oxide resulting in profound hypotension, MI, and even death.

Ranolazine

Ranolazine is indicated for the treatment of patients with chronic angina who have not achieved an adequate response with other antianginal drugs. In 2007 the American College of Cardiology Foundation (ACCF) and the American Heart Association (AHA) suggested that ranolazine may be safely administered for symptomatic relief after unstable angina or non–ST segment elevation MI, but it does not seem to reduce significantly cardiovascular death, MI, or recurrent ischemia. Ranolazine provides antiischemic effects that complement the benefits of CCBs, β blockers, and nitrates. Although the exact mechanism of how ranolazine exerts its

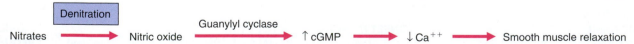

Figure 22-3 Mechanism of action of nitrates on smooth muscle relaxation. Nitrates are converted intracellularly (denitration) to nitric oxide and 5-nitrosothiol. Nitric oxide interacts with and activates guanylyl cyclase to increase intracellular concentrations of cyclic guanosine 3′,5′-monophosphate *(cGMP)*. Increased cGMP results in phosphorylation of various proteins, which reduces calcium *(Ca++)* release from the sarcoplasmic reticulum, subsequently causing smooth muscle relaxation.

TABLE 22-13 Pharmacokinetics and Dosage Guidelines for Nitrates

NAME	DOSAGE FORMS	ONSET OF ACTION (min)	DURATION OF ACTION (hr)	INITIAL DOSAGE
Nitroglycerin	Buccal tablet, ER Oral capsule, ER Oral tablet, ER Sublingual spray Sublingual tablet Intravenous solution Topical ointment Transdermal patch	Angina pectoris • Oral ER: 20-45 • Sublingual: 1-3 • Topical ointment: 30-60 • Transdermal patch: 30-60 • Translingual spray: 2 • Perioperative hypertension • IV: 1-5	Oral ER: 3-8 Sublingual: up to 1 Topical ointment: 7 Transdermal patch: 8-10 Transdermal spray: up to 1	*Angina pectoris* • IV: 5-25 mcg/min to response • Oral capsule, ER: 2.5-9 mg every 12 hr; may increase to every 8 hr if needed and if tolerated • Topical ointment: 7.5-30 mg applied twice daily to a 36-square-inch area of truncal skin • Transdermal patch: 0.2-0.4 mg/hr • Sublingual tablet: 0.3-0.6 mg every 5 min, 3 times • Sublingual spray: 1-2 metered sprays onto or under the tongue; may repeat in 3-5 min, with no more than 3 metered sprays in 15 min • Chronic heart failure • IV: non-PVC tubing, 5 mcg/min, initial titration should be in 5-mcg/min increments at intervals of 3-5 min guided by patient response • Perioperative hypertension • IV: 5 mcg/min, initial titration should be in 5-mcg/min increments at intervals of 3-5 min, guided by patient response
Isosorbide dinitrate	Oral capsule, ER Oral tablet Oral tablet, chewable Oral tablet, ER Sublingual tablet	Oral: 60 Oral tablet, chewable: 2-3 Sublingual tablet: 2-10	Oral: 8 Oral tablet, chewable: 2 Sublingual tablet: 1-2	*Angina pectoris* • Oral tablet (immediate release): 5-20 mg two or three times daily • Oral tablet/capsule, ER: 40 mg once or twice daily • Oral tablet, chewable: 5-10 mg every 2-3 hr or as needed; titrate to effect • Chronic heart failure • Sublingual tablet: 5-15 mg every 2-3 hr • Oral: 30-160 mg/day in divided doses
Isosorbide mononitrate	Oral tablet Oral tablet, ER	45-60	6-12	*Angina pectoris* • Oral tablet (immediate release): 5-20 mg twice or three times daily • Oral tablet: 20 mg every morning, then 20 mg 7 hr later • Oral tablet, ER: 30-60 mg once daily *Myocardial infarction* • Oral tablet: 20 mg once to three times daily

ER, Extended release; *IV*, intravenous; *PVC*, polyvinyl chloride.

antianginal and antiischemic effects is unknown, it is speculated that it selectively inhibits the late phase of the inward sodium channel in ischemic myocytes, resulting in decreased myocardial oxygen consumption.[22] Ranolazine increases exercise tolerance, which reduces angina frequency and the need for emergent nitroglycerin interventions. In contrast to standard antianginal medications, ranolazine does not alter blood pressure or heart rate. The initial adult dose of ranolazine extended release tablets is 500 mg twice daily, with a maximal dose of 1 g twice daily.

Adverse reactions observed with ranolazine include dizziness, palpitations, headache, constipation, nausea, abdominal pain, and peripheral edema. Small, reversible increases in serum creatinine and BUN have also been observed without the incidence of renal toxicity. Ranolazine is excreted primarily in the urine (75%) and to a lesser extent in the feces (25%); however, the manufacturer suggests that no dosage adjustments are needed in patients with renal impairment. Nevertheless, patients with renal impairment taking ranolazine were observed to have a 15-mm Hg increase in blood pressure—frequent blood pressure monitoring is prudent in such patients. Ranolazine can prolong the cardiac Q–T_c interval (Q–T interval [duration of ventricular electrical activity], corrected for heart rate) and place patients at risk of torsades de pointes; this effect is dose-dependent. A dose of 1 g twice daily prolongs the Q–T$_c$ by 6 msec and is more pronounced with hepatic dysfunction. Ranolazine is contraindicated in patients with any degree of hepatic dysfunction or who are receiving other agents that prolong the Q–T$_c$. Baseline and follow-up electrocardiography (ECG) should be completed during ranolazine therapy.

Ranolazine is extensively metabolized in the gut and liver by CYP3A4 and to a lesser extent by CYP2D6. CYP3A4 inhibitors, such as ketoconazole, fluconazole, macrolides, diltiazem, and verapamil, can significantly increase the plasma levels of ranolazine and are contraindicated. Ranolazine is a substrate of P-gp, and it should not be taken with verapamil, a known inhibitor of P-gp. Ranolazine is a P-gp inhibitor and has been shown to increase the plasma concentration of digoxin by 1.5-fold. Ranolazine is also an inhibitor of CYP3A4 and CYP2D6, plausibly increasing the plasma levels of drugs that are substrates of these enzymes, such as statins, tricyclic antidepressants, and antipsychotics.

ANTITHROMBOTIC AGENTS

KEY POINT

Antithrombotic agents include anticoagulants (e.g., heparin, low-molecular-weight heparin [LMWH], direct thrombin inhibitors [DTIs], factor Xa inhibitors, and coumarins); antiplatelet agents (e.g., aspirin, dipyridamole, cilostazol, pentoxifylline, ticlopidine, clopidogrel, prasugrel, ticagrelor, glycoprotein [GP] IIb/IIIa inhibitors, and vorapaxar); and thrombolytic agents (i.e., agents that lyse clots, such as streptokinase and alteplase).

Antithrombotics may be defined as agents that prevent or break up blood clots in conditions such as thrombosis or embolism. Three categories of antithrombotic agents are currently available in the United States: anticoagulants, antiplatelets, and thrombolytics. Anticoagulant agents work by preventing the formation of the fibrin clot and preventing further clot formation in already existing thrombi. Antiplatelet agents inhibit the action of platelets in the initial stage of the clotting process. Thrombolytics break up thrombi by degrading fibrin. Box 22-1 lists currently available antithrombotic agents.[23]

Formation and Elimination of Acute Coronary Thrombus

Under normal conditions, the body maintains an equilibrium state between clot formation (thrombosis) and clot breakdown (fibrinolysis).[24] Thromboses are initiated by an injury to the endothelial wall of a coronary vessel. When injury occurs, the anticoagulated endothelial surface is disrupted, and the highly procoagulant subendothelial surface is exposed. Instantaneously platelets aggregate in response to the release of chemotactic substances, such as

---

BOX 22-1   List of Antithrombotic Agents

Anticoagulant Agents
Parenteral Anticoagulants
- High-molecular-weight heparin
  - Unfractionated heparin
- Low-molecular-weight heparins
  - Dalteparin (Fragmin)
  - Enoxaparin (Lovenox)
- Selective factor Xa inhibitor
  - Fondaparinux (Arixtra)
- Direct thrombin inhibitors
  - Argatroban
  - Bivalirudin (Angiomax)
  - Desirudin (Iprivasc)
  - Lepirudin (Refludan)

Oral Anticoagulants
- Warfarin sodium (Coumadin)
- Direct thrombin inhibitor
  - Dabigatran (Pradaxa)
- Selective factor Xa inhibitors
  - Apixaban (Eliquis)
  - Rivaroxaban (Xarelto)

Antiplatelet Agents
- Aspirin
- Clopidogrel (Plavix)
- Prasugrel (Effient)
- Ticagrelor (Brilinta)
- Cilostazol (Pletal)
- Dipyridamole (Persantine)
- Aspirin and extended-release dipyridamole (Aggrenox)
- Ticlopidine HCl (Ticlid)
- Vorapaxar (Zontivity)
- Glycoprotein IIb/IIIa inhibitors
  - Abciximab (ReoPro)
  - Eptifibatide (Integrilin)
  - Tirofiban (Aggrastat)

Thrombolytic Agents
- Alteplase (Activase)
- Reteplase (Retavase)
- Streptokinase (Streptase)
- Tenecteplase (TNKase)

---

thromboxane A$_2$; this is followed by platelet adhesion to the subendothelial vessel surface, representing the initial step in clot formation. Platelet adhesion is mediated mainly by von Willebrand factor. von Willebrand factor is present in the subendothelium and is actively recruited when the subendothelium is injured. Adhered platelets are exposed to many subendothelial proteins, such as collagen and thrombin. Collagen and thrombin also promote platelet activation. Activated platelets release platelet agonists such as adenosine diphosphate (ADP), norepinephrine, serotonin, and arachidonic metabolites, mitigating and amplifying platelet aggregation and forming an unstable thrombus or platelet plug.

The most important consequence of platelet activation is the expression of platelet receptor glycoprotein (GP) IIb/IIIa on the platelet's surface, allowing binding to fibrinogen.

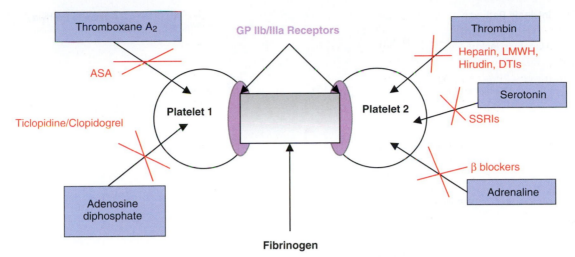

Figure 22-4 Triggers affecting platelet aggregation and their antagonists. Numerous agonists can mitigate platelet activation, which can be inhibited by drugs with corresponding mechanisms of action. Expression of the platelet receptor glycoprotein *(GP)* IIb/IIIa on the platelet surface causes fibrinogen to bind to the platelet and subsequent linking of the two platelets (aggregation). This is the final common pathway to platelet aggregation. *ASA,* Aspirin; *DTIs,* direct thrombin inhibitors; *LMWH,* low-molecular-weight heparin; *SSRIs,* selective serotonin reuptake inhibitors.

Fibrinogen binds to the two GP IIb/IIIa molecules, causing a cross-linking of receptors on adjacent platelets and initiating platelet aggregation. Triggers affecting platelet aggregation and their antagonists are depicted in Figure 22-4. Fibrinogen is converted into fibrin monomers by the action of thrombin; this is the final step in clot formation. Homeostasis is complete when the fibrin clot becomes insoluble within the vessel. This stable fibrin clot is the end result of the coagulation cascade. Under normal conditions, multiple inhibitors and control mechanisms keep these reactions localized to the site of the injury.

The fibrin clot ultimately must be removed for hemostasis to be maintained. Activation of the fibrinolytic system by tissue plasminogen activators (tPAs), which are present in most body fluids and tissues, results in the conversion of plasminogen to plasmin, initiating the dissolution of fibrin and fibrinogen. The breakdown of fibrinogen and fibrin results in polypeptides termed **fibrin split** or **fibrinogen degradation products (FDPs)**. FDPs are anticoagulant substances that can cause bleeding if fibrinolysis becomes uncontrolled and excessive. **D-dimers** are fragments of plasmin-digested, cross-linked fibrin that increase in concentration after the onset of fibrinolysis. Blood testing for D-dimer fragments may assist in the diagnosis of pathogenic venous thromboembolism (VTE). The extrinsic and intrinsic pathways of the coagulation system[25] are depicted and described in Figure 22-5.

Anticoagulant Agents

Heparins: Unfractionated Heparin and Low-Molecular-Weight Heparin

Heparin is a nonionic sulfated glycosaminoglycan anticoagulant naturally present in the secretory granules of human mast cells. When heparin is released from mast cells, it is ingested and destroyed by macrophages. Heparin is not detectable in plasma except in pathologic circumstances (e.g., mastocytosis). Commercially available unfractionated heparin (UFH), or simply *heparin,* is indicated for prevention and treatment of VTE, prevention and treatment of pulmonary embolism (PE), treatment of atrial fibrillation with embolization, diagnosis and treatment of disseminated intravascular coagulation, and prophylaxis and treatment of peripheral arterial embolism.

Heparin is extracted from porcine intestinal mucosa or bovine lungs; however, because of the high propensity of thrombocytopenia with the bovine lung derivative, only the porcine derivative is routinely employed in practice. Heparin serves as a catalyst that accelerates the rate of the thrombin-to-antithrombin III reaction by at least 1000-fold by serving as a catalytic template to which both bind, resulting in a ternary complex (heparin, thrombin, and antithrombin). Antithrombin III is a large protein (58,000 Da) that is synthesized in the liver and is known as a *suicide substrate.* Heparin is a high-molecular-weight complex mucopolysaccharide containing specific pentasaccharide units and approximately 45 monosaccharide side chains with a mean molecular mass of 12,000 Da (range 5,000 to 30,000 Da).[26,27,28]

Most of the monosaccharide side chains of UFH are more than 18 monosaccharides long and are necessary to form the ternary complex. Heparin molecules that possess less than 18 monosaccharide units (less than 5400 Da) do not catalyze the thrombin-to-antithrombin III reaction. However, the heparin molecules that include less than 18 monosaccharides catalyze a conformational change on antithrombin III that inhibits the effects of factor Xa (Stuart factor) and does not require a ternary complex. LMWHs are generally about 4500 Da (range 1,000 to 10,000 Da) and contain 15 monosaccharide units and do not form a ternary complex. Their anticoagulant activity is exhibited via factor Xa inhibition. Because factor Xa occurs earlier in the

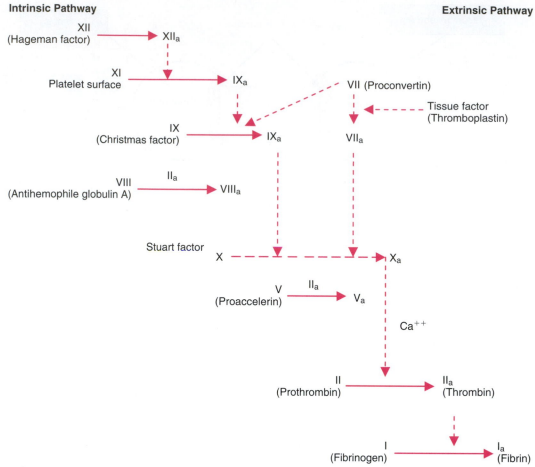

Figure 22-5 Extrinsic and intrinsic pathways of the coagulation system. The coagulation system is divided into the intrinsic pathway and extrinsic pathway. The intrinsic or contact activation pathway is activated by trauma or infection, which causes inflammatory proteins to be released in the circulation. The main role of the extrinsic pathway is to initiate coagulation during hemostasis. In the presence of calcium, the activated forms of factors X and V catalyze the conversion of prothrombin to thrombin.

coagulation cascade, the inhibition of a single molecule of factor Xa prevents thousands of thrombin molecules from forming. The antifactor Xa/antifactor IIa ratio of UFH is 1:1; the antifactor Xa/antifactor IIa ratio of LMWH ranges from 2:1 (dalteparin) to 3.8:1 (enoxaparin). Heparin also inhibits the conversion of fibrinogen to fibrin and inhibits the activation of factor XIII, preventing the formation of a stable fibrin clot. LMWH is postulated to suppress von Willebrand factor, which increases platelet aggregation, and to stimulate the release of tissue factor pathway inhibitor, which inhibits factor Xa.

LMWHs include dalteparin (Fragmin) and enoxaparin (Lovenox). In contrast to LMWHs, UFH binds extensively to plasma proteins such as GPs, vitronectin, lipoproteins, fibrinogen, platelet proteins, acute-phase reactant proteins, and endothelial cells, yielding poor UFH bioavailability and an unpredictable effect. The predictable bioavailability of LMWHs allows for subcutaneous administration for all indications. UFH is administered subcutaneously for VTE prophylaxis but must be administered as a continuous infusion for serious indications such as MI and to minimize the risk of hemorrhage.

Heparin (UFH) is cleared faster and requires more frequent dosing or an intravenous continuous infusion. The half-life of UFH is approximately 30 to 60 minutes, whereas the half-life of LMWH is 4 to 5 hours, allowing for once-daily or twice-daily LMWH administration. The onset of action of heparin is within 6 hours of initiation of a continuous infusion. LMWH time to peak antifactor Xa activity is 2 to 5 hours. Each commercially available LMWH is synthesized by different mechanisms, possesses moderately different pharmacokinetic and pharmacodynamic characteristics, and has different FDA-approved indications and dose regimens; these agents are not interchangeable. Table 22-14 presents the pharmacokinetic properties and dose parameters for all heparins.

Activated partial thromboplastin time (aPTT) is used to monitor the effects of heparin because it is sensitive to the inhibitory effects of thrombin, factor Xa, and factor IXa, and correlates with heparin levels. When the concentration of plasma heparin is 0.1 to 1 U/mL, aPTT and thrombin time are prolonged. The goal of heparin therapy is to prevent unwanted clotting without an increased risk of hemorrhage. This goal may be accomplished by

TABLE 22-14 Pharmacokinetic Properties and Dosage Guidelines of Heparins

HEPARIN FORMULATION	MOLECULAR WEIGHT (Da)	ANTI-XA/ANTI-IIA RATIO	HALF-LIFE (min)	DOSAGE: PROPHYLAXIS	DOSAGE: TREATMENT
Dalteparin (Fragmin)	4000-6000	2:1	119-139	*General surgery:* 5000 U every 24 hr *Hip/knee orthopedic surgery:* Postoperative start: 2500 U 4-8 hr after surgery, then 5000 U every 24 hr Preoperative start, day of surgery: 2500 U within 2 hr before surgery, 2500 U 4-8 hr after surgery, then 5000 U every 24 hr Perioperative start, evening before surgery: 5000 U until 14 hr before surgery, 5000 U 4-8 hr after surgery, then 5000 U every 24 hr *Acute medical illness:* 5000 U every 24 hr	200 U/kg every 24 hr or 100 U/kg every 12 hr *Kidney impairment:* No specific dosage adjustment recommended *Extended VTE treatment in patients with cancer:* Days 1-30: 200 U/kg every 24 hr Months 2-6: 150 U/kg every 24 hr *Unstable angina or non-Q wave MI:* 120 U/kg (maximum of 10,000 U) every 12 hr with concurrent aspirin therapy until clinically stable
Enoxaparin (Lovenox)	3500-5500	3.8:1	129-180	*General surgery:* 40 mg every 24 hr; for CrCl <30 mL/min use 30 every 24 hr *Hip orthopedic surgery:* 30 mg every 12 hr (TKR/THR); 40 mg every 24 hr (THR only); if CrCl <30 mL/min, use 30 mg every 24 hr *Acute medical illness:* 40 mg every 24 hr; if CrCl <30 mL/min use 30 mg every 24 hr	*Acute DVT:* 1 mg/kg every 12 hr or 1.5 mg/kg every 24 hr *Kidney impairment:* CrCl <30 mL/min use 1 mg/kg every 24 hr *STEMI:* Age <75 years: 30 mg IV bolus plus 1 mg/kg SQ every 12 hr Age ≥75 years: 0.75 mg/kg SQ every 12 hr *NSTEMI:* 1 mg/kg SQ every 12 hr in conjunction with oral aspirin
Fondaparinux (Arixtra)	1728	NA		*General surgery (adults ≥50 kg):* 2.5 mg daily beginning 6-8 hr after surgery *Hip or knee orthopedic operations:* 2.5 mg every 24 hr beginning 6-8 hr after surgery *Acute medical illness:* 2.5 mg every 24 hr	Weight ≤ 50 kg: 5 mg every 24 hr Weight 50-100 kg: 7.5 mg every 24 hr Weight >100 kg: 10 mg every 24 hr *Kidney impairment:* CrCl <30 mL/min: contraindicated
Unfractionated Heparin (UFH)	10,000-15,000	1:1	30-150*	5000 U every 8 hr	*DVT/PE:* IV: 80 units/kg (or 5000 units) IV push followed by continuous infusion of 18 units/kg/hr (or 1300 units/hr) SQ: Monitored dosing: initial 17,500 units or 250 units/kg then 250 units every 12 hr Unmonitored dosing: Initial: 333 units/kg then 250 units/kg every 12 hr *STEMI:* Bolus of 60 units/kg (maximum: 4000 units), then 12 units/kg/hr (maximum: 1000 units/hr) as continuous infusion, with target aPTT of 1.5-2 times upper limit of control (50-70 sec) *NSTEMI:* Initial bolus of 60 units/kg (maximum of 4000 units) followed by 12 units/kg/hr (maximum of 1000 units/hr). Dosage adjustment to correspond to therapeutic range equivalent with target aPTT of 1.5-2 times upper limit of control (50-70 sec)

aPTT, Activated partial thromboplastin time; *CrCl,* creatinine clearance; *DVT,* deep vein thrombosis; *IV,* intravenous administration; *MI,* myocardial infarction; *NA,* not available; *NSTEMI,* non–ST segment elevation myocardial infarction; *PE,* pulmonary embolism; *SQ,* subcutaneous administration; *STEMI,* ST segment elevation myocardial infarction; *THR,* total hip replacement; *TKR,* total knee replacement; *VTE,* venous thromboembolism.

*Half-life of UFH has saturable binding, and half-life increases with doses more than 400 U/kg.

maintaining aPTT between 1.5 and 2 times the upper limit of the control value. aPTT should not be used to monitor LMWHs. The effect of LMWHs may be monitored on the basis of antifactor Xa levels; however, because the relationship between antifactor Xa levels and clinical outcomes is tenuous, routine measurement is not indicated and should be reserved for special populations, such as patients with renal disease, obese patients, and underweight patients.[27]

More recently, there has been a major change in the *United States Pharmacopeia* (USP) monograph of UFH. As a result of the heparin contamination problem encountered from 2007 to 2009, a new reference standard for heparin and a new test to determine potency were established by the FDA. These changes have resulted in an estimated 10% reduction in anticoagulant activity of UFH, which was validated. Because of this decrease in potency, the intravenous dose of UFH may need to be increased to achieve target aPTT, and more frequent or intensive aPTT monitoring may be required. No dose adjustment is needed for subcutaneous administration of UFH.[28]

Adverse effects induced by UFH and LMWHs include bleeding, hematoma, early thrombocytopenia, delayed thrombocytopenia with or without white clot syndrome, hyperkalemia, osteoporosis (with prolonged use), and increase in liver enzyme tests (LETs). An increase in LETs may occur in 10% to 30% of patients receiving LMWHs or high molecular weight heparins. However, the increase in LETs seems benign and has not been associated with any cases of hepatic sequelae. Early-onset heparin-induced thrombocytopenia type 1 (HIT-1) manifests with a decrease in platelets of approximately 50,000/mm^3. The decrease in platelets is transient and inconsequential. Delayed-onset heparin-induced thrombocytopenia type 2 (HIT-2) is due to the formation of antiplatelet antibodies between days 6 and 12.

If a patient has heparin-dependent antibodies present in plasma from previous heparin exposure, HIT-2 may occur at any time. HIT-2 is dependent on platelet factor-4 binding. These platelet antibodies aggregate and form the basis for the paradoxical heparin-induced white clot syndrome. The white clot syndrome is a medical emergency that may manifest as PE, MI, stroke, renal or hepatic thrombosis, or skin necrosis and gangrene. The diagnosis of HIT-2 is clinical and may be confirmed by several laboratory tests. Clinical diagnosis of HIT-2 includes a significant reduction in the platelet count of greater than 50%, a decrease in the platelet count to less than 100,000/mm^3, or both. Ostensibly the risk of thrombocytopenia is greatest with UFH and lowest with LMWHs; however, LMWHs cannot be administered as an alternative to heparin because of greater than 95% cross-reactivity.[29]

Fondaparinux (Arixtra), a pentasaccharide-selective antifactor Xa inhibitor agent, does not possess a risk of cross-reactivity and is currently being studied in clinical trials as a treatment modality for HIT-2 and white clot syndrome. Current treatment options for HIT-2 include the direct thrombin inhibitors (DTIs) argatroban, lepirudin

(Refludan), and bivalirudin, or selective factor Xa inhibitor fondaparinux.[29]

The antidote for heparin is protamine sulfate. Protamine sulfate is derived from the sperm of mature testes of salmon and related species. Protamine is electropositive and rapidly binds to the electronegative heparin to form salts that have no anticoagulant effect. Protamine also causes a dissociation of heparin–antithrombin III complexes in favor of a heparin-protamine complex. The recommended neutralizing dose of protamine is 1 mg for every 100 U of heparin, up to a total of protamine 50 mg per dose. Protamine should be administered by slow intravenous infusion over at least 1 to 3 minutes to prevent hypotension, bradycardia, or dyspnea. Patients who have previously received protamine-containing insulin, have undergone a vasectomy, or have a known sensitivity to fish or medications derived from fish (calcitonin-salmon, cold water fish oils containing omega-3 fatty acids, and oyster shell–derived calcium supplements) are at an increased risk for experiencing allergic reactions such as anaphylaxis and developing antiprotamine antibodies.[24] Excessive protamine may act as an anticoagulant, resulting in bleeding complications; a careful underdose strategy is suggested. There is no proven method for neutralizing LMWHs. Protamine seems to neutralize approximately 60% of the antifactor Xa activity of LMWHs. UFH may be the preferred parenteral anticoagulant in patients who are at risk for clinically significant bleeding, such as patients with end-stage renal disease receiving hemodialysis treatments.

Direct Thrombin Inhibitors

There are four commercially available highly specific parenteral DTIs and one orally available DTI. Dabigatran (Pradaxa), the only orally available DTI, is used for deep vein thrombosis (DVT) postoperative prophylaxis in knee and kip surgery patients, treatment of DVT and PE, and prevention of stroke and systemic embolism in patients with nonvalvular atrial fibrillation. Desirudin (Iprivasc) is indicated for DVT prophylaxis, bivalirudin (Angiomax) is indicated for unstable angina, and argatroban and lepirudin (Refludan) are indicated for prophylaxis or treatment of thrombosis in patients with HIT-2 and are used for anticoagulation against thromboembolic conditions in patients with or at risk for HIT-2. Argatroban and lepirudin are considered first-line options. DTIs exert their anticoagulant effects by directly inhibiting the effects of thrombin on a sustained fibrin clot. One molecule of a DTI binds to one molecule of thrombin. DTIs are independent of antithrombin III reactions and are not inhibited by platelet factor IV. aPTT is used to monitor the effects of DTIs and is generally maintained at about 1.5 to 2.5 times the upper limit of the control.

The most common adverse effects of DTIs are minor and major hemorrhage. DTIs may cause allergic skin reactions and anaphylactic reactions manifesting with bronchospasm, stridor, and dyspnea. There are no proven antidotes for DTIs. However, there may be a role for recombinant human factor VIIa (rFVIIa; NovoSeven) in DTI bleeding toxicities. rFVIIa is cloned from hamster kidney cells; it is a vitamin K–dependent GP (molecular mass 50 Da) structurally similar to human plasma–derived factor VIIa. rFVIIa can activate factor IX to IXa and factor X to Xa, converting prothrombin to thrombin and fibrinogen to fibrin and forming a hemostatic plug.

Natural hirudin is produced in trace amounts by the salivary glands of the leech *Hirudo medicinalis*. Lepirudin is a recombinant hirudin derived from yeast cells. FDA-approved dosage recommendations include an initial bolus dose of 0.4 mg/kg body weight followed by 0.15 mg/kg/hr continuous infusion. Current American College of Chest Physicians (ACCP) guidelines have a slightly different recommendation. The ACCP recommends a starting dose of no more than 0.10 mg/kg/hr and a lower bolus dose of 0.2 mg/kg to be administered only in the setting of life-threatening or limb-threatening thrombosis. These new recommendations were introduced because of the high rates of bleeding associated with the FDA-approved dosage.[29]

Lepirudin has a half-life of 1.3 hours. aPTT should be obtained about 4 hours after the start of the infusion. Lepirudin is almost exclusively renally eliminated, requiring careful dosage adjustments in mild to moderate renal dysfunction, and it is contraindicated in patients with severe renal impairment. The anticoagulant effects may be enhanced in patients with hepatic disease, and close monitoring in these patients is recommended. The formation of lepirudin–antihirudin antibody complexes has been observed in 40% of patients receiving lepirudin and may enhance the effect of lepirudin by delaying its renal elimination. An advantage of lepirudin is its lack of effect on the international normalized ratio (INR) value, facilitating accurate warfarin monitoring and dosage (see the next section for more details on the INR).

Argatroban is a synthetic agent, derived from L-arginine, that reversibly binds to the thrombin active site. It is administered through continuous intravenous infusion. The half-life of argatroban is 30 to 50 minutes. The route of elimination is primarily via the hepatic CYP3A4/5 isoenzyme system, and the potential for drug interactions exists with CYP3A4/5 inhibitors and inducers. There are four argatroban hepatic metabolites; only M1 is active. It is about threefold to fivefold weaker than the parent drug and is present at 0% to 20% relative to the parent. The recommended initial dose of argatroban is 2 mcg/kg/min of body weight up to 130 kg. aPTT should be attained 1 to 3 hours after initiation. The dose should be adjusted until steady-state aPTT is 1.5 to 3 times the initial baseline value but does not exceed 100 seconds at a maximum of 10 mcg/kg/min. In critically ill patients or patients with hepatic dysfunction, the initial dose of argatroban should be reduced to 0.2 mcg/kg/min or 0.5 mcg/kg/min. The effects of argatroban are not significantly influenced by renal impairment, and dosage adjustments are unnecessary in this setting.

When used in combination with warfarin, especially at doses exceeding 2 mcg/kg/min, argatroban has the potential to prolong the INR beyond that of warfarin alone.

However, argatroban exerts no additional effects on vitamin K–dependent factor Xa activity. Special warfarin dosing considerations are required when concomitantly using argatroban and warfarin.

New Oral Anticoagulant Agents

Although warfarin is very effective in preventing thromboembolic events, its narrow therapeutic index and pharmacogenomic variability impose the need for routine monitoring and diet restrictions. Therefore the quest continues for the development of an ideal anticoagulant of similar promising attributes of warfarin, but without the undesirable aspects, such as the risk of bleeding. Within a decade, three oral anticoagulants (OACs) have been made available on the American market: a DTI, dabigatran (Pradaxa), and two direct Xa inhibitors, rivaroxaban (Xarelto) and apixaban (Eliquis). An overview of the pharmacology of the new OACs[30,31,32] is provided in Table 22-15.

Dabigatran etexilate is a DTI. As a prodrug, dabigatran etexilate is rapidly converted to dabigatran upon oral administration and achieves a maximum plasma concentration (T_{max}) within 2 to 3 hours. When administered orally dabigatran etexilate has relatively low bioavailability of 7.2%, accounting for the high doses that are needed to maintain therapeutic plasma concentrations. The half-life of dabigatran is 14 to 17 hours. Dabigatran is predominantly excreted in the kidneys (up to 80%) and in the feces.[30] Although its metabolism is independent of CYP, potential drug interactions with quinine, quinidine, verapamil, and with P-gp inhibitors and/or inducers have been reported. When dabigatran is used for stroke prevention in nonvalvular atrial fibrillation patients, the recommended dose is 150 mg twice daily. However, patients should receive 50% of the recommended dose (75 mg twice daily) for stroke prevention if CrCl falls between 15 to 30 mL/min to avoid dabigatran accumulation and potential risk of bleeding.[30] The dose should be also reduced to 75 mg twice daily if the CrCl is 30 to 50 mL/min and the patient is on concomitant dronedarone or ketoconazole, and it should be avoided in patients who are taking any P-gp inhibitors with CrCl <30 mL/min or any patients who are taking any P-gp inducers such as rifampin. In patients who are diagnosed with acute DVT or PE and have received 5 to 10 days of appropriate parenteral anticoagulant, the dabigatran dose in patients with CrCl >30 mL/min is 150 mg twice daily and is not recommended for patients with CrCl <30 mL/min or patients with CrCl <50 mL/min who are taking concomitant P-gp inhibitor, or any patients that are taking P-gp inducers. It should be avoided in patients on hemodialysis in all indications. Unlike warfarin, dabigatran does not require routine blood test monitoring and dietary restrictions. In the RE-LY trial comparing the efficacy and safety of dabigatran and warfarin, both drugs demonstrated a similar efficacy and safety profile. The rate of serious bleeding was similar between the two drugs and dabigatran was associated with fewer strokes than warfarin.[33] After dabigatran's approval, a large number of reports of bleeding

TABLE 22-15 New Oral Anticoagulants Indications, Dosage Guidelines, Pharmacokinetics, Cautions, and Reversal for Elective Surgery

	APIXABAN	RIVAROXABAN	DABIGATRAN
Brand name	Eliquis	Xarelto	Pradaxa
FDA indication(s)	Postoperative DVT prophylaxis, stroke prevention in nonvalvular atrial fibrillation	Thromboembolism treatment and prophylaxis, stroke prevention in nonvalvular atrial fibrillation	Thromboembolism treatment and prophylaxis, stroke prevention in nonvalvular atrial fibrillation
Dosage			
Stroke prevention in nonvalvular atrial fibrillation	5 mg twice daily (2.5 mg twice daily if two of the following: age ≥80 years, body weight ≤60 kg, or serum creatinine ≥1.5 mg/dL)	20 mg daily with evening meal	150 mg twice daily
DVT/PE treatment	10 mg twice daily for 7 days then 5 mg twice daily for 6 mo (non–FDA approved dosage)	15 mg twice daily for 3 wk then 20 mg daily with food	150 mg twice daily (after 5-10 days IV anticoagulation)
DVT/PE prophylaxis	2.5 mg twice daily	20 mg daily with food	N/A
Pharmacokinetics/Pharmacodynamics			
Cmax (hr)	3-4	2-4	1-2
Bioavailability	50%	80%-100%	7%
Volume of distribution (L)	21	50	50-70
Protein binding	87%	92%-95%	35%
Half-life (hr)	12	5-9; 11-13 elderly	12-17; 14-17 elderly
Clearance	25% renal, 75 % biliary	60% renal, 33% biliary	80% renal
Metabolism	CYP3A4	CYP3A4, CYP2J2	Hepatic glucuronidation
P-glycoprotein substrate	Yes	Yes	Yes
Drug interactions	Avoid with strong dual inhibitors of P-gp and CYP3A4 if already taking 2.5 mg twice daily	Avoid with strong CYP3A4 inhibitors or inducers; avoid with strong dual inducers of P-gp and CYP3A4; avoid with dual strong inhibitors of P-gp and CYP3A4	Avoid with P-gp inducers; avoid with P-gp inhibitors
Cautions			
Boxed warning	D/c therapy increases risk of thrombotic events	D/c therapy increases risk of thrombotic events; epidural or spinal hematomas may occur if used while receiving neuraxial anesthesia or spinal puncture	D/c therapy increases risk of thrombotic events
Contraindications	Active bleed, hypersensitivity, prosthetic heart valve	Active bleed, hypersensitivity	Active bleed, hypersensitivity, prosthetic heart valve
Reversal for elective surgery	High bleeding risk procedure: d/c at least 48 hr prior Low bleeding risk procedure: d/c at least 24 hr prior	D/c at least 24 hr prior	CrCl≥ 50 mL/min, d/c 1-2 days prior CrCl< 50 mL/min, d/c 3-5 days prior

CrCl, Creatinine clearance; *CYP,* cytochrome P450; *d/c,* discontinue; *DVT,* deep vein thrombosis; *FDA,* U.S. Food and Drug Administration; *IV,* intravenous administration; *N/A,* not available; *P-gp,* p-glycoprotein; *PE,* pulmonary embolism.

were submitted to the FDA's Adverse Events Reporting System (AERS) database, a postmarketing surveillance program. In the data assessment, dabigatran was associated with a lower risk of clot-related strokes, bleeding in the brain, and death than warfarin. However, the study found an increased risk of major gastrointestinal bleeding with use of dabigatran compared with warfarin. The MI risk was similar for warfarin and dabigatran. This latest finding indicated that the observed bleeding rates associated with new use of dabigatran did not appear to be higher than the bleeding rates associated with the use of warfarin, which resonated with the RE-LY study.[34] Dabigatran is contraindicated in patients with active bleeding, patients with mechanical prosthetic heart valves, and patients with serious hypersensitivity to any components of its formulation.[30] An overview of dabigatran pharmacology is provided in Table 22-15.

Rivaroxaban is a direct factor Xa inhibitor with a competitive and reversible binding to factor Xa. Unlike dabigatran, rivaroxaban has a high oral bioavailability of 60% to 80% and a Tmax of 3 hours upon oral ingestion. Interestingly studies had shown that rivaroxaban exhibited a slightly lower antiXa activity in fasting patients compared with patients who were fed; therefore it is recommended to administer with food for a rivaroxaban dose equal or greater than 15 mg. For patients who cannot swallow whole tablets, the manufacturer's labeling states the 15 mg and 20 mg tablets may be crushed and mixed with applesauce immediately before use. The half-life of rivaroxaban is between 5 to 9 hours, with approximately 33% of the drug excreted unchanged renally and 66% metabolized in the liver primarily via CYP. Because of its association with the CYP system, it is subjected to drug interactions of CYP3A4 enzymes, and it is also affected by P-gp inhibitors and/or inducers. For treatment of VTEs, the recommended dosage is 15 mg twice daily with food for 3 weeks followed by 20 mg once daily with food for a total duration of 3 months in patients with provoked DVT or ≥3 months with unprovoked DVT depending on the patient's bleeding risk. In selected patients, rivaroxaban can be used for up to 6 to 12 months after the initial treatment for further reduction of recurrent DVT or PE. Initiation of rivaroxaban for postoperative DVT prophylaxis should start within 6 to 10 hours postoperatively with 10 mg daily for 12 to 14 days in knee replacement and 35 days in hip replacement. Lastly for patients with nonvalvular atrial fibrillation requiring anticoagulation for stroke prevention, the manufacturer recommends taking 20 mg daily of rivaroxaban with the evening meal. Similar to dabigatran, rivaroxaban requires dosage adjustment in patients with renal impairment. In patients who are treated for DVT or PE or in patients with postoperative prophylaxis, the use of rivaroxaban should be avoided if CrCl is less than 30 mL/min. In patients with nonvalvular atrial fibrillation the dosage should be reduced to 15 mg once daily if CrCl is between 15 and 50 mL/min and avoided in patients with CrCl less than 15 mL/min. It should be avoided in patients on hemodialysis in all indications. Caution should be exhibited when rivaroxaban is administered with a strong CYP3A4 and P-gp inhibitor or inducer.[31] In the ROCKET-AF trial comparing the efficacy and safety profile of rivaroxaban and warfarin in patients with atrial fibrillation, rivaroxaban was noninferior to warfarin for the prevention of stroke or systemic embolism. In the study, both drugs demonstrated similar risk of major bleeding that required blood transfusion. However, rivaroxaban was associated with less frequent intracranial hemorrhage and fatal bleeding compared with warfarin.[35] Rivaroxaban is contraindicated in patients with active bleeding or patients with hypersensitivity to any components of its formulation.[31] The manufacturer's recommended dosages regarding different indications is outlined in Table 22-15.

Apixaban is an oral direct factor Xa inhibitor with a reversible binding. Upon oral administration, it achieves Tmax approximately within 3 hours with an oral bioavailability of 50%. Apixaban has a half-life of 9 to 14 hours. Similar to rivaroxaban, the drug is metabolized in the liver via a CYP-dependent pathway, followed by elimination of 25% through the kidneys and the remainder into the feces. It is affected by CYP3A4 and P-gp inducers and/or inhibitors. For stroke prevention in patients with nonvalvular atrial fibrillation, the manufacturer recommends to administer apixaban 5 mg twice daily unless the patient has any two of the following patient-specific characteristics, including age ≥80 years, body weight ≤60 kg, or serum creatinine ≥1.5 mg/dL; then reduce dosage to 2.5 mg twice daily. For postoperative VTE prophylaxis, it is recommended to administer apixaban 2.5 mg twice daily beginning 12 to 24 hours postoperatively for 35 days in hip replacement and 12 days in knee replacement. At the time of publication, apixaban is not approved for the treatment of DVT and PE in the United States. If apixaban is administered concomitantly with a strong CYP3A4 and P-gp inhibitor such as clarithromycin, ketoconazole, itraconazole, or ritonavir the dosage should be reduced to 2.5 mg twice daily unless the dose had been previously reduced to 2.5 mg twice daily or if the patient meets two of the dose reduction criteria mentioned earlier. In addition, apixaban should not be administered with strong CYP3A4 and P-gp inducers because of the risk of subtherapeutic concentrations.[32] Compared with warfarin in patients with nonvalvular atrial fibrillation and prior history of stroke in the ARISTOTLE trial, apixaban was shown to be superior to warfarin. As illustrated in the study, apixaban was associated with a significant reduction of stroke and systemic embolism compared with warfarin[36]. In addition to its efficacy, apixaban demonstrated a safety profile superior to that of warfarin, such that apixaban was associated with less frequent intracranial bleeding, major or nonmajor bleeding, and mortality of any cause. Similar to all anticoagulants, apixaban is contraindicated in patients with active bleeding and patients with hypersensitivity to any components of its formulation. A list of the recommended dosages for different indications is provided in Table 22-15.

Warfarin (Coumadin)

Warfarin (Coumadin) is an OAC indicated for prophylaxis and treatment of venous thrombosis, PE, thromboembolic complications associated with atrial fibrillation and cardiac valve replacement, and as an adjunct in the treatment of coronary occlusion. Warfarin is also used to reduce the risk of death, reinfarction, and thromboembolic events such as stroke or systemic embolization after MI. Warfarin is a racemic mixture; the (S)-isomer has a half-life of 2 days, and the less potent (R)-isomer has a half-life of 1.3 days; warfarin is administered once daily. The full anticoagulant effect of warfarin has a delayed onset of 5 days, necessitating overlap with a parenteral heparin agent when rapid anticoagulation is preferred for at least 5 days and a therapeutic INR.

The initial dose of warfarin for a majority of patients should be the expected maintenance dose, which is usually 5 to 10 mg. Loading doses of 10 mg for 2 days are only recommended for sufficiently healthy patients who are treated as outpatients followed by dosage based on INR.[27] Warfarin starting doses of less than 5 mg may be most appropriate in elderly patients. Warfarin interferes with the hepatic synthesis of vitamin K–dependent clotting factors II, VII, IX, and X and endogenous anticoagulant proteins C and S. The time to complete anticoagulation with warfarin is not immediate. Inhibition of coagulation factors begins 12 to 24 hours after administration; however, the complete antithrombotic effects of warfarin may not occur until 5 to 7 days after initiation of therapy.

The INR is the standard for monitoring warfarin therapy. Prothrombin time (PT) as a tool for monitoring warfarin therapy is problematic because thromboplastin reagents vary in their responsiveness to warfarin-induced reduction in clotting factors, a variability that depends on their method of preparation. The INR is a *mathematical correction* of the results of the one-stage PT that standardizes the reporting of PT determinations worldwide. The INR takes into account the sensitivity of the thromboplastin used in each specific laboratory to determine the PT. The target INR range for warfarin in most clinical scenarios is 2 to 3. The INR should be used exclusively to indicate doses of warfarin clinically; however, the PT should be reviewed in conjunction with the INR to aid in detecting laboratory errors in calculation or assay methodology.

Hemorrhage is the most common adverse effect associated with warfarin and ranges from minor to life-threatening major bleeding. Bleeding manifestations may include ecchymoses, petechiae, purpura, melena, hematochezia, hematuria, hemoptysis, hematemesis, epistaxis, or gingival bleeding. Because warfarin inhibits protein C (half-life 8 hours) and protein S (half-life 30 hours), which have shorter half-lives than factors II (half-life 60 hours), IX (half-life 24 hours), and X (half-life 72 hours), there is a risk of a paradoxical hypercoagulability, thrombus formation, and skin necrosis with gangrene. The procoagulant effect of warfarin can be enhanced in patients who have protein C and protein S deficiency. To minimize the immediate procoagulant effect of warfarin, an overlap of 5 days with a parenteral anticoagulant is warranted. Purple toe syndrome, caused by the release of atheromatous plaque emboli and cholesterol-rich microembolization, occurs approximately 3 to 10 weeks after initiation of coumarin therapy. Purple toe syndrome is reversible and is typically characterized by a purplish or mottled discoloration of the plantar surfaces and sides of the toes that blanches on moderate pressure and fades with elevation of the legs. Oral or parenteral vitamin K_1 (phytonadione) may be administered to reverse the anticoagulation effects of warfarin.

Many factors such as diet, disease states, and drugs can alter the pharmacologic characteristics and effects of warfarin.[27] Patients should be counseled to eat a healthy and consistent diet. An increased intake of vitamin K–containing supplements and foods, such as green leafy vegetables, may result in a reduced anticoagulant response, decreased INR, and subsequently treatment failure such as an embolism. Conversely, abrupt decreases in vitamin K dietary intake may result in an increased anticoagulant response with an increased INR and subsequent risk of hemorrhage. Hepatic disease and, to a lesser extent, renal disease may decrease elimination of warfarin and increase the effects of warfarin. A plethora of drugs can increase or decrease the effects of warfarin. It is prudent to measure the INR frequently when factors that interact with warfarin are added to a patient's regimen. Table 22-16 lists selected significant warfarin drug interactions.

The role of genetic polymorphism in the management of warfarin has been the focus of interest in more recent studies. CYP2C9, which plays an integral role in the metabolism of the S-isomer of warfarin, and VKOR complex subunit 1 (VKORC1), the gene that determines the activity of vitamin K epoxide reductase, both undergo genetic polymorphism leading to variances in warfarin responses

TABLE 22-16	Selected Significant Drug Interactions With Warfarin
PRECIPITANT DRUG	**MECHANISM**
Amiodarone Cimetidine Lovastatin Metronidazole Omeprazole Quinidine TMP-SMX	These agents may increase anticoagulant effect of warfarin by inhibiting hepatic cytochrome P450 isozymes (CYP2C9, CYP3A4, or CYP1A2) involved in its metabolism; risk of bleeding may be increased
Chloral hydrate Loop diuretics Nalidixic acid NSAIDs	These agents may increase anticoagulant effect of warfarin by displacement from protein-binding sites (albumin); risk of bleeding may be increased
Antimicrobials NSAIDs Salicylates	These agents may increase anticoagulant effect of warfarin by inhibiting gastrointestinal vitamin K or by inhibiting platelet aggregation; risk of bleeding may be increased
Barbiturates Carbamazepine Oxcarbazepine Etretinate Glutethimide Rifampin Rifabutin	These agents may decrease anticoagulant effect of warfarin by induction of hepatic cytochrome P450 isozymes (CYP2C9, CYP3A4, or CYP1A2) involved in its metabolism; lack of warfarin efficacy and thrombosis may occur
Cholestyramine Estrogens Oral contraceptives Spironolactone Sucralfate Thiazide diuretics Vitamin K	These agents may decrease anticoagulant effect of warfarin by various mechanisms; lack of warfarin efficacy and thrombosis may occur

NSAIDs, Nonsteroidal antiinflammatory drugs; *TMP-SMX,* trimethoprim-sulfamethoxazole.

between patients. Studies have shown that testing for a patient's genetic type can lead to decreased major bleeding or thromboembolic events resulting in hospital admission; however, current guidelines recommend against the *routine use* of pharmacogenetic testing for guiding dose administration of vitamin K antagonists (VKAs).[27] Genetic test kits (e.g., GeneMedRx) are available for purchase, FDA approved, and covered by insurance plans; dosage guidelines are available in the product package insert.

Because warfarin is a high-risk medication that can significantly interact with many medications, requires frequent INR monitoring, and is pharmacokinetically challenging to determine correct dose, pharmacist-based warfarin clinics with physician supervision and collaboration have become a standard of best practice. More than 1500 such clinics are active in the United States today.

New Oral Anticoagulants and Drug Interactions

Warfarin, as mentioned previously, presents the potential for several drug interactions because of its metabolism via CYP2C9, CYP1A2, CYP3A4, and CYP2C19. In addition to CYP metabolism involving rivaroxaban and apixaban, all three new OACs (i.e., dabigatran, rivaroxaban, and apixaban) are P-gp substrates. P-gp is a drug transporter found in the gastrointestinal enterocytes and hepatocytes. P-gp works by pumping the drug back into the intestinal lumen, which consequently reduces the bioavailability and the plasma concentration of orally administered drugs. These drug transporters are also found in the kidneys and participate in drug elimination via this route. Therefore P-gp inhibitors can significantly increase the bioavailability and plasma concentrations, and inducers can significantly decrease the bioavailability and plasma concentrations of drugs metabolized via this pathway. Other substrates of P-gp include colchicine, cyclosporine, digoxin, fexofenadine, indinavir, morphine, and sirolimus. Inhibitors of the P-gp include amiodarone, clarithromycin, erythromycin, ketoconazole, quinidine, saquinavir, verapamil, and grapefruit juice. P-gp inducers include carbamazepine, dexamethasone, phenobarbital, phenytoin, rifampin, St. John's wort, tipranavir, and trazodone. It is important for the clinician to be aware of any concomitant P-gp inhibitors or inducers when a patient is taking one of the new OACs because of the risk of toxicity or ineffectiveness, depending on inhibition or induction of this transporter system.[37-40] Table 22-17 shows the most common P-gp substrates, inhibitors, and inducers.

Potential Reversal Agents for New Oral Anticoagulants

The advent of the new OACs (i.e., dabigatran etexilate, rivaroxaban, and apixaban) heralds the discussion for potential reversal agents in the event of clinically severe bleeding. To date, no specific agent has been studied in large-scale randomized trials for the reversal of the new OACs. However, nonspecific hemostatic agents, including recombinant factor VIIa (Novo Seven), prothrombin complex concentration (PCC) products, and activated PCC (FEIBA) have been

TABLE 22-17	P-Glycoprotein Substrates, Inhibitors, and Inducers	
SUBSTRATES	**INHIBITORS**	**INDUCERS**
Apixaban	Amiodarone	Carbamazepine
Colchicine	Clarithromycin	Rifampin
Cyclosporine	Erythromycin	St. John's wort
Dabigatran	Grapefruit juice	Tipranavir
Digoxin	Ketoconazole	
Fexofenadine	Quinidine	
Indinavir	Saquinavir	
Morphine	Verapamil	
Rivarixoban		
Sirolimus		

suggested for the reversal of major bleeding attributed by the new OACs in addition to supportive care and administration of blood products and plasma.[41,42,43] An important advantage of warfarin over the new OACs is the availability of an FDA-approved oral and parenteral vitamin K antidote with well-established dose guidelines, and the FDA-approved four-factor PCC (Kcentra) for urgent reversal of warfarin-induced major bleeding.

Recombinant factor VIIa (Novo Seven) initiates thrombin generation by activating factor X, thus promulgating the coagulation cascade. PCCs are concentrated pooled plasma products that typically contain clotting factors. These factors are generally not activated and will require activation via the coagulation cascade. In addition, some PCC products also contain proteins C and S, and in some cases, a minimal amount of heparin and antithrombin to prevent thrombotic complications. Three-factor PCC (Bebulin and Profilnine) contains trace or subtherapeutic amounts of nonactive factor VII relative to factors II, IX, and X. Four-factor PCC (Kcentra) contains relatively large amounts of four nonactive vitamin K-dependent procoagulant factors II, VII, IX, and X. Unlike previously mentioned PCC products, activated PCC (FEIBA) contains activated factor VII and factors II, IX, X, albeit mainly in nonactivated form. Therefore activated PCC (FEIBA) combines the effect of both recombinant factor VIIa (Novo Seven) and four-factor PCC (Kcentra).[44,45,46] These agents are not considered antidotes and not approved by the FDA for the reversal of the new OACs. An overview of different hemostatic agents for reversal of new OACs is summarized in Table 22-18.

If nonurgent reversal is required due to an elective surgery or invasive procedure, it is recommended to hold the new OACs for a certain period of time before the procedure depending on the patient's risk for bleeding and the patient's renal function. Dabigatran should be discontinued 1 to 2 days before elective surgery in patients with CrCl >50 mL/min and 3 to 5 days in patients with CrCl <50 mL/min. Longer times should be considered for patients undergoing major surgery, spinal surgery, or insertion of spinal or epidural catheter or port.[30] The rivaroxaban package insert recommends holding rivaroxaban for 24 hours before a procedure; however, some have recommended holding rivaroxaban for minimum of 3 days before surgery in

TABLE 22-18	Potential Reversal Agents for New Oral Anticoagulants			
	RECOMBINANT ACTIVATED FACTOR VIIA	**THREE-FACTOR PCC**	**FOUR-FACTOR PCC**	**ACTIVATED PCC**
Brand name	Novo Seven	Bebulin or Profilnine	Kcentra	FEIBA
Onset	10 min	10 min	10 min	10 min
Duration of action	2-6 hr	12-24 hr	6-8 hr	12-24 hr
Recommended dosage	Hemophilia with inhibitors: 90 mcg/kg/2 hr. Factor VII deficiency: 15-30 mcg/kg/4-6 hr. Acquired hemophilia: 70-90 mcg/kg/2-3 hr	Hemorrhage: Minor: 25-35 units/kg. Moderate: 40-55 units/kg. Major: 60-70 units/kg	INR 2 to <4: 25 units/kg. INR 4-6: 35 units/kg. INR >6: 50 units/kg	50-100 units/ kg/6-12 hr
Monitoring	Control of bleeding	Factor IX level, PT, PTT, INR (in warfarin reversal)	INR	Control of bleeding
Cost in a 70-kg patient	$2,000-$10,000, varies with indications	$2000-$5000, varies with severity of bleeding	$2000-$4000, varies with level of INR	$6,000-$12,000

INR, International normalized ratio; *PCC,* prothrombin complex concentration.

patients with CrCl >50 mL/hr and 5 days in patients with CrCl <50 mL/min. The risk of bleeding should be weighed against the urgency of the procedure.[31,47] For patients who are taking apixaban and are scheduled for surgery or invasive procedure with moderate-to-high risk of bleeding, it is recommended for apixaban to be held for 48 hours before the procedure. If the procedure carries a low risk of bleeding then apixaban can be held for 24 hours before the procedure.[32]

Four-Factor Prothrombin Complex Concentrate (Kcentra) for Warfarin Reversal

Recently in 2013, the FDA approved the four-factor PCC (Kcentra) for the urgent reversal of warfarin anticoagulation in adults with acute major bleeding. Like plasma, Kcentra is used in conjunction with the administration of vitamin K to reverse the anticoagulation effect and stop the bleeding. Unlike the plasma counterpart, Kcentra does not require blood group typing or thawing, adding the additional advantage for dosage convenience and ease. Kcentra dosage is individualized based on the pretreatment INR. For pretreatment INR of 2 to <4, Kcentra is to be administered at 25 units/kg to a maximum dose of 2500 units. For pretreatment INR of 4 to 6, Kcentra is to be administered at 35 units/kg to a maximum dose of 3500 units. For pretreatment INR of >6, Kcentra is to be administered at 50 units/kg to a maximum dose of 5000 units. In addition to administration ease, Kcentra is given in a significantly lower volume than plasma, providing an alternative for those patients who may not tolerate the volume of plasma required for warfarin anticoagulation reversal. Similar to all procoagulants, Kcentra is associated with the occurrence of blood clots; therefore it carries a boxed warning regarding the risk of thromboembolic events, requiring close monitoring for signs and symptoms of blood clotting complications.[48,49]

2012 CHEST Anticoagulation Guidelines Update

The CHEST Guideline is a publication compiled by the ACCP and provides evidence-based recommendations on various CVD states, including atrial fibrillation and VTEs, which include PE and DVT. The most recent edition of the guidelines was published in 2012.[27] Though warfarin has been the mainstay of anticoagulant treatment for many years, newer OACs that do not require therapeutic drug monitoring have become available. These include dabigatran (Pradaxa), rivaroxaban (Xarelto), and apixaban (Eliquis).

Atrial fibrillation is a common arrhythmia that predisposes patients to stroke and embolism. For patients with moderate to high risk as determined by the $CHADS_2$ score (score >1), anticoagulation is recommended. OACs are preferred over antiplatelet therapy. Dabigatran is the only OAC in addition to warfarin suggested to be used by the guidelines for atrial fibrillation because at the time it was the only one possessing approval for this use. The guideline provides a weak suggestion to use dabigatran over warfarin.[50]

For acute VTE, the guidelines recommend initial treatment with parenteral anticoagulation or rivaroxaban.[27] LMWH such as enoxaparin or dalteparin, or DTIs such as fondaparinux, are recommended over unfractionated heparin for parenteral anticoagulation. The guideline offers a weak recommendation for the use of warfarin and LMWH over rivaroxaban because of the lack of safety data available at the time of publishing. Apixaban is not mentioned in the guidelines and it has not been approved for use in VTE. For a provoked DVT or PE, the duration of treatment recommended is 3 months. For an unprovoked event, extended treatment is recommended if bleeding risk is not moderate to high.[50]

Benefits for the use of the newer OACs include the fast onset of action, lack of need for continuous drug therapy monitoring, and the convenience of not requiring bridging with rivaroxaban and apixaban. Barriers to their use include the lack of evidence in use for renally impaired patients, lack of specific antidotes for reversal of effect, drug interactions, and cost. In patients with mechanical valves or valvular atrial fibrillation, liver dysfunction, or severe renal impairment, warfarin would generally be the drug of choice.[37]

Antiplatelet Agents

Aspirin

In platelets, the prostaglandin derivative thromboxane A_2 is a major inducer of platelet aggregation and vasoconstriction. Aspirin is hydrolyzed to salicylic acid and inhibits prostaglandin production by acetylating cyclooxygenase, the initial enzyme in the prostaglandin biosynthesis pathway. This inhibition of platelet aggregation lasts for the life of the platelet, which is approximately 7 to 10 days. By inhibiting platelet aggregation, aspirin increases bleeding times. Low doses of aspirin inhibit platelet aggregation, whereas larger doses inhibit cyclooxygenase in arterial walls, which interferes with PGI_2 production. PGI_2 is a potent vasodilator and inhibitor of platelet aggregation. Lower doses plausibly may be more effective than higher doses in preventing coronary heart disease; however, this has not been proven clinically.

Aspirin has many indications including fever and pain associated with headaches, neuralgias, myalgias, and arthralgias. Antithrombotic indications for aspirin include reducing the risk of thrombosis, such as in the primary and secondary prevention of nonfatal or fatal MI in patients with or without previous MI or unstable angina, and preventing recurrent transient ischemic attacks (TIAs) or stroke. The dose of aspirin for its analgesic, antiinflammatory, and antipyretic effects is considered high dose and may be 325 to 650 mg up to every 4 hours daily as needed. The dose of aspirin for its antithrombotic indications is considered low dose; the range for prevention of MI is 81 to 325 mg daily and for TIA or stroke is 50 to 325 mg daily. Of patients taking aspirin as an antithrombotic, 25% may be genetically prone to aspirin resistance, and higher doses may be necessary to overcome resistance (e.g., 500 mg to 1.5 g daily). Aspirin resistance is best detected via bleeding time tests; however, these tests are not yet validated or standardized, and they are not routinely employed in clinical practice.

Aspirin-induced adverse effects are dose-dependent and include peptic ulcer disease, renal dysfunction, increased blood pressure, tinnitus, pulmonary dysfunction, and bleeding. The risk of clinically significant hemorrhage with aspirin (e.g., gastrointestinal bleeds) is dose-dependent. However, any dose of aspirin carries a risk of major bleeding compared with placebo controls. Patients should be counseled on the signs and symptoms of bleeding, which may include anemia, abnormal bruising, epistaxis, bleeding of the gums, dizziness and lightheadedness associated with

low blood pressure, and rapid heart rate. Aspirin, especially at high doses, can induce or exacerbate asthma by inhibiting bronchodilatory prostaglandins (PGE_2 and PGI_2) and can exacerbate dyspnea in patients with chronic obstructive pulmonary disease. Aspirin is contraindicated in patients who have a history of allergy, especially anaphylaxis to NSAIDs. Patients with rhinorrhea, nasal polyps, and aspirin-induced or NSAID-induced dyspnea are at greatest risk of aspirin-induced or NSAID-induced anaphylaxis. Aspirin should not be administered to children or teenagers with viral infections because of the risk of Reye syndrome.

An important drug-drug interaction between ibuprofen and aspirin has been identified. Ibuprofen interferes with aspirin access to the platelet serine-binding site and inhibits the pharmacologic effect of aspirin. This drug interaction occurs during single ingestion when ibuprofen is administered before aspirin or with long-term use of ibuprofen and aspirin regardless of whether ibuprofen is administered before or after aspirin. Diclofenac (Voltaren) and celecoxib (Celebrex) do not seem to interact with aspirin; other NSAIDs have not been studied. The combination of aspirin and NSAIDs may lead to a high risk of life-threatening gastropathy, especially in elderly patients or patients using concomitant antithrombotic agents. Aspirin and NSAIDs inhibit gastrointestinal vasodilatory prostaglandins (PGE_2 and PGI_2), increasing the accumulation of aggressive factors (acid) and decreasing the supply of defensive factors (sodium bicarbonate). Patients should be immediately placed on gastropathy prophylaxis with proton pump inhibitors (PPIs) (e.g., omeprazole, pantoprazole, esomeprazole, or lansoprazole) or misoprostol (Cytotec).

Dipyridamole

Dipyridamole is a vasodilator and platelet adhesion inhibitor. It has been postulated that patients with prosthetic heart valves have abnormally shortened platelet survival time. Dipyridamole lengthens the abnormally shortened platelet survival time in a dose-dependent manner. The primary effect of dipyridamole is to inhibit cGMP-specific phosphodiesterase, increasing cGMP levels and augmenting the effects of nitric oxide. Dipyridamole weakly inhibits red blood cell, endothelial cell, and platelet uptake of the platelet activity inhibitor adenosine and inhibits the formation of thromboxane A_2; this effect occurs in a dose-dependent manner (0.5 to 1.9 mcg/mL). This uptake inhibition results in dipyridamole inhibiting platelet function by inhibiting cyclic adenosine 3',5'-monophosphate (cAMP)–specific phosphodiesterase, which leads to increased cellular concentrations of cAMP within platelets, preventing platelet aggregation by stimuli such as collagen and ADP. Dipyridamole does not alter PT levels but can increase the platelet bleeding time.

Dipyridamole (Persantine) is indicated only as an adjunct to warfarin in the prevention of postoperative thromboembolic complications of cardiac valve replacement. Intravenous dipyridamole, occasionally used for cardiac exercise stress testing, may decrease blood pressure and increase heart rate and cardiac output; this effect is generally not seen with the oral dosage form. Dipyridamole is eliminated via hepatic conjugation and glucuronidation; it does not undergo hepatic CYP elimination. Dipyridamole has a weak metabolite and undergoes negligible renal elimination. The half-life of dipyridamole is 13 hours. Adverse reactions are transient and include headache, dizziness, hypotension, and abdominal distress. Rarely, dipyridamole has aggravated angina symptoms; the intravenous form has precipitated acute myocardial ischemia. Dipyridamole can potentiate the effects of intravenous adenosine, causing fatal asystole or sustained ventricular tachycardia; a decreased dose of adenosine should be used when treating paroxysmal supraventricular tachycardia.

Aggrenox is a combination gelatin capsule containing 200 mg of extended-release dipyridamole with 25 mg of aspirin and is indicated to reduce the risk of stroke for patients who have had TIAs or complete ischemic strokes. Steady-state dipyridamole peak and trough plasma levels are 2 and 0.5 mcg/mL, allowing for dipyridamole to achieve its effects on cAMP and cGMP throughout the dosing interval; this is not likely to occur with prompt-release dipyridamole. Dipyridamole requires an acidic environment for gut absorption; Aggrenox contains tartaric acid, allowing for maximal bioavailability in patients who have gut hypochlorhydria or achlorhydria (e.g., elderly patients).

The second European Stroke Prevention Study (ESPS-2) showed that dipyridamole modified-release formulation, 200 mg given twice daily, is effective in the secondary prevention of stroke and TIA compared with a placebo and that coadministration with aspirin, 25 mg twice daily, provides an additional benefit.[51] ESPS-2 showed that the relative risk reduction for stroke with aspirin administration compared with a placebo was 18.1% ($P = .013$); for modified-release dipyridamole, the relative risk reduction was 16.3% ($P = .039$); and with the combination, it was 37% ($P < .001$). Aggrenox must not be substituted with prompt-release dipyridamole and aspirin. The recommended dosage of Aggrenox is one capsule twice daily, swallowed whole. Because of increased risk of headache, it may be advisable to start with one capsule daily at bedtime and low-dose aspirin in the morning for up to 1 week until tolerated before increasing the Aggrenox dose to twice daily.[52]

Clopidogrel (Plavix)

Clopidogrel (Plavix) is a prodrug thienopyridine derivative platelet aggregation inhibitor that interferes with platelet membrane function by inhibiting ADP-induced platelet-fibrinogen binding and subsequent platelet-platelet interactions. Indications for clopidogrel include the reduction of atherosclerotic events in patients with a history of MI, stroke, or peripheral arteriolar disease and acute coronary syndrome (ACS) regardless of whether a patient is managed medically, by percutaneous coronary intervention (PCI), or by coronary artery bypass grafting. Clopidogrel is slightly more effective than aspirin in reducing the combined risk of ischemic stroke, MI, or vascular death in patients with atherosclerotic vascular disease.[53] For patients with ACS, clopidogrel plus aspirin was found to be superior to aspirin

alone in reducing composite endpoints of MI, stroke, and cardiovascular death. Clopidogrel has not shown superiority to aspirin for stroke prophylaxis except in patients with peripheral vascular disease.

Clopidogrel is extensively metabolized by the liver; its metabolites are eliminated equally via the kidneys and the feces. The half-life of clopidogrel metabolites is 8 hours; steady state is reached in 3 to 7 days. The onset of action of clopidogrel can be seen in 2 hours. The average platelet inhibition seen with clopidogrel is between 40% and 60%. Platelet aggregation and bleeding time return to normal within 5 days after clopidogrel discontinuation. The dose of clopidogrel in ACS is a 300-mg loading dose followed by 75 mg once daily (plus aspirin). A higher loading dose of 600 mg is recommended for patients undergoing PCI. For the prevention of cardiovascular events such as ACS, stroke, and peripheral arterial disease, the dose is 75 mg of clopidogrel once daily.

Because clopidogrel is a prodrug, it must undergo a two-step hepatic conversion to be activated. Only about 15% of the drug is converted to its active form, mainly through CYP2C19 and CYP3A4. Several trials have evaluated the possible interactions between clopidogrel and other drugs that can inhibit or competitively bind to these same isoenzymes, potentially inhibiting the conversion of clopidogrel to its active form and rendering the drug ineffective. PPIs, which are commonly prescribed for prophylaxis of stress ulcer, gastrointestinal reflux disease, and prophylaxis of gastrointestinal bleeding, are metabolized by CYP2C19 at varying degrees. Studies have reported that there is a significant increase in clinical event rates (e.g., MI, death) or greater platelet reactivity with concurrent use of clopidogrel and a PPI. Pantoprazole (Protonix) is the only PPI that does not undergo CYP2C19 metabolism and may potentially be devoid of this interaction, but more studies need to be conducted to confirm this. Other medications such as cimetidine, etravirine, felbamate, fluconazole, fluvoxamine, fluoxetine, ketoconazole, voriconazole, and ticlopidine should also be avoided because they can reduce antiplatelet activity of clopidogrel.

Statins or reductase inhibitors have also been an area of interest with regard to clopidogrel drug interactions. Similar to clopidogrel, statins are CYP3A4 substrates. In vivo studies that examined the degree of platelet inhibition by clopidogrel in patients taking a statin have shown that there is a significant decline in platelet inhibition with the use of statins. However, no large clinical trials have shown that this interaction can lead to negative clinical outcomes. Despite the lack of clinical trials evaluating the interaction between statins and clopidogrel, caution is advised when combining these two medications. If statin therapy is required, pravastatin (Pravachol) or rosuvastatin (Crestor) should be considered because these drugs do not undergo CYP3A4 metabolism and potentially are devoid of any significant drug interactions.[54]

Testing for genetic polymorphism has also received considerable emphasis in the FDA boxed warning for clopidogrel. Although genetic polymorphism for CYP2C19 has been shown in several studies to reduce antiplatelet activity and increase major adverse cardiac events (MACEs), prospective studies show clinical efficacy of personalizing antiplatelet therapy based on genotype analysis. The recommendation issued by the FDA to clinicians is to consider alternative treatment strategies, such as combining clopidogrel with cilostazol or using high-dose clopidogrel (600 mg loading dose followed by 150 mg daily for ACS) in patients identified as poor CYP2C19 metabolizers.

Unrelated to genetic polymorphisms and clopidogrel resistance, a study of 25,086 patients evaluated the dose of clopidogrel plus the dose of aspirin for patients with ACS and those undergoing PCI.[55] There was no difference in the primary endpoint of CV death, MI, or stroke at 30 days between the double-dose clopidogrel (600 mg on day 1, followed by 150 mg for 6 days, then 75 mg daily) versus a standard-dose clopidogrel 75 mg daily with either low-dose or high-dose aspirin. The secondary endpoint of definite stent thrombosis in those undergoing PCI was reduced in the clopidogrel higher-dose group for both drug eluting stent (DES) versus non-DES subtypes, but this benefit was offset by increased major bleeding in the higher-dose clopidogrel group. The efficacy and safety of these approaches remain uncertain and more studies are necessary.[55] Alternatively one may consider switching to another antiplatelet agent, such as prasugrel or ticagrelor, which does not undergo CYP2C19 metabolism.

The most common adverse effect of clopidogrel is hemorrhage, manifesting with purpura and epistaxis; other adverse effects include headaches, dizziness, abdominal pain, diarrhea, rash, and pruritus. In contrast to ticlopidine, clopidogrel has a lower incidence of rash, gastrointestinal disturbances, neutropenia, and thrombotic thrombocytopenic purpura (TTP), and cholestatic jaundice has not been reported with clopidogrel.

Ticlopidine (Ticlid)

Ticlopidine (Ticlid), a thienopyridine, is a platelet aggregation inhibitor that interferes with platelet membrane function by inhibiting ADP-induced platelet-fibrinogen binding and subsequent platelet-platelet interactions. The effect of ticlopidine on platelet function is irreversible and lasts for the life of the platelet. Ticlopidine is indicated for stroke. In the Ticlopidine Aspirin Stroke Study (TASS), the ticlopidine group had a 21% greater relative risk reduction for stroke compared with the aspirin group and a 9% greater reduction in stroke, MI, or vascular death at 3 years.[56] The Canadian-American Ticlopidine Study (CATS) showed that ticlopidine reduced the relative risk of stroke, MI, or vascular death by 30% compared with a placebo (10.8%; $P = .006$).[57] The half-life of ticlopidine is 14 hours; however, with repeat doses it approaches 4 to 5 days. Steady state is achieved within 14 to 21 days. Platelet aggregation is inhibited 50% within 4 days and 60% to 70% within 10 days. Platelet aggregation and bleeding time return to normal within 14 days after ticlopidine discontinuation. Ticlopidine is extensively metabolized by the liver; active metabolites have not been elucidated.

Because of the risk of life-threatening blood dyscrasias such as TTP and neutropenia and agranulocytosis, ticlopidine is a refractory agent reserved for patients who are intolerant or allergic to aspirin or clopidogrel or who have failed therapy with these agents. The onset of TTP occurs after 3 to 4 weeks of therapy, and the onset of neutropenia occurs after 4 to 6 weeks of therapy. TTP rarely occurs after 3 months of therapy. The incidence of TTP may be 1 case in every 1600 to 4000 patients. Signs and symptoms of TTP include microangiopathic hemolytic anemia (schistocytes on peripheral smear), purpura, petechiae, pallor, renal dysfunction, fever, weakness, difficulty speaking, seizures, jaundice, and dark or bloody urine. With proper detection, ticlopidine discontinuation, and management by plasmapheresis, 80% of patients survive. Because of the risk of ticlopidine-induced TTP and neutropenia, patients should have a complete blood count monitoring neutrophils, platelets, and hemoglobin and hematocrit biweekly for the first 3 months.

Rarely, ticlopidine can cause thrombocytopenia not induced by TTP. Ticlopidine may cause gastrointestinal disturbances such as diarrhea, nausea, and vomiting in one third of patients. Similar to clopidogrel, it does not directly cause peptic ulcer disease. Rare cases of rash that may progress to Stevens-Johnson syndrome and cholestatic jaundice have occurred with ticlopidine use. Ticlopidine may persistently increase total cholesterol levels by 10%.

Prasugrel (Effient)

Prasugrel (Effient) is a prodrug thienopyridine-derivative platelet aggregation inhibitor that interferes with platelet membrane function by inhibiting ADP-induced platelet-fibrinogen binding and subsequent platelet-platelet interactions. When prasugrel is compared with other agents in the same class, it has a very limited scope; it is indicated only for the prevention of thrombosis in patients with ACS undergoing PCI. Prasugrel in combination with aspirin decreases nonfatal MI slightly more than clopidogrel in combination with aspirin but with an increased risk of bleeding. Prasugrel is contraindicated in patients who have had history of a TIA or stroke. In patients older than 75 years or in patients who weigh less than 60 kg, prasugrel was shown to have a greater risk of bleeding, which outweighs its benefit.[58] Prasugrel is extensively metabolized by hydrolysis in the liver followed by CYP3A4 and CYP2D6; its metabolites are eliminated via the kidneys and feces. The half-life of the active metabolite of prasugrel is 7 to 8 hours. The onset of action of prasugrel can be seen in 30 minutes. The average platelet inhibition observed with prasugrel is 50% to 80%. Platelet aggregation and bleeding time return to normal approximately 5 to 9 days after prasugrel discontinuation. The dose of prasugrel in ACS is a 60-mg loading dose followed by 10 mg once daily (plus aspirin). In patients who weigh less than 60 kg, a decreased dose of 5 mg is recommended, although there have not been any clinical trials to support this practice.

The most common adverse effect of prasugrel is hemorrhage, which is greater than that observed with clopidogrel.

Other adverse effects are similar to clopidogrel. A higher incidence of colonic neoplasm was seen during the trial for its approval.[59,60]

Ticagrelor (Brilinta)

Ticagrelor (Brilinta) is a reversible and noncompetitive inhibitor of the ADP P2Y12 receptor on the platelet surface.[61] It prevents ADP-mediated activation of the GPIIb/IIIa receptor complex, resulting in decreased platelet aggregation. Ticagrelor is indicated to reduce the rate of thrombotic cardiovascular events in patients with ACS and the rate of stent thrombosis in patients treated with PCI, and is an appropriate alternative to clopidogrel or prasugrel for these indications. Ticagrelor has been shown to decrease the combined rate of cardiovascular death, MI, and stroke compared with clopidogrel, though no difference in rate of stroke was evident. However, ticagrelor has been associated with increased noncoronary artery bypass graft (CABG)-related bleeding and discontinuation caused by adverse effects compared with clopidogrel.[61-62] Similarly, prasugrel has also been shown to reduce the combined rate of cardiovascular death, nonfatal MI, and nonfatal stroke compared with clopidogrel, but it too has an increased bleeding risk.[60,62] Although there is a plethora of data comparing ticagrelor or prasugrel to clopidogrel, there is a dearth of data regarding the efficacy and safety of ticagrelor compared with prasugrel.[21] When ticagrelor is used, it should be initiated with a loading dose of 180 mg and continued with a dose of 90 mg twice daily. Ticagrelor should be used together with an initial loading dose of aspirin 325 mg followed by aspirin 75 to 100 mg daily. Ticagrelor's most significant adverse effect is hemorrhage and its use is contraindicated in patients with active pathologic bleeding and a history of intracranial hemorrhage; it should also not be used in patients with severe hepatic impairment or hypersensitivity to ticagrelor or any of its components. The risk for bleeding with ticagrelor is increased in patients with a recent trauma or surgery, recent gastrointestinal bleeding, peptic ulcer disease, moderate to severe hepatic impairment, surgical procedure, advanced age, or concomitant use of drugs that increase bleeding risk, including anticoagulants, antiplatelets, NSAIDs, selective serotonin reuptake inhibitors, and serotonin norepinephrine reuptake inhibitors. Other adverse effects that may occur with ticagrelor use include dyspnea, headache, bradyarrhythmias, and increased serum creatinine. Ticagrelor is a CYP3A4 substrate and should not be used together with strong CYP3A4 inhibitors such as ketoconazole, itraconazole, posaconazole, clarithromycin, nefazodone, ritonavir, nelfinavir, saquinavir, or indinavir; this may increase the serum concentration of ticagrelor. It should also not be used with strong CYP3A4 inducers such as rifampin, carbamazepine, St. John's wort, and phenytoin, which may decrease the serum concentration of ticagrelor. Additionally, although ticagrelor is used together with aspirin, aspirin maintenance doses greater than 100 mg reduce the effectiveness of ticagrelor and should be avoided.[61,62]

Cilostazol (Pletal) and Pentoxifylline (Trental)

Cilostazol (Pletal) is a quinolinone derivative that selectively and reversibly inhibits cellular phosphodiesterase III by increasing the levels of cAMP, resulting in vasodilation and inhibition of platelet aggregation. Cilostazol is indicated for intermittent claudication in patients with peripheral arterial disease. Cilostazol allows for increased walking distances and improves symptoms and quality of life in patients with intermittent claudication. The clinical benefits may not be noticed for at least 2 to 4 weeks, and may take 12 weeks. The only alternative to cilostazol for intermittent claudication is pentoxifylline (Trental); however, it has been proven inefficacious. Pentoxifylline is a xanthine agent with rheologic properties that decrease blood viscosity and improve erythrocyte flexibility.

Cilostazol is associated with a high incidence of transient adverse effects, such as headache, diarrhea, dizziness, and palpitations. In patients with heart failure, oral phosphodiesterase inhibitors such as milrinone have been associated with increased mortality resulting from arrhythmias; cilostazol and several of its metabolites are contraindicated in patients with heart failure and should be used prudently in patients with CAD. Cilostazol has been associated with increases in heart rate and reductions in P–R, QRS, and Q–T intervals on ECG. In the dog model, cilostazol has been associated with cardiac lesions and endocardial hemorrhage, similar to toxicities noted with milrinone; the risk of developing cardiac lesions with long-term cilostazol use is unknown. Cilostazol is a CYP3A4 and CYP2C19 substrate and has been associated with significantly elevated levels when combined with the CYP3A4 inhibitors ketoconazole, diltiazem, and erythromycin. Smokers exhibited 20% lower levels of cilostazol. Cilostazol is administered at 100 mg twice daily; the dose should be reduced in the presence of CYP3A4 inhibitors to 50 mg twice daily. Food increases the bioavailability of cilostazol by 90%; cilostazol should be administered on an empty stomach to circumvent this interaction. Grapefruit juice inhibits gut CYP3A4 and may increase plasma cilostazol levels and should be avoided during cilostazol use.

Vorapaxar (Zontivity)

Vorapaxar (Zontivity) is the only protease-activated receptor-1 (PAR-1) antagonist currently on the market. Vorapaxar inhibits PAR-1 on the platelet surface, resulting in inhibition of thrombin-induced and thrombin receptor agonist peptide (TRAP)-induced platelet aggregation.[63] Although its antiplatelet activity is reversible, because of its prolonged half-life it is effectively irreversible. Vorapaxar is indicated for the reduction of thrombotic cardiovascular events in patients with peripheral arterial disease or a history of MI.[63] Vorapaxar has been shown to decrease the combined rate of cardiovascular death, MI, stroke, and urgent coronary revascularization. Vorapaxar is given at a dose of 2.08 mg once daily together with aspirin and/or clopidogrel. Vorapaxar should generally not be used as the sole antiplatelet agent or with other antiplatelet agents besides aspirin and clopidogrel because of limited data regarding efficacy and safety. Because of risk for bleeding with vorapaxar, use is contraindicated in patients with active pathologic bleeding or a history of stroke, transient ischemic attack, or intracranial hemorrhage. Risk for bleeding is highest in patients who are older in age, have a low body weight, have reduced renal or hepatic function, have a history of bleeding disorders, or are using vorapaxar together with other drugs that increase bleeding risk, including anticoagulants, antiplatelets, NSAIDs, selective serotonin reuptake inhibitors, and serotonin norepinephrine reuptake inhibitors. Vorapaxar is a substrate of CYP3A4 and CYP2J2. Vorapaxar should not be used together with strong CYP3A4 inhibitors, which may increase the serum concentration of vorapaxar, or with strong CYP3A4 inducers, which may decrease the serum concentration of vorapaxar.[63]

Glycoprotein IIb/IIIa Inhibitors

GP IIb/IIIa inhibitors are indicated for the treatment of patients with ACS—unstable angina or non–ST segment elevation acute MI—and patients who are medically managed and patients undergoing PCI. Abciximab (ReoPro) is the GP IIb/IIIa inhibitor of choice for PCI. The management of unstable angina or non–ST segment elevation acute MI includes the use of aspirin, heparin, and a GP IIb/IIIa inhibitor. This combination has led to a decrease in the composite endpoints of new MI or death.[64] In patients who are being managed medically for a non–ST segment elevation ACS, the use of GP IIb/IIIa inhibitors has been marginalized to patients with moderate to high risk based on a risk assessment score and continued ischemia or patients with diabetes. GP IIb/IIIa inhibitors are administered via continuous intravenous infusions. Oral formulations of GP IIb/IIIa inhibitors failed to display efficacy in clinical trials and are unavailable.

The most common adverse effect reported during therapy was bleeding. The incidence of major bleeding manifesting as gastrointestinal, genitourinary, or intracranial hemorrhage with the three-drug combination was only slightly greater than with aspirin and heparin alone,

illustrating the safety of the GP IIb/IIIa inhibitors. Although minor bleeding with GP IIb/IIIa inhibitors is common (10%), it is generally inconsequential. Because these agents may cause thrombocytopenia, monitoring of the daily platelet, hemoglobin, and hematocrit is required. Abciximab has been implicated as a cause of immune-mediated thrombocytopenia in 5% of patients. Table 22-19 presents the pharmacologic characteristics of GP IIb/IIIa inhibitors.

Thrombolytic Agents

Thrombolytics are indicated for the management of PE, ischemic stroke, and acute ST segment elevation MI—the most extensive and life-threatening type of heart attack. Thrombolytics reduce the incidence of heart failure and death associated with acute MI and restore coronary blood flow by dissolving the thrombus, limiting the extent of ischemia and necrosis. Thrombolytics convert plasminogen to plasmin. Subsequently, the proteolytic enzyme plasmin initiates clot lysis and produces FDPs.

For the treatment of ST segment elevation ACS manifesting with at least 1 mm of ST segment elevation in two or more contiguous ECG leads, all available thrombolytics (streptokinase, alteplase, reteplase, and tenecteplase) are indicated; however, streptokinase is considered a second-line agent because of its lack of fibrin specificity. Eligible patients should receive thrombolytic therapy within 12 hours of symptom onset; however, a benefit can be realized for 24 hours. Thrombolytics are preferred to primary PCI when patients present within 3 hours of symptom onset and the *door to primary PCI time* would be greater than 90 minutes. For acute massive PE, alteplase is the only thrombolytic indicated. Alteplase is reserved for patients with acute massive PE who present with symptoms within 2 weeks but optimally within 5 days. Alteplase is the only thrombolytic indicated for the management of acute ischemic stroke for patients who present within 3 hours of symptom onset and no later than 6 hours after onset.[62] The use of thrombolytics is often precluded because of their

TABLE 22-19	Characteristics of Glycoprotein IIb/IIIa Inhibitors		
	ABCIXIMAB	**TIROFIBAN**	**EPTIFIBATIDE**
Brand name	Reopro	Aggrastat	Integrilin
Common uses	Adjunct to PCI	Management of ACS, medically or with PCI	Management of ACS, medically or with PCI; adjunct to PCI
Pharmacology	Chimeric human-murine monoclonal antibody Fab fragment GP IIb/IIIa inhibitor	Nonpeptide GP IIb/IIIa inhibitor	Cyclic heptapeptide GP IIb/IIIa inhibitor
Origin	Antibodies from immunized mice	Chemically derived	Active component of snake venom peptides
Binding to platelets	Irreversible	Reversible	Reversible
Elimination half-life	30 min	2 hr	2.5 hr
Platelet function recovery	Approximately 48 hr	Approximately 4 hr	Approximately 4 hr
Elimination	Renal, lymphatic system	65% renal, 25% biliary	50% renal, 30% metabolized in plasma into amino acids

ACS, Acute coronary syndrome; *PCI,* percutaneous coronary intervention.

extensive list of contraindications.[65] The absolute and relative contraindications for the use of thrombolytics are listed in Box 22-2.

The most common adverse effect associated with these agents is major and minor bleeding. Major bleeding includes gastrointestinal, genitourinary, respiratory tract, retroperitoneal, and intracranial hemorrhage. Minor bleeding often manifests as superficial or surface bleeding as a result of arterial punctures and surgical intervention. Thrombolytic-induced hemorrhagic stroke in patients older than 75 years occurs more often with alteplase than with streptokinase. Patients older than 75 years should receive streptokinase rather than alteplase. Alteplase and tenecteplase are known to be fibrin specific because they promote the conversion of plasminogen into plasmin in the presence of clot-bound fibrin only, with limited systemic proteolysis. The increased fibrin specificity is believed to induce less extensive systemic depletion of clotting factors such as fibrinogen and plasminogen. The clinical relevance of thrombolytic fibrin specificity has not been elucidated. Thrombolytics have rarely been associated with cholesterol embolization manifesting as purple toe syndrome, livido reticularis, acute renal failure, gangrene, MI, bowel infarction, stroke, and rhabdomyolysis. When thrombolytics are used for ACS, they can cause reperfusion arrhythmias manifesting as bradycardia or ventricular tachyarrhythmias. Table 22-20 presents the pharmacologic properties of thrombolytic agents.[66]

BOX 22-2   Thrombolytic Contraindications in Acute Treatment of Stroke

Absolute
- History or evidence of intracranial hemorrhage
- Clinical presentation suggestive of subarachnoid hemorrhage
- Known arteriovenous malformation
- SBP greater than 185 mm Hg or DBP greater than 110 mm Hg despite repeated measurements and treatment
- Platelet count less than 100,000/mm³
- Prothrombin time greater than 15 seconds or INR greater than 1.7
- Active internal bleeding or acute trauma (fracture)
- Head trauma or stroke within previous 3 months
- Arterial puncture at noncompressible site within 1 week
- Active internal bleeding
- Concurrent use of direct thrombin inhibitors (DTIs) or direct factor Xa inhibitors with elevated sensitive laboratory tests (such as activated partial thromboplastin time [aPTT],

international normalized ratio [INR], platelet count, and ecarin clotting time [ECT]; thrombin time [TT]; or appropriate factor Xa activity assays)
- Blood glucose concentration less than 50 mg/dL (2.7 mmol/L)
- Heparin received within 48 hours, resulting in abnormally elevated aPTT greater than the upper limit of normal
- Recent intracranial or intraspinal surgery

Relative
- Rapidly improving stroke symptoms
- Myocardial infarction in the previous 3 months
- Recent gastrointestinal or urinary tract hemorrhage (within previous 21 days)
- Major surgery or serious trauma within previous 14 days
- Seizure with postictal residual neurologic impairment
- Pregnancy

TABLE 22-20   Pharmacologic Properties of Thrombolytic Agents

	STREPTOKINASE	ALTEPLASE (rtPA)	RETEPLASE (rPA)	TENECTEPLASE (TNK-tPA)
Brand name	Streptase	Activase	Retavase	TNKase
Source	Streptococcal culture	Recombinant DNA technology using heterologous mammalian tissue culture	Recombinant DNA technology using Escherichia coli	Recombinant DNA technology using Chinese hamster ovary cells
Common uses	Pulmonary embolism, deep vein thrombosis, peripheral arterial occlusion, clearance of occluded central venous access devices, ST segment elevation	Pulmonary embolism, stroke, clearance of occluded central venous access device, ST segment elevation	Myocardial infarction, ST segment elevation	Myocardial infarction, ST segment elevation
Type of agent	Bacterial proactivator	Tissue plasminogen activator	Tissue plasminogen activator	Tissue plasminogen activator
Plasma half-life (min)	12-18	2-6	13-16	90-130
Fibrinolytic activation	Systemic	Systemic	Systemic	Systemic
Antigenic	Yes	No	No	No
Fibrin specific	+	+++	++	++++
Systemic bleeding risk	+++	++	++	+
ICH risk	+	++	++	++

ICH, Intracranial hemorrhage; *rPA,* recombinant plasminogen activator; *rtPA,* recombinant tissue-type plasminogen activator; *TNK,* tenecteplase; *tPA,* tissue-type plasminogen activator.

SELF-ASSESSMENT QUESTIONS

Answers can be found in Appendix A.

1. What is the systolic and diastolic blood pressure goal for patients older than 60 years without any comorbidities?
2. List adverse effects associated with angiotensin-converting enzyme inhibitors (ACEIs).
3. Which antihypertensive agents are preferred in the treatment of blacks without any comorbidities?
4. Which of the β blockers possess intrinsic sympathomimetic activity (ISA)?
5. Which of the β blockers possess selective β_1-blocker activity?
6. List adverse effects associated with α_1-adrenergic antagonists.
7. What are the most common side effects of nitrates?
8. List metabolic effects associated with thiazide diuretics.
9. Name five medications that may cause drug-induced increases in blood pressure.
10. Which calcium channel blocker is most likely to cause constipation?
11. Identify the best available parameter to monitor the effects of warfarin.
12. What is the antidote for heparin?
13. What is the mechanism of action of warfarin?
14. List the commercially available oral factor Xa inhibitors.
15. Identify the commercially available oral direct thrombin inhibitor.
16. List the common CYP3A4 and P-glycoprotein inhibitors.
17. Name the pharmacologic class responsible for inhibiting the final pathway in platelet aggregation.
18. Which thrombolytic is recommended for patients older than 75 years who present with ST segment elevation myocardial infarction?
19. Name the only ACEI that is available in a parenteral dosage form.
20. Identify the best available parameter to monitor the effects of heparin.
21. Is clopidogrel or ticlopidine superior to aspirin for stroke prevention?

CLINICAL SCENARIO

Answers can be found in Appendix A.

A 75-year-old man presents to the emergency department complaining of chest pain of 1 hour in duration. He has had intermittent chest pain for the past week. He describes experiencing substernal pain that radiates down his left arm. The pain is associated with diaphoresis and is not relieved by change in body position. He has had a history of hypertension for the past 10 years. He has no history or family history of coronary artery disease. He is currently taking labetalol, 200 mg twice daily, and an enteric-coated aspirin, 81 mg daily. He has no known allergies.

On physical examination, he appears anxious and is complaining of chest pain. His vital signs are as follows: blood pressure (BP) of 140/70 mm Hg, pulse (P) of 74 beats/min, and respiratory rate (RR) of 20 breaths/min. His heart sounds are normal, with no murmurs or gallops present. His lungs are clear on auscultation, and his abdomen, extremities, and funduscopic examination are unremarkable. His skin is cool and clammy.

Electrocardiography (ECG) shows evidence of sinus bradycardia with a heart rate of 49 beats/min. His cardiac enzymes all are elevated (creatine kinase [CK] of 200 U/L, CK-MB [CK isoenzymes found in muscle and brain fractions] of 20 U/L, and troponin I of 2 mcg/mL).

Based on his history, physical examination, and ECG, this 75-year-old man is diagnosed with non–ST segment elevation myocardial infarction (MI).

Using the SOAP method, assess this clinical scenario.

REFERENCES

1. Go AS, Mozaffarian D, Roger VL, et al: Heart disease and stroke statistics—2013 update: a report from the American Heart Association. *Circulation* 127:e6–e245, 2013.
2. CDC: Vital signs: awareness and treatment of uncontrolled hypertension among adults—United States, 2003–2010. *MMWR* 61(35):703–709, 2012.
3. Vasan RS, Beiser A, Seshadri S, et al: Residual lifetime risk for developing hypertension in middle-aged women and men: the Framingham Heart Study. *JAMA* 287:1003, 2002.
4. James PA, Oparil S, Carter BL, et al: 2014 evidence-based guideline for the management of high blood pressure in adults report from the panel members appointed to the eighth Joint National Committee (JNC8). *JAMA* 311(5):507–520, 2014.
5. *Drugs facts and comparisons*, St Louis, 2000, Facts & Comparisons, Wolters Kluwer Health.
6. Oates J: Antihypertensive agents and the drug therapy of hypertension. In Hardman J, Limbrid L, editors: *Goodman & Gilman's the pharmacological basis of therapeutics*, ed 9, New York, 1995, McGraw-Hill.
7. Chobanian AV, Bakris GL, Black HR, et al: Joint National Committee on Prevention, Detection, Evaluation, and Treatment of High Blood Pressure National Heart, Lung, and Blood Institute, National High Blood Pressure Education Program Coordinating Committee: Seventh Report of the Joint Committee on Detection, Evaluation, and Treatment of High Blood Pressure [JNC-VII]. *Hypertension* 42:1206, 2003.
8. Weber M, Messerli F, Bruner H: Angiotensin II receptor inhibition. *Arch Intern Med* 156:1996, 1957.
9. *Drug facts and comparisons*, St Louis, 2009, Facts & Comparisons, Wolters Kluwer Health.
10. Tekturna package insert, East Hanover, N.J., 2010, Novartis Pharmaceuticals Corp.
11. Grossman E, Messerli FH, Grodzicki T, et al: Should a moratorium be placed on sublingual nifedipine capsules given for hypertensive emergencies and pseudoemergencies. *JAMA* 276:1328, 1996.
12. Veelken R: Schimieder R: Overview of α_1-adrenergic antagonism and recent advances in hypertensive therapy. *Am J Hypertens* 9:139S, 1996.
13. Furberg C, Wright J, Davis B, et al: ALLHAT Officers and Coordinators for the ALLHAT Collaborative Research Group:

Major cardiovascular events in hypertensive patients randomized to doxazosin vs chlorthalidone: the Antihypertensive and Lipid Lowering Treatment to Prevent Heart Attack Trial (ALLHAT). *JAMA* 283:1967, 2000.

14. Yancy CW, Jessup M, Bozkurt B, et al: 2013 ACCF/AHA guideline for the management of heart failure: a report of the American College of Cardiology Foundation/American Heart Association task force on practice guideline. *Circulation* 128:e240–e327, 2013.

15. Hydralazine [package insert]. Sellersville, Pa., Teva Pharmaceuticals USA; 2012.

16. Minoxidil [package insert]. Corona, Calif., Watson Pharma, Inc; 2009.

17. Lloyd-Jones D, Adams RJ, Brown TM, et al: Heart disease and stroke statistics—2010 update: a report from the American Heart Association Statistics Committee and Stroke Statistics Subcommittee. *Circulation* 121:e1–e170, 2010.

18. Chaitman BR, Pepine CJ, Parker JO, et al: Combination Assessment of Ranolazine In Stable Angina (CARISA) Investigators: Effects of ranolazine with atenolol, amlodipine, or diltiazem on exercise tolerance and angina frequency in patients with severe chronic angina: a randomized controlled trial. *JAMA* 291:309, 2004.

19. Thandani U: Treatment of stable angina. *Curr Opin Cardiol* 14:349, 1999.

20. Williams G: Hypertensive vascular disease. In Fauci AS, Braunwald E, Isselbacher KJ, et al, editors: *Harrison's principles of internal medicine,* ed 14, New York, 1998, McGraw-Hill.

21. Jneid H, Anderson JL, Wirght RS, et al: 2012 ACCF/AHA Focused Update of the Guideline for the Management of Patients with Unstable Angina/Non-ST-Elevation Myocardial Infarction (Updating the 2007 Guideline and Replacing the 2011 Focused Update) developed in collaboration with the American College of Emergency Physicians, the Society for Cardiovascular Angiography and Interventions, and the Society of Thoracic Surgeons. *Circulation* 126:875–910, 2012.

22. Lexi-Drugs Online: Ranolazine monograph, Hudson, Ohio, Lexi-Comp Inc. Available at <http://www.crlonline.com/crlonline>. Accessed August 31, 2010.

23. Mathis AS: Newer antithrombotic strategies in the initial management of non-ST-segment elevation acute coronary syndromes. *Ann Pharmacother* 34:208, 2000.

24. Heesen M, Winking M, Kemkes-Matthes B, et al: What the neurosurgeon needs to know about the coagulation system. *Surg Neurol* 47:32, 1997.

25. Miesbach W, Seifried E: New direct oral anticoagulants—Current therapeutic options and treatment recommendations for bleeding complications. *Thromb Haemost* 108:1–8, 2012.

26. Hirsh J, Raschke R: Heparin and low-molecular-weight heparin: the Seventh ACCP Conference on Antithrombotic and Thrombolytic Therapy. *Chest* 126:188S, 2004.

27. Kearon C, Akl EA, Comerota AJ, et al: Antithrombotic Therapy and Prevention of Thrombosis, ed 9: American College of Chest Physicians Evidence-Based Clinical Practice Guidelines. *Chest* 141(2_suppl):e419S–e494S, 2012.

28. Lexi-Drugs Online: Heparin monograph, Hudson, Ohio, Lexi-Comp Inc. Retrieved from <www.online.lexi.com>.

29. Linkins LA, Dans AL, Moores LK, et al: Treatment and prevention of heparin-induced thrombocytopenia: American College of Chest Physicians evidence-based clinical practice guidelines, ed 9. *Chest* 141(2, Suppl):e495S–e530S, 2012.

30. Pradaxa [package insert]. Ridgefield, Conn., Boehringer Ingelheim Pharmaceuticals, Inc.; 2014.

31. Xarelto [package insert]. Titusville, N.J., Janssen Pharmaceuticals, Inc.; 2014.

32. Eliquis [package insert]. Princeton, N.J., Bristol-Myers Squibb Company; 2014.

33. Connolly SJ, Ezekowitz MB, Yusuf S, et al: Dabigatran versus warfarin in patients with atrial fibrillation. *N Engl J Med* 361:1139–1151, 2009.

34. FDA Drug Safety Communication: FDA study of Medicare patients finds lower risk of stroke and death but higher for gastrointestinal bleeding with Pradaxa (dabigatran) compared to warfarin. Retrieved from <http://www.fda.gov/Drugs/DrugSafety/ucm396470.htm>.

35. Patel MR, Mahaffey KW, Garf J, et al: Rivaroxaban versus warfarin in nonvalvular atrial fibrillation. *N Engl J Med* 365:883–891, 2011.

36. Granger CB, Alexander JH, McMurray JJV, et al: Apixaban versus warfarin in patients with atrial fibrillation. *N Engl J Med* 365:981–992, 2011.

37. Weitz JI, Gross PL: New oral anticoagulants: which one should my patient use? *Hematology Am Soc Hematol Educ Program* 2012:536–540, 2012.

38. Bailey DG, Dresser GK: Natural products and adverse drug interactions. *CMAJ* 170(10):1531–1532, 2004.

39. Horn JR, Hansten P: Drug Transporters: The Final Frontier for Drug Interactions. *Pharm Times* 2008. Published online.

40. Kiani J, Imam SZ: Medicinal importance of grapefruit juice and its interaction with various drugs. *Nutr J* 30(6):33, 2007.

41. Mancl EE, Crawford AN, Voils SA: Contemporary anticoagulation reversal: Focus on direct thrombin inhibitors and factor Xa inhibitors. *J Pharm Pract* 26(1):43–51, 2012.

42. Eerenberg ES, Kamphuisen PW, Sijpkens MK, et al: Reversal of rivaroxaban and dabigatran by prothrombin complex concentrate: A randomized, placebo-controlled, crossover study in healthy subjects. *Circulation* 124:1573–1579, 2011.

43. Perzborn E, Heitmeier S, Laux V, et al: Reversal of rivarobaban-induced anticoagulation with prothrombin complex concentrate, activated prothrombin complex concentrate and recombinant activated factor VII in vitro. *Thromb Res* 133:671–681, 2014.

44. Nitzki-George D, Wozniak I, Caprini JA: Current state of knowledge on oral anticoagulant reversal using procoagulant factors. *Ann Pharmacother* 47:841–855, 2013.

45. Fawole A, Daw HA, Crowther MA: Practical management of bleeding due to the anticoagulants dabigatran, rivaroxaban, and apixaban. *Cleve Clin J Med* 80(7):443–451, 2013.

46. Siegal DM, Crowther MA: Acute management of bleeding in patients on novel oral anticoagulants. *Eur Heart J* 23:489–500, 2013.

47. Wysokinski WE, McBane RD: Periprocedural bridging management of anticoagulation. *Circulation* 24:486–490, 2012.

48. Thigpen JL, Limdi NA: Reversal of oral anticoagulation. *Pharmacotherapy* 33(11):1199–1213, 2013.

49. Kcentra [package insert]. Marburg, Germany, CSL Behring GmbH; 2013.

50. You JJ, Singer DE, Howard PA, et al: Antithrombotic therapy for atrial fibrillation, ed 9: American College of Chest Physicians Evidence-Based Clinical Practice Guidelines. *Chest* 141(2_suppl):e531S–e575S, 2012.

51. Diener HC, Cunha L, Forbes C, et al: European Stroke Prevention Study. 2. Dipyridamole and acetylsalicylic acid in the secondary prevention of stroke. *J Neurol Sci* 143:1, 1996.

52. Aggrenox [package insert]. Boehringer Ingelheim Pharmaceuticals, Ridgefield, Conn.; 2012.

53. CAPRIE Steering Committee: A randomized, blinded, trial of clopidogrel versus aspirin in patients at risk of ischaemic events (CAPRIE). *Lancet* 348:1329, 1996.

54. Holmes DR, Jr, Dehmer GJ, Kaul S, et al: ACCF/AHA clopidogrel clinical alert: approach to the FDA "Boxed Warning": a report of the American College of Cardiology Foundation Task Force on clinical expert consensus documents and the American Heart Association. *Circulation* 122:537, 2010.

55. Mehta SR, Bassand JP, Chrolavicius S, et al: Dose comparison of clopidogrel and aspirin in acute coronary syndromes. *N Engl J Med* 363:930–942, 2010.

56. Hass WK, Easton JD, Adams HP, Jr, et al: A randomized trial comparing ticlopidine hydrochloride with aspirin for the

prevention of stroke in high-risk patients (TASS). *N Engl J Med* 321:501, 1989.

57. Gent M, Blakely JA, Easton JD, et al: The Canadian-American Ticlopidine Study (CATS) in thromboembolic stroke. *Lancet* 1:1215, 1989.

58. Wiviott SD, Braunwald E, McCabe CH, et al: TRITON-TIMI 38 investigators: Prasugrel versus clopidogrel in patients with acute coronary syndromes. *N Engl J Med* 357:2001–2015, 2007.

59. Micromedex Healthcare Series. Available at: <http://www.thomsonhc.com>. Accessed July 25, 2014.

60. Effient [package insert]. Indianapolis, Ind., Eli Lilly and Company; 2013.

61. Brilinta [package insert]. Wilmington, Del., AstraZeneca LP; 2013.

62. O'Gara PT, Kushner FG, Ascheim DD, et al: ACCF/AHA guideline for the management of ST-elevation myocardial infarction. *J Am Coll Cardiol* 61(4):2013, 2013.

63. Zontivity [package insert]. Whitehouse Station, N.J., Merck & Co., Inc.; 2014.

64. Latour-Perez J: Risk and benefits of glycoprotein IIb/IIIa antagonists in acute coronary syndrome. *Ann Pharmacother* 35:472, 2001.

65. Jauch EC, Saver JL, Adams HP, et al: Guidelines for the early management of patients with acute ischemic stroke: A guideline for the healthcare professionals from the American Heart Association/American Stroke Association. *Stroke* 44:870–947, 2013.

66. Ohman EM, Harrington RA, Cannon CP, et al: Intravenous thrombolysis in acute MI. *Chest* 119:253S, 2001.

CHAPTER 23

Sleep and Sleep Pharmacology

Ahmed S. BaHammam, David N. Neubauer,
Seithikurippu R. Pandi-Perumal

OBJECTIVES

After reading this chapter, the reader will be able to:

1. Define terms that pertain to sleep and sleep pharmacology
2. Describe sleep, its individual stages, and their electrophysiologic correlates
3. Comprehend the basic neurophysiologic mechanisms that promote brain arousal and wakefulness
4. Comprehend the basic neurophysiologic mechanisms that promote sleep onset and maintenance
5. Describe basic circadian processes and their interaction with the sleep-wake cycle
6. Recognize several sleep disorders that are amenable to pharmacotherapy
7. Describe the rationale for using certain classes of drugs to treat specific sleep-related disorders

KEY TERMS AND DEFINITIONS

Barbiturates Compounds whose parent structure is uric acid. These compounds depress central nervous system activity. Long-acting barbiturates such as pentobarbital have been used to treat epilepsy. Barbital was used during the early twentieth century to facilitate sleep in individuals with insomnia.

Benzodiazepines Compounds whose parent structure is a fusion of a diazepine ring with a benzene ring. Benzodiazepines enhance activity of the inhibitory neurotransmitter γ-aminobutyric acid (GABA). Benzodiazepines, which reduce anxiety and promote muscle relaxation, also promote sleep. The earliest benzodiazepines were chlordiazepoxide (Librium) and diazepam (Valium). Benzodiazepines for insomnia are now being replaced by nonbenzodiazepines such as zolpidem (Ambien), eszopiclone (Lunesta), and others.

Circadian rhythms *"Circa"* is Latin for "about," and *"diem"* is Latin for "day." Circadian rhythms refer to the approximately 24-hour cycle of biochemical, physiologic, and behavioral processes.

Electroencephalography (EEG) Measurement and recording of the gross electrical activity of the brain. During EEG recordings, electrodes are typically placed across multiple scalp regions. The electrodes are connected to amplifiers and filters that detect, magnify, and record the electrical activity of the brain.

Hypersomnia Presence of excessive sleepiness. Daytime sleepiness is so great that it leads to inappropriate daytime napping or sleep. Excessive sleepiness is not alleviated by prolonged sleep times or by napping.

Hypnotic Class of drugs used to induce sleep.

Parasomnias Group of sleep disorders manifested by undesirable motor, sensory, or behavioral phenomena that occur during sleep. The *International Classification of Sleep Disorders, Revised (ICSD-3)* lists 24 parasomnias.[1] More commonly encountered parasomnias include confusional arousals, sleep terrors, and sleepwalking.

Polysomnography Measurement and recording of EEG activity during sleep, typically coupled with measurement and recording of cardiorespiratory activity and eye movements.

The origins of sleep and the meaning of dreams have fascinated people for centuries—from philosophers to poets, ideas of the significance of sleep abound. Edgar Allen Poe described sleep as "little slices of death," whereas William Shakespeare regarded it to be the "chief nourisher in life's feast." Until more recently, sleep was considered to be a passive, dormant counterpart to waking life. We now know that sleep is an active process that may look similar to, but is very different from, either anesthesia or coma.

HISTORY OF TREATMENT OF SLEEP DISORDERS

Humans spend about a third of their life sleeping, and sleep disorders, which affect a large proportion of the general population and occur in all age groups, represent a major public health and global economic burden.[2] It is estimated that 50 million to 70 million adults in the United States have a chronic sleep disorder that interferes with their daily functioning and adversely affects their health and quality of life. Until the mid-1960s, the field of sleep medicine focused primarily on describing and treating insomnia, parasomnias (e.g., sleep walking, night terrors) and **hypersomnia**, such as narcolepsy. Patients experiencing these symptoms typically sought consultations from neurologists, psychiatrists, psychologists, or their family physician. Until more recently, treatments were generally based on empiric pharmaceutical intervention, behavioral modification protocols, or psychotherapy.

The role of the respiratory therapist in sleep medicine is still emerging, and areas of necessary proficiency and expertise are yet to be fully defined. An authoritative knowledge about sleep, sleep disorders, pharmacology, and the therapeutic actions of drugs on sleep architecture is required, together with knowledge of associated side effects or adverse drug reactions and toxicities. In the future respiratory therapists may be involved with the attending physician in determining appropriate pharmacotherapy for sleep-related disorders, such as narcolepsy or periodic limb movement disorder (PLMD). At a minimum, it is highly probable that during the course of performing sleep diagnostic procedures, the respiratory therapist will assess the patient's current therapeutic regimen and, after consultation with the physician, determine whether medications should be temporarily suspended before diagnostic procedures. Chapter 23 provides basic knowledge about sleep medicine for both the respiratory therapist who is still developing clinical skills and the experienced therapist who is actively participating in patient care with physicians.

KEY POINT

The *International Classification of Sleep Disorders, Revised (ICSD-3)*, published in 2014 by the American Academy of Sleep Medicine (AASM), classifies sleep disorders and diagnostic criteria. Diagnostic codes for each disorder are also provided. Currently, more than 80 sleep disorders are described in the *ICSD-3*.

It is beyond the scope of this chapter to address the entire spectrum of sleep disorders classified in the *International Classification of Sleep Disorders (ICSD-3)* or to provide an exhaustive summary of all the pharmacologic, neutraceutical, or cognitive behavioral therapies employed in this field. This chapter describes the classes of drugs that are likely to be encountered when treating patients with sleep disorders. First, a broad but brief overview of the history and evolution of sleep research and sleep pharmacology is presented followed by a brief overview of the brain mechanisms underlying the processes of wakefulness and sleep, including circadian aspects. Some key sleep-related disorders are described, and typical compounds that may be used to treat those disorders are reviewed. Adult sleep apnea syndrome, which is primarily treated with mechanical devices such as oral appliances or application of continuous positive airway pressure (CPAP), are not discussed. Apnea and bradycardia of prematurity, which are treated primarily with respiratory stimulants, are discussed in Chapter 8.

The onset and duration of sleep are orchestrated through multiple brain structures and neurotransmitter substrates, and pathology within those structures or neurotransmitter systems manifest as a sleep disorder. For example, loss of orexin/hypocretin-producing neurons in the lateral hypothalamus (LH) is associated with the inability to maintain prolonged periods of wakefulness or sleep and the intrusion of rapid eye movement (REM) sleep, or the signs of REM sleep, into wakefulness. Sleep pharmacotherapeutics evolved with the understanding that normalization of activity within perturbed brain regions, neurotransmitter systems, or both, leads to a reduction of the signs and symptoms of specific sleep disorders.

KEY POINT

Compounds to induce and sustain sleep have been in use for almost 5000 years. The oldest may perhaps be opium (which contains morphine), whereas the most recent are nonbenzodiazepines and orexin receptor antagonists.

As a result of increased public awareness about sleep disorders and scientific advances, sales of sleep-related drugs have increased markedly. Sales of medications to treat insomnia in the United States increased from $1.3 billion in 2001 to approximately $4.6 billion in 2006. However, the interest in pharmaceutical sleep aids is not new; sleep-inducing compounds were discovered and used thousands of years ago. Perhaps the first compound to be used as a sleep-inducing aid was the juice from the opium poppy. Some of the earliest written descriptions of the opium poppy have been found on Sumerian clay tablets dating to approximately 3000 BC. At that time, the juice of the poppy was harvested and consumed because of its ability to induce a euphoric state; this led to the plant being considered a *Gil Hul*, or "joy plant." Descriptions of the opium poppy have also appeared in writings of the Assyrians and Persians. The Greeks eventually were introduced to the opium poppy, which may represent the first time it was used expressly for sleep induction. Greek mythology depicts many sleep-related deities, including Hypnos (sleep), Morpheus (dreams), Nyx (night), and Thanatos (death, the twin brother of Hypnos) in association with opium extracted from the poppy. Homer described the properties of opium in both *The Iliad* and *The Odyssey* as an intoxicating, pain-relieving, and sleep-inducing substance.

More recent literature also expounds the sleep-inducing power of opium; in the *Wizard of Oz*, Dorothy, her dog Toto, and the Cowardly Lion fall into a deep sleep as they pass through a field of poppies on their approach to the Emerald City. The sleep-inducing effects of the opium poppy can be attributed to numerous alkaloids contained within the plant, including morphine and codeine. Both are central nervous system (CNS) depressants and opioid pain relievers.

Development of sleep-inducing compounds was revolutionized in the early nineteenth century by the synthesis of opium. Shortly after this, chloral hydrate and the bromides were developed. Chloral hydrate, a CNS depressant, rapidly induces deep sleep. Bromides, invented in the mid-nineteenth century, are also CNS depressants and induce sleep relatively quickly. Their popularity as sleep aids increased through the late nineteenth century and into the early twentieth century. Also during the nineteenth century, nitrous oxide was rediscovered, and ether and nitrous oxide were inhaled as "party favorites" of upper-class Europeans and Americans. The initial discoveries of ether by the Spanish alchemist Raymundus Lullius in 1275 and nitrous oxide by the English chemist Joseph Priestly in 1772 were lost to medical science until their reintroduction in 1842.[3] At that time, Crawford W. Long (1815–1878), a surgeon in Georgia, employed the recreational drug ether in surgical procedures because of its incredibly rapid induction of "sleep, amnesia and pain relief." In doing so, he unknowingly ushered in the modern era of anesthesia.[3]

Barbiturates, first discovered in the mid-nineteenth century, soon replaced bromides as the "sleeping pills" of choice in the early twentieth century. This class of drugs comprises more than 25,000 compounds that were synthesized by combining various compounds with barbituric acid. Although multiple barbituric acid compounds were developed, only a select few (including a diethyl derivative) resulted in sleep-promoting properties. Barbiturates, such as phenobarbital, are very effective at inducing sleep. However, they also have multiple side effects, not the least of which is the potential risk for barbiturate addiction, and if taken with alcohol, they can result in respiratory suppression and death. These hypnotic agents have now been replaced by newer, more effective, and safer compounds.

Benzodiazepines such as diazepam (Valium), temazepam (Restoril), and clonazepam (Klonopin) were first marketed in the 1970s. Early formulations of these CNS depressants shared similar side effect profiles to the barbiturates, although their margin of safety was much greater. However, benzodiazepines possess the potential for addiction, and because of the long half-life and the duration

needed to eliminate some benzodiazepines from the body (more than 12 to 24 hours), next-day "hangover" sleepiness effects and memory impairments are common. Since the introduction in the 1990s of nonbenzodiazepine and analogs of these compounds (e.g., zopiclone, zolpidem, zaleplon, and eszopiclone), the use of benzodiazepines for insomnia has declined.

The "ideal **hypnotic**" should possess the following principal characteristics. It should induce sleep rapidly (in about 10 to 15 minutes); maintain sleep over prolonged periods (about 7 to 8 hours); and be devoid of daytime residual side effects on memory, cognition, or alertness. It should also possess additional characteristics such as rapid absorption; optimal half-life; receptor-specific binding; no active metabolite; no potential for abuse, tolerance, or dependence; no respiratory depressive effect; and no interaction with alcohol or other CNS depressants.

In addition to "sleeping pills," many nondepressant medications are used in sleep medicine. In disorders such as restless legs syndrome (RLS) and PLMD, sleep onset is often delayed and fragmented. First-line therapy for these disorders includes dopamine agonists and in some cases, opiates. Respiratory stimulants are another class of medications sometimes employed in the treatment of sleep disorders. Medroxyprogesterone and acetazolamide have been used in an effort to enhance ventilation in patients with high altitude–induced central sleep apnea or obesity-hypoventilation syndrome. More recently, the antidepressant mirtazapine has been shown to reduce apnea severity in animal models emulating sleep apnea and in some patients.[4] An effective pharmaceutical treatment for obstructive sleep apnea does not yet exist.

KEY POINT

Manifestations of sleep disorders can emerge from within different sleep states. REM sleep behavior disorder occurs only during REM sleep. Confusional arousals tend to occur when awakening from slow wave sleep (SWS) (stage N3). Somnambulism (sleep walking) is also known to occur during the first third of the night, the sleep period predominated by SWS (stage N3).

PROGRESSION OF SLEEP

Sleep was originally thought to be a passive rather than an active process. Richard Canton (1842–1926), a physiologist at the Royal Infirmary in Liverpool, is credited with the discovery of **electroencephalography (EEG)**, an important milestone in the understanding of sleep as an active process. His experimental observations on cortical currents in rabbits and monkeys were published in the *British Journal of Medicine*.[5] Using a mirror galvanometer, Canton observed an increase in the amplitude of waves measured from the cortex during states of sleep as opposed to a decrement in cortical amplitudes during wakefulness. Canton was the first to perform sleep EEG on mammals.[6] Subsequently several observations including those of Constantin von Economo (1876–1931) and the experiments by Giuseppe Morruzi and colleagues clearly showed that sleep is not a passive phenomenon but involves several brain regions, especially the diencephalon and the brainstem, which actively control sleep and states of arousal.[7,8] In 1957 William Dement and Nathaniel Kleitman (Father of sleep research) reported the cyclical alternating pattern of non–rapid eye movement (NREM) and REM sleep.[9]

When determining the most appropriate pharmaceutical intervention for a sleep disorder, it is important to first consider how sleep is defined and measured, and the normative values of time spent in sleep and in each sleep stage (i.e., sleep architecture). Mammalian sleep can be defined as a cyclical, reversible behavioral state of perceptual disengagement from, and unresponsiveness to, the external environment. Within normal human monophasic sleep, sleep is polygraphically characterized into two distinct stages based on a constellation of behavioral and electrophysiologic parameters. These two stages are NREM and REM sleep. NREM sleep is categorized further into stages N1 to N3 (formerly known as stages 1 to 4); N1 is the lightest and stage N3 is the deepest sleep stage. Figures 23-1 to 23-4 show examples of EEG-defined wakefulness followed by examples of stages N1 to N3.

The term for REM sleep is derived from the periodic bursts of REMs during sleep. REM sleep has both *tonic* (persistent) and *phasic* (episodic) components. During tonic REM sleep, the EEG tracing shows a similar pattern to that of N1, but it may also exhibit increased activity in the theta frequency range (3 to 7 Hz) and sawtooth type of waves. REM sleep is also accompanied by a generalized muscle atonia, with the exception of the extraocular muscles and the diaphragm. Figure 23-5 shows an example of EEG-defined REM sleep.

Eugene Aserinsky and Nathaniel Kleitman were the first to observe the electrophysiologic characteristics of REM sleep and in particular, the rapid, jerky, and binocularly symmetric eye movements in this sleep stage.[10] EEG patterns similar to wakefulness were noted, showing the characteristic fast, desynchronized rhythms in the cortical EEG, and the term *paradoxical sleep* was introduced by Michel Valentin Marcel Jouvet and Michel in 1960; the term *active sleep* was used by other researchers. These terms are used interchangeably in the literature, although subtle differences exist. Additionally, autonomic activation occurs during this state as respiratory and heart rates are increased. Dream recall is also common when subjects are awakened during this stage, whereas dream recall during NREM sleep is relatively rare (Table 23-1).

Sleep stages occur in cycles that repeat approximately every 90 to 120 minutes. A normal sleep cycle begins with N1 and proceeds through N3. Sleep rapidly passes through the same stages in reverse order before REM sleep is initiated, usually first occurring about 90 minutes after sleep onset. Although significant interindividual variation in sleep need is noted, adult humans typically sleep about 7 to 9 hours per night and spend almost one-third of their lives sleeping. Figure 23-6 provides a graphic representation of the cyclical distribution of sleep stages across a single night in a normal healthy adult (sleep hypnogram).

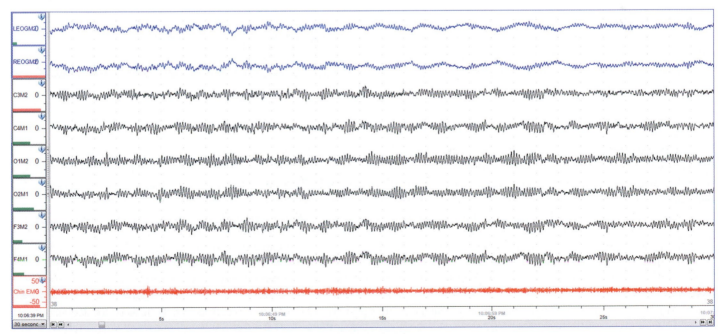

Figure 23-1 Wakefulness. A 30-second Epoch consisting of the parameters of staging sleep (electroencephalogram [EEG], electrooculogram [EOG], and chin electromyogram [EMG]) showing stage wake (W). The record shows alpha rhythm and increased chin EMG tone.

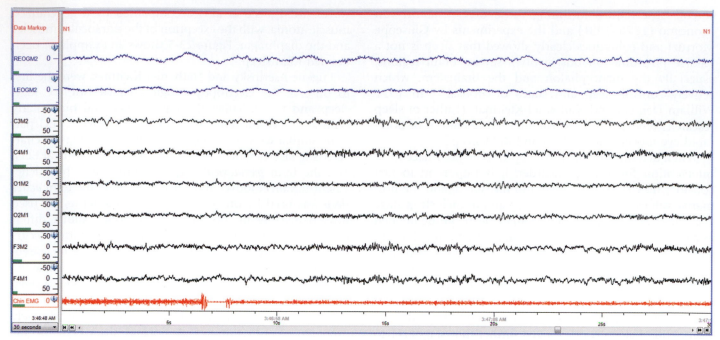

Figure 23-2 A 30-second Epoch consisting of the parameters of staging sleep (electroencephalogram [EEG], electrooculogram [EOG], and chin electromyogram [EMG]) showing stage N1. The EOG shows presence of slow eye movements (SEM) which is conjugate, reasonably regular and sinusoidal eye movements and the EEG shows low amplitude, mixed frequency activity, predominantly of 4-7 Hz (theta waves).

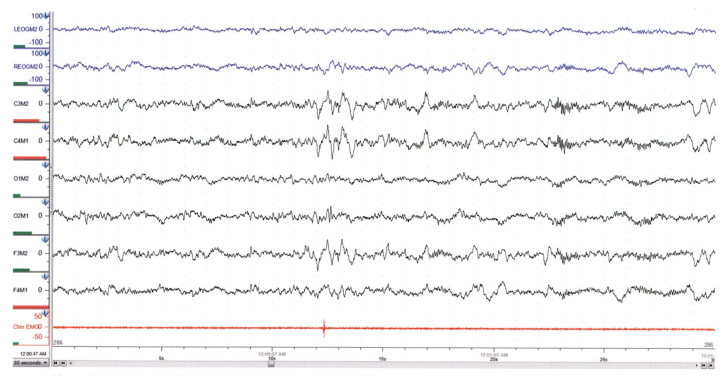

Figure 23-3 A 30-second Epoch consisting of the parameters of staging sleep (electroencephalogram [EEG], electrooculogram [EOG], and chin electromyogram [EMG]) showing stage N2. EEG demonstrates sleep spindles (short rhythmic waveform clusters of 11-16 Hz, often showing a waxing and waning appearance with a duration ≥0.5 second and K complexes (negative sharp waves immediately followed by a slower positive component with total duration ≥0.5 second shown maximally in the frontal leads).

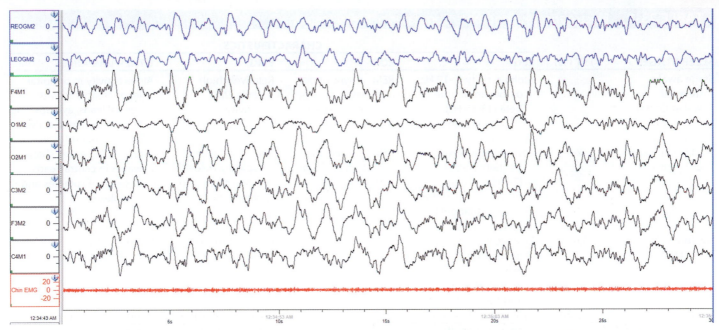

Figure 23-4 A 30-second Epoch consisting of the parameters of staging sleep (electroencephalogram [EEG], electrooculogram [EOG], and chin electromyogram [EMG]) showing stage N3. The EEG shows slow wave activity, which are waves of a frequency of 0.5-2 Hz with a peak-to-peak amplitude >75 μV.

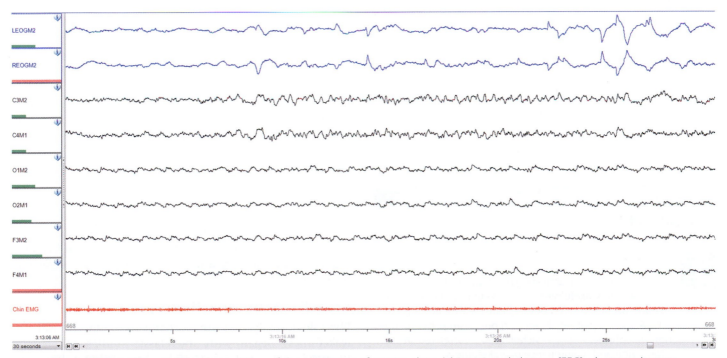

Figure 23-5 A 30-second Epoch consisting of the parameters of staging sleep (electroencephalogram [EEG], electrooculogram [EOG], and chin electromyogram [EMG]) showing stage R (rapid eye movement [REM] sleep). The EOG shows rapid eye movements and the EEG shows mixed-frequency, low-amplitude waves. Chin EMG is absent.

TABLE 23-1   Electroencephalographic Correlates of Sleep Stages

SLEEP STAGES	TST (%)	CHARACTERISTICS			
		EEG	EOG	EMG	OTHER VARIABLES
Stage awake (relaxed wakefulness)		Alpha activity (8-12 Hz) or low-amplitude beta (13-35 Hz), mixed-frequency waves	REM (in sync or out of sync deflections), eye blinks	Relatively high tonic EMG activity	Alpha activity in occipital leads compared with central leads, eye opening suppresses alpha activity, movement artifacts
N1, formerly known as stage 1	2-5	Low-voltage, mixed-frequency waves (2-7 Hz range), mainly irregular theta activity, triangular vertex waves	SEMs, waxing and waning of alpha rhythm	Tonic EMG levels typically below range of relaxed wakefulness	Alpha ≤50%, vertex sharp waves in central leads, absence of spindles and K complexes
N2, formerly known as stage 2	45-55	Relatively low-voltage, mixed-frequency waves, some low-amplitude theta and delta activity	No eye movement	Low chin muscle activity	Sleep spindles (7-14 Hz) and K complexes occur intermittently
N3, formerly known as stages 3 and 4	5-20	≥20%-50% of epoch consists of delta (0.5-2 Hz) activity	No eye movement	Chin muscle activity is lower than N1 and N2	Sleep spindles may be present
Stage REM	20-25	EEG is relatively low voltage with mixed frequency resembling N1 sleep	Episodic rapid, jerky, and usually lateral eye movements in clusters	EMG tracing almost always reaches its lowest levels owing to muscle atonia	Phasic and tonic components, presence of sawtooth waves, alpha waves are 1-2 Hz slower than waves occurring during wakefulness and non-REM sleep

EEG, Electroencephalography; *EMG,* electromyography; *EOG,* electrooculography; *REM,* rapid eye movement; *SEMs,* slow eye movements; *TST,* total sleep time.

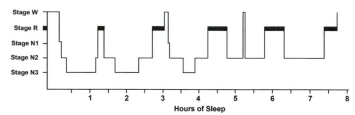

Figure 23-6 A sleep hypnogram showing normal distribution of sleep stages.

NEUROPHYSIOLOGIC MECHANISMS

Arousal and Wakefulness

KEY POINT

The neural arousal or activating mechanisms that produce the state of wakefulness reside within multiple brain regions, and each region uses a different neurotransmitter. Activities within brain regions using histamine, norepinephrine, and acetylcholine are correlated in the production and maintenance of wakefulness.

In a series of postmortem examinations of the brains of patients who had died as a result of the outbreak of *encephalitis lethargica* after World War I, von Economo[8] observed that lesions in the rostral midbrain and posterior hypothalamus had a profound effect on sleep and wakefulness. He derived two significant correlates from his observations. The first was that lesions in the preoptic and basal forebrain (BF) areas caused severe insomnia. The second was that lesions in the posterior and LH caused severe hypersomnia. On the basis of these data, von Economo hypothesized the existence of a group of sleep-promoting neurons around the hypothalamic optic chiasm and conversely a group of wake-promoting neurons in the area of the posterior hypothalamus. Both observations have been proved to be essentially correct, but it was only toward the end of the twentieth century that the hypothalamic influences on sleep and wakefulness were integrated into the mechanisms of vigilance state control. Before that, the emphasis had been on brainstem mechanisms and the *ascending reticular activating system (ARAS).*

Ascending Reticular Activating System

Physiologic analysis of the mechanisms of EEG arousal and wakefulness began with the classic studies of Frédéric Bremer (1892–1982); in 1935 he showed that if the brainstem of a cat was completely transected at the level of the midbrain (i.e., to produce the *cerveau isolé* [isolated brainstem]), the result was that the cat maintained a persistent state of sleep. Different interpretations of this result were possible until Moruzzi and Magoun[11] demonstrated the existence of an active arousal center below the level of the transaction, in the pons (i.e., the brainstem). Subsequent lesion and electrical stimulation studies identified the brainstem core, or pontine reticular system, as a critical component of arousal and wakefulness. This system was termed the *ascending reticular activating system (ARAS)* and was morphologically defined by cell bodies that projected from the brainstem to innervate the midbrain and cortex.

A more recent advance has been the identification of the importance of a cholinergic activating system in EEG arousal. This is one of the major components of the ARAS, and its identification depended on methods that were developed for labeling neurons that contain specific neurotransmitters. Steriade and colleagues[12] identified cells located near the pons-midbrain junction that increased their discharge rate about 60 seconds before the first change to an aroused state was noted on the EEG. These neurons were found to project to the thalamus, and the change in their discharge rate was the first indication of arousal. Subsequent work identified these neurons as containing the neurotransmitter acetylcholine and being localized to the laterodorsal pontine tegmentum/pedunculopontine tegmentum (LDT/PPT) region.

Cholinergic systems are not the exclusive substrate of EEG arousal, however, and evidence that multiple systems are involved in arousal and wakefulness came from the inability of lesions of any single one of these systems to disrupt EEG arousal on a permanent basis.[13] Other brainstem reticular neuronal projections to the thalamus using glutamate neurotransmission and noradrenergic and serotoninergic projections from the locus caeruleus and raphe nuclei also play important roles in maintaining wakefulness. In addition to brainstem nuclei, a cholinergic input to the cortex that ascends from the BF nuclei, especially the nucleus basalis of Meynert, plays an important role. Histaminergic neurons localized in the tuberomammillary nucleus (TMN) of the posterior hypothalamus also promote wakefulness. Discovery of the orexin/hypocretin system in 1999 (see section on Narcolepsy later) led to another CNS arousal system being identified. It is probably the latter hypothalamic systems that were affected in the brains examined by von Economo.[8]

The current conception of the mechanisms of arousal and wakefulness can be summarized by noting that wakefulness and the concomitant EEG arousal is a state of brain activation resulting from the influence of several excitatory neurotransmitters. The term ARAS has been replaced by *ascending activating system (AAS)*. NREM sleep is the absence of such excitatory drive, and from the onset of sleep through to the deep stages of slow wave sleep (SWS) (N3), NREM sleep is marked by the gradual reduction of this arousing influence. REM sleep then occurs as a different aroused state, but one that is still modulated by some of the same excitatory pathways that are active during wakefulness. Wakefulness is supported by several apparently redundant parallel neurotransmitter pathways, which include glutamate, acetylcholine (projecting from both the LDT/PPT nuclei in the brainstem and the BF), and the monoamines

(i.e., norepinephrine, serotonin, and histamine). With the exception of the hypothalamic TMN and LH projections, which also innervate the cortex, and the cholinergic BF projection, which exclusively innervates the cortex, these ascending projections of the AAS innervate the thalamus.

Thalamic Mechanisms of Arousal

Most AAS projections that mediate EEG arousal and wakefulness have their synapses in the thalamus, which is an essential center for the organization of EEG arousal and for maintaining activation at a cortical level. Thalamic mechanisms at a cellular level influence the differences between wakefulness and NREM sleep. A detailed consideration of these thalamic mechanisms is beyond the scope of this chapter; they depend primarily on the cells in the thalamus that project to the cortex (i.e., thalamocortical neurons).[14] Thalamocortical neurons differ in their rate and pattern of discharge depending on the vigilance state. When the arousal-related glutamatergic, cholinergic, noradrenergic, and serotoninergic projections are active, they drive the thalamocortical neurons to discharge in single spike mode. This discharge keeps the EEG in an active state, which contributes to arousal and wakefulness.

In contrast, in the absence of activating or arousing inputs, thalamocortical cells modify their discharge rate to a burst mode. This bursting drives oscillations in thalamic and cortical loop circuits, and these oscillations are the substrate of the slowing and increasing amplitude of the EEG that characterizes NREM sleep. The gradual and continuing reduction in the arousing input results in the gradual deepening of NREM sleep until delta waves dominate the EEG during SWS.

Sleep Onset and Processes That Maintain Sleep

KEY POINT

The neural mechanisms that produce the state of sleep also reside within several brain regions, and each region uses a different neurotransmitter. Onset of activity within the ventrolateral preoptic (VLPO) nuclei orchestrates the onset and maintenance of NREM sleep.

An important consideration is the mechanism that begins this process of reducing the drive from the activating (wakefulness) systems.[15] In other words, how does sleep begin? Electrophysiologic recordings of cells in the BF and anterior hypothalamic regions showed that some of these neurons discharge only during sleep, and this was hypothesized to be an active sleep-promoting mechanism. Confirmation came from studies by Sherin and colleagues,[16] who used anatomic techniques to detect neurons in the ventrolateral preoptic (VLPO) area that were selectively active during NREM sleep. Subsequent immunohistochemical studies identified the neurotransmitters contained in these cells as inhibitory γ-aminobutyric acid (GABA) and glycine. Anatomic work showed neurons containing GABA and glycine projected not only to wakefulness-promoting histaminergic neurons in the TMN and other hypothalamic centers including the BF, but also to all the brainstem nuclei important in EEG arousal.[17] This group of cells coordinates the *inhibition of activity* in all components of the AAS to facilitate sleep onset. Current studies continue to investigate the interaction of these neurons with other systems that are important in sleep and in particular how other cells within a region around the VLPO area, named the extended VLPO area, are involved with initiating the onset of REM sleep.

Two-Process Model of Sleep Regulation

Homeostatic sleep drive. Sleep propensity is determined by homeostatic and circadian sleep drives. The homeostatic component of sleep need is the sleepiness that follows prolonged wakefulness, and there is now considerable evidence to support the role of adenosine as a mediator of this component. This role of adenosine seems to depend primarily on its inhibitory action on the BF wakefulness-promoting neurons. Commonsense evidence for a sleep-enhancing effect of adenosine comes from the ubiquitous use of coffee and tea to increase alertness because these beverages contain caffeine, an adenosine receptor antagonist.[18] McCarley and colleagues[19] hypothesized that during prolonged wakefulness adenosine accumulates selectively in the BF and promotes the transition from wakefulness to sleep by inhibiting the wakefulness-promoting BF neurons through its action at the adenosine A1 receptor. Regulation of the levels of extracellular adenosine depends primarily on metabolic rate: Increased metabolism leads to reduced high-energy phosphate stores and increased adenosine, which, via an equilibrative transporter, leads to increased extracellular adenosine. The BF wakefulness-promoting neurons inhibit the VLPO area, and the adenosine-mediated inhibition of BF cells is one mechanism by which the VLPO cells begin to discharge as sleepiness increases and the sleep episode begins.

! KEY POINT

The suprachiasmatic nuclei (SCN) are the neuroanatomic sites of the primary mammalian biologic clock. Subpopulations of SCN neurons exhibit spontaneous patterns of discharge activity and are described as self-sustaining neural oscillators, or pacemakers. When maintained in culture and devoid of afferent input, these neural pacemakers follow a "free-running" activity pattern that is slightly less than 24 hours.

Circadian process. In addition to the homeostatic need for sleep, sleepiness depends on a second major influence: circadian phase. Humans, similar to many other species, continue to show regular, circadian sleep-wake cycles and other physiologic and hormonal rhythms in the absence of a 24-hour light/dark (LD) cycle. These rhythms must depend on an internal "clock" or pacemaker that is self-sustaining in the absence of external time cues and can be reset by changes in the environment. The mechanisms of this internal clock have been subject to research over many

years, and significant progress has been made using genetic data obtained from a wide variety of species, including the bread mold *Neurospora*, the fruit fly *Drosophila*, and the mouse.[20] The diversity of the species from which these results have been obtained emphasizes a remarkable conservation of function in time-keeping in biologic systems during evolution.

This circadian influence on sleep also acts through the VLPO area to work in concert with the homeostatic drive to maintain sleep by consolidating the sleep period. The circadian pacemaker achieves this consolidation by a mechanism that at first sight seems to be in a paradoxical phase relationship to the normal timing of the sleep period. This assumption follows from the fact that the circadian drive for wakefulness is strongest in the evening hours, just before the normal time of sleep onset. Conversely, the circadian drive for sleepiness is strongest in the morning hours, just before the usual waking time. This process helps to consolidate the sleep phase despite the homeostatic drive for sleepiness in the evening and homeostatic drive for wakefulness in the morning.

Combining the characteristics of the endogenous sleep-wake rhythm with those of a circadian oscillator has led to testable mathematical models of sleep propensity. One of the most significant of these models was developed by Borbely,[21] who based his model on a two-process single oscillator model. In this model, sleep is seen as the net result of two processes. One, *process S*, or sleep propensity, builds during wakefulness and declines exponentially during sleep and is indexed by the delta power of the EEG. As noted earlier, adenosine is a likely candidate for the endogenous mediator of process S. The second process, *process C*, is an endogenous circadian oscillator that closely parallels core body temperature. The output from the endogenous clock is probably the mediator of process C.

Circadian sleep-wake and physiologic rhythms are treated as sinusoidal variables in this model, assumptions that are not supported by actual data. The sleep-wake state is essentially a binary process, and the actual shape of the variation in physiologic variables across the nychthemeron is asymmetric and is modulated under normal conditions by changes related to activity and sleep onset. The recording of core body temperature under several different conditions, including normal expression of the sleep-wake cycle, sleep deprivation with constant activity over 24 hours, and continuous bed rest with minimal activity but normal sleep-wake behavior, might provide more accurate modeling data after appropriate subtractive manipulation.[22] This point is addressed in more detail subsequently.

Circadian Processes and Chronobiology

The circadian processes of sleep and wakefulness are also important for considerations related to pharmacotherapy. The basic underlying biologic oscillators affect the response to a drug in addition to driving the biologic rhythms such as sleep propensity and core body temperature.

Circadian Timing System

Biologic rhythms vary systematically across the 24 hours of the nychthemeron. In particular, **circadian rhythms** are driven by endogenous pacemakers that have periods (τ, tau) approximating 24 hours.[23] As noted previously, these are self-sustained, internally generated biologic signals that in the natural environment are normally synchronized or entrained to the 24-hour LD cycle. Both sleep and temporal organization are evolutionarily conserved behaviors, although they can change during the life span of an organism.[24] Such evolutionarily conserved, intrinsic temporal order is crucial for human health and well-being, and disturbances in these rhythms result in behavioral, physiologic, psychological, biochemical, and endocrinologic abnormalities.

Studies over many years have attempted to derive an accurate estimation of the period of the endogenous pacemaker. To do so required the subjects not only to be placed under "free-running" conditions in which the environment was completely devoid of any time cues, but also under conditions in which the period of the endogenous pacemaker could not be entrained to the rest-activity cycle. These considerations led to the adoption of the forced desynchrony protocol, originally developed by Kleitman in 1938.[9] In this type of study, subjects were kept on a rest-activity cycle that was sufficiently long (e.g., 28 hours) to prevent the entrainment of the endogenous pacemaker to this rhythm. Results were variable, however, until Czeisler and colleagues[25] in 1999 changed the protocol so that their subjects were exposed to very dim light (about 10 to 15 lux) throughout. In this way, Czeisler and colleagues were able to determine the period of the human circadian pacemaker at 24.18 hours; they also reported that healthy older subjects had the same periodicity, with the same stability and precision, as younger subjects.

Under normal circumstances, circadian rhythms become synchronized or entrained to the environmental LD cycle, which acts as a pervasive and prominent synchronizer, or *zeitgeber*.[26] Light signals are perceived in the retina and are transmitted via a monosynaptic pathway, the retinohypothalamic tract (RHT), to the SCN. Non–image forming effects of retinal light exposure range from effects on various physiologic measures, such as shifts in the circadian rhythms of melatonin and body temperature, to effects on psychological measures—for example, high environmental light intensity increases arousal and alertness.

Although the mechanism by which light exerts these alerting effects is unknown, a more recently discovered network of blue light–sensitive retinal ganglion cells (RGCs)[27,28] is likely part of the input system for the physiologic effects. In animals[29] and in humans,[30] the suppression of melatonin and shifts in circadian rhythms are particularly sensitive to a short-wavelength, blue component of light. The blue light–sensitive RGCs express the photopigment melanopsin and a neuropeptide—pituitary adenylate cyclase activating polypeptide (PACAP).[27,28,31] Significantly, the RGCs project to brain regions implicated in sleep mechanisms, including the SCN and the VLPO area.[28,32] This finding suggests that they might mediate the effect of light on sleepiness.[33]

Suprachiasmatic Nucleus: The Central Oscillator

The SCN, which is localized to the anterior hypothalamus, acts as the "biologic clock" to coordinate the circadian rhythm.[34,35] The SCN receives photic information via the glutamatergic RHT and the geniculohypothalamic tract (GHT), which contains neuropeptide Y (NPY) and non-photic information via serotoninergic neurons originating in the dorsal raphe nucleus (DRN). SCN neurons, which project to the dorsomedial and posterior hypothalamic areas and the VLPO area, actively promote and maintain wakefulness during the day and sleep at night (Figure 23-7). The SCN is involved in the regulation of the timing of sleep-wake states and in the expression of the sleep-wake cycle and may play a role in the coordination of specific sleep stages.[35,36] The role of the SCN in the control of sleep has been studied extensively in several species. In squirrel monkeys, a diurnal species similar to humans, the circadian signal produced by the SCN promotes wakefulness during the subjective day and consolidation of sleep at night. Lesions of the SCN have been found to disrupt the consolidation of both sleep and wakefulness as a result of a disrupted circadian rhythm.[37] Neurons in the SCN express two melatonin receptors (MT1 and MT2) that have different functional roles.

Chronopharmacology

Chronobiology is concerned with the mechanisms of periodic biologic influences on health and disease[38]; pharmacology refers to the medical discipline concerned with the biochemical and physiologic aspects of drug effects, including absorption, distribution, metabolism, elimination, toxicity, and specific mechanisms of drug action. The effectiveness of drugs, also a critical aspect of pharmacology, depends on pharmacodynamics (i.e., what the drug does to the body) and pharmacokinetics (i.e., what the body does to the drug). These considerations involve the quantitative aspects of drug absorption, distribution, and excretion that are crucial for the design of rational dosage regimens.

Chronopharmacology, or the study of time-dependent variations in pharmacology,[39] was developed from the inclusion of chronobiologic principles in the study of pharmacology. Traditionally, drug delivery has assumed that a chemical is absorbed predictably from the site of administration. A second-generation drug delivery goal has been the achievement of a continuous constant rate (i.e., zero-order) delivery of drugs. However, living organisms are not "zero-order" in their response to drugs. As mentioned earlier, living organisms are predictable resonating dynamic systems governed by intrinsic oscillators, so they require different amounts of a drug at different times within the circadian cycle to maximize the desired and undesired (i.e., chronotoxicity) effects of the drug. Two concepts are important when considering changes in drug efficacy over the 24-hour period. The first is circadian changes in drug

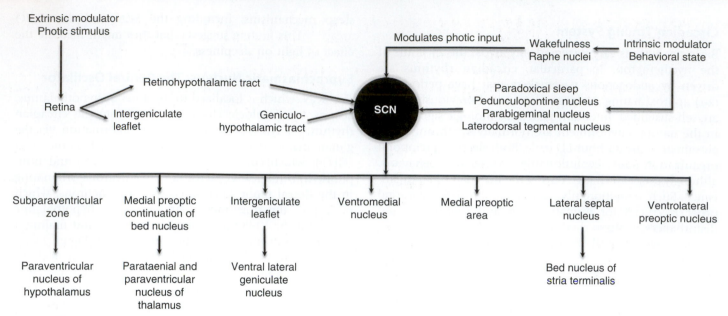

Figure 23-7 Primary afferent and efferent pathways of suprachiasmatic nuclei *(SCN)*. In addition to the well-described retinohypo-thalamic tract, which provides SCN with extrinsic stimuli (light), the lesser described serotoninergic afferent pathway arising from the raphe nuclei and cholinergic afferent pathways originating in the pedunculopontine, parabigeminal, and laterodorsal tegmen-tum nuclei *(LDT)* are illustrated. This figure graphically illustrates a conceptual model through which intrinsic behavioral state–related stimuli could affect neuronal activity in SCN. (From Decker MJ, Lee SY, Rye DB, et al: *Front Neurol* 1:122, 2010.)

bioavailability (i.e., chronokinetics), and the second is circadian changes in the susceptibility to the drug (i.e., chronesthesy). In brief, clinical chronopharmacology, or chronotherapeutics, is the purposeful alteration of drug levels to match biologic rhythms and to optimize therapeutic outcomes and minimize side effects.

Melatonin as a Chronobiotic and Chronohypnotic Agent

Drugs that directly influence circadian mechanisms are often referred to as *chronobiotics*.[40] The prototype for this type of drug is melatonin (*N*-acetyl-5-methoxytryptamine), a pineal hormone that has been identified as an important endogenous regulatory factor, with levels that vary with circadian time. In humans, melatonin is an important signal for maintaining endogenous rhythms in synchrony with the environmental LD cycle. Melatonin is exclusively secreted during the subjective night, and its plasma level increases during the evening and declines in the early morning.[41] The finding that melatonin is secreted primarily during the night and the close relationship between the nocturnal increase in endogenous melatonin and the timing of human sleep have suggested that melatonin might be important in sleep regulation. The onset of melatonin secretion occurs approximately 2 hours before bedtime and has been shown to correlate with the onset of evening sleepiness. In other words, the transition phase from wakefulness and arousal to high sleep propensity coincides with the nocturnal increase in endogenous melatonin. As noted earlier, SCN neurons express high concentrations of both melatonin receptors (MT1 and MT2), although both receptors are also found widely expressed throughout the CNS.

Signaling via MT1 leads primarily to inhibition of activity in SCN neurons.[42] In contrast, the principal MT2-mediated actions in the SCN are related to circadian phase shifts and constitute activation of protein kinase C and increased cell activity.[43]

It is possible that melatonin contributes to sleep initiation by inhibiting the circadian wakefulness-generating mechanisms, an effect that could be mediated by MT1 receptors in the SCN. Melatonin release is pulsatile during light sleep, and the hormone could function to induce deeper sleep and prevent awakening by continuing to inhibit arousal at the level of the SCN. Overall, the hypnotic and chronobiotic effects of melatonin might be mediated in the SCN and possibly through the MT1 receptor.[44] Induction and maintenance of sleep at the appropriate circadian phase, which could be MT1-mediated, is different from shifting the phase of sleep, which could be MT2-mediated, as a result of exogenous change in the *zeitgeber*.

It is relevant that the hypnotic effect of melatonin depends on the circadian phase of administration. Stone and coworkers,[45] using a double-blind placebo-controlled study, found that melatonin administered at night (23:30 hours) had no significant effect on sleep in healthy individuals, whereas melatonin administered in the evening (18:00 hours) exerted a hypnotic activity. Despite such evidence for the hypnotic action of melatonin, its efficacy in promoting sleep is still controversial, especially because most results show only borderline significance or are otherwise difficult to evaluate because of methodologic inconsistencies.[46] However, the relatively poor outcomes in these studies in terms of sleep efficiency or total sleep time may be due to the short half-life of melatonin in plasma (less than 30 minutes). It is possible that a melatonin receptor agonist with a longer half-life and occupying receptors in the SCN for a longer duration could be more effective than melatonin in promoting sleep in insomniac patients.[47]

Ramelteon is a melatonin receptor agonist that has been shown to be selective for MT1 and MT2 receptors but without affinity for the melatonin-binding site, quinone reductase 2, previously denoted as MT3.[48] Ramelteon has no affinity for other major CNS receptors, including binding sites for neurotransmitters, neuropeptides, regulatory enzymes, or ion channels.[48] However, various additional non–membrane binding sites of melatonin remain to be tested.[49]

The ability of a melatonin receptor agonist to stabilize circadian rhythms is evident with tasimelteon (Hetlioz), which recently has been approved by the U.S. Food and Drug Administration (FDA) for the treatment of the non-24 type of circadian rhythm sleep-wake disorder. It was developed for totally blind individuals who experience repeated episodes of difficulty with nighttime sleep and daytime sleepiness.

SLEEP DISORDERS: CAUSES AND TREATMENTS

As noted at the beginning of this chapter, there are more than 80 identified sleep disorders. Epidemiologic data reveal that the incidence and prevalence of these disorders vary in the general population. Although some of these disorders can be effectively managed by non-pharmacologic therapies or medical management (e.g., CPAP for obstructive sleep apnea), others are treated effectively with pharmacologic agents. Available pharmacologic treatment options for some of these disorders are outlined in this section.

Insomnia

Insomnia is characterized by difficulty in falling asleep (i.e., a sleep latency of greater than 30 minutes), insufficient sleep (i.e., total sleep time of less than 5.5 to 6 hours), multiple nocturnal awakenings, early morning awakening with inability to resume sleep, or nonrestorative sleep. Common daytime complaints include somnolence, fatigue, irritability, and difficulty concentrating and performing everyday tasks. In addition, subjects with a diagnosis of insomnia are at higher risk for illness and for injury caused by drowsiness while driving. Because insomnia is associated with difficulty in concentration, it is a major risk factor for accidents.[50] Insomnia is a common disorder that affects 30% to 35% of the U.S. adult population and is chronic in about 10%.[51] The risk of insomnia is greatest in elderly adults. The adverse physiologic and psychological sequelae of insomnia have a major negative effect on the quality of life in affected individuals.[52] Almost 10% of people with chronic insomnia have daytime consequences of fatigue, irritability, and impaired concentration that affect health,

mood, and normal functioning. With reduced productivity and an increased risk of accidents, the overall economic burden of insomnia is estimated to be 1% of gross domestic product.[53] Insomnia is also experienced as a stressor by patients who have major depressive disorders, and disturbed sleep has been identified as a hallmark of depression; this is not always recognized in clinical practice.

Pharmacologic treatment of insomnia in the last few decades has been based on several classes of medication (Table 23-2). Benzodiazepines were introduced in the 1970s and rapidly increased in popularity because of their efficacy and relative safety compared with barbiturates, carbamates, chloral derivatives, and methaqualone. In recent years, however, prescriptions for benzodiazepines have declined because of the associated side effect profile, including the tendency of benzodiazepines to promote dependence, the occurrence of rebound insomnia after withdrawal of short-acting and intermediate-acting derivatives, and the loss of efficacy after a few weeks of treatment. The reduction in benzodiazepine use has also coincided with the introduction of a structurally dissimilar group of nonbenzodiazepine derivatives, including the cyclopyrrolone agents zopiclone and eszopiclone, the imidazopyridine derivative zolpidem, and the pyrazolopyrimidine compound zaleplon. Recently, the FDA approved Belsomra (suvorexant) tablets for use as needed to treat insomnia. Suvorexant promotes sleep through the binding inhibition of orexin A and B, neuropeptides that promote wakefulness.[54]

Restless Legs Syndrome and Periodic Limb Movement Disorder

The first clinical description of RLS was made in the seventeenth century by Willis, an English physician, who stated, "Wherefore to some, when being abed they betake themselves to sleep, presently in the Arms and Legs, leaping and Contractions of the tendons, and so great a Restlessness and Tossing of their members ensue, that the diseased are no more able to sleep, than if they were in a Place of greatest torture."[55] More than 200 years later, the physician Ekbom coined the phrase "restless legs" and stated that "the syndrome is so common and causes such suffering that it should be known to every physician."[56]

RLS is now recognized as a chronic and progressive neurologic disorder characterized by unpleasant sensations in the legs and a compelling urge to move them while the patient is awake. These symptoms occur most frequently during the evening or at night, as well as during periods of rest. Approximately 5% to 15% of European and American populations are affected by RLS. Adverse outcomes associated with RLS include hypertension, alcohol abuse, neurocognitive deficits, and decrements in mental and physical health. Patients with RLS report an urge to move their limbs during the daytime if they become confined in a delineated space for extended periods, for example, having to sit at a desk. Unpleasant sensations in the limbs typically combined with urges to move the legs occurring in the evening often lead to difficulties with sleep onset or sleep

TABLE 23-2	Medications Approved by U.S. Food and Drug Administration for Treatment of Insomnia			
MEDICATION	**TRADE NAME**	**DOSE (mg)**	**HALF-LIFE (hr)**	**DEA SCHEDULE**
BZD Receptor Agonists				
Immediate-Release BZDs				
Estazolam	ProSom	1, 2	8-24	IV
Flurazepam	Dalmane	15, 30	48-120	IV
Quazepam	Doral	7.5, 15	48-120	IV
Temazepam	Restoril	7.5, 15, 22.5, 30	8-20	IV
Triazolam	Halcion	0.125, 0.25	2-4	IV
Immediate-Release Non-BZDs				
Eszopiclone	Lunesta	1, 2, 3	5-7	IV
Zaleplon	Sonata	5, 10	1	IV
Zolpidem	Ambien	5, 10	1.5-2.4	IV
Modified-Release Non-BZDs				
Zolpidem CR	Ambien CR	6.25-12.5	2.8-2.9	IV
Selective Melatonin Receptor Agonist				
Ramelteon	Rozerem	8	1-2.6	None
Histamine Receptor Antagonist				
Doxepin	Silenor	3, 6	15.3	None
Orexin Receptor Antagonist				
Suvorexant	Belsomra	5, 10, 15, 20	12	IV

BZD, Benzodiazepine; *CR*, controlled release; *DEA*, Drug Enforcement Administration.

maintenance. When these symptoms are experienced by children, they have often been incorrectly identified as "growing pains."

PLMD is frequently associated with RLS. PLMD is defined as periodic episodes of spontaneous, repetitive, and highly stereotyped involuntary limb movements that occur during sleep. Four or more repetitive muscle contractions lasting 0.5 to 5 seconds and separated by 4 to 90 seconds are conventionally regarded as indicative of PLMD. The night-to-night variability in their occurrence and variability in the intensity of daytime and evening sensory symptoms often lead to PLMD being underappreciated or missed during a clinical evaluation. Chronic sleep restriction and sleep fragmentation is one adverse outcome attributed to both RLS and PLMD; this is believed to contribute to the deleterious physical, mental, and social effects associated with the disorders. Consequently, the negative effect of RLS on quality of life is similar to that observed with other chronic disorders such as depression, heart failure, and diabetes.

More recent epidemiologic and genetic linkage studies distinguish two forms of RLS: early onset, or primary, RLS, and late onset, or secondary, RLS. The early onset form typically begins in childhood or young adulthood with gradual progression in symptom severity. Early onset RLS is inherited in an autosomal dominant fashion, shows genetic anticipation, is twice as prevalent in females, and is associated with at least two separate genetic loci.[57] In addition, PLMD is more typically associated with this form of RLS.

Late onset RLS is characterized by a later age of symptom onset, usually older than 45 years; an equal female to male ratio; a rapidly progressive course; and a relationship with anemia and other associated identifiable causes such as diabetes, kidney disease, neuropathy, and even nervous system trauma.[57] In addition to these intrinsic pathophysiologic mechanisms, certain extrinsic factors are associated with increased frequency and severity of symptoms. H_2 histamine antagonists such as ranitidine or cimetidine have been reported to worsen symptoms of RLS.[58] Caffeine, alcohol, and some antidepressants, including fluoxetine, also are reported to worsen the frequency and severity of RLS or PLMD symptoms.[59] Epidemiologic studies suggest that the onset of RLS increases with age, with a prevalence rate of 2% in children, 3% in 30-year-olds, and up to 20% in 80-year-olds. Genetic studies and linkage analyses also show that early onset RLS is a heritable trait, but the pathophysiologic mechanisms of RLS remain unclear.[57]

Because of the essential motor component of the disorder, dopamine deficiencies may contribute to the etiology of RLS and PLMD. Research has focused on determining whether reductions in extracellular dopamine levels within the CNS or deficiencies in postsynaptic responsivity to dopamine might contribute to the symptoms of RLS and PLMD. Reduced levels of extracellular dopamine are central to several hypotheses regarding neurochemical substrates contributing to RLS. However, elucidation of any actual dopaminergic dysfunction has remained enigmatic. It is possible that reduced synthesis or increased sequestration of dopamine within cell bodies and terminals leads to diminished extracellular dopamine. Alternatively, dopamine production and release may be normal, but the number or type, or both, of postsynaptic dopamine receptors may be altered and so result in the symptoms.

The first link made between dopamine and RLS was based on the observation that many patients derived relief from dopamine-augmenting drugs. This was acknowledged in the "Practice Parameters for the treatment of RLS and PLM,"[60] which stated that dopaminergic agents are the best-studied and most successful agents for treatment of RLS and PLMD. After multiple clinical trials with dopamine-enhancing compounds, levodopa with decarboxylase inhibitors and dopamine agonists such as pergolide were found to be the most effective for treatment of RLS and PLMD.[60] Despite the promise that dopamine-enhancing compounds can reduce the symptoms of RLS, it should be noted that their use for RLS is currently approved only for adults; data are lacking with regard to their use for RLS in pediatric populations and during pregnancy. When prescribing any type of dopaminergic medication for RLS symptom relief, the potential for side effects, such as nausea, gastrointestinal distress, reduced blood pressure, and sleepiness, should be taken into account and discussed with a sleep medicine physician. In addition, because dopamine modulates mood, cognition, wakefulness, and sleep, any dopamine precursor, agonist, or antagonist can feasibly result in acute thought and behavioral changes. Given that most RLS patients need very low doses of dopaminergic medications for symptomatic relief, the likelihood of a serious or adverse outcome is remote (Table 23-3).

Narcolepsy

The earliest clinical descriptions of narcolepsy were documented by the German physician Westphal in 1877 and by Fisher in 1878. However, the French physician Gelineau, writing in 1880, is generally acknowledged as the first clinician to recognize narcolepsy as a distinct clinical entity. Initial descriptions included characterization of excessive daytime sleepiness and "sleep attacks." Although all three of these early descriptions documented the appearance of sleep attacks, they did not discern the symptoms of sudden muscle weakness triggered by an emotional event (i.e., cataplexy) as separate from the sleep attack event. This is most evident from the first description of narcolepsy as a clinical entity: "I propose to give the name of narcolepsy (narco, somnolence; lepsy, seized by) to a rare neurosis or at least little known until now, characterized by a mandatory need to sleep, sudden and of short duration, that recurs at more or less close intervals."[61] In 1902, Loewenfeld recognized that the emotion-induced muscle weakness was a separate feature of the disorder and first used the term cataplexy to describe it.

Today narcolepsy is characterized by a tetrad of clinical symptoms. Two features of the tetrad—persistent excessive daytime sleepiness and cataplexy—were documented in the original descriptions of the disorder and remain the only two clinical features essential for diagnosis. The recognition of two additional features—hypnagogic hallucinations (the onset of dreams while still awake) and sleep paralysis (a temporary loss of muscle tone or an inability to perform voluntary movements either at sleep onset or on awakening)—were added later.[62] Another common symptom of narcolepsy is fragmented sleep with multiple arousals and awakenings at night.

Narcolepsy may not be as rare a disorder as once thought; according to the National Institute of Neurological Disorders and Stroke (NINDS), narcolepsy is an underrecognized and underdiagnosed condition. Nevertheless, in the United States, narcolepsy is the third most frequently diagnosed primary sleep disorder after sleep apnea and RLS. Current estimates suggest that 1 in about 2000 Americans are narcoleptic. The prevalence of narcolepsy is apparently significantly greater in Japan, affecting 1 in 600 people, but substantially less in Israel, affecting only 1 in 500,000, although differences in diagnosis may account for at least part of this variation. There is no gender difference in the prevalence of the disorder.

The onset of narcoleptic symptoms typically occurs between the ages of 15 and 30, although there are reports of symptom onset occurring in very young children and in adults older than 30. In addition, it is not unusual for 12 years to elapse between the initial onset of symptoms and a definitive diagnosis. Up to 10% of patients diagnosed with narcolepsy report that a close relative has similar symptoms. The familial association of narcolepsy was recognized in the early descriptions, as noted in the mother of the narcoleptic patient first examined by Westphal and the sister of the first narcoleptic patient described by Fisher. Such familial clustering suggests a genetic origin for this disorder. Although immediate family members of narcoleptics are at a statistically greater risk of developing the disorder, this risk is low compared with purely genetic disorders and indicates that other factors must be involved.

TABLE 23-3	Pharmacologic Management of Restless Legs Syndrome			
DRUG	**DOSE (mg/day)**	**TIME TO PEAK PLASMA LEVEL (min)**	**HALF-LIFE (hr)**	**MODE OF ELIMINATION**
Levodopa	100-400	30	1.5-3	Hepatic
Carbidopa/Levodopa	10/100-25/250	120	6-8	Hepatic
Bromocriptine	2.5-10	45-60	3-4 (up to 40)	Hepatic
Pergolide	0.1-0.75	60	27	Renal
Cabergoline	0.25-3.0	120	63-68	Hepatic
Pramipexole	0.25-1.5	120	8-12	Renal
Ropinirole	0.5-4.0	60-120	Approximately 6	Hepatic

Most cases of narcolepsy are sporadic and occur without evidence of genetic inheritance. Until more recently, the etiology of narcolepsy was unknown, but it was associated with the specific human leukocyte antigen (HLA) allele, DQB10602, and often in combination with HLA-DR2 (DRB115). In 1998 two research groups first described, clustered around the lateral and perifornical hypothalamus, a group of cells that contained a previously unknown neurotransmitter.[63] These cells contained orexin/hypocretin; based on the neuroanatomy they were hypothesized to be involved in the regulation of sleep and wakefulness. However, the physiology suggested a major role in food intake and energy balance, which was the focus of research during the first 12 months. Within 1 year of the discovery, however, two independent groups discovered in 1999 that the clinical symptoms of narcolepsy were associated with a loss or dysfunction of orexin/hypocretin-containing cells.[64]

After the initial descriptions of narcolepsy, various empiric treatments were tried with little success. Among these were spinal fluid taps, intrathecal air injection, x-ray irradiation of portions of the hypothalamus, and later, ephedrine administration. In 1935 Prinzmetal and Bloomberg synthesized a new compound, benzedrine, the original drug in the class later known as amphetamines. Although originally developed to treat nasal congestion, it had no effect on the nasal mucosa, but when given orally, benzedrine led to a reduction in weight, and it was soon routinely used as an appetite suppressant. Subsequently the CNS-stimulating effect of the amphetamines was recognized, leading to their use to treat hypersomnolence. For many years, a regimen of amphetamines in conjunction with a tricyclic antidepressant such as imipramine, which reduces REM sleep, was the standard pharmaceutical intervention for narcolepsy. Then modafinil, a nonamphetamine wake-promoting agent, was developed.

With a side effect profile free from addiction, tolerance, and other adverse outcomes associated with amphetamines, modafinil soon became the treatment of choice for alleviating the symptoms of excessive daytime sleepiness associated with narcolepsy. In 2002 sodium oxybate, (Xyrem), a CNS depressant, gained FDA approval for the treatment of excessive daytime sleepiness and cataplexy in narcoleptic patients. The use of a CNS depressant may seem counterintuitive as a strategy for treating excessive daytime sleepiness. However, sodium oxybate, taken immediately before sleep and again 2 to 4 hours later, causes an increase in SWS, a reduction in the number of nocturnal awakenings, and enhanced sleep continuity. The result is a reduction in daytime sleepiness and cataplexy and a less fragmented sleep period. The mechanism by which sodium oxybate reduces excessive daytime sleepiness and cataplexy is unknown, but it may involve activation of $GABA_B$ receptors.

Determining the most appropriate treatment for a narcoleptic patient is influenced by several factors, including age, severity of symptoms, presence or absence of cataplexy, other medical conditions, and concomitant medications. Conservative treatment of narcolepsy involves administration of two or more medications with a stimulant for excessive daytime sleepiness, a tricyclic antidepressant for cataplexy, and a hypnotic for insomnia and fragmented nocturnal sleep. A young narcoleptic patient without cataplexy may achieve some relief of symptoms by maintaining a fixed schedule of sleep time combined with prescheduled daytime naps, if feasible. This approach ensures an adequate opportunity for sleep, and coupled with an alerting compound such as modafinil or armodafinil (the R-enantiomer of modafinil with a longer half-life of 10-15 hours) it may help to restore a functional level of daytime alertness.

In contrast, a patient presenting with more severe symptoms including cataplexy, hypnagogic hallucinations, and sleep fragmentation may require aggressive treatment. In addition to good sleep hygiene, an amphetamine such as methylphenidate might be prescribed to help sustain daytime wakefulness, together with sodium oxybate. This regimen could be combined with a selective serotonin reuptake inhibitor (SSRI) or a tricyclic antidepressant to treat cataplexy and the other symptoms of REM sleep dysregulation, including hypnagogic hallucinations. In a patient with sleep fragmentation, sodium oxybate is often useful because sleep continuity is enhanced and excessive daytime sleepiness and cataplexy are controlled. Cataplexy and hypnagogic hallucinations require additional agents such as sodium oxybate, an SSRI, or a tricyclic antidepressant. Nonpharmacologic therapies, such as scheduled naps, regular sleep and wake schedules, and proper sleep hygiene are essential elements for any successful treatment regimen.

Parasomnias

Parasomnias are undesirable motor, sensory, or behavioral phenomena that occur primarily during sleep.[65] These phenomena range from normal to abnormal and from benign to potentially lethal and can be associated with normal developmental processes or neurodegeneration. The *ICSD-3* lists 24 parasomnias encompassing NREM sleep or arousal disorders, REM sleep-related disorders, sleep-wake transition disorders, and other parasomnias.[1] The focus here is on more common NREM and REM sleep parasomnias. NREM sleep parasomnias, also termed *arousal disorders*, include confusional arousals, sleep terrors, and sleepwalking. Arousal disorders can be either primary or secondary if they are associated with an identifiable pathology such as a seizure disorder, obstructive sleep apnea, nocturnal cardiac ischemia, or nocturnal paroxysmal dystonia. The pathophysiologic mechanisms underlying arousal disorders are still unknown, but current hypotheses suggest that they may result from the brain being simultaneously in a state of partial wakefulness and NREM sleep. This state leads to an ability to perform complex motor or verbal actions without conscious awareness of the actions.

Primary arousal disorders share several common factors including familial clustering, which suggests a genetic predisposition; childhood predominance; and a tendency to occur during NREM sleep. Confusional arousals are characterized by episodes of marked mental confusion during or after an arousal from sleep. They usually occur during the first third of the night, last 30 seconds to 5 minutes, and may be accompanied by mumbling, automatic behaviors, or both. During the event, the person does not leave the bed, and there are no signs of fear or terror. After a confusional arousal, the individual usually falls back to sleep with no recollection of the event (i.e., retrograde amnesia) on awakening. Triggers for confusional arousals include anything that either fragments sleep or enhances SWS. Examples include environmental factors such as noise or temperature, stress, fever, pain, pregnancy, recovery from sleep deprivation, and CNS-active medications. As noted earlier, youth, a family history, and a history of being a deep sleeper are predisposing factors.

Sleep terrors, which are observed primarily in children, are similar to confusional arousals and occur during the first third of the night. They also begin in NREM sleep, typically during SWS at a time when an episode of REM sleep would be expected and last 30 seconds to 5 minutes. The triggers for sleep terrors are similar to those for confusional arousals; the principal difference is that sleep terrors are accompanied by an abrupt awakening, intense vocalization, and inconsolable fear or terror. Sleep terrors most frequently occur in children 5 to 7 years old and appear with equal prevalence in boys and girls. Most children with sleep terrors outgrow them by 8 years of age, although about 30% may continue to experience them into adolescence; only about 1% experience sleep terrors as adults.

Another parasomnia, somnambulism or sleepwalking, also occurs during NREM sleep but is characterized by the presence of automatic behaviors of varying complexity, including walking, eating, mumbling, and rarely, violence. The duration of these episodes can be 15 minutes to several hours. The episode is usually self-limiting and terminates with a return to sleep. Clinical evidence shows that attempts to intervene may be met with resistance and outbursts.

As with other NREM sleep parasomnias, the familial clustering of somnambulism suggests a genetic predisposition. Triggers for somnambulism, such as sleep fragmentation and increased depth or duration of SWS, are similar to those of the other arousal disorders. The age of onset for somnambulism is about 5 years with the highest prevalence at about 12 years of age. Somnambulism can occur in 15% to 30% of children and young adolescents, with boys and girls equally affected. Most children who are sleepwalkers typically outgrow the events by age 15, but 1% may continue to experience episodes in adulthood.

Another clinically identifiable category of parasomnias occurs during REM sleep and for this reason typically in the second half of the night. These include REM sleep behavior disorder (RBD), nightmare disorder, and isolated sleep paralysis. In contrast to NREM arousal disorders, REM sleep parasomnias usually affect adults more frequently than children, and they do not exhibit a genetic pattern of inheritance. RBD, in particular, is associated with neurodegenerative disorders such as Parkinson disease and multiple systems atrophy and usually occurs in older men.

Symptoms include violent dream enactment behavior owing to a loss of atonia during REM sleep. If left untreated, RBD can cause serious injury to the patient and the sleeping partner.

Treatment for NREM and REM sleep parasomnias frequently includes avoidance of potential triggers, and in the case of somnambulism and RBD necessitates a safe, well-monitored sleeping environment. The most common pharmaceutical treatment for REM and NREM sleep parasomnias is usually a longer-acting benzodiazepine. Through reduction of both SWS and REM sleep time and the number of transitions between sleep states, benzodiazepines essentially reduce the occurrence of the state in which an arousal disorder or RBD episode can occur. Benzodiazepines were initially developed as anxiolytics and subsequently as hypnotics. The success of the first compounds led to further research and development, and many compounds of this class eventually became available. Notable hypnotic benzodiazepine compounds are nitrazepam (Mogadon), temazepam (Restoril), flurazepam (Dalmane), and midazolam (Versed); others, such as clonazepam (Klonopin), are frequently used in treatment of parasomnias and as antiseizure medications.

Considerations for employing benzodiazepine compounds in treatment include their half-life (i.e., the time required for one-half of the active drug to be metabolized or eliminated from the body). Short-acting benzodiazepines have half-lives of 12 hours or less, but long-acting benzodiazepines have half-lives that often exceed 24 hours. A gradual increase in the blood levels of a longer-acting drug has the potential to cause residual effects. A benzodiazepine taken in the evening to reduce the likelihood of experiencing an arousal event may induce residual sleepiness the next day. With regard to their use for the treatment of arousal disorders, apart from their role in the reduction of the overall duration of time in states as noted earlier, no definitive conclusions are yet possible concerning their mechanism of action. Clonazepam, as a longer-acting benzodiazepine, is a frequent first choice, although careful selection of the appropriate benzodiazepine for a particular patient is essential to reduce the likelihood of residual daytime sleepiness. This is especially important to consider when treating parasomnias because many patients are children or elderly adults.

? SELF-ASSESSMENT QUESTIONS

Answers can be found in Appendix A.

1. What is the International Classification of Sleep Disorders, (ICSD-3), and what information does it contain?
2. What are the electroencephalographic correlates of wakefulness and sleep stages N1, N2, N3, and REM?
3. What type of drug had been used for centuries to promote sleep onset and maintenance?
4. What class or classes of drugs have replaced opium?

Continued

5. How many people in the United States experience chronic sleep disorders?
6. Who was von Economo, and what theories guided his neuroanatomic exploration of brain regions involved in the processes of initiating and maintaining wakefulness and sleep?
7. What is the reticular activating system?
8. How do neurons within the ventrolateral preoptic (VLPO) area affect sleep?
9. What are the suprachiasmatic nuclei (SCN), and what are intrinsic discharge properties exhibited by many of its neurons?
10. Define chronobiology and chronopharmacology.
11. Describe pharmacologic treatments for insomnia.
12. What is the difference between restless legs syndrome (RLS) and periodic limb movement disorder (PLMD)?
13. What is the tetrad of clinical symptoms that defines narcolepsy, and what types of drugs are used to treat this disorder?
14. Give two examples of a parasomnia, and name the class of drugs routinely used in the treatment of these sleep disorders.
15. Insomnia is characterized by what types of principal complaint, and what drug classes are used to treat this disorder?

CLINICAL SCENARIO

Answers can be found in Appendix A.

A 59-year-old white man with a body mass index of 27 and a history of hypertension, arthritis, and depression presents to the sleep clinic with chief complaints of excessive daytime sleepiness, awakening from nocturnal sleep after 2 to 3 hours, and prickly sensations in the legs that coincide with nocturnal awakenings but are temporarily relieved by walking. He also reports experiencing the same prickly sensations in his legs during long trips in the car, regardless of the time of day. The sensations in his legs also occur spontaneously two to three times a week during the evening hours.

The patient underwent full overnight **polysomnography** during which the following parameters were monitored: electroencephalography (EEG), electrooculography (EOG), submental and leg electromyography (EMG), electrocardiography (ECG), oxyhemoglobin saturation, respiratory effort, and nasal and oral airflow. Analysis of data revealed a sleep efficiency of 94% with a sleep latency of 5 minutes. The arousal index was 15 arousals per hour of sleep. Distribution of sleep stages was notable for an increased amount of N2 and rapid eye movement (REM) sleep with a reduced amount of N3 sleep. The REM latency was normal.

Periodic leg movements occurred 41 times per hour of sleep and resulted in 11 arousals per hour of sleep. No arrhythmias were noted on ECG. No snoring was noted with the patient in the lateral position. The apnea/hypopnea index (number of apneas and hypopneas per hour of sleep) was mildly elevated at 8.2 with a further increase to 13.6 events per hour during REM sleep. Oxyhemoglobin desaturation reached a nadir of 82% in REM sleep and 86% in non-REM sleep.

Using the SOAP method, assess this clinical scenario.

REFERENCES

1. American Academy of Sleep Medicine: *International classification of sleep disorders (ICSD)*, ed 3, Darien, IL, 2014, American Academy of Sleep Medicine.
2. Léger D, Pandi-Perumal SR: *Review of Sleep Disorders: Their Impact on Public Health*, Sleep Med Rev. Vol. 30. Oxford, 2007, OUP, p 7.
3. Askitopoulou H, McGoldrick KE, Westhorpe RN, Wilkinson DJ: History of Anaesthesia VII. Proceedings of the 7th International Symposium on the History of Anaesthesia, 2012: Crete University Press HERAKLEION.
4. Carley DW, Olopade C, Ruigt GS, Radulovacki M: Efficacy of mirtazapine in obstructive sleep apnea syndrome. *Sleep* 30(1):35–41, 2007.
5. Canton R: The electric current of the brain. *BMJ* 278:2, 1875.
6. Brazier MA: The history of the electrical activity of the brain as a method for localizing sensory function. *Med Hist* 7:199–211, 1963.
7. Dourmashkin RR: What caused the 1918-30 epidemic of encephalitis lethargica? *J R Soc Med* 90(9):515–520, 1997.
8. Von Economo C: Sleep as problem of localization. *J Nerv Ment Dis* 71(3):249:259, 1930.
9. Kleitman N: *Sleep and wakefulness*, Chicago, 1987, University of Chicago Press.
10. Aserinsky E, Kleitman N: Regularly occurring periods of eye motility, and concomitant phenomena, during sleep. *Science* 118(3062):273–274, 1953.
11. Moruzzi G, Magoun HW: Brain stem reticular formation and activation of the EEG. *Electroencephalogr Clin Neurophysiol* 1(4):455–473, 1949.
12. Steriade M, Datta S, Pare D, et al: Neuronal activities in brain-stem cholinergic nuclei related to tonic activation processes in thalamocortical systems. *J Neurosci* 10(8):2541–2559, 1990.
13. Jones BE: From waking to sleeping: neuronal and chemical substrates. *Trends Pharmacol Sci* 26(11):578–586, 2005.
14. McCormick DA, Bal T: Sleep and arousal: thalamocortical mechanisms. *Annu Rev Neurosci* 20:185–215, 1997.
15. Pace-Schott EF, Hobson JA: The neurobiology of sleep: genetics, cellular physiology and subcortical networks. *Nat Rev Neurosci* 3(8):591–605, 2002.
16. Sherin JE, Shiromani PJ, McCarley RW, Saper CB: Activation of ventrolateral preoptic neurons during sleep. *Science* 271(5246):216–219, 1996.
17. Sherin JE, Elmquist JK, Torrealba F, Saper CB: Innervation of histaminergic tuberomammillary neurons by GABAergic and galaninergic neurons in the ventrolateral preoptic nucleus of the rat. *J Neurosci* 18(12):4705–4721, 1998.
18. Fredholm B: Adenosine receptors in the central nervous system. *News Physiol Sci* 10:122, :128, 1995.
19. McCarley RW: Adenosine and 5-HT as regulators of behavioural state. In Borbely AA, et al, editors: *The regulation of sleep*, Strasbourg, 2000, Human Frontier Science Program; Strecker, RE, S Morairty, MM Thakkar, T Porkka-Heiskanen, R Basheer, LJ Dauphin, et al: Adenosinergic modulation of basal forebrain and preoptic/anterior hypothalamic neuronal activity in the control of behavioral state. *Behav Brain Res* 115(2):183–204, 2000.

20. Lakin-Thomas PL: Circadian rhythms: new functions for old clock genes. *Trends Genet* 16(3):135–142, 2000.
21. Borbely AA: A two process model of sleep regulation. *Hum Neurobiol* 1(3):195–204, 1982.
22. Folkard S: The pragmatic approach to masking. *Chronobiol Int* 6(1):55–64, 1989.
23. Halberg F: Physiologic 24-hour periodicity in human beings and mice, the lighting regimen and daily routine. In Withrow R, editor: *Photoperiodism and related phenomena in plants and animals*, Washinton,DC, 1959, p 903.
24. Pandi-Perumal SR, Seils LK, Kayumov L, et al: Senescence, sleep, and circadian rhythms. *Ageing Res Rev* 1(3):559–604, 2002.
25. Czeisler CA, Duffy JF, Shanahan TL, et al: Stability, precision, and near-24-hour period of the human circadian pacemaker. *Science* 284(5423):2177–2181, 1999.
26. Morin LP: The circadian visual system. *Brain Res Brain Res Rev* 19(1):102–127, 1994.
27. Berson DM, Dunn FA, Takao M: Phototransduction by retinal ganglion cells that set the circadian clock. *Science* 295(5557):1070–1073, 2002.
28. Hattar S, Liao HW, Takao M, et al: Melanopsin-containing retinal ganglion cells: architecture, projections, and intrinsic photosensitivity. *Science* 295(5557):1065–1070, 2002.
29. Hattar S, Lucas RJ, Mrosovsky N, et al: Melanopsin and rod-cone photoreceptive systems account for all major accessory visual functions in mice. *Nature* 424(6944):76–81, 2003; Boulos, Z: Wavelength dependence of light-induced phase shifts and period changes in hamsters. *Physiol Behav* 57(6):1025–1033, 1995.
30. Lewy AJ, Wehr TA, Goodwin FK, et al: Light suppresses melatonin secretion in humans. *Science* 210(4475):1267–1269, 1980.
31. Melyan Z, Tarttelin EE, Bellingham J, et al: Addition of human melanopsin renders mammalian cells photoresponsive. *Nature* 433(7027):741–745, 2005.
32. Gooley JJ, Lu J, Fischer D, Saper CB: A broad role for melanopsin in nonvisual photoreception. *J Neurosci* 23(18):7093–7106, 2003.
33. Lu J, Shiromani P, Saper CB: Retinal input to the sleep-active ventrolateral preoptic nucleus in the rat. *Neuroscience* 93(1):209–214, 1999.
34. Moore RY, Speh JC, Leak RK: Suprachiasmatic nucleus organization. *Cell Tissue Res* 309(1):89–98, 2002.
35. Welsh DK, Takahashi JS, Kay SA: Suprachiasmatic nucleus: cell autonomy and network properties. *Annu Rev Physiol* 72:551–577, 2010.
36. Mistlberger RE: Circadian regulation of sleep in mammals: role of the suprachiasmatic nucleus. *Brain Res Brain Res Rev* 49(3):429–454, 2005; Decker, MJ, DB Rye, SY Lee, and KP Strohl: Paradoxical sleep suppresses immediate early gene expression in the rodent suprachiasmatic nuclei. *Front Neurol* 1:122, 2010.
37. Edgar DM, Dement WC, Fuller CA: Effect of SCN lesions on sleep in squirrel monkeys: evidence for opponent processes in sleep-wake regulation. *J Neurosci* 13(3):1065–1079, 1993.
38. Cardinali DP, Pandi-Perumal SR: Chronopharmacology and its implications to the pharmacology of sleep. In Pandi-Perumal SR, Monti JM, editors: *Clinical pharmacology of sleep*, Basel, 2006, Birkhäuser Verlag.
39. Lemmer B: *Chronopharmacology: cellular and biochemical interactions*, New York, 1989, Dakker, M.
40. Dawson D, Armstrong SM: Chronobiotics—drugs that shift rhythms. *Pharmacol Ther* 69(1):15–36, 1996.
41. Arendt J, Skene DJ: Melatonin as a chronobiotic. *Sleep Med Rev* 9(1):25–39, 2005.
42. Liu C, Weaver DR, Jin X, et al: Molecular dissection of two distinct actions of melatonin on the suprachiasmatic circadian clock. *Neuron* 19(1):91–102, 1997; Jin, X, C von Gall, RL Pieschl, VK Gribkoff, JH Stehle, SM Reppert, et al: Targeted disruption of the mouse Mel(1b) melatonin receptor. *Mol Cell Biol* 23(3):1054–1060, 2003.
43. McArthur AJ, Hunt AE, Gillette MU: Melatonin action and signal transduction in the rat suprachiasmatic circadian clock: activation of protein kinase C at dusk and dawn. *Endocrinology* 138(2):627–634, 1997; Hunt, AE, WM Al-Ghoul, MU Gillette, and ML Dubocovich: Activation of MT(2) melatonin receptors in rat suprachiasmatic nucleus phase advances the circadian clock. *Am J Physiol Cell Physiol* 280(1):C110–C118, 2001.
44. von Gall C, Stehle JH, Weaver DR: Mammalian melatonin receptors: molecular biology and signal transduction. *Cell Tissue Res* 309(1):151–162, 2002; Pandi-Perumal, SR, I Trakht, V Srinivasan, DW Spence, GJ Maestroni, N Zisapel, et al: Physiological effects of melatonin: role of melatonin receptors and signal transduction pathways. *Prog Neurobiol* 85(3):335–353, 2008.
45. Stone BM, Turner C, Mills SL, Nicholson AN: Hypnotic activity of melatonin. *Sleep* 23(5):663–669, 2000.
46. Mendelson WB: A critical evaluation of the hypnotic efficacy of melatonin. *Sleep* 20(10):916–919, 1997.
47. Turek FW, Gillette MU: Melatonin, sleep, and circadian rhythms: rationale for development of specific melatonin agonists. *Sleep Med* 5(6):523–532, 2004.
48. Kato K, Hirai K, Nishiyama K, et al: Neurochemical properties of ramelteon (TAK-375), a selective MT1/MT2 receptor agonist. *Neuropharmacology* 48(2):301–310, 2005; Miyamoto, M: Pharmacology of ramelteon, a selective MT1/MT2 receptor agonist: a novel therapeutic drug for sleep disorders. *CNS Neurosci Ther* 15(1):32–51, 2009.
49. Hardeland R, Poeggeler B, Srinivasan V, et al: Melatonergic drugs in clinical practice. *Arzneimittelforschung* 58(1):1–10, 2008.
50. Pandi-Perumal SR, Verster JC, Kayumov L, et al: Sleep disorders, sleepiness and traffic safety: a public health menace. *Braz J Med Biol Res* 39(7):863–871, 2006.
51. Summers MO, Crisostomo MI, Stepanski EJ: Recent developments in the classification, evaluation, and treatment of insomnia. *Chest* 130(1):276–286, 2006.
52. Vgontzas AN, Kales A: Sleep and its disorders. *Annu Rev Med* 50:387–400, 1999.
53. Stoller MK: Economic effects of insomnia. *Clin Ther* 16(5):873–897, discussion 854, 1994; Walsh, JK, Clinical and socioeconomic correlates of insomnia. *J Clin Psychiatry* 65(Suppl 8):13–19, 2004.
54. Bennett T, Bray D, Neville MW: Suvorexant, a dual orexin receptor antagonist for the management of insomnia. *P T* 39(4):264–266, 2014.
55. Coccagna G, Vetrugno R, Lombardi C, Provini F: Restless legs syndrome: an historical note. *Sleep Med* 5(3):279–283, 2004.
56. Pearce JM: Restless leg syndrome. *Eur Neurol* 53(4):206–207, 2005.
57. Karroum E, Konofal E, Arnulf I: [Restless-legs syndrome]. *Rev Neurol (Paris)* 164(8–9):701–721, 2008.
58. O'Sullivan RL, Greenberg DB: H2 antagonists, restless leg syndrome, and movement disorders. *Psychosomatics* 34(6):530–532, 1993.
59. Ryan M, Slevin JT: Restless legs syndrome. *Am J Health Syst Pharm* 63(17):1599–1612, 2006; Hoque, R and AL Chesson, Jr: Pharmacologically induced/exacerbated restless legs syndrome, periodic limb movements of sleep, and REM behavior disorder/REM sleep without atonia: literature review, qualitative scoring, and comparative analysis. *Journal of clinical sleep medicine: JCSM: official publication of the American Academy of Sleep Medicine* 6(1):79–83, 2010.
60. Littner MR, Kushida C, Anderson WM, et al: Practice parameters for the dopaminergic treatment of restless legs syndrome and periodic limb movement disorder. *Sleep* 27(3):557–559, 2004.
61. Gelineau J: De la narcolepsie. *Gazette des Hôpitaux (Paris)* 53:626–628, 1981.
62. Yoss RE, Daly DD: Criteria for the diagnosis of the narcoleptic syndrome. *Proc Staff Meet Mayo Clin* 32(12):320–328, 1957.

63. Sakurai T, Amemiya A, Ishii M, et al: Orexins and orexin receptors: a family of hypothalamic neuropeptides and G protein-coupled receptors that regulate feeding behavior. *Cell* 92(4):573–585, 1998; de Lecea, L, TS Kilduff, C Peyron, X Gao, PE Foye, PE Danielson, et al: The hypocretins: hypothalamus-specific peptides with neuroexcitatory activity. *Proc Natl Acad Sci U S A* 95(1):322–327, 1998.

64. Chemelli RM, Willie JT, Sinton CM, et al: Narcolepsy in orexin knockout mice: molecular genetics of sleep regulation. *Cell* 98(4):437–451, 1999; Lin, L, J Faraco, R Li, H Kadotani, W Rogers, X Lin, et al: The sleep disorder canine narcolepsy is caused by a mutation in the hypocretin (orexin) receptor 2 gene. *Cell* 98(3):365–376, 1999.

65. Pandi-Perumal SR: Parasomnias. In Stoleman I, editor: *Encyclopaedia of psychopharmacology*, London, 2010, Springer-Verlag.

Answers to Self-Assessment Questions and Clinical Scenarios

CHAPTER 1

Self-Assessment Questions

1. What is the definition of the term *drug?*

   Answer: A drug may be defined as any chemical that alters an organism's function.

2. What is the difference between the generic name and trade name of a drug?

   Answer: The generic name of a drug is nonproprietary, whereas the brand name is the name given by a particular manufacturer of the drug. If a physician prescribes a particular brand of a drug, the pharmacist must sell that brand unless generic substitution is indicated on the prescription.

3. What part of a prescription contains the name and amount of the drug being prescribed?

   Answer: The inscription.

4. A physician's order reads as follows: "gtt iv of racemic epinephrine, c̄3 cc of normal saline, q4h, while awake." What has been ordered?

   Answer: Four drops of racemic epinephrine with 3 cc of normal saline, to be given intravenously every 4 hours while the patient is awake.

5. The drug salmeterol was released for general clinical use in the United States in 1994. Where would you look to find information about this drug, such as the available dose forms, dosages, properties, side effects, and action?

   Answer: Several sources of information would be available on a new drug in addition to research reports in the journal literature: the package insert with the drug, the *Physician's Desk Reference* (PDR), and the United States Pharmacopeia–National Formulary (USP–NF). Usually a new drug release is accompanied by marketing literature from the manufacturer that is available from drug representatives or at conferences.

Clinical Scenario

Subjective: He played golf on a newly mown course. He had exhibited allergies in the past few years and was diagnosed as having asthma. He began to experience difficulty breathing later in the day, with wheezing and some shortness of breath on mild exertion. His heart rate increased from 66 to 84 beats/min, and he felt shaky. By midnight his wheezing had returned. He continued using the Primatene Mist through the next morning. A friend found him later that evening audibly wheezing, gasping for air, and in severe respiratory distress.

Objective: No objective data were presented in the scenario. Although some information may be misconstrued as objective, it is not. All objective data must be obtained by a health care professional during the physical examination.

Assessment: Failure to seek medical help while self-treating with an over-the-counter (OTC) drug product. He probably did not realize that (1) Primatene Mist is epinephrine, which is short-acting (1 to 2 hours in duration) and will not control the full development of an asthma exacerbation, termed the *late-phase* reaction; and (2) a progressive asthma episode can cause serious obstruction of the airway and often worsens in the evening or night. Given his continued symptoms, he required more aggressive therapy than Primatene Mist.

Plan: Intubate and ventilate the patient. Place the patient on inhaled albuterol or levalbuterol. Inhaled anticholinergic may be of benefit. Start the patient on IV steroids.

CHAPTER 2

Self-Assessment Questions

1. If a drug is in liquid solution, what routes of administration are available for its delivery, considering only its dose form?

   Answer: Oral, injection, inhalation (nebulization), and topical (possibly). The type of drug, pharmacokinetics, and intended effect will further narrow the choice of route of administration.

2. Although generic drug equivalents all have the same amount of active drug, do formulations of the same drug from different manufacturers all have the same ingredients?

   Answer: No, not necessarily. Ingredients other than the active drug may differ. For example, in a tablet preparation, the substances used to form the active drug into a molded tablet may vary.

3. If 200 mg of a drug results in a plasma concentration of 10 mg/L, what is the calculated volume of distribution (V_D)?

   Answer: $V_D = 200 \text{ mg}/(10 \text{ mg/L}) = 20$ L.

4. If the V_D of a drug, such as phenobarbital, is 38 L/70 kg, and an effective concentration is 10 mg/L, what loading dose would be needed for an average adult (assuming total bioavailability)?

   Answer: Dose = V_D × concentration = 38 L × 10 mg/L = 380 mg.

5. If an inhaled aerosol has zero gastrointestinal absorption of active drug and only lung absorption, what is the L/T ratio?

   Answer: 1; L/T = lung availability/(lung + stomach availability); and stomach = 0.

6. True or False: A patient uses a reservoir device with an inhaled aerosol and there is no swallowed portion of the drug; therefore there are no systemic side effects.

   Answer: False. Systemic drug levels are caused by *total* drug absorbed from the gastrointestinal tract and lungs. Sufficient lung absorption of the active drug could produce extrapulmonary side effects.

7. Which receptor system signal mechanism is responsible for the effects caused by β-receptor activation, such as those seen with adrenergic bronchodilators (e.g., albuterol)?

   Answer: G protein–linked receptors.

Clinical Scenario

Subjective: A 67-year-old man with a history of chronic obstructive pulmonary disease (COPD), hospitalized for a respiratory infection. An aerosol treatment of racemic epinephrine is ordered qid.

Objective: After the aerosol treatment, his heart rate (HR) decreased from 26 to 18 breaths/min. Adequate breath sounds were auscultated with a decrease in wheezing. It is noted that accessory muscle use has lessened and shortness of breath has been reduced after treatment at 8:00 AM. At 10:00 AM, accessory muscle use, wheezing, and shortness of breath return.

Assessment: After reviewing the pharmacokinetics of the drug, it is not suitable for a qid schedule. The duration of the drug's effect is too short. The improvement in airway resistance has declined, and the patient is working harder to breathe again.

Plan: You could administer racemic epinephrine more frequently, on a q2h schedule instead of the qid schedule. However, a better choice might be to identify a longer-acting bronchodilator with a duration of 4 to 6 hours, such as albuterol or levalbuterol. Both are noncatecholamine agents (see Chapter 6) that could be used in a qid schedule. Less-frequent dosing is also more cost effective for an in-hospital patient.

CHAPTER 3

Self-Assessment Questions

1. What are the three most common aerosol-generating devices used to deliver inhaled drugs?

   Answer: Small volume nebulizer (SVN), metered dose inhaler (MDI) with or without a reservoir device, and dry powder inhaler (DPI).

2. Describe the inspiratory pattern you would instruct a patient to use with an MDI.

   Answer: Exhale to end-tidal volume; begin to inhale slowly through the mouth and simultaneously actuate the MDI; continue to inhale to total lung capacity and hold the breath for 5 to 10 seconds.

3. What are three advantages offered by using a reservoir device with an MDI?

   Answer: Reservoir devices can modify the aerosol plume from an MDI in three ways: (1) allow time/distance between actuation and inhalation for particle evaporation and reduced particle size; (2) allow distance for the high initial particle velocity to slow; and (3) somewhat simplify the hand-breathing coordination required with MDI use. The net effect of the first two influences reduces oropharyngeal impaction and loss.

4. Would a DPI be appropriate for a 3-year-old child with asthma?

   Answer: No. These devices require an inspiratory flow rate of 60 L/min or more for optimal use. This probably exceeds the capability of most 3-year-old children. DPIs are not recommended for children younger than 5 years.

5. What is meant by the term *dead volume* in an SVN?

   Answer: The dead volume is the residual amount of solution left in a nebulizer when the nebulizer "sputters" and is no longer able to generate aerosol. This is usually around 0.5 to 1 mL in most disposable nebulizers.

6. What is the optimal filling volume and power gas flow rate to use with an SVN?

   Answer: For most disposable nebulizers, the optimal filling volume is 3 to 5 mL and the power gas flow rate is 8 to 10 L/min. A flow rate of 8 L/min probably gives the maximal particle size penetration into the lower respiratory tract and therefore produces the maximal drug mass able to reach the airway. However, a flow rate of 10 L/min will reduce particle size further and decrease the treatment time.

7. How does the electrostatic charge affect an MDI when used with a holding chamber?

   Answer: The electrostatic charge pulls the particles out of suspension, thereby decreasing the amount of drug available to the patient. At present, some manufacturers produce "antistatic" chambers; however, it has been found that washing a standard holding chamber with household detergent and allowing it to air dry will decrease the static. Decreasing static increases the available drug to the patient.

8. Which device would be better to deliver a β agonist to an adult patient in the emergency department—SVN, MDI, or DPI?

   Answer: It really depends on a number of factors, including drug availability, patient or clinical preference, practicality, and convenience. The best choice would be an SVN or MDI with a holding chamber. An MDI without a holding chamber or a DPI would not be good selections because of the patient not being able to coordinate and decreased inspiratory flow.

Clinical Scenario

Subjective: A 17-year-old adolescent male with a history of allergic asthma complains that he can feel drug in the canister when he shakes it before using, but it feels as if "very little spray" is coming out when he inhales a puff. He believes the MDI is not functioning properly and that he is not getting the regular inhaled dose.

Objective: Not available.

Assessment: Check MDI for correct use and educate patient on new hydrofluoroalkane (HFA) formulation.

Plan: First check to be sure there are in fact no obstructions in the mouthpiece of the actuator. After shaking well, discharge a dose to room air (away from everyone) to see whether there is a visible plume. If possible, you might compare the aerosol plume from his canister with another MDI to see whether they appear comparable. If you have a laboratory (i.e., in the hospital), try to have the canister weighed to ensure adequate fullness. Short of analyzing the aerosol, you cannot guarantee a correct dose of albuterol, but you can measure the person's peak expiratory flow with a peak flow meter or his FEV_1 with a portable spirometry screening unit before and after use. If he exhibits his usual amount of reversibility, this is indirect evidence of drug delivery. Also, ask him if he obtains relief when he uses the MDI during wheezing or chest tightness. The HFA formulation of albuterol has a higher plume temperature and a lower plume force on actuation. It is a softer and gentler spray. Patients who may have used a chlorofluorocarbon (CFC) formulation of albuterol by MDI often think they are not getting the usual dose because they cannot feel the colder, forceful blast they experienced with the CFC formulation.

CHAPTER 4

Self-Assessment Questions

Prepared-Strength Dose Calculations

1. A bottle is labeled Demerol (meperidine) 50 mg/cc. How many cubic centimeters are needed to give a 125-mg dose?
   Answer: 50 mg/1 cc = 125 mg/x cc; x = 2.5 cc.

2. An agent comes as 500 mg/10 mL. How many milliliters are needed to give a 150-mg dose?
   Answer: 500 mg/10 mL = 150 mg/x mL; x = 3 mL.

3. Hyaluronidase comes as 150 U/cc. How many cubic centimeters are needed for a 30-U dose?
   Answer: 150 U/cc = 30 U/x cc; x = 0.2 cc.

4. Morphine sulfate 4 mg is ordered; you have a vial with 10 mg/mL. How much do you need?
   Answer: 10 mg/mL = 4 mg/x mL; x = 0.4 mL.

5. A dosage schedule for the surfactant poractant calls for 2.5 mL/kg birth weight. How much drug will you need for an infant weighing 800 g?
   Answer: 800 g × 1 kg/1000 g = 0.8 kg; 2.5 mL/kg × 0.8 kg = 2 mL.

6. Diphenhydramine (Benadryl) elixir contains 12.5 mg of diphenhydramine HCl in each 5 mL of elixir. How many milligrams are there in a ½-teaspoonful dose (1 tsp = 5 mL)?
   Answer: ½ teaspoon = 2.5 mL.
   12.5 mg/5 mL = x mg/2.5 mL; x = 6.25 mg.

7. A pediatric dose of 100 mg of a syrup is ordered. The dosage form is an oral suspension containing 125 mg/5 cc. How much of the suspension contains a 100-mg dose?
   Answer: 125 mg/5 cc = 100 mg/x cc; x = 4 cc.

8. How many units (U) of heparin are found in 0.2 mL if you have 1000 U/mL?
   Answer: 1000 U/mL = x units/0.2 mL; x = 200 U.

9. Albuterol syrup is available as 2 mg/5 mL. If a dosage schedule of 0.1 mg/kg is used, how much syrup is needed for a 30-kg child? How many teaspoons is this?
   Answer: 30 kg × 0.1 mg/kg = 3 mg
   2 mg/5 mL = 3 mg/x mL; x = 7.5 mL
   7.5 mL × 1 tsp/5 mL = 1.5 tsp

10. Terbutaline is available as 2.5-mg tablets. How many tablets do you need for a 5-mg dose?
    Answer: 2.5 mg/1 tab = 5 mg/x tab; x = 2 tablets.

11. If a cough syrup is available as 120 mg/5 mL, how much dose is there in ½ tsp?
    Answer: ½ tsp = 2.5 mL; 120 mg/5 mL = x mg/2.5 mL; x = 60 mg.

12. Theophylline is available as 250 mg/10 mL and is given intravenously at 6 mg/kg body weight. How much solution do you give for a 60-kg woman?
    Answer: 60 kg × 6 mg/kg = 360 mg; 250 mg/10 mL = 360 mg/x mL; x = 14.4 mL.

13. Terbutaline sulfate is available as 1 mg/mL in an ampule. How many milliliters are needed for a 0.25-mg dose?
    Answer: 1 mg/mL = 0.25 mg/x mL; x = 0.25 mL.

14. A patient is told to take 4 mg of albuterol four times daily. The medication comes in 2-mg tablets. How many tablets are needed for one 4-mg dose?
    Answer: 2 mg/tab = 4 mg/x tab; x = 2 tablets.

15. An agent is available as a syrup with 10 mg/5 mL. How many teaspoons should be taken for a 20-mg dose?
    Answer: 1 tsp = 5 mL.
    10 mg/5 mL = 20 mg/x mL; x = 10 mL.
    10 mg × 1 tsp/5 mL = 2 tsp.

16. If an agent is available at 3 mg/mL, how many milliliters are needed for a dose of 9 mg?
    Answer: 3 mg/mL = 9 mg/x mL; x = 3 mL.

17. If a dosage schedule requires 0.25 mg/kg of body weight, what dose is needed for an 88-kg person?
    Answer: 0.25 mg/kg × 88 kg = 22 mg.

18. If theophylline is available as 80 mg/15 mL, how much is needed for a 100-mg dose?
    Answer: 80 mg/15 mL = 100 mg/x mL; x = 18.75 mL.

19. How much drug is needed for a 65-kg adult, using 0.5 mg/kg?
    Answer: 0.5 mg/kg × 65 kg = 32.5 mg.

20. The pediatric dosage of an antibiotic is 0.5 g/20 lb body weight, not to exceed 75 mg/kg/24 hr.
    a. What is the dose for a 40-lb child?
    b. If this dose is given twice in 1 day, has the maximal dose been exceeded?
    Answers
    a. 0.5 g/20 lb × 40 lb = 1.0 g.
    b. 2 doses = 2 × 1.0 g = 2.0 g = 2000 mg
    40 lb × 1 kg/2.2 lb = 18 kg
    2000 mg/18 kg = 111.1 mg/kg
    Yes, the maximal dose has been exceeded: two doses give 2000 mg/40 lb, which is 2000 mg/18 kg, or 111.1 mg/kg/day.

Percentage-Strength Solutions

1. How many grams of calamine are needed to prepare 120 g of an ointment containing 8% calamine?
   Answer: $0.08 = x$ g/120 g; $x = 9.6$ g.
2. In 147 mL of solution, there is 1 mL of active enzyme. What is the percentage strength of active enzyme in the solution?
   Answer: $x = 1$ mL/147 mL; $x = 0.0068 = 0.68\%$.
3. If theophylline is available in a 250 mg/10 mL solution, what percentage strength is this?
   Answer: $x = 0.25$ g/10 mL; $x = 0.025 = 2.5\%$.
4. You have epinephrine 1:100. How many milliliters of epinephrine would be needed to contain 30 mg of active ingredient?
   Answer: $0.01 = 0.03$ g/x mL; $x = 3$ mL.
5. A dose of 0.4 mL of epinephrine HCl 1:100 is ordered. How many milligrams of epinephrine HCl (the active ingredient) does this dose contain?
   Answer: $0.01 = x$ g/0.4 mL; $x = 0.004$ g $= 4$ mg.
6. If you administer 3 mL of a 0.1% strength solution, how many milligrams of active ingredient have you given?
   Answer: $0.001 = x$ g/3 mL; $x = 0.003$ g $= 3$ mg.
7. A drug is available as a 1:200 solution, and the maximal dose that may be given by aerosol for a particular patient is 3 mg. What is the maximal amount of solution (in milliliters) that may be used?
   Answer: $1:200 = 0.5\% = 0.005$; 3 mg $= 0.003$ g; $0.005 = 0.003$ g/x mL; $x = 0.6$ mL.
8. Epinephrine 1:1000 contains how many milligrams per milliliter?
   Answer: $1:1000 = 0.1\% = 0.001$; $0.001 = x$ g/1 mL; $x = 0.001$ g $= 1$ mg.
9. How many milligrams per milliliter are there in 0.3 mL of 5% strength agent?
   Answer: $0.05 = x$ g/0.3 mL; $x = 0.015$ g $= 15$ mg.
10. How many milligrams of sodium chloride are needed for 10 mL of a 0.9% solution?
    Answer: $0.009 = x$ g/10 mL; $x = 0.09$ g $= 90$ mg.
11. If you have lidocaine (Xylocaine) at 5 mg/mL, what percentage strength is this?
    Answer: $x = 0.005$ g/mL; $x = 0.005 = 0.5\%$.
12. A 0.5% strength solution contains how many milligrams in 1 mL?
    Answer: $0.005 = x$ g/mL; $x = 0.005$ g $= 5$ mg.

13. Cromolyn sodium contains 20 mg in 2 mL of water. What is the percentage strength?
    Answer: $x = 0.02$ g/2 mL; $x = 0.01 = 1\%$.
14. How much active ingredient of acetylcysteine have you given with 4 cc of a 20% solution?
    Answer: $0.2 = x$ g/4 cc; $x = 0.8$ g $= 800$ mg.
15. You have 20% acetylcysteine; how many milliliters of this do you need to form 4 mL of an 8% solution?
    Answer: $0.08 = 0.2(x)$ mL/4 mL; $0.2(x) = 0.32$; $x = 1.6$ mL, and saline qs for 4 mL.
16. The recommended dose of an agent with a percent strength of 5% is 0.3 cc. How many milligrams of solute are there in this amount?
    Answer: $0.05 = x$ g/0.3 cc; $x = 0.015$ g $= 15$ mg.
17. Acetylcysteine was marketed as 10% acetylcysteine with 0.05% isoproterenol. How many milligrams of each ingredient were in a 4-cc dose of solution? (Isoproterenol: $0.0005\ x$ g/4 cc; $x = 0.002$ g $= 2$ mg.)
    Answer: Acetylcysteine: $0.10 = x$ g/4 cc; $x = 0.4$ g $= 400$ mg.
18. Which contains more drug: ½ cc of a 1% drug solution with 2 mL of saline or ½ of a 1% drug solution with 5 mL of saline?
    Answer: They each contain the same amount of drug: 5 mg ($0.01 = x$ g/0.5 cc; $x = 0.005$ g $= 5$ mg). The different amounts of diluent (2 mL, 5 mL) will change the resulting percentage strength and the total amount of new solution but not the amount of drug.
19. How many milligrams per milliliter are in a 20% solution?
    Answer: $0.20 = x$ g/mL; $x = 0.2$ g $= 200$ mg.

Clinical Scenario

You have a 1 normal (N) solution of saline (NaCl) and you need isotonic saline 0.9%, also called "normal saline," for diluent in a nebulizer solution. *Can you use the 1 N solution as diluent, unchanged?*

Answer: A 1 normal (N) solution contains 1 g equivalent weight (GEW) of solute per liter of solution. If we calculate the percentage strength of a 1 N solution of NaCl, we can compare this with 0.9% to determine equivalence or lack of equivalence. The molecular weights of sodium (Na) and chlorine (Cl) are 23 and 35.5, respectively. A GEW is the molecular weight divided by the valence of the elements:

1 GEW, NaCl $= 23.0$ g $+ 35.5$ g $= 58.5$ g. 1 N solution $= 1$ GEW/L $= 58.5$ g/L or 5.85 g/100 mL $= 5.85\%$.

Therefore, a 1 N solution of NaCl is 5.85% strength and is not the same concentration as normal saline, which is 0.9% strength. A 0.9% solution would be 0.9 g/100 mL, not 5.85 g/100 mL. Use of the more concentrated 1 N solution, which is hypertonic relative to body fluid, may cause bronchial irritation in a nebulizer solution for inhalation.

CHAPTER 5

Self-Assessment Questions

1. Which portion of the nervous system is under voluntary control: the autonomic or the skeletal muscle motor nerve portion?
   Answer: The skeletal muscle motor nerve portion.
2. What is the neurotransmitter at each of the following sites: neuromuscular junction; autonomic ganglia; and most sympathetic end sites?
   Answer: Neuromuscular junction—acetylcholine; autonomic ganglia—acetylcholine; most sympathetic end sites—norepinephrine.
3. Where are muscarinic receptors found?
   Answer: At parasympathetic nerve terminal sites.
4. What is the effect of cholinergic stimulation on airway smooth muscle?
   Answer: Bronchoconstriction.
5. What is the effect of adrenergic stimulation on the heart?
   Answer: Increased rate and force of contraction.
6. Classify the drugs pilocarpine, physostigmine, propranolol, and epinephrine.
   Answer: Pilocarpine—direct-acting cholinergic; physostigmine—indirect-acting cholinergic; propranolol—adrenergic-blocking agent (β_1 and β_2); epinephrine—adrenergic agonist (stimulates α and β receptors).
7. How do indirect-acting cholinergic agonists (parasympathomimetics) produce their action?
   Answer: Indirect-acting parasympathomimetics, such as neostigmine, inhibit the enzyme cholinesterase, which increases the amount of acetylcholine available to stimulate postsynaptic sites at the nerve terminal.
8. What effect would the drug atropine have on the eye and on airway smooth muscle?
   Answer: Atropine is a competitive blocking agent for muscarinic receptors. The drug would block the eye circular iris muscle to dilate the pupil (mydriasis), paralyze the ciliary muscle to flatten the lens (cycloplegia), and antagonize cholinergically induced bronchoconstriction in the airway.
9. What is the general difference between α and β receptors in the sympathetic nervous system?
   Answer: The α receptors generally cause an excitatory effect (e.g., vasoconstriction), and β receptors generally produce inhibition (e.g., airway smooth muscle relaxation).
10. What is the primary mechanism for terminating the neurotransmitters acetylcholine and norepinephrine?
    Answer: Acetylcholine is metabolized by cholinesterase enzymes; norepinephrine is reabsorbed back into the presynaptic neuron.
11. What is the predominant sympathetic receptor type found on airway smooth muscle?
    Answer: The β_2 receptor.
12. Identify the adrenergic receptor preference for phenylephrine, norepinephrine, and epinephrine.
    Answer: Phenylephrine—α receptors (α_1 specifically); norepinephrine—$\alpha > \beta$ receptors; epinephrine—α and β receptors equally.
13. What is the autoregulatory receptor on the sympathetic presynaptic neuron?
    Answer: α_2 Receptors.
14. Classify the following drugs by autonomic class and receptor preference: dopamine, ephedrine, albuterol, phentolamine, propranolol, and prazosin.
    Answer: Dopamine—sympathomimetic (dopamine receptors, α, and β); ephedrine—sympathomimetic (α and β); albuterol—sympathomimetic (β_2 preferential); phentolamine—α sympatholytic (α_1 and α_2); propranolol—β sympatholytic (β_1 and β_2); prazosin—α_1 sympatholytic.
15. What is the autoregulatory receptor on the parasympathetic presynaptic neuron at the terminal nerve site?
    Answer: The muscarinic receptor subtype M_2.
16. Contrast, in general, α_1-receptor and α_2-receptor effects.
    Answer: α_1-Receptor effects are generally excitatory (e.g., vasoconstriction of peripheral blood vessels). α_2-Receptor effects are generally inhibitory (e.g., inhibition of norepinephrine release from nerve terminals).
17. What substance may be the neurotransmitter in the nonadrenergic, noncholinergic (NANC) inhibitory nervous system in the lung?
    Answer: Vasoactive intestinal peptide (VIP) or possibly nitric oxide (NO).
18. What substance is the neurotransmitter in the NANC excitatory nervous system in the lung?
    Answer: Substance P.

Clinical Scenario

Subjective: A 42-year-old white female with a long-standing history of asthma presents to the emergency department (ED). She states that she has been feeling as if her "heart were racing" today. She currently uses a β-adrenergic bronchodilator (albuterol) as needed and inhales an anticholinergic bronchodilator (ipratropium bromide) before bedtime.

Objective: On admission to the ED, she has the following vital signs: pulse (P), 155 beats/min and regular; blood pressure (BP), 146/90 mm Hg; and respiratory rate (RR), 22 breaths/min, with mild distress. Her breath sounds are clear to auscultation and a chest radiograph (posteroanterior [PA]) shows no abnormalities. A lead II electrocardiogram (ECG) reveals supraventricular tachycardia (SVT). Oxygen saturation as revealed by pulse oximetry (SpO_2) is 90%.

Assessment: This is an example of altering the balance of autonomic control in the lung. Propranolol (Inderal) is a nonspecific β blocker (β_1 and β_2). As a β_1-blocking agent the drug will slow the heart rate. However, the blockade of β_2 receptors in the airway prevents endogenous epinephrine and exogenous adrenergic agents from stimulating those receptors. The intravenous dose directly antagonizes the effect of the β-receptor stimulation in the airways with the adrenergic bronchodilator albuterol, and it inhibits the degree of bronchodilation achieved in this asthmatic, whose airways tend to react to stimuli and constrict. The balance between adrenergic relaxation of the airway and cholinergic constriction is tipped in favor of unbalanced cholinergic activity. She begins to exhibit symptoms of bronchoconstriction (wheezing, dyspnea).

Plan: Prevention is the best approach. In a patient such as an asthmatic, β-receptor stimulation is an important property to preserve. The use of a drug other than a β-blocking agent would be indicated for the supraventricular tachycardia (SVT) to avoid the undesirable side effect of β blockade in the lung. Alternative drugs for tachycardia are discussed in subsequent chapters; these would include a calcium channel–blocking agent such as verapamil or an agent such as amlodipine. Her use of the β-adrenergic bronchodilator albuterol, which is a β_2 agonist, should also be reviewed to ensure proper dosage and frequency of use. Although it is β_2 specific, an adrenergic agonist can stimulate the heart.

CHAPTER 6

Self-Assessment Questions

1. Identify an adrenergic bronchodilator used clinically that is a catecholamine.
   Answer: Racemic epinephrine.
2. Which catecholamine has been used as a bronchodilator and is commonly given to treat allergic reaction by self-injection?
   Answer: Epinephrine.
3. What is the duration of action of the catecholamine bronchodilators?
   Answer: Approximately 1.5 hours; up to 3 hours at most.
4. Identify two advantages introduced with the modifications of the catecholamine structure in adrenergic bronchodilators.
   Answer: Increased β_2 specificity and longer duration of action.
5. Identify the usual dose by aerosol for an SVN for levalbuterol and albuterol.
   Answer: Levalbuterol—0.63 to 1.25 mg; albuterol—0.5 cc of a 0.5% concentration.
6. What is an extremely common side effect with β_2-adrenergic bronchodilators?
   Answer: Muscle tremor.
7. Identify the approximate duration of action for racemic epinephrine, albuterol, salmeterol, and olodaterol.
   Answer: Racemic epinephrine—1 to 3 hours; albuterol—4 to 6 hours; salmeterol—12 hours; olodaterol—24 hours.

8. Identify the generic drug for each of the following brand names: Brovana, Arcapta, Serevent Diskus, and Ventolin HFA.
   Answer: Brovana—arformoterol; Arcapta—indacaterol; Serevent Diskus—salmeterol; and Ventolin HFA—albuterol.
9. Which route of administration is more likely to have greater severity of side effects with a β agonist, oral or inhaled aerosol?
   Answer: Oral (tremor is more severe).
10. You notice a pinkish tinge to aerosol rainout in the large-bore tubing connecting a patient's mouthpiece to a nebulizer after a treatment with racemic epinephrine; what has caused this?
    Answer: The catecholamine epinephrine will be broken down by light and air to the adrenochrome form, producing a pinkish or pinkish-brown residue in tubing.
11. A patient exhibits paradoxic bronchoconstriction from the propellant when using an HFA MDI. Suggest an alternative for the patient.
    Answer: Consider trying the liquid formulation, DPI, or a Respimat depending on availability of the drugs and devices.
12. If you are working with an asthmatic with occasional symptoms of wheezing and chest tightness that respond well to an inhaled β agonist, would you suggest using salmeterol?
    Answer: No; salmeterol is indicated for maintenance therapy of asthmatics needing regular use of a β agonist or step 2 therapy (regular β agonist and inhaled corticosteroid or other agents); it also should be used in conjunction with an inhaled corticosteroid.
13. Suggest a β agonist that would be appropriate for the patient in question 12.
    Answer: Any of the following: albuterol, levalbuterol, or metaproterenol.

Clinical Scenario

Subjective: A 24-year-old white male presents with a complaint of difficulty in breathing. He has no history of asthma or other previous pulmonary disease. He is an accountant with a medium-size firm. He noticed a few "chest colds" from October through January, but these resolved with over-the-counter cold medications such as decongestants and cough suppressants. During a round of golf in late May, he had difficulty breathing. He described a tightness in his chest and the sound of wheezing on interview. The course had recently been mown. The pollen count was quite high at the time, and there was an increased ozone concentration, leading to a smog alert on the day of his round. He also complained of waking up several times during the night with mild shortness of breath.

Objective: His respiratory rate (RR) is 14 breaths/min with no obvious distress at rest; blood pressure (BP) is

128/74 mm Hg; heart rate (HR) is 76 beats/min; and temperature (T) is within normal limits. His oxygen saturation by pulse oximetry (SpO_2) is 93% on room air. On auscultation you detect mild expiratory wheezing bilaterally.

Assessment: Asthma exacerbation.

Plan: Administer a peak flow. Alternatively office spirometry would provide more complete information on his FEV_1 and midmaximal flow rates. A "before and after" bronchodilator study would further determine if he has *reversible* obstruction; however, his history and symptoms suggest this. If low, treatment with a short-acting bronchodilator, such as albuterol or levalbuterol, would be appropriate. Because he will be going home, an HFA MDI would be best. Correct education on its use is a must.

CHAPTER 7

Self-Assessment Questions

1. What was the first FDA-approved anticholinergic bronchodilator for aerosol inhalation?
   Answer: Ipratropium (Atrovent).
2. What is currently the only FDA-approved long-acting anticholinergic combination product on the market?
   Answer: Umeclidinium and vilanterol (Anoro Ellipta).
3. What is the usual recommended dose of ipratropium by MDI and by SVN?
   Answer: MDI: 34 mcg, two actuations, each 17 mcg (from the mouthpiece). SVN: 500 mcg, 2.5 mL of a 0.02% solution.
4. Identify a long-acting anticholinergic bronchodilator and give its duration of action.
   Answer: Tiotropium (Spiriva), aclidinium (Tudorza Pressair), or umeclidinium (Incruse Ellipta); all up to 24 hours.
5. What is the usual clinical indication for use of an anticholinergic bronchodilator such as ipratropium?
   Answer: Maintenance treatment of chronic obstructive pulmonary disease (COPD).
6. Which disease state, asthma or COPD, may show greater response to an anticholinergic bronchodilator rather than a β agonist?
   Answer: COPD patients are likely to have a greater response to an anticholinergic agent rather than a β agonist in reversibility of airflow obstruction.
7. With which type of anticholinergic agent are you more likely to observe systemic side effects: tertiary ammonium or quaternary ammonium compounds?
   Answer: Tertiary; these are less ionized and are better absorbed and distributed through body tissues.
8. What are the most common side effects seen with inhaled ipratropium and tiotropium?
   Answer: Dry mouth and cough.
9. Can ipratropium be used with subjects who have glaucoma?
   Answer: Yes. However, use with caution, have the patient notify his or her ophthalmologist, and monitor intraocular pressures.
10. Can ipratropium be alternated with or combined with a β agonist in the treatment of COPD and asthma?
    Answer: Yes. The two types of agents may have additive effects in reversing airflow obstruction. In addition, they have complementary sites and mechanisms of action, and the time to peak effect is later for ipratropium compared with that of a β agonist, resulting in more sustained peak bronchodilation.
11. What precautions should you observe if administering ipratropium by SVN?
    Answer: Protect the eyes from exposure to the nebulized drug by using a mouthpiece instead of a mask whenever possible or covering the eyes if a facemask is used for administration. This is done to avoid the ocular effects of mydriasis and cycloplegia.
12. What is the clinical indication for the use of an anticholinergic intranasal spray?
    Answer: Rhinorrhea associated with nonallergic perennial rhinitis, colds, and allergic rhinitis if unresponsive to intranasal corticosteroids.

Clinical Scenario

Subjective: In the interview, he states that he has increasingly noticed exertional dyspnea with mild physical activity over the past few months. With questioning, he admits to occasional social alcohol intake of either 1 or 2 beers or a couple of mixed drinks several times a week. He has been happily married to the same woman since he was 24. He also admits to regular cigarette smoking of about 1 pack/day since he was 20 years old. He leads a sedentary life with no physical exercise. He states that he does have a chronic cough, which is worse in the morning, although he denies much productivity.

Objective: Physical examination reveals very mild digital clubbing, a slightly increased anteroposterior (AP) diameter, diminished and distant breath sounds bilaterally with some rhonchi, mildly hyperresonant percussion notes, no jugular venous distention upright or supine, and no peripheral edema. His vital signs are as follows: blood pressure (BP), 146/90 mm Hg; temperature (T), 37.2° C; pulse (P), 88 beats/min; and respiratory rate (RR), 16 breaths/min with no laboring. His arterial blood gas (room air) results are as follows: pH, 7.40; arterial carbon dioxide pressure ($PaCO_2$), 42.5 mm Hg; arterial oxygen pressure (PaO_2), 62 mm Hg; base excess, 1.9 mEq/L; and hemoglobin (Hgb), 14.5 g/dL. Chest radiograph (PA, lateral) shows some loss of lung markings, mild flattening of the hemidiaphragms, and increased AP diameter. His electrolytes and white cell count are normal. Moderate airflow obstruction is present as evidenced by the FEV_1 of 1.94 L, an FEV_1/FVC of 65%, and an increased RV/TLC ratio. Gas exchange is impaired, as seen in the below-normal DL_{CO}.

Assessment: COPD, probably bronchitis and emphysema.

Plan: First and foremost, quit smoking. Give smoking cessation material and program information to him. Second, consider a rehabilitation or disease management educational program to incorporate knowledge of the disease, its treatment options, exercise, and nutrition. A bronchodilator should be considered after assessing the degree of reversibility of his airflow obstruction by spirometry after bronchodilator administration. Furthermore, the use of both a β agonist and anticholinergic may be warranted. If the postassessment of spirometry is positive a short-β agonist should be prescribed on a PRN basis. More notable would be to place the patient on a long-acting β-agonist and anticholinergic. The addition of "triple" therapy may also be considered.

CHAPTER 8

Self-Assessment Questions

1. What drug in the xanthine group is used most often therapeutically?
   Answer: Theophylline (aminophylline).
2. What is the difference between aminophylline and theophylline?
   Answer: Aminophylline is a salt of theophylline, designed to increase aqueous solubility for intravenous administration.
3. What is the recommended therapeutic plasma level for theophylline in asthma and chronic obstructive pulmonary disease (COPD)?
   Answer: 5 to 15 mcg/mL, asthma; 5 to 10 mcg/mL, COPD.
4. How do you know whether a given dose of theophylline would produce a satisfactory treatment effect in an asthmatic?
   Answer: The most exact method is to monitor the plasma level of theophylline and adjust the dose to maintain a therapeutic plasma level. Alternatively, and less precisely, the dose can be adjusted to control symptoms and side effects.
5. Identify at least three adverse side effects seen with theophylline.
   Answer: Gastric irritation, insomnia, anxiety/shakiness, tachycardia, nausea, loss of appetite, and headache.
6. What is meant by a "narrow therapeutic margin"?
   Answer: For a drug with a narrow therapeutic margin, the dose required to produce a therapeutic effect is close to the dose that begins to produce toxic side effects.
7. Although theophylline is a weak bronchodilator, what other effects make it useful in treating chronic airflow obstruction?
   Answer: (1) Stimulation of ventilatory drive in the central nervous system and (2) strengthening of diaphragmatic contractile force.
8. True or False: Theophylline causes bronchodilation and improved airflow solely by inhibiting phosphodiesterase, which breaks down cAMP.
   Answer:

Clinical Scenario

Subjective: A 70-year-old white male arrived to the hospital emergency department complaining of dyspnea. He reported coughing up thick, greenish sputum with some tinges of blood in the last few days. In the interview, he admitted to smoking two packs of cigarettes a day since age 18, stopping about 2 years ago. He has had six hospitalizations within the last 2 years. Current medications include ipratropium bromide by MDI, 2 puffs four times daily, with a $β_2$ agonist by MDI as needed, 1 to 3 puffs. He reports he has been using the $β_2$ MDI regularly during the last month, at least four times daily.

Objective: On physical examination, he was very short of breath (SOB), even at rest, and used accessory muscles with a respiratory rate (RR) of 22 breaths/min. There was little discernible chest expansion. His breath sounds were distant in all areas with expiratory wheezes and air movement appeared poor. He was afebrile with a pulse (P) of 120 beats/min and blood pressure (BP) of 170/112 mm Hg. He appeared oriented, coherent, and somewhat malnourished, with thin arms. Laboratory values on admission showed normal electrolytes, but his white blood cell (WBC) count was 15.2×10^3/cc and his hemoglobin was 10.6 g/dL. Arterial blood gas values on room air were as follows: pH, 7.40; arterial carbon dioxide pressure ($PaCO_2$), 42.4 mm Hg; arterial oxygen pressure (PaO_2), 64 mm Hg; base excess, +1.9 mEq/L; and arterial oxygen saturation (SaO_2), 90%. A chest radiograph (posteroanterior [PA]) shows hyperinflation of the lung fields with flattened diaphragms.

Assessment: He has an exacerbation of COPD.

Plan: Administer oxygen. Although a PO_2 of 64 mm Hg on room air with a saturation of 90% appears to be satisfactory, this is achieved by a labored pattern of respiration with tachypnea (respiratory rate [RR], 22 breaths/min) and is accompanied by increased blood pressure (170/112 mm Hg) and tachycardia (120 beats/min). In addition, he is mildly anemic. Relieving his hypoxemia, and thereby reducing his work of breathing and myocardial work, may prevent the need for ventilatory support. Administer a short-acting β agonist and anticholinergic. Consider use of IV steroids with possible consideration of theophylline. After exacerbation is relieved, consider tiotropium bromide to replace ipratropium bromide at home.

CHAPTER 9

Self-Assessment Questions

1. Identify the mucolytic agents approved for inhalation as an aerosol in the United States—give the generic and brand names.
   Answer: Dornase alfa (Pulmozyme), given 2.5 mg daily by jet nebulization; hypertonic (7%) saline, 4 mL by jet nebulization up to four times daily, and *N*-acetylcysteine (NAC; or Mucomyst), 4 mL of a 10% solution by jet nebulization (however, the latter is not of proven benefit for airway disease).
2. What is the mode of action for dornase alfa?
   Answer: Depolymerizes extracellular DNA, decreasing sputum tenacity.

3. What is the clinical indication for use of dornase alfa?

Answer: To promote secretion clearance in persons with cystic fibrosis.

4. What are contraindications to the use of mucolytic medications?

Answer: Poor or absent cough reflex, weakness, inability to protect the airway, and allergy or documented sensitivity to the medication used.

5. How do macrolide antibiotics affect mucus and what are their indications for use?

Answer: Low-dose macrolide antibiotics are mucoregulatory medications that decrease mucus hypersecretion caused by inflammation and also preserve the normal or constitutive secretion.

6. How should dornase alfa be administered when high-frequency compression is used?

Answer: It may be at least as effective, and probably easier to administer, when given concomitant with high-frequency chest wall compression (HFCWC).

7. What is a common side effect seen with NAC by aerosol?

Answer: Bronchospasm, airway inflammation, and decreased pulmonary function.

8. What are the indications for the use of acetylcysteine?

Answer: Acetylcysteine is approved for systemic use in treating acetaminophen overdose. There are no indications for giving this as an aerosol.

9. How and when should bicarbonate aerosol or instillation be used?

Answer: It should not be used as a mucoactive drug

Clinical Scenario

Subjective: A 17-year-old woman with cystic fibrosis (CF) was admitted to your hospital with an acute respiratory infection (pulmonary exacerbation). She is pleasant, mature, and well informed concerning her disease. She complains of an increased cough, increased sputum production with some hemoptysis, and weight loss over the past 2 weeks.

Objective: She was diagnosed with CF at the age of 2 years because of failure to thrive and did well clinically until age 12. She had a nasal polypectomy and a G-tube placed for night feeding several years ago, which resulted in a weight gain of 30 pounds (13.6 kg). She is chronically infected with resistant *Pseudomonas* and *Stenotrophomonas* and she has grown atypical *Mycobacterium* in the past. She has been admitted with exacerbations of CF twice in the past year. She has been taking 300 mg of tobramycin (TOBI) bid by aerosol at home regularly this year, with courses of oral ciprofloxacin when symptoms of respiratory infection surfaced. Vital signs are as follows: temperature (T), 37.5° C; pulse (P), 110 beats/min and regular; respiratory rate (RR), 26 breaths/min; and blood pressure (BP), 110/50 mm Hg. Oxygen saturation by pulse oximetry (SpO_2) is 0.92 in ambient air. She has mild dyspnea while walking. Auscultation of the chest revealed crackles in all fields, with more in the right upper lobe. Extremities showed clubbing with no cyanosis. She has a cough productive of greenish, thick sputum. No nasal polyps are visible to examination. Chest radiograph (posteroanterior [PA] and lateral) shows diffuse chronic changes with thick interstitial markings consistent with bronchiectasis, and a normal cardiac silhouette. There is an infiltrate in the right upper lobe. Her pulmonary function test results show a decrease in airflow and hyperinflation of the lung consistent with an obstructive disease state.

Assessment: Exacerbation of CF airway disease.

Plan: Her pulmonary function tests indicate moderate airway obstruction, accompanied by the usual problematic secretions seen in CF. Her history also suggests increased bronchiectasis with purulent sputum production and a need for intravenous antibiotic therapy and hospitalization. She may benefit either from dornase alfa (Pulmozyme), 2.5 mg daily by nebulizer, or hyperosmolar (7%) saline. She may also find use of a β agonist, such as albuterol, helpful to improve or maintain lung function and secretion clearance. Finally, continued use of aerosolized antibiotic should be considered to reduce the bacterial burden of her respiratory secretions. Continue to assess the following to determine effectiveness of her dornase alfa treatment: (1) the use of parenteral antibiotics over the coming year; (2) the use of oral antibiotics over the next year; (3) the need for hospitalizations for acute exacerbations; and (4) maintenance or hopefully even improvement in her pulmonary function.

CHAPTER 10

Self-Assessment Questions

1. What is the definition of a *surface-active substance?*

Answer: An agent that can change surface tension at liquid-air interfaces.

2. In general what is the clinical indication for use of exogenous surfactants?

Answer: Prevention (prophylaxis) of respiratory distress syndrome (RDS) in premature newborns with immature lungs or newborns with evidence of immature lung development, and treatment (rescue) of infants who have developed RDS.

3. State the type (category) of exogenous surfactant for each of the following: beractant, calfactant, poractant alfa, and lucinactant.

Answer: Beractant (Survanta)—modified natural bovine extract; calfactant (Infasurf)—natural bovine extract; poractant alfa (Curosurf)—natural porcine extract; lucinactant (Surfaxin)—synthetic.

4. What are the major ingredients of natural pulmonary surfactant?

Answer: Lipids (about 90%), including dipalmitoylphosphatidylcholine (DPPC); proteins, 10%.

5. Give the dosage schedule of each of the current exogenous surfactants.

Answer: Survanta—4 mL/kg;   Infasurf—3 mL/kg; Curosurf—2.5 mL/kg; Surfaxin—5.8 mL/kg.

6. What is the difference between "rescue" and "prophy-laxis" treatment with surfactants?
   Answer: Rescue—drug given in the presence of RDS. Prophylaxis—drug given *before* the onset of RDS.
7. Identify at least three possible adverse effects with the use of exogenous surfactant treatment.
   Answer: Apnea, overventilation, overoxygenation, airway occlusion, desaturation, and bradycardia.
8. Why does the improvement in lung mechanics last after only one or two administrations of exogenous surfactant?
   Answer: Apparently, exogenous surfactant enters the recycling pool in alveolar cells.
9. How would you assess the effectiveness of exogenous surfactant treatment in a premature newborn with respiratory distress?
   Answer: Monitor vital signs, including color and activity, for evidence of airway occlusion, desaturation, and bradycardia. Be prepared to manually ventilate and suction the airway. Assess changes in level of ventilation and oxygenation: chest rise, arterial oxygen saturation (SaO_2) or transcutaneous oxygen pressure ($tcPO_2$), exhaled volumes, and compliance. Modify ventilator settings and fraction of inspired oxygen (FIO_2) on the basis of changes.

Clinical Scenario

Subjective: A 16-year-old female gave birth to a 25-week, 515-g baby girl by vaginal delivery. The mother had no prenatal care and she had premature rupture of the membranes 12 days before delivery.

Objective: Apgar scores after intubation and application of positive-pressure ventilation with a bag and mask were 7 and 9 at 1 and 5 minutes, respectively. Physical examination revealed the following: pulse (P), 140 beats/min; blood pressure (BP), 34/22 mm Hg; temperature (T), 99.6° F; and oxygen saturation by pulse oximetry (SpO_2), 85 to 90%. Laboratory results revealed glucose, 39 mg/dL; white blood cell (WBC) count, 11,900/mm³; hematocrit, 47%; and platelets, 297,000/mm³. Chest radiograph showed respiratory distress syndrome, stage II.

Assessment: The gestational age and low birth weight indicate prematurity, which is associated with lung immaturity and lack of endogenous surfactant. The chest radiograph confirms the presence of neonatal RDS.

Plan: Administer an exogenous surfactant to the baby at the proper dose prescribed. Consider a second dose of surfactant if subsequent decline in lung function is indicated by the decrease in compliance, deteriorating vital signs, and oxygenation. Ventilation and oxygenation should be monitored after a repeat dose, and adjustments made to avoid overventilation and overoxygenation.

CHAPTER 11

Self-Assessment Questions

1. Identify all corticosteroids using generic names approved for clinical use by oral inhalation in the United States.
   Answer: Beclomethasone, flunisolide, fluticasone, budesonide, mometasone, and ciclesonide.
2. What is the major therapeutic effect of corticosteroids?
   Answer: Their antiinflammatory effect.
3. Name two common respiratory diseases in which inhaled corticosteroids are prescribed.
   Answer: Asthma, and (less frequently) chronic obstructive pulmonary disease (COPD).
4. What is the rationale for administering corticosteroids by the inhalation route, rather than by the oral route, in asthma?
   Answer: By targeting the lung directly with corticosteroids that have high topical potency, systemic levels can be minimized and systemic side effects decreased or avoided.
5. Contrast the effects of β agonists with the effects of corticosteroids on the early phase and late phase of asthma.
   Answer: β Agonists may relieve the early phase of bronchoconstriction, whereas corticosteroids can reduce airway inflammation, preventing both the early and late phases of asthma.
6. What is the effect of orally administered corticosteroids on growth, bone density, and adrenal function?
   Answer: Growth is decreased in children; bone density is decreased, causing osteoporosis; normal adrenal steroid secretion is suppressed, and in general the hypothalamic-pituitary-adrenal (HPA) axis activity is suppressed.
7. What is the purpose of alternate-day steroid therapy?
   Answer: To reduce exposure of the body to exogenous corticosteroids and thereby reduce systemic side effects, such as adrenal suppression.
8. Can you transfer an asthmatic patient from oral steroid use to inhaled steroid use? Explain the precautions or reasons, as appropriate.
   Answer: Transfer can be accomplished; however, the patient should be weaned from the oral dose, using tapering doses while initiating inhaled steroids to allow adequate recovery of adrenal function because inhaled steroids will not maintain significant plasma levels at the recommended doses.
9. State two common side effects with inhaled steroids.
   Answer: Oral thrush (candidiasis) and dysphonia.
10. Identify two methods of minimizing the side effects identified in question 9.
    Answer: (1) Use of a reservoir device with MDI orally inhaled corticosteroids; (2) rinsing of the throat by gargling after inhaling a corticosteroid.
11. Have inhaled corticosteroids traditionally been used with an asthmatic during an acute episode?
    Answer: No; there is no acute bronchodilating effect and the dose of inhaled steroids is too low for acute management of airway inflammation. However, inhaled corticosteroids have been investigated for emergency department treatment of acute severe asthma, along with aggressive bronchodilator therapy.

Clinical Scenario

Subjective: A 55-year-old white female presents to the emergency department (ED) with a chief complaint of cough, wheezing, shortness of breath, and chest pain. Two days earlier, she reported rhinorrhea, sore throat, sinus congestion, and subsequent increase in dyspnea and wheeze.

Objective: Physical examination on admission to the ED exhibited wheezing on auscultation, use of accessory muscles, no cyanosis or diaphoresis, and mild respiratory distress. Vital signs were as follows: temperature (T), 98.4° F; pulse (P), 96 beats/min and regular; respiratory rate (RR), 22 breaths/min; and blood pressure (BP), 92/68 mm Hg. Chest radiograph showed hyperinflation but no infiltrates or other abnormalities. Electrocardiogram revealed sinus tachycardia. Arterial blood gas determination on room air indicated the following: pH, 7.44; arterial carbon dioxide pressure ($PaCO_2$), 38 mm Hg; arterial oxygen pressure (PaO_2), 54 mm Hg; base excess (BE), 2.2; bicarbonate (HCO_3^-), 25.9 mEq/L; and arterial oxygen saturation (SaO_2), 89.4%. Hemoglobin was 13.3 g/dL, and the white blood cell (WBC) count was $8.8 \times 10^3/mm^3$. Administration of metered dose inhaler (MDI) albuterol by reservoir showed little improvement in her peak flow rates.

Assessment: Pulmonary exacerbation.

Plan: Admitted to the hospital. Administer 2.5 mg albuterol and 0.5 mg ipratropium bromide via small volume nebulizer (SVN); place on oxygen at 3 L/min by nasal cannula. Administer 40 mg of intravenous methylprednisolone and a brand of phenylephrine for nasal decongestion and sinus clearance.

CHAPTER 12

Self-Assessment Questions

1. Identify four nonsteroidal antiasthma drugs used in the management of chronic asthma; give generic and brand names.
   Answer: Cromolyn sodium, montelukast (Singulair), zafirlukast (Accolate), and zileuton (Zyflo).

2. Which immunoglobulin is implicated in allergy and is termed *cytophilic?*
   Answer: Immunoglobulin E (IgE).

3. Which type of asthma involves allergic reaction to an antigenic stimulus?
   Answer: Extrinsic, or atopic.

4. Which type of helper T cell, Th1 or Th2, is involved primarily in the atopic allergic response?
   Answer: Th2 cells (helper type 2 lymphocytes).

5. A resident wishes to order nebulized cromolyn sodium for a young asthmatic patient in the emergency department who is wheezing and in moderate distress. Would you agree?
   Answer: No. Cromolyn sodium, as a mediator antagonist, is a prophylactic agent to *prevent* mast cell degranulation and mediator release; the drug has no bronchodilating properties.

6. Which of the following could be recommended as possible choices for the asthmatic patient in question 5: inhaled albuterol, inhaled salmeterol, inhaled ipratropium bromide, or theophylline either orally or intravenously?
   Answer: All the agents listed could be used in an acute asthma episode except for salmeterol because its pharmacokinetics are not useful for an acute attack.

7. An asthmatic patient has been taking 40 mg of oral prednisone for 1 week after an acute asthma attack and an emergency department visit. His physician now wants to switch him to inhaled cromolyn and discontinue the oral prednisone. What is the risk in doing this, and what would you recommend?
   Answer: There is a risk of adrenal insufficiency caused by the steroid therapy and hypothalamic-pituitary-adrenal (HPA) suppression and by the fact that cromolyn is not a steroid. A tapered dose regimen of the oral prednisone while the cromolyn is started could be recommended.

8. How does the mechanism of action of zafirlukast and montelukast differ from that of zileuton?
   Answer: Zafirlukast and montelukast act by competitive antagonism of leukotriene receptors ($CysLT_1$ receptors), whereas zileuton acts by inhibition of the 5-lipoxygenase enzyme.

9. What is the recommended dosage and route of administration for zafirlukast, montelukast, and zileuton?
   Answer: Zafirlukast—20 mg twice daily, by the oral route; montelukast—10 mg once daily, orally; zileuton—600 mg four times daily, or two 600 mg extended release (Zyflo CR) twice daily, orally.

10. Which of the three antileukotriene agents in question 9 offers the most convenient dosing and the fewest drug interactions?
    Answer: Montelukast (Singulair), with once-daily dosing, and no significant drug interactions such as what can occur with zileuton or zafirlukast.

11. When would you recommend using omalizumab?
    Answer: In a patient with uncontrolled moderate to severe asthma, especially uncontrolled by corticosteroids.

12. A 17-year-old asthmatic patient has been treated for symptoms for the last 12 months. His symptoms have not improved despite the use of the highest inhaled corticosteroid dose and regular use of salmeterol; in addition, trials on montelukast, cromolyn sodium, and oral theophylline have been unsuccessful. What would you recommend for this patient?
    Answer: Omalizumab would be a great recommendation. The use of omalizumab may be able to decrease the use of corticosteroids being administered.

Clinical Scenario

Subjective: A 45-year-old white female is seen in the emergency department with a complaint of chest tightness, shortness of breath, and wheezing for the past 1.5 days.

She also complains of a cough, with only occasional thin whitish sputum during that period. She denies any fever or chills. She was diagnosed with adult-onset asthma 3 years ago and is aspirin sensitive. She has no history of tobacco use. She has been using over-the-counter (OTC) racemic epinephrine as needed and, since about 4 months ago, has been taking oral theophylline 300 mg twice daily. She is alert but mildly anxious. On questioning, she states that she has been using OTC racemic epinephrine almost every 2 hours over the past 24 hours with little improvement. She states that she has been experiencing many headaches, upset stomach, some lack of appetite, and insomnia often during the week. It has been 2 to 3 hours since she last had an OTC racemic epinephrine treatment.

Objective: The patient's vital signs are as follows: temperature (T), 97° F; pulse (P), 112 beats/min and regular; blood pressure (BP), 135/90 mm Hg; and respiratory rate (RR), 22 breaths/min with no laboring. Expiration is slightly prolonged, but there is no use of accessory muscles. No cyanosis is evident. Auscultation reveals diffuse wheezes, greater on expiration than inspiration, and rhonchi bilaterally. Routine blood work later showed the following: hemoglobin, 13.5 g/dL; and white blood cell (WBC) count, $6.1 \times 10^3/mm^3$ with 13% eosinophils. Electrolytes were also found to be within normal limits except for a plasma glucose level of 281 mg/dL. A chest radiograph showed some hyperinflation bilaterally, with no infiltrates, no pneumothorax, and normal heart size. An arterial blood gas measurement on room air revealed the following: pH, 7.38; arterial carbon dioxide pressure ($PaCO_2$), 42 mm Hg; arterial oxygen pressure (PaO_2), 72 mm Hg; base excess, +0.3 mEq/L; and arterial oxygen saturation (SaO_2), 96%.

Assessment: Asthma exacerbation; increased heart rate and blood pressure secondary to asthma and use of racemic epinephrine.

Plan: Place patient on oxygen at 2 L/min by nasal cannula because of her hypoxemia (PaO_2, 72 mm Hg) and give 4 actuations of albuterol using an MDI with a holding chamber every 20 minutes. A plasma theophylline level draw. If she is better after therapy dismiss to home on oral prednisone, tapered dose for 1 week. Consider removing theophylline because of her headaches and replacing with low dose inhaled corticosteroid; however, given her recent cough symptoms and aspirin sensitivity, she may be a good candidate for use of an antileukotriene agent. Continue a short-acting β agonist PRN and monitor daily with a peak flow meter. Insist that she not use OTC racemic epinephrine.

CHAPTER 13

Self-Assessment Questions

1. Identify the disease states for which each of these drugs is used when inhaled as an aerosol: pentamidine, ribavirin, tobramycin, aztreonam, and zanamivir.

Answer: Pentamidine—*Pneumocystis jiroveci* pneumonia (PJP) prophylaxis in acquired immunodeficiency syndrome (AIDS) (last option); Ribavirin—respiratory syncytial virus (RSV) treatment with risk of severe or complicated infection; Tobramycin—management of *Pseudomonas aeruginosa* in cystic fibrosis; Aztreonam—management of *Pseudomonas aeruginosa* in cystic fibrosis; Zanamivir—treatment of acute influenza infection.

2. Briefly explain the rationale for aerosolizing an antibiotic such as tobramycin or aztreonam in cystic fibrosis.

Answer: The oral route gives inadequate lung levels; inhaled and intravenous routes give higher lung tissue levels.

3. What is the brand name of aerosolized pentamidine?
Answer: NebuPent.

4. What is the dose and frequency for aerosolized pentamidine?
Answer: 300 mg q4wk.

5. What device is approved for aerosolization of pentamidine?
Answer: Respirgard II.

6. Identify the common airway effects with aerosolized pentamidine and suggest a method for preventing or lessening these effects.
Answer: Cough, bronchoconstriction; pretreat with a β agonist.

7. What is a major risk to the caregiver when aerosolizing pentamidine to a patient with AIDS?
Answer: Contraction of tuberculosis (TB) infection.

8. What is the current Centers for Disease Control and Prevention (CDC) recommended prophylactic treatment for PJP in AIDS patients?
Answer: Use trimethoprim-sulfamethoxazole (TMP-SMX) orally as long as side effects are tolerated and acceptable. The use of inhaled pentamidine is an option.

9. What is the brand name and dose for aerosol ribavirin?
Answer: Virazole 6 g/300 mL (2%), 12 to 18 hr/day for 3 to 7 days.

10. What is the mechanism of action of ribavirin?
Answer: Virostatic; as a nucleoside analog, ribavirin interferes with viral transcription and replication.

11. Name two serious hazards when ribavirin is given to a patient undergoing mechanical ventilation.
Answer: (1) Occlusion of endotracheal tube; (2) expiratory valve and sensor occlusion.

12. In general, how can you prevent environmental contamination when delivering ribavirin to an oxygen hood?
Answer: A containment/scavenging system around the hood.

13. What is the recommended dosage for inhaled tobramycin?
Answer: Aerosolize 300 mg twice daily, alternating 28 days on/28 days off.

14. Identify common side effects that have been observed with aerosolized tobramycin.

    Answer: Tinnitus and voice changes.

15. Name two potential hazards to family members with aerosolized tobramycin at home.

    Answer: Exposure to aerosolized drug in ambient air may lead to (1) allergic reactions in those sensitive to the drug and (2) fetal harm in a pregnant female.

16. What is the recommended dosage for inhaled aztreonam?

    Answer: 75 mg by Altera Nebulizer System TID, alternating 28 days on/28 days off.

17. What should be done before a patient is prescribed inhaled aztreonam?

    Answer: Collect baseline pulmonary function results to monitor FEV_1 and pretreat with a bronchodilator.

18. Give the brand name and dosage for zanamivir.

    Answer: Relenza; 2 inhalations (10 mg) twice daily 12 hours apart, for 5 days.

19. In one sentence, describe the mechanism of action of zanamivir.

    Answer: Zanamivir inhibits the viral enzyme neuraminidase, causing viral aggregation and clumping, hence preventing viral release and spreading.

20. Identify common hazards in the use of inhaled zanamivir.

    Answer: Pulmonary function deterioration, including bronchospasm in those with reactive airway disease, and inappropriate treatment or undertreatment of nonviral bacterial infections.

21. What factors cause debate over the use of zanamivir in treating influenza?

    Answer: Essentially cost versus efficacy—small reduction in symptoms; no inexpensive, easily available test to confirm influenza infection; and increased possible risk in airway disease.

Clinical Scenario

Subjective: Brody Hendrix is a 29-year-old adult male with cystic fibrosis. He has been admitted to the hospital with complaints of increasing cough, shortness of breath, and sputum production. He reports that his sputum is greenish. His recent history reveals that his last admission for exacerbation of cystic fibrosis was approximately 6 months ago. He has used albuterol by metered dose inhaler (MDI), with 2 puffs qid, and recently began to use salmeterol, 2 puffs bid. He maintains himself on a regular regimen of cystic fibrosis medications, including iron and vitamin supplements and pancrelipase (Pancrease). Approximately 3 weeks ago, he complained of increasing pulmonary secretions and noted a mild elevation of his temperature. At that time, his physician prescribed ciprofloxacin, 500 mg orally bid, and he completed a course of 14 days, ending 5 days ago.

Objective: He is alert, oriented, and in no acute distress at this time. His skin is warm and dry. His vital signs are as follows: blood pressure (BP), 106/66 mm Hg; pulse (P),

88 beats/min and regular; respiratory rate (RR), 20 breaths/min; and temperature (T), 98.9° F. His respiratory pattern is normal, and there is no use of accessory muscles. Auscultation reveals scattered rales and wheezes bilaterally, both anteriorly and posteriorly. His cough is nonproductive during the examination. Chest radiograph shows hyperexpanded lung fields with linear fibrotic changes bilaterally over the lung fields. Cardiac silhouette shows mild right atrial hypertrophy. No consolidation or pleural effusion is seen. Complete blood count (CBC) results are as follows: hemoglobin, 13.2 g/dL; hematocrit, 38.6%; and white blood cell (WBC) count, $13.5 \times 10^3/mm^3$. Remaining blood values are within normal limits. Pulse oximetry measures 89% saturation on room air. His pulmonary function, measured approximately 2 months ago, shows FVC, 67% of predicted; FEV_1, 40% of predicted; FEF25-75, 17% of predicted; RV, 260% of predicted; and TLC, 115% of predicted.

Assessment: Mr. Hendrix has an acute exacerbation of cystic fibrosis.

Plan: Continue with his usual cystic fibrosis medications (vitamins, iron supplement, Pancrease enzymes). *Oxygen* is indicated by his SpO2 (oxygen saturation by pulse oximetry) value. *Antibiotic therapy* will be needed to reduce his bacterial burden, as indicated by his temperature and WBC count. Because he has completed a course of ciprofloxacin and symptoms are now recurring, there is the possibility of resistance to the ciprofloxacin. A different, or at the least an additional, antibiotic may be needed. Recommend administering aerosolized tobramycin or aztreonam. An aggressive program of bronchial hygiene is usual to clear his secretions and would include *chest physiotherapy* with postural drainage and percussion as tolerated for mobilization of secretions; β_2 *agonist* by aerosol to maintain airway patency; possible administration of the anticholinergic bronchodilator *ipratropium* by either SVN or MDI; and, finally, adequate fluid intake and balanced nutrition.

CHAPTER 14

Self-Assessment Questions

1. What is the difference between bacteriostatic and bactericidal antimicrobial agents?

    Answer: Bacteriostatic agents inhibit the growth of bacteria, whereas bactericidal agents kill bacteria.

2. Give an example of a class of antimicrobials that kill in a concentration dependent and concentration independent manner.

    Answer: Concentration dependent antimicrobials include: aminoglycosides, fluoroquinolones, and daptomycin. Concentration independent antimicrobials include: β-lactams, tetracyclines, glycopeptides, and macrolides.

3. Describe at least three parameters that may indicate antibiotic failure in a patient.

    Answer: Continued fever spikes, elevated WBC count, repeated positive cultures, and nonresolution or worsening of symptoms (such as hypotension or mental status change) may indicate antibiotic failure.

4. Why is combination antibiotic therapy useful? (Be specific.)

    Answer: Antimicrobial combinations can provide broad-spectrum activity as part of an empiric regimen. Certain infections are polymicrobial and so require a combination of antimicrobials to be therapeutically effective. Antimicrobial combinations can be used for their synergistic effect and to reduce the emergence of resistance.

5. Describe the mechanism of action of penicillin antibiotics. Name at least two additional antibiotic classes with similar mechanisms of action.

    Answer: Penicillins bind to cell wall proteins to inhibit the cross-linkage of peptidoglycan, which reduces the structural integrity of the cell wall, resulting in lysis. Cephalosporins, carbapenems, and monobactams have a similar mechanism of action.

6. Which β-lactam antibiotic is least likely to cause an allergic reaction in a patient with a penicillin allergy?

    Answer: Aztreonam.

7. Name three antimicrobial agents that would be useful in the treatment of community-acquired pneumonia.

    Answer: Macrolide (azithromycin or clarithromycin), Ketolide (telithromycin), Fluoroquinolone (levofloxacin or moxifloxacin), β-lactam (amoxicillin-clavulanate), or doxycycline.

8. What is the antimicrobial agent of choice for treatment of *Pneumocystis* pneumonia (PCP)?

    Answer: Trimethoprim-sulfamethoxazole.

9. What agents are considered first-line therapy for treatment of pulmonary tuberculosis?

    Answer: Isoniazid, Rifamycin (rifampin, rifabutin, or rifapentine), pyrazinamide, and ethambutol.

10. Which antimicrobial agents are useful for the treatment of nosocomial pneumonia caused by *Pseudomonas aeruginosa*?

    Answer: Carbapenem (excluding ertapenem), cefepime, ceftazidime, or piperacillin/tazobactam plus an aminoglycoside (gentamicin, tobramycin, or amikacin) or fluoroquinolone (ciprofloxacin or levofloxacin).

Clinical Scenario

Subjective: This is a 64-year-old white male with a history of chronic obstructive pulmonary disease (COPD) and recurrent pneumonia. The patient complains of productive cough with green sputum, fever, and worsening shortness of air (SOA). He also has gastroesophageal reflux disease (GERD) and chronic alcohol abuse.

Objective: Physical examination revealed the following vital signs: temperature (T), 102.2° F; blood pressure (BP), 150/85 mm Hg; heart rate (HR), 105 beats/min; respiratory rate (RR), 29 breaths/min; and oxygen saturation by pulse oximetry (SpO₂), 90% on 2 L O₂, 82% on room air. The patient is an elderly male in acute distress; tachycardic, with a regular rhythm; bilateral crackles, with decreased breath sounds over lower left lobe. His white blood cell (WBC) count is 18.4×10^3 cells/mm³. Sputum demonstrated many WBCs, few epithelial cells, many gram-positive cocci in clusters with culture pending. His chest x-ray (CXR) film revealed left lower lobe (LLL) infiltrate.

Assessment: Because of the patient's past medical history of multiple hospitalization with recurrent pneumonia (including methicillin-resistant *Staphylococcus aureus* [MRSA]) and symptoms consistent with a diagnosis of health care–associated pneumonia (HCAP) including productive cough, fevers, and shortness of air (SOA). The signs of infection include his elevated temperature, elevated heart and respiratory rates, bilateral wheezing, elevated WBC count, many WBCs in his sputum gram stain, and LLL infiltrate on CXR. The Gram stain revealed gram-positive cocci in clusters, which is consistent with the most likely pathogen in this patient, MRSA.

Plan: Antimicrobial therapy should be initiated immediately with either intravenous (IV) vancomycin or IV linezolid. Although daptomycin also has excellent activity again MRSA, it cannot be used for pneumonia because this agent is inactivated by lung surfactants. After appropriate response to IV therapy, the patient could be discharged on oral (PO) linezolid to finish his course of treatment. Prior to discharge, the patient needs to be counselled on the importance of smoking cessation and decreased alcohol consumption.

CHAPTER 15

Self-Assessment Questions

1. Identify the four classes of ingredients found in cold medications.

    Answer: Adrenergic decongestants, antihistamines (H₁ blockers), expectorants, and antitussives. *Note:* An analgesic may be added.

2. For each of the following agents, identify the category (e.g., adrenergic, antitussive): codeine, chlorpheniramine, phenylephrine, dextromethorphan, and pseudoephedrine.

    Answer: Codeine—antitussive; chlorpheniramine—antihistamine; phenylephrine—adrenergic; dextromethorphan—antitussive; pseudoephedrine—adrenergic.

3. What is the intended purpose of α-adrenergic agents in cold medications?

    Answer: Topical vasoconstriction to open the upper (nasal) airway.

4. What is the intended effect of antihistamines (H₁ blockers) in cold medications?

    Answer: To dry secretions (rhinitis) produced by histamine release and stimulation of H₁ receptors.

5. Are antihistamines in cold remedies H₁ or H₂ blockers?

    Answer: H₁ blockers. (H₂ blockers, e.g., ranitidine [Zantac], are antiulcer drugs.)

6. You drink several beers at a friend's house after taking a dose of Benadryl. Should you drive home, and why or why not?

   Answer: No. Antihistamines cause drowsiness and alcohol produces an additive effect on this—reflexes are decreased.

7. Identify the most common expectorant in over-the-counter (OTC) cold remedies.

   Answer: Guaifenesin (glyceryl guaiacolate).

8. Briefly explain how guaifenesin stimulates mucus production.

   Answer: Probably through stimulation of vagal receptors in the stomach.

9. List some specific fluids you would recommend to someone with a cold.

   Answer: Water, juices, or milk.

10. Differentiate a "cold" from the "flu."

    Answer: Cold—nonbacterial upper respiratory infection with mild malaise and runny, stuffy nose (more localized than the flu); flu—systemic viral infection with fever, chills, headache, muscle ache, and extreme fatigue.

Clinical Scenario

Subjective: A 24-year-old student, a previously healthy male, is within normal weight limits and performs mild but irregular physical activity. He complains of mild malaise, a runny stuffy nose, sneezing, and a slight sore throat. He denies headache or muscle ache, describes the malaise as a very mild fatigue, and states that he noticed a gradually increasing rhinitis over a period of hours, with sneezing beginning during the first 6 hours of these symptoms.

Objective: He has no fever.

Assessment: His symptoms indicate a cold rather than the flu.

Plan: Point out that there is no "cure" if this is a rhinovirus infection. He should treat his symptoms, however. An adrenergic *decongestant* may be helpful in opening his nasal passages and reducing some of the rhinitis. The use of a topical agent will give fewer systemic effects, such as a feeling of shakiness, and central nervous system stimulation than an oral agent. Caution him to use the decongestant sparingly to avoid rebound nasal congestion; treating the rebound congestion with additional sprays can produce a self-sustaining congestion. An antitussive agent, such as dextromethorphan, can be helpful if he has a nonproductive, dry, irritating cough, particularly if this prevents adequate rest at night. The use of an antihistamine should be avoided if possible to prevent impaction of secretions and subsequent sinus problems. However, if an antihistamine is used, it should be taken only at night or when alert activity (including driving) is not needed. Rest and good nutrition, including juices, will assist his own immune response to recover from the infection.

CHAPTER 16

Self-Assessment Questions

1. For which disease state is an α_1-proteinase inhibitor (API) indicated?

   Answer: Congenital α_1-antitrypsin deficiency.

2. What is the route of administration for an α_1-proteinase inhibitor?

   Answer: Intravenous.

3. What is the mode of action of α_1-proteinase inhibitors in treating emphysema associated with inadequate API levels?

   Answer: Intravenous administration of exogenous α_1-proteinase inhibitor increases blood levels and diffuses into the lung tissue to increase epithelial fluid levels, where the API inactivates the enzyme neutrophil elastase (NE), which can destroy lung tissue.

4. Is treatment with an α_1-proteinase inhibitor indicated for age-related emphysema or in general for individuals who smoke and have emphysema later in life?

   Answer: No. Use of API is recommended only for those who have congenital α_1-antitrypsin (α_1-AT) deficiency and severe COPD. Such individuals often are smokers, which is a risk factor for development of COPD in α_1-AT deficiency, usually at an early age (third or fourth decade).

5. Identify three pharmaceutical formulations of nicotine that are used as smoking cessation aids.

   Answer: The transdermal patch, chewing gum, lozenge, nasal spray, and inhaler.

6. What is the usual effect of nicotine, whether in a smoking cessation aid or in cigarettes, on blood pressure?

   Answer: Nicotine acts at the ganglionic synapses to increase blood pressure, with peripheral vasoconstriction; epinephrine is released from the adrenal medulla, contributing to hypertension, tachycardia, and vasoconstriction.

7. Name two nonnicotine agents used in the treatment of smoking cessation.

   Answer: Varenicline (CHANTIX) and bupropion (Zyban, Wellbutrin).

8. What is the effect of inhaled nitric oxide?

   Answer: Relaxation of the pulmonary vascular endothelium and reduction of pulmonary hypertension.

9. Identify two potentially toxic by-products of inhaled nitric oxide.

   Answer: Methemoglobin and nitrogen dioxide.

10. What is the usual dose of inhaled nitric oxide?

    Answer: The recommended dose is 20 ppm, maintained up to 14 days or until the underlying oxygen desaturation has resolved and weaning from inhaled nitric oxide can be accomplished.

11. Identify two disease states in which nitric oxide has been used to reverse pulmonary hypertension.

    Answer: Persistent pulmonary hypertension of the newborn and acute respiratory distress syndrome.

12. What is the greatest hazard in terms of pulmonary health with the delivery of Ventavis?

    Answer: Ventavis is known to cause bronchospasm.

13. What is the initial dose of Tyvaso?

    Answer: 3 breaths per treatment session (18 mcg), four times daily during waking hours.

Clinical Scenario

Subjective: The patient complaints of shortness of breath on exertion and increasing fatigue during her usual activities. She reported that she had an uncle who had died "many years previously" in middle age with lung disease. She admitted that she had been a heavy smoker (around a pack per day) for 5 or 6 years but quit more than 8 years ago. She described having several attacks of "bronchitis" in the past year. She also described a small, but increasing, production of sputum during the past year, usually clear unless she had an episode of bronchitis.

Objective: Auscultation of her chest reveals expiratory wheezing, diminished breath sounds bilaterally, and a somewhat prolonged expiratory phase. There is no digital clubbing, cyanosis, pedal edema, or jugular distention. Vital signs are as follows: temperature (T), 37.1° C; blood pressure (BP), 110/76 mm Hg; pulse (P), 76 beats/min; and respiratory rate (RR), 24 breaths/min and regular. On room air, her reading on pulse oximetry is 91%. There is a mild elevation of her white blood cell (WBC) count ($13.1 \times 10^3/mm^3$), normal hemoglobin and hematocrit, normal electrolytes, and *Pseudomonas* and normal flora was found in her sputum. Chest radiograph showed some hyperlucency; hyperinflation with moderately lowered, somewhat flattened hemidiaphragms on full inspiration; and an infiltrate in the right lower lobe. ABG values on room air were as follows: pH, 7.35; $PaCO_2$, 54 mm Hg; PaO_2, 66 mm Hg; HCO_3^-, 30 mEq/L; and SaO_2, 92%. Pulmonary function tests revealed an FEV_1 that was 60% of predicted, with an elevated residual volume (RV) and RV/total lung capacity (TLC) ratio, an increased TLC above predicted, and a decreased DL_{CO} (diffusing capacity of the lung for CO).

Assessment: Her clinical and laboratory findings support a diagnosis of chronic obstructive pulmonary disease (COPD). However, her smoking history is not sufficient to produce the degree of severity seen, and her age is incompatible with the usual presentation of COPD.

Plan: Obtain an α_1-proteinase inhibitor blood level because of suspicion of congenital α_1-antitrypsin deficiency.

CHAPTER 17

Self-Assessment Questions

1. Can an aerosol formulation for oral inhalation be legally administered to neonates, infants, and pediatric patients?

   Answer: Yes, using appropriate devices and techniques and with a duly licensed physician's order.

2. Can an adrenergic bronchodilator such as albuterol reduce airway resistance when used in neonates and children?

   Answer: Yes. Multiple studies have found improved airway mechanics with aerosolized albuterol delivered by either metered dose inhaler (MDI)/reservoir system or nebulizer.

3. According to the data reviewed in this chapter, does the adult dose of an aerosol drug need to be reduced with neonatal and pediatric patients, based on weight?

   Answer: No. Because of multiple factors in neonatal and pediatric patients, the actual dose of an inhaled aerosol reaching the lungs is proportionately less than an adult lung dose and increases/decreases with increasing/decreasing age.

4. What aerosol delivery devices could be used with a 2-year-old child?

   Answer: A nebulizer (with mask if necessary) or an MDI with a reservoir and mask.

Clinical Scenario

Subjective: A 24-month-old boy who was born at 27 weeks' gestation presents to the emergency room in respiratory distress. His medical history is significant for bronchopulmonary dysplasia.

Objective: Vital signs are as follows: temperature, 37.5° C; pulse, 175 beats/min; respiratory rate, 76 breaths/min; blood pressure, 85/55 mm Hg; SpO_2, 85% on room air. The physical examination reveals the presence of intercostal retractions, increased anteroposterior diameter, nasal flaring, and bilateral diffuse expiratory wheezing.

Assessment: The patient receives 1.25 mg unit dose via small volume nebulizer (SVN). While receiving the aerosol, the patient's pulse rate climbs to 220 beats/min and he becomes cyanotic despite the O_2 used to nebulize the drug. The patient is promptly intubated and mechanically ventilated.

Plan: Although the patient receives albuterol throughout his stay, one may recommend levalbuterol. Although the case did not detail the dose of albuterol given during the child's stay, it would be safe to say that it was a lower dose. The patient was prescribed albuterol syrup at discharge; however, other choices may include MDI formulations of albuterol or levalbuterol with a spacer device with attached mask or SVN formulation with mask.

CHAPTER 18

Self-Assessment Questions

1. List four general uses of skeletal muscle relaxants.

   Answer:
   - To facilitate endotracheal intubation.
   - For muscle relaxation during surgery, particularly of the thorax and abdomen.
   - To enhance patient-ventilator synchrony.

- To reduce intracranial pressure in intubated patients with uncontrolled intracranial pressure.
- To reduce oxygen consumption.
- To terminate convulsive *status epilepticus* and *tetanus* in patients refractory to other therapies.
- To facilitate procedures or diagnostic studies.
- For selected patients who must remain immobile (e.g., trauma patients).

2. What are the two classifications of neuromuscular blocking agents?
   Answer: Nondepolarizing and depolarizing.

3. Identify each of the following agents by classification type: vecuronium, succinylcholine, and pancuronium.
   Answer: Vecuronium—nondepolarizing; succinylcholine—depolarizing; pancuronium—nondepolarizing.

4. Which type of neuromuscular blocker can be reversed?
   Answer: Nondepolarizing.

5. What type of drug would you use to reverse vecuronium?
   Answer: Cholinesterase inhibitor (e.g., neostigmine).

6. Identify another drug that you would want to give before you reverse vecuronium.
   Atropine or glycopyrrolate (i.e., antimuscarinic agents).

7. Briefly explain why you might need to paralyze a patient receiving mechanical ventilation.
   Answer: To relax the chest wall and prevent spontaneous breathing efforts that are out of phase with the ventilator, causing increased intrathoracic pressure and decreased alveolar ventilation.

8. Neuromuscular blocking agents do not block consciousness; what two types or classes of drugs would be indicated in a paralyzed patient on mechanical ventilation?
   Answer: Analgesics and sedatives.

9. Identify at least two neuromuscular blocking agents that would be preferred for paralysis in a patient receiving mechanical ventilation (assume normal renal and hepatic function).
   Answer: Vecuronium has minimal histamine release and cardiovascular effects; atracurium and rocuronium are also alternatives.

10. You are called to the recovery room to set up a ventilator for an elderly patient who has just undergone a total hip replacement and has failed to breathe after a single dose of succinylcholine. What might the problem be?
    Answer: Atypical plasma cholinesterase.

11. What would you do first to assess a ventilated patient who is restless and "fighting" the ventilator before using a paralyzing agent?
    Answer: Assess ventilator function and patient status: (1) ventilator—possible malfunction; inappropriate settings (flow, F_{IO_2}, volume, inspiratory:expiratory [I:E] ratio); (2) patient-airway patency, SaO_2 or SpO_2, possible pain or anxiety requiring analgesia and sedation rather than paralysis.

Clinical Scenario

Subjective: A 64-year-old white female presents with a complaint of shortness of breath and congestion along with fatigue and lethargy over the last 3 days. She has a history of diabetes mellitus, hypertension, and chronic obstructive pulmonary disease (COPD) secondary to smoking. She has had a productive cough of yellow-greenish sputum and states she has had fever and chills over the past several days.

Objective: Pulse (P), 130 beats/min; blood pressure (BP), 100/72 mm Hg; temperature (T), 38.5° C; and respiratory rate (RR), 30 breaths/min, with a moderate amount of respiratory distress. On auscultation, breath sounds are diminished bilaterally. An electrocardiogram shows sinus tachycardia. Chest radiograph shows bilateral interstitial infiltrates. Her white blood cell (WBC) count is $23.7 \times 10^3/mm^3$ with 35% bands, hemoglobin is 11.2 g/dL and hematocrit is 33.2%, and electrolytes are within normal limits, except for glucose, which is 250 mg/dL. Arterial blood gas values on a 100% nonrebreather mask are as follows: pH, 7.2; arterial carbon dioxide pressure ($PaCO_2$), 50 mm Hg; arterial oxygen pressure (PaO_2), 55 mm Hg; and arterial oxygen saturation (SaO_2), 82%.

Assessment: The patient is not effectively oxygenating. As a result, the patient has a PaO_2/FIO_2 ratio of 55. The patient is very tachypneic and has impending ventilatory failure.

Plan: Intubate and ventilate.

CHAPTER 19

Self-Assessment Questions

1. What is a diuretic?
   Answer: A diuretic is any substance that increases urine output.

2. Identify the five major groups of diuretics used clinically.
   Answer: Osmotic, carbonic anhydrase inhibitors, thiazide, loop, and potassium sparing.

3. If an agent such as one of the loop diuretics causes a loss of potassium, how would this lead to a metabolic alkalosis?
   Answer: Sodium that is still reabsorbed will exchange for either potassium or hydrogen. Low potassium, resulting from excretion, forces reabsorbed sodium to exchange for hydrogen, depleting hydrogen ions and raising pH. Hydrogen is also excreted as a result of the diuretic, adding to the alkalosis. Potassium replacement is usually necessary to prevent hypokalemia.

4. Which diuretics would preserve potassium?
   Answer: The potassium-sparing agents, such as amiloride, triamterene, or spironolactone.

5. What is the potential effect of a carbonic anhydrase inhibitor on acid-base balance?
   Answer: A loss of bicarbonate, leading to metabolic acidosis.

6. Explain how a diuretic such as furosemide can be helpful in acute congestive heart failure with pulmonary and vascular edema.

Answer: A potent diuretic such as furosemide will cause excretion of volume from the circulatory system by limiting sodium and therefore water retention. This will decrease the amount of volume leaking from the vasculature both in the lung and in the periphery, as well as venous return to the heart. Reduced pulmonary edema will improve oxygenation, which will also improve oxygen available to the heart. Reduced preload also reduces the work of the myocardium. Reduced preload and improved oxygenation are beneficial to restoring heart function.

7. Which diuretic agent has a vasodilatory effect when used for long-term treatment?
   Answer: Hydrochlorothiazide (HCTZ).

8. In an otherwise healthy adult with mild hypertension, what diuretic agent should be considered as the first line of treatment?
   Answer: HCTZ.

9. Which diuretic agent has been successfully used in the management of acute respiratory distress syndrome (ARDS)?
   Answer: Furosemide.

10. Match each of the following sets of drugs on the left with the most likely interaction on the right.
    Answer:

Gentamicin *PLUS* furosemide	Hyperglycemia
Hydrochlorothiazide *PLUS* prednisone	Ototoxicity and nephrotoxicity
Spironolactone *PLUS* enalapril	Hyperkalemia
Hydrochlorothiazide *PLUS* carbamazepine	Hyponatremia

Clinical Scenario

Subjective: A 73-year-old white male presents to the emergency department with a chief complaint of severe dyspnea that began about 8 hours before presentation. The patient's history is significant for long-standing hypertension and coronary artery disease. He states that he began feeling dyspneic the night before presentation and then awoke at about 5:00 AM severely dyspneic and coughing up white, foamy phlegm. When queried about his compliance with his medicines, he admits that he sometimes forgets to take his clonidine. The patient has chronic renal insufficiency and has had right inguinal hernia repair. He denies any allergies. The patient is taking the following medications: clonidine 0.1 mg PO bid; atenolol 50 mg PO hs each night; aspirin 325 mg PO qd; transdermal nitroglycerin 0.4 mg qh (he places a patch on in the morning and takes it off at bedtime); and furosemide 40 mg PO q AM.

Objective: Physical examination reveals an elderly white male in obvious respiratory distress. His vital signs are as follows: pulse (P), 120 beats/min and regular; respiratory rate (RR), 32 beats/min; blood pressure (BP), 230/140 mm Hg, and he is afebrile. His neck shows positive jugular venous distension. Heart auscultation reveals a regular rate, with a systolic ejection murmur (I/VI), negative S_3, and positive S_4. His lungs demonstrate bibasilar inspiratory crackles half of the way up the thorax. His abdomen is flat and bowel sounds are present; no masses or tenderness are identified. His extremities are slightly cool, and pulses are felt in all extremities, but are somewhat thready.

The patient's laboratory results are as follows: Na, 138 mEq/L; K, 3.6 mEq/L; blood urea nitrogen (BUN), 40 mg/dL; and creatinine, 2.8 mg/dL. His electrocardiogram (ECG) shows sinus tachycardia with inferior Q waves and lateral Q waves of questionable significance. A chest radiograph shows mild cardiomegaly with bilateral infiltrates consistent with pulmonary edema.

Assessment: This is a 73-year-old white male with ischemic heart disease, hypertension, and chronic renal insufficiency. His history, physical examination, and diagnostic data are consistent with acute pulmonary edema. His blood pressure is markedly elevated. There is a history of possible medical noncompliance, which would make one suspicious that he has not taken his clonidine. Acute hypertension in the face of already impaired left ventricular systolic function is a common cause of acute pulmonary edema. Of note, the patient does have some evidence of renal insufficiency with an elevated creatinine level. His potassium is at the lower end of normal, probably secondary to his furosemide.

Plan: This patient is currently taking furosemide 40 mg daily; thus, an acceptable approach would be to double the oral dose and give it intravenously. Therefore, furosemide 80 mg intravenously would be a reasonable choice. If within 30 to 45 minutes of receiving intravenous furosemide the patient has not begun to increase urine output, another loop diuretic would be reasonable. However, typically the preceding dose of furosemide would be doubled (to 160 mg in this case) and administered. The patient does have mild renal insufficiency and is taking a β blocker. Both of these probably attenuate the normal potassium wasting seen with diuretics; however, with vigorous diuresis, he would most certainly become hypokalemic without potassium replacement. This can lead to dangerous arrhythmias, particularly in patients with ischemic cardiomyopathy. The potassium should be monitored closely and administered to a level of 4.0 mEq/L or greater.

CHAPTER 20

Self-Assessment Questions

1. What is the difference between sedation and analgesia?
   Answer: Sedation—decreased response to stimuli, relaxation; analgesia—relief of pain.

2. Identify the general class (sedative-hypnotic, analgesic, tranquilizer, anesthetic, or antipsychotic) of each of the following agents: lorazepam, phenobarbital, doxapram, chloral hydrate, thiopental, midazolam, nitrous oxide, chlorpromazine, halothane, morphine, and ibuprofen.

Answer: Lorazepam—minor tranquilizer (antianxiety); phenobarbital—sedative-hypnotic; doxapram—respiratory stimulant; chloral hydrate—nonbarbiturate sedative-hypnotic; thiopental—general (intravenous) anesthetic; midazolam—general anesthetic; nitrous oxide—general anesthetic (gas); chlorpromazine—antipsychotic; halothane—general anesthetic (liquid-gas); morphine—narcotic analgesic; ibuprofen—nonsteroidal antiinflammatory drug (NSAID) and analgesic.

3. You are planning to extubate and remove a patent from the ventilator. However, the nurse administers a large dose of lorazepam (Ativan) for anxiety. What problem may occur if you proceed?

    Answer: Hypoventilation, depressed ventilatory drive.

4. What is the most serious side effect of tranquilizers, sedatives, or analgesics (especially opioids)?

    Answer: Central nervous system depression resulting in respiratory depression—hypoventilation or respiratory arrest.

5. You have two patients, both of whom have overdosed on central nervous system depressants: *Patient 1 is comatose, cyanotic, with dilated pupils. Patient 2 is comatose, cyanotic, with pinpoint pupils.* Which patient may have taken a barbiturate and which may have taken a narcotic analgesic?

    Answer: Barbiturate—Patient 1; narcotic—Patient 2.

6. Identify your initial priorities as a respiratory therapist in caring for a patient with an overdose of tranquilizers.

    Answer: (1) Maintenance or establishment of airway; (2) provide ventilation; and (3) supplemental O_2 as needed to maintain PaO_2.

7. What is the mode of action of the benzodiazepines?

    Answer: Benzodiazepines bind to benzodiazepine receptors in the central nervous system and facilitate the action of γ-aminobutyric acid in inhibiting neuronal transmission through increased chloride ion flow.

8. Identify an agent that can reverse the effects of benzodiazepines such as midazolam and triazolam.

    Answer: Flumazenil.

9. Would barbiturates be helpful in managing pain in a ventilated patient?

    Answer: No, unless a dose capable of producing unconsciousness is used. There is no direct effect on pain transmission.

10. Would meperidine be helpful to prevent or lessen perception of pain?

    Answer: Yes; meperidine (Demerol) is a morphine-like narcotic and will occupy opiate receptors to block nerve transmission of pain.

11. Suggest an analgesic for minor pain for a patient with a bleeding disorder such as hemophilia or a patient who is taking an anticoagulant such as warfarin.

    Answer: Acetaminophen would be the drug of choice. Aspirin and NSAIDs can both inhibit platelet aggregation and prolong bleeding times, even in normal subjects, and should be avoided in those with bleeding disorders.

12. Are there any serious side effects to use of a ventilatory stimulant such as doxapram?

    Answer: Yes; central nervous system stimulation to the point of seizures.

Clinical Scenario

Subjective: A 35-year-old black male was admitted to the hospital with lethargy after being found in his apartment by a friend. An empty bottle of amitriptyline pills was lying next to the man. In the emergency room (ER), the patient became more lethargic to the point of unresponsiveness and developed hypopnea and bradypnea. He was intubated and mechanically ventilated with a volume-cycled ventilator. The patient had a history of depression but had been in good physical health. He was taking amitriptyline, which was prescribed by his psychiatrist for his depression. He has no allergies, and his past medical history and family history were unremarkable.

Objective: Physical examination revealed a mesomorphic male appearing to be his stated age. His vital signs were as follows: temperature (T), 39° C rectally; pulse (P), 140 beats/min; respiratory rate (RR), 12 breaths/min on an assist/control (A/C) rate of 12 breaths/min; blood pressure (BP), 110/60 mm Hg, right arm, supine. Head, eyes, ears, nose, and throat (HEENT) were unremarkable except for oral endotracheal tube (ETT) in place. His chest was normoresonant to percussion and his lungs had clear breath sounds bilaterally. Cardiovascular examination revealed that on palpation, the point of maximal impulse was located normally in the fifth intercostal space in the midclavicular line. Auscultation revealed normal S_1 and S_2 without murmurs, gallops, or rubs. He had normal jugular venous pressure, and his pulses were 2+ throughout. The man's abdomen was mildly distended with absent bowel sounds. No masses or organomegaly were present. His extremities were unremarkable, and his skin was very warm and dry. He was unresponsive to visual, auditory, or tactile stimuli, and his pupils were equally dilated and sluggishly responsive to light. All of his extremities were flaccid, and his reflexes were 1+ throughout. His plantar reflexes were downgoing. Laboratory results revealed normal hemogram, electrolytes, blood urea nitrogen (BUN), creatinine, and liver function test results. The tricyclic antidepressant (TCA) level was in the toxic range. His chest radiograph was normal. The ETT was approximately 2 cm above the carina. The electrocardiogram (ECG) showed sinus tachycardia at 140 beats/min with prolonged PR and QRS intervals. Arterial blood gas (ABG) on A/C ventilation at 12 breaths/min, with a tidal volume (V_T) of 800 mL and a fraction of inspired oxygen (FIO_2) of 1, resulted in the following: pH, 7.44; arterial carbon dioxide pressure ($PaCO_2$), 38 torr; arterial oxygen pressure (PaO_2), 550 torr.

Assessment: The patient has had a TCA overdose. Confirmed by subjective data submitted by his friend finding an empty bottle of amitriptyline pills and objective data found from the toxicology screen showing high levels of tricyclic antidepressant (TCA) in his blood. The patient is being mechanically ventilated because of depression of his respiratory drive from the TCA.

Plan: Treat with activated charcoal via nasogastric tube, properly hydrate with intravenous fluids, and monitor. Wean FIO_2, as PaO_2 is within normal range at 100% O_2. Extubate after respiratory status has been restored. Get a psychiatric evaluation after extubation.

CHAPTER 21

Self-Assessment Questions

1. In which phase of the cardiac cycle does ventricular contraction occur?
   Answer: Systolic phase.
2. Identify three functions that regulate mean arterial pressure.
   Answer: Heart rate, stroke volume, and systemic ventricular resistance
3. Which measurements, taken by a pulmonary artery catheter, are estimates of intravascular volume?
   Answer: Central venous pressure and pulmonary capillary wedge pressure.
4. Hypotension is first managed by what mode of therapy?
   Answer: Fluid administration.
5. What vasopressor acts only on the α receptors within the vasculature?
   Answer: Phenylephrine.
6. Which agents exert an inotropic effect on the heart?
   Answer: Dobutamine, isoproterenol, digoxin, and milrinone.
7. What electrolyte abnormality may potentiate the adverse effects of digoxin?
   Answer: Hypokalemia.
8. What drug should be given for the management of extravasation caused by vasopressors?
   Answer: Phentolamine.
9. What Vaughan Williams class of antiarrhythmics acts on the fast sodium channels in the myocardium?
   Answer: Class I (IA, IB, and IC).
10. What antiarrhythmic agent is structurally similar to amiodarone but has an improved side-effect profile?
    Answer: Dronedarone.
11. In patients taking dofetilide, at what Q–T_c interval should the drug be discontinued because the risk for torsades de pointes becomes too great?
    Answer: Q_{Tc} interval > 500 msec.
12. Which antiarrhythmic agent is highly associated with the development of lupus erythematosus?
    Answer: Procainamide.
13. Identify the four categories of sudden cardiac death.
    Answer: Ventricular fibrillation (VF), pulseless ventricular tachycardia (PVT), pulseless electrical activity (PEA), and asystole.

14. What medication is indicated for treatment of asystole and PEA but not VF or pulseless VT during cardiac arrest?
    Answer: Atropine.
15. What are the two alternative routes of medication administration during cardiac arrest when an intravenous route is not available?
    Answer: Intraosseous and endotracheal routes.
16. In a patient with septic shock, what is the pH in which the Surviving Sepsis Guidelines recommend utilizing sodium bicarbonate therapy?
    Answer: A pH less than 7.15.
17. When medications are administered via the endotracheal route during cardiac arrest, the dose should be increased by how many times the usual intravenous dose?
    Answer: 2 to 2.5 times.

Clinical Scenario 1

Subjective: A 28-year-old female was rushed to the emergency department of a local hospital by paramedic staff after she collapsed suddenly at work. When she collapsed the staff in her office called for an ambulance although basic life support was not started. It was reported that she was in ventricular fibrillation when the paramedic staff arrived at the scene.

Objective: The paramedics promptly administered two shocks with a defibrillator and after the second shock a pulse could be felt. On arrival to the hospital, the patient's blood pressure dropped to 85/42 mm Hg and the cardiac monitor showed a supraventricular tachycardia of 170 beats/min.

Assessment: The patient is hypotensive and in supraventricular tachycardia.

Plan: Fluids should be initiated before any vasopressors. Fluids are the mainstays for improving hypotensive episodes. Rapid administration of adenosine is implemented to terminate SVTs. Because of its ultrashort half-life adenosine is best administered through a central line for rapid arrival at the site of action or, if given through a brachial line, the arm should be held in the upright position followed almost instantly by a saline flush.

Clinical Scenario 2

Subjective: A 49-year-old man is visiting his mother, who was admitted to a nursing home for long-term rehabilitation because of a spinal cord injury. He goes to the bathroom and a few minutes later his mother hears a loud thud; she calls out to him, but there is no response. After an additional 3 minutes, the head nurse and the clinical pharmacist initiate cardiopulmonary resuscitation (CPR) and obtain the code cart.

Objective: The initial electrocardiogram (ECG) reading reveals pulseless electrical activity (PEA).

Assessment: PEA.

Plan: Administer both epinephrine and atropine at a dose of 1 mg rapid IV push followed by a 20-mL normal saline flush. Defibrillate the patient. Administer amiodarone 300 mg. After administration of the 300-mg IV bolus, all patients should be started on continuous infusion, delivering amiodarone at a rate of 1 mg/min for 6 hours and then decreased to 0.5 mg/min for 18 hours, and eventually converted to the oral formulation.

CHAPTER 22

Self-Assessment Questions

1. What is the systolic and diastolic blood pressure goal for patients older than 60 years of age without any co-morbidities?
   Answer: Less than 150/90 mm Hg.
2. List adverse effects associated with angiotensin-converting enzyme inhibitors (ACEIs).
   Answer: The most common ACEI-induced adverse effect is a persistent nonproductive dry cough, with an incidence of 20% to 30%. ACEI-induced adverse effects include rash, dysgeusia, hyperkalemia, orthostatic hypotension, blood dyscrasias, angioedema, and proteinuria.
3. Which antihypertensive agents are preferred in the treatment of African Americans without any co-morbidities?
   Answer: Thiazide-type diuretics and calcium channel blockers.
4. Which of the β blockers possesses intrinsic sympathomimetic activity (ISA)?
   Answer: The β blockers with ISA are acebutolol, carteolol, penbutolol, and pindolol.
5. Which of the β blockers possess selective β_1-blocker activity?
   Answer: Acebutolol, atenolol, betaxolol, bisoprolol, and metoprolol.
6. List adverse effects associated with α_1-adrenergic antagonists.
   Answer: α_1-Adrenergic antagonist adverse effects include orthostatic hypotension, dizziness, syncope, reflex tachycardia, palpitations, and headaches. These adverse effects are generally a manifestation of the first-dose phenomenon.
7. What are the most common side effects of nitrates?
   Answer: The most common side effects of nitrates include tachycardia, palpitations, headaches, dizziness, and flushing.
8. List metabolic effects associated with thiazide diuretics.
   Answer: The metabolic effects of thiazide diuretics include hypokalemia, hypomagnesemia, hypercalcemia, hyperuricemia, and hyperglycemia.
9. Name five medications that may cause drug-induced increases in blood pressure.
   Answer: Five drugs that may cause drug-induced increases in blood pressure are venlafaxine, cyclosporine, ma huang, ibuprofen, and rofecoxib.
10. Which calcium channel blocker is most likely to cause constipation?
    Answer: Verapamil is the calcium channel blocker most likely to cause constipation.
11. Identify the best available parameter to monitor the effects of warfarin.
    Answer: The international normalized ratio is the best parameter available to monitor the effects of warfarin.
12. What is the antidote for heparin?
    Answer: Protamine is the antidote for heparin.
13. What is the mechanism of action of warfarin?
    Answer: Warfarin exerts its effect by interfering with the hepatic synthesis of vitamin K–dependent clotting factors II, VII, IX, and X.
14. List the commercially available oral factor Xa inhibitors.
    Answer: Apixaban and rivaroxaban.
15. List the commercially available oral direct thrombin inhibitor.
    Answer: Dabigatran.
16. List the common CYP3A4 and P-glycoprotein inhibitors.
    Answer: Amiodarone, clarithromycin, erythromycin, and ketoconazole.
17. Name the pharmacologic class responsible for inhibiting the final pathway in platelet aggregation.
    Answer: The glycoprotein IIb/IIIa inhibitors are responsible for inhibiting the final pathway in platelet aggregation.
18. Which thrombolytic is recommended for patients older than 75 years of age who present with ST segment elevation myocardial infarction?
    Answer: Streptokinase is the thrombolytic recommended for patients greater than 75 years of age who present with ST segment elevation myocardial infarction.
19. Name the only ACEI that is available in a parenteral dosage form.
    Answer: Enalaprilat is the only ACEI that is available in a parenteral dosage form.
20. Identify the best available parameter to monitor the effects of heparin.
    Answer: Activated partial thromboplastin time (APTT) is the best parameter available to monitor the effects of heparin.
21. Is clopidogrel or ticlopidine superior to aspirin for stroke prevention?
    Answer: Clopidogrel has no demonstrated superiority to aspirin except for patients who have peripheral vascular disease. Both clopidogrel and aspirin are first-line therapies for stroke prevention. Ticlopidine has demonstrated superiority to aspirin; however, because of its deleterious side effect profile, ticlopidine is a second-line therapy for stroke prevention. Stroke prevention pharmacotherapy is lifelong.

Clinical Scenario

Subjective: A 75-year-old male presents to the emergency department complaining of chest pain of 1 hour in duration. He has had intermittent chest pain for the past week. He describes experiencing substernal pain that radiates down his left arm. The pain is associated with diaphoresis and is not relieved by change in body position. He has had a history of hypertension for the past 10 years. He has no history or family history for coronary artery disease.

Objective: The patient is currently taking labetalol, 200 mg twice daily, and an enteric-coated aspirin, 81 mg daily. He has no known allergies. On physical examination, he appears anxious and is complaining of chest pain. His vital signs are as follows: blood pressure (BP), 140/70 mm Hg; pulse (P), 74 beats/min; and respiratory rate (RR), 20 breaths/min. His heart sounds are normal, with no murmurs or gallops present. His lungs are clear on auscultation, and his abdomen, extremities, and funduscopic examination are unremarkable. His skin is cool and clammy. Electrocardiography displays evidence of sinus bradycardia with a heart rate of 49 beats/min. His cardiac enzymes all were elevated (creatine kinase [CK], 200 U/L; CK-MB [CK isoenzymes found in muscle and brain fractions], 20 U/L; and troponin I, 2 mcg/mL).

Assessment: A non–ST segment elevation myocardial infarction (MI).

Plan: This patient does not have ST segment elevation myocardial infarction and therefore is not a candidate for thrombolytic therapy. However, glycoprotein IIb/IIIa inhibitors would provide a benefit by inhibiting platelet aggregation and thrombus formation after an atherosclerotic plaque rupture. The use of glycoprotein IIb/IIIa inhibitors reduces the risk of death or nonfatal myocardial infarction.

CHAPTER 23

Self-Assessment Questions

1. What is the *International Classification of Sleep Disorders, Revised* (ICSD-R), and what information does it contain?
   Answer: The ICSD-R, published in 2005 by the American Academy of Sleep Medicine (AASM), provides classification of sleep disorders and diagnostic criteria. Diagnostic codes for each disorder are also provided. Currently, more than 80 sleep disorders are described within this manual.

2. What are the electroencephalographic correlates of wakefulness and sleep stages N1, N2, N3, and rapid eye movement (REM)?
   Answer: See electroencephalogram (EEG) column in Table 23-1:
   N1, formerly known as Stage 1: Low voltage, mixed frequency waves (2 to 7 Hz range), mainly irregular theta activity, triangular vertex waves.
   N2, formerly known as Stage 2: Relatively low voltage, mixed frequency waves, some low amplitude theta and delta activity.
   N3, formerly known as Stages 3 and 4: ≥20% to 50% of the epoch consists of delta (0.5 to 2 Hz) activity.

Stage REM: EEG is relatively low voltage with mixed frequency resembling N1 sleep.

3. What type of drug had been used for centuries to promote sleep onset and maintenance?
   Answer: Opium.

4. What class or classes of drugs have replaced opium?
   Answer: Barbiturates, then benzodiazepines, then nonbenzodiazepines.

5. How many people in the United States experience chronic sleep disorders?
   Answer: Approximately 50 to 70 million adults in the United States suffer chronically from sleep disorders.

6. Who was von Economo and what theories guided his neuroanatomic exploration of brain regions involved in the processes of initiating and maintaining wakefulness and sleep?
   Answer: He was a physician who, in a series of postmortem examinations on the brains of patients who had succumbed to encephalitis lethargica, observed that lesions in the rostral midbrain and posterior hypothalamus had a profound effect on sleep and wakefulness.

7. What is the reticular activating system?
   Answer: A system of cell bodies that originate in the brainstem and innervate the midbrain and cortex.

8. How do neurons within the ventrolateral preoptic (VLPO) area affect sleep?
   Answer: Onset of activity within the VLPO nuclei orchestrates the onset and maintenance of NREM sleep.

9. What are the suprachiasmatic nuclei (SCN) and what are intrinsic discharge properties exhibited by many of its neurons?
   Answer: The SCN are the neuroanatomical sites of the primary mammalian biologic clock. Subpopulations of SCN neurons exhibit spontaneous patterns of discharge activity, and accordingly, are described as self-sustaining neural oscillators, or pacemakers.

10. Define chronobiology and chronopharmacology.
    Answer: Chronobiology is the study of mechanisms contributing to the periodicity of biologic processes. Chronopharmacology is the study of time-dependent variations in pharmacology.

11. Describe pharmacologic treatments for insomnia.
    Answer: See Table 23-2. Benzodiazepine (BZD) receptor agonists: Estazolam, Flurazepam, Quazepam, Temazepam, Triaolam, Eszopiclone, Zaleplon, Zolpidem, Zolpidem CR; and selective melatonin receptor agonist: Ramelteon.

12. What is the difference between restless legs syndrome (RLS) and periodic limb movement disorder (PLMD)?
    Answer: Restless legs syndrome is a chronic neurologic disorder characterized by unpleasant sensations in the legs and a compelling urge to move them while the patient is awake.
    Periodic limb movement disorder is defined as periodic episodes of spontaneous, repetitive and highly stereotyped involuntary limb movements that occur during sleep.

13. What is the tetrad of clinical symptoms that defines narcolepsy and what types of drugs are used to treat this disorder?

    Answer: Narcolepsy is characterized by a tetrad of clinical symptoms: (1) persistent excessive daytime sleepiness, (2) cataplexy, (3) hypnagogic hallucinations, and (4) sleep paralysis.

14. Give two examples of a parasomnia and name the class of drugs routinely used in the treatment of these sleep disorders.

    Answer: REM sleep behavior disorder and somnambulism. A common pharmaceutical treatment for both REM and NREM sleep parasomnias is a long-acting benzodiazepine.

15. Insomnia is characterized by what types of principal complaint, and what drug classes are used to treat this disorder?

    Answer: Insomnia is characterized by difficulty in falling asleep or staying asleep, insufficient sleep, multiple nocturnal awakenings, early morning awakening with inability to resume sleep, or nonrestorative sleep. Table 23-2 describes some of the primary drugs used to treat insomnia. See answer for Question 11.

Clinical Scenario

Subjective: The patient was a 59-year-old white male with a body mass index (BMI) of 27 and a history of hypertension, arthritis, and depression. He presents to the sleep clinic with chief complaints of excessive daytime sleepiness, awakening from nocturnal sleep after 2 to 3 hours, and prickly sensations in the legs that coincide with nocturnal awakenings but are temporarily relieved by walking. He also reports experiencing the same prickly sensations in his legs during long trips in the car, regardless of the time of day. The sensations in his legs also spontaneously occur 2 to 3 evenings per week during the evening hours.

Objective: Analysis of polysomnography data revealed a sleep efficiency of 94% with a sleep latency of 5 minutes. The arousal index was 15 arousals per hour of sleep. Distribution of sleep stages was notable for an increased amount of N2 and REM sleep with a reduced amount of N3 sleep. The REM latency was normal. Periodic leg movements occurred 41 times per hour of sleep and resulted in 11 arousals per hour of sleep. There were no arrhythmias noted on the ECG. No snoring was noted with the patient in the lateral position. The apnea/hypopnea index (number of apneas and hypopneas per hour of sleep) was mildly elevated at 8.2 with a further increase to 13.6 events per hour during REM sleep. Oxyhemoglobin desaturation reached a nadir of 82% in REM sleep and 86% in nonREM sleep.

Assessment: The patient suffers from periodic limb movement disorder and obstructive sleep apnea (OSA).

Plan: Treatment for the both restless legs syndrome and nocturnal periodic limb movements should be considered. Treatment is usually undertaken with a dopaminergic agent, benzodiazepine, or opiate and reduction of medications and behaviors known to provoke symptoms. Treatment for the patient's mild sleep apnea could include weight loss, upper airway surgery, dental devices, or continuous positive airway pressure (CPAP).

Units and Systems of Measurement

OUTLINE

SCIENTIFIC NOTATION

Scientific notation is a method for expressing very large or very small numbers, using a single digit multiplied by a whole number power of 10.

Use of Scientific Notation

Place the decimal point of the number to the right of the first non-zero digit.

Multiply the number by 10 raised to a power equal to the number of places moved by the decimal point.

The exponent of 10 is positive for moves to the left and negative for moves to the right.

Example of a large number: 2292.0 is the same as 2.292×10^3.

Example of a small number: 0.002292 is the same as 2.292×10^{-3}.

ABBREVIATIONS OF MEASURES

cc or cu. cm	= cubic centimeters (1/1000 L)
cL	= centiliter (1/100 L)
dr	= dram or drachm
fl. oz	= fluid ounces
ft	= foot or feet
g	= gram
gal or gals	= gallons
gr	= grains
gtt	= drops
hr	= hour
IU	= International Units (SI)
kg	= kilogram (1000 g)
L or l	= liter
lb or lbs	= pounds
m	= meter
m or min	= minims
mcg or µg	= microgram (1/1,000,000 g)
meq or mEq	= milliequivalent
mg	= milligram (1/1000 g)
min	= minutes
mL	= milliliter (1/1000 L)
mm	= millimeter 1/1000 m)
O, pt, or pts	= pints
oz or ozs	= ounces
sc	= scruple
sec	= seconds
st	= stones
T or tbsp	= tablespoon
t or tsp	= teaspoon
µL	= microliter (1/1,000,000 L)

METRIC SYSTEM

The metric system is based on multiples or fractions of 10.

PREFIX	SCALE
Kilo-	10^3
Hecto-	10^2
Deca-	10^1
Base Unit	$10^0 = 1$
Deci-	10^{-1}
Centi-	10^{-2}
Milli-	10^{-3}
Micro-	10^{-6}
Nano-	10^{-9}
Pico-	10^{-12}

INTERNATIONAL SYSTEM OF UNITS (SYSTÈME INTERNATIONAL D'UNITÈS [SI UNITS])

SI Base Units

Length	meter, m
Mass	kilogram, kg
Time	second, s
Temperature	Kelvin, K
Amount of substance	mole, mol

SI-Derived Units

Area	square meter, m^2
Volume	cubic meter, m^3
Concentration	mole per cubic meter, mol/m^3

TEMPERATURE SCALES AND TEMPERATURE CONVERSIONS

SCALE	ABSOLUTE ZERO	FREEZING (WATER)	BOILING (WATER)
Kelvin	0°	273°	373°
Centigrade	−273°	0°	100°
Fahrenheit	−460°	32°	212°

Conversion: Centigrade/Fahrenheit

To convert from Fahrenheit to Centigrade:

$$\text{Centigrade (degrees)} = 0.55 \times (\text{Fahrenheit} - 32)$$

To convert from Centigrade to Fahrenheit:

$$\text{Fahrenheit (degrees)} = (1.8 \times \text{Centigrade}) + 32$$

LIQUID METRIC CONVERSIONS

UNITED STATES		UNITED KINGDOM	
1 gallon (gal)	= 3785 mL	1 gallon	= 4546 mL
1 pint (pt)	= 473.18 mL	1 pint	= 568.26 mL
16 fluid ounces	= 473.18 mL	20 fluid ounces	= 568.26 mL
8 fluid ounces	= 236.49 mL	10 fluid ounces	= 284.14 mL
4 fluid ounces	= 118.29 mL	5 fluid ounces	= 142.07 mL
1 fluid ounce	= 29.57 mL	1 fluid ounce	= 28.41 mL

HOUSEHOLD/APOTHECARY

1 tablespoon	= 15 mL (approx.)	
1 teaspoon	= 5 mL (approx.)	
1 cc	= 1 g	= 1 mL (approx.)
15 to 16 drops (gtt)	= 1 cc	= 1 mL
10 minims	= 0.616 mL	
1 drop	= 1 minim (approximate)	

Note: Spoon and drop conversions should be regarded as approximations because of the different surface tensions and specific gravity of various liquids.

SOLID METRIC CONVERSIONS

IMPERIAL	METRIC
Avoirdupois	
1 stone	6.35 kg
2.2 pounds	1 kg
1 pound	453.592 g, 0.45 kg
1 ounce	28.35 g
Apothecary	
1 pound	373.242 g
1 ounce	31.10 g
1 dram/drachm	28.8 g
1 scruple	1.2 g
15 grains	1 g
10 grains	600 mg
$7\frac{1}{2}$ grains	500 mg
5 grains	300 mg
$1\frac{1}{2}$ grains	100 mg
1 grain	65.79891 mg
$\frac{1}{2}$ grain	30 mg
$\frac{1}{4}$ grain	15 mg
$\frac{1}{8}$ grain	8 mg
$\frac{1}{12}$ grain	5 mg
$\frac{1}{100}$ grain	600 mcg
$\frac{1}{150}$ grain	400 mcg
$\frac{1}{200}$ grain	300 mcg
$\frac{1}{250}$ grain	250 mcg
$\frac{1}{300}$ grain	200 mcg

HOUSEHOLD UNITS

The metric system of measure generally is used for drug amounts. However, household measures such as teaspoons or tablespoons are used for administering medications in the home environment. For example, a cough syrup may have a label giving a usual adult dose as "1 teaspoon every

6 hours." Household measures are not consistent; a teaspoon may vary from 3 to 5 mL. Although the metric system, which is more exact and consistent with milligrams, micrograms, and milliliters, is recommended in place of household measures, the following equivalences may be helpful. Use of household measures such as teaspoons can be very helpful in discussing amounts of substance with a patient.

1 teaspoon = 5 mL = 60 drops

1 tablespoon = 15 mL (or 3 teaspoons)

1 cup = 240 mL (or 8 fluid ounces)

RATIOS AND PERCENT SOLUTIONS

1:100	= 1 g/100 mL (10 mg/mL)	= 1%
1:200	= 500 mg/100 mL (5 mg/mL)	= 0.5%
1:1000	= 100 mg/100 mL (1 mg/mL)	= 0.1%
1:5000	= 20 mg/100 mL (200 mcg/mL)	= 0.02%
1:10,000	= 10 mg/100 mL (100 mcg/mL)	= 0.01%

CALCULATION OF MILLIEQUIVALENTS (mEq)

$$\text{mEq} = \text{Weight in grams}/\text{mEq Weight in grams}$$

ION OR COMPOUND	mEq WEIGHT (g)	ION OR COMPOUND	mEq WEIGHT (g)
Mg^{++}	0.012	HCO_3^-	0.061
NH_4^+	0.018	Citrate	0.063
Ca^{++}	0.020	CaCl dihydrate	0.0735
Na^+	0.023	KCl	0.0745
Phosphorus	0.031	$NaHCO_3^-$	0.084
Cl	0.0355	Lactate	0.089
K^+	0.039	$MgSO_4$ heptahydrate	0.123
NH_4Cl	0.0535		
NaCl	0.0585	Calcium gluconate	0.224
Acetate	0.059		

For milliequivalent weights not shown, use the formula: Milliequivalent weight (mEq W.) = atomic weight (g)/(valence) × 1000.

DRUG ADMINISTRATION TIMES

Standardized medication administration times should be followed as much as possible. The following table shows the hours of the day that are to be used as standardized times of medication administration. If the prescriber wishes the first dose to be administered before the earliest available standardized time, the prescriber should state "expedite" or "first dose now" with the drug order. In intensive care units, the first dose of a newly ordered parenteral antibiotic regimen should be administered within 2 hours unless specified otherwise by the prescriber.

ORDERED TIME	HOUR(S) TO BE GIVEN	MILITARY TIME
qam	8:00 AM	0800
qd	8:00 AM	0800
qhs	9:00 PM	0900
qprn	5:00 PM	1700
bid	8:00 AM and 5:00 PM	0800 and 1700
q12h	8:00 AM and 8:00 PM	0800 and 2000
q8h	8:00 AM, 6:00 PM, and 12:00 AM	0800, 1800, and 2400
tid	8:00 AM, 12:00 PM, and 5:00 PM	0800, 1200, and 1700
tid ac	7:00 AM, 12:00 PM, and 5:00 PM	0700, 1200, and 1700
tid w/m	7:30 AM, 12:30 PM, and 5:30 PM	0730, 1230, and 1730
qid	8:00 AM, 12:00 PM, 5:00 PM, and 9:00 PM	0800, 1200, 1700, and 2100
q6h	6:00 AM, 12:00 PM, 6:00 PM, and 12:00 AM	0600, 1200, 1800, and 2400
ac and hs	7:00 AM, 12:00 PM, 5:00 PM, and 9:00 PM	0700, 1200, 1700, and 2100
pc and hs	8:00 AM, 1:00 PM, 6:00 PM, and 9:00 PM	0800, 1300, 1800, and 2100
1 hr ac and hs	6:30 AM, 11:30 AM, 4:30 PM, and 9:00 PM	0630, 1130, 1630, and 2100
1 hr pc and hs	8:30 AM, 1:30 PM, 6:30 PM, and 9:00 PM	0830, 1330, 1830, and 2100
5×/day	6:00 AM, 10:30 AM, 3:00 PM, 7:30 PM, and 11:00 PM	0600, 1030, 1500, 1930, and 2300
q4h	4:00 AM, 8:00 AM, 12:00 PM, 4:00 PM, 8:00 PM, and 12:00 AM	0400, 0800, 1200, 1600, 2000, and 2400

ESTIMATING LEAN BODY WEIGHT

Lean Body Weight Calculation

Males: 50 kg + 2.3 kg per each inch over 5 feet of height
Females: 45 kg + 2.3 kg per each inch over 5 feet of height

HEIGHT		ESTIMATED LEAN BODY WEIGHT		HEIGHT		ESTIMATED LEAN BODY WEIGHT	
IMPERIAL	METRIC	MALES (kg)	FEMALES (kg)	IMPERIAL	METRIC	MALES (kg)	FEMALES (kg)
4 ft 8 in	142 cm	40.8	36.3	5 ft 9 in	175 cm	70.7	66.2
4 ft 9 in	145 cm	43.1	38.6	5 ft 10 in	178 cm	73.0	68.5
4 ft 10 in	147 cm	45.4	40.9	5 ft 11 in	180 cm	75.3	70.8
4 ft 11 in	150 cm	47.7	43.2	6 ft 0 in	183 cm	77.6	73.1
5 ft 0 in	152 cm	50.0	45.5	6 ft 1 in	185 cm	79.9	75.4
5 ft 1 in	155 cm	52.3	47.8	6 ft 2 in	188 cm	82.2	77.7
5 ft 2 in	157 cm	54.6	50.1	6 ft 3 in	191 cm	84.5	80.0
5 ft 3 in	160 cm	56.9	52.4	6 ft 4 in	193 cm	86.8	82.3
5 ft 4 in	163 cm	59.2	54.7	6 ft 5 in	196 cm	89.1	84.6
5 ft 5 in	165 cm	61.5	57.0	6 ft 6 in	198 cm	91.4	86.9
5 ft 6 in	168 cm	63.8	59.3	6 ft 7 in	201 cm	93.7	89.2
5 ft 7 in	170 cm	66.1	61.6	6 ft 8 in	203 cm	96.0	91.5
5 ft 8 in	173 cm	68.4	63.9				

Acceptable Mixtures of Most Commonly Prescribed Respiratory Care Drugs

| TABLE C-1 | Admixture Advices for Commonly Used Drug Solutions/Suspensions in Nebulizers |

	ALBUTEROL	IPRATROPIUM	CROMOLYN	BUDESONIDE	TOBRAMYCIN	COLISTIN	DORNASE ALFA
Albuterol/Levalbuterol	Not applicable	Possible*	Possible*	Possible*	Possible*	Possible*	Not recommended
Ipratropium	Possible*	Not applicable	Possible*	Possible*	Possible*	No information	Not recommended
Cromolyn	Possible*	Possible*	Not applicable	Possible*	Not recommended	No information	Not recommended
Budesonide	Possible*	Possible*	Possible*	Not applicable	Not recommended	No information	Not recommended
Tobramycin	Possible*	Possible*	Not recommended	Not recommended	Not applicable	No information	Not recommended
Colistin	Possible*	No information	No information	No information	Not reasonable	Not applicable	Not recommended
Dornase alfa	Not recommended	Not recommended	Not recommended	Not recommended	Not recommended	Not recommended	Not applicable

*Mixtures are compatible, if preservative-free solutions (no benzalkonium chloride) are used.
From Kamin W, Schwabe A, Krämer I: Inhalation solutions—which one are allowed to be mixed? Physico-chemical compatibility of drug solutions in nebulizers, *J Cyst Fibros* 5:205-213, 2006. European Cystic Fibrosis Society. Published by Elsevier B.V.

GLOSSARY OF SELECTED TERMS

An eclectic glossary of terms encountered in pharmacology, many from the basic sciences, is offered for convenience in using the text as a study source. This glossary is not intended to substitute for a comprehensive dictionary of medical terms. Selection of terms for inclusion is based on the author's experience in reading the literature of drug actions and effects. Terms that are frequently found or used in discussing drugs but may be less well known to the practicing clinician are included.

Abhesive Coating that reduces adhesion. (Chapter 9)

Acetylcholine (Ach) Chemical produced by the body that is used in transmission of nerve impulses. It is destroyed by the enzyme cholinesterase. (Chapter 5)

Acetylcholinesterase (AchE) Enzyme that breaks down the neurotransmitter acetylcholine at the synaptic cleft so that the next nerve impulse can be transmitted across the synaptic gap. (Chapter 18)

Acute respiratory distress syndrome (ARDS) Respiratory disorder characterized by respiratory insufficiency. This disorder may occur as a result of trauma, pneumonia, oxygen toxicity, gram-negative sepsis, or systemic inflammatory response. (Chapter 1)

Adrenal cortical hormone Chemicals secreted by the adrenal cortex. An adrenal cortical hormone is also referred to as a *steroid*. (Chapter 11)

Adrenergic (adrenomimetic) Refers to a drug stimulating a receptor for norepinephrine or epinephrine. (Chapter 5)

Adrenergic bronchodilator Agent that stimulates sympathetic nervous fibers, which allow relaxation of smooth muscle in the airway. Also known as a *sympathomimetic bronchodilator* or β_2 *agonist*. (Chapter 6)

Aerodynamic diameter of a particle Diameter of a unit-density (1 g/cc) spherical particle having the same terminal settling velocity as the measured particle. (Chapter 3)

Aerosol Suspension of liquid or solid particles, between 0.001 and 100 micrometers (μm) in diameter, in a carrier gas. (Chapter 3)

Aerosol therapy Delivery of aerosol particles to the lungs. (Chapter 3)

Aerosolized agents Group of aerosol drugs for pulmonary applications that includes adrenergic, anticholinergic, mucoactive, corticosteroid, antiasthmatic, and antiinfective agents and surfactants instilled directly into the trachea. (Chapter 1)

Afferent Signals that are transmitted to the brain and spinal cord. (Chapter 5)

Agonist Chemical or drug that binds to a receptor and creates an effect on the body. (Chapter 2)

Airway resistance (R_{aw}) Measure of impedance to ventilation caused by movement of gas through the airway. (Chapter 1)

Alkaloids Group of alkaline substances taken from plants, which react with acids to form salts (e.g., theophylline). (Chapter 8)

α_1-Antitrypsin (α_1-AT) Inhibitor of trypsin that may be deficient in patients with emphysema. Also known as α_1-*proteinase inhibitor (API)*. (Chapter 16)

α-Receptor stimulation Causes vasoconstriction and vasopressor effect; in the upper airway (nasal passages), this can provide decongestion. (Chapter 6)

Amnestic properties Having the ability to cause total or partial loss of memory. (Chapter 18)

Analgesics Drugs that provide pain relief. Analgesics can be subdivided into narcotic and nonnarcotic medications. *Narcotic drugs* are derivatives of opium, such as morphine and codeine. *Nonnarcotic medications* are useful in treating pain and inflammation. They also have antipyretic activity. (Chapter 20)

Anesthetics Drugs that depress the nervous system. Anesthetics can be divided into local and general anesthetics. *General anesthetics* cause total loss of consciousness and reflexes, which results in the absence of pain perception. *Local anesthetics* are applied to a specific site, decrease pain perception at the specific site, and do not affect level of consciousness. Both types of anesthetics are often used during surgical procedures. (Chapter 20)

Antagonism Antibiotic combination in which the activity of one antibiotic interferes with the activity of the other (block receptor site, enzymatic inactivation), resulting in less activity with the combination than with the individual drugs (i.e., $1 + 1 < 1$). (Chapter 14)

Antagonist Chemical or drug that binds to a receptor but does not create an effect on the body; it actually blocks the receptor site from accepting an agonist. (Chapter 2)

Antiadrenergic Refers to a drug blocking a receptor for norepinephrine or epinephrine. (Chapter 5)

Antiarrhythmics Group of cardiac medications that are classified according to mechanism of action; in some instances, they may have multiple mechanisms of action. The most common classification system of antiarrhythmics is the Vaughan Williams classification system, which is divided into four distinct categories and a miscellaneous section. (Chapter 21)

Antibiotics Substance derived or produced from a microorganism that inhibits or kills other microorganisms. (Chapter 14)

Anticholinergic Refers to a drug blocking a receptor for acetylcholine. (Chapter 5)

Anticholinergic bronchodilator Agent that blocks parasympathetic nervous fibers, which allows relaxation of smooth muscle in the airway. (Chapter 7)

Antidepressants Drugs that can alter levels of certain neurotransmitters, in particular norepinephrine and serotonin, within the brain. Depending on the class of antidepressant, they can either inhibit the reuptake of neurotransmitters or decrease their degradation, ultimately allowing for increased levels of neurotransmitter at the nerve terminal. (Chapter 20)

Antihistamine Drugs that reduce the effects mediated by histamine, a chemical released by the body during allergic reactions. Antihistamine is often administered to reduce secretions (e.g., runny nose and sneezing), but they can cause drowsiness and impaired responses. (Chapter 15)

Antileukotriene Agents that blocks the inflammatory response in asthma. (Chapter 12)

Antimicrobials Natural and synthetic compounds that either inhibit or kill microorganisms. (Chapter 14)

Antimuscarinic bronchodilator Same as an *anticholinergic bronchodilator:* an agent that blocks the effect of acetylcholine at the cholinergic site. (Chapter 7)

Antipsychotics Drugs used to treat psychotic disorders, such as schizophrenia. These drugs primarily affect the neurotransmitter dopamine. (Chapter 20)

Antithrombotic Drug that prevents or breaks up blood clots in such conditions as thrombosis or embolism; antithrombotics include anticoagulants, antiplatelets, and thrombolytics. (Chapter 22)

Antitussive Drugs that suppress the cough reflex. *Note:* Productive coughs should not be suppressed; the logic of an expectorant-antitussive combination is questionable. (Chapter 15)

Anxiolytics Drugs used to treat several conditions, including anxiety disorders and insomnia; also known as *minor tranquilizers*. The most common class of anxiolytics is the benzodiazepines. They bind to the γ-aminobutyric acid receptor to increase the inhibitory actions of this neurotransmitter. (Chapter 20)

API deficient Refers to an individual who has low serum levels of API possessing altered electrophoretic properties. (Chapter 16)

API dysfunctional Refers to an individual who has normal serum levels of API that does not function normally. (Chapter 16)

API normal Refers to an individual who has normal serum levels of API that functions normally. (Chapter 16)

API null Refers to an individual who has undetectable serum levels of API. (Chapter 16)

Arrhythmia (dysrhythmia) Irregular (faster or slower) heartbeat; the term *arrhythmia* is used more frequently than *dysrhythmia*. (Chapter 21)

Arterial blood pressure (blood pressure) Defined hemodynamically as the product of cardiac output (heart rate × stroke volume) and total peripheral resistance. (Chapter 22)

Aspiration Accidental inhalation of food particles, fluids, or gastric contents into the lungs. (Chapter 18)

Asthma paradox Refers to the increasing incidence of asthma morbidity and especially asthma mortality, despite advances in the understanding of asthma and availability of improved drugs to treat asthma. (Chapter 6)

Atrioventricular (AV) node Link between atrial depolarization and ventricular depolarization. (Chapter 21)

Barbiturates Compounds whose parent structure is uric acid. These compounds depress central nervous system activity. Long-acting barbiturates such as pentobarbital have been used to treat epilepsy. Barbital was used during the early twentieth century to facilitate sleep in individuals with insomnia. (Chapter 23)

Benzodiazepines Compounds whose parent structure is a fusion of a diazepine ring with a benzene ring. Benzodiazepines enhance activity of the inhibitory neurotransmitter γ-aminobutyric acid. Benzodiazepines, which reduce anxiety and promote muscle relaxation, also promote sleep. The earliest benzodiazepines were chlordiazepoxide (Librium) and diazepam (Valium). Benzodiazepines for insomnia are now being replaced by nonbenzodiazepines such as zolpidem (Ambien) and eszopiclone (Lunesta). (Chapter 23)

β_1-Receptor stimulation Causes increased myocardial conductivity and increased heart rate and increased contractile force. (Chapter 6)

β_2-Receptor stimulation Causes relaxation of bronchial smooth muscle, with some inhibition of inflammatory mediator release and stimulation of mucociliary clearance. (Chapter 6)

Bioavailability Amount of drug that reaches the systemic circulation. (Chapter 2)

Bohr effect Presence of carbon dioxide aiding in the release and delivery of oxygen from hemoglobin. (Chapter 21)

Brand name See *Trade name*. (Chapter 1)

Bronchospasm Narrowing of the bronchial airways caused by contraction of smooth muscle. (Chapter 6)

Cardiac output (CO) Amount of blood that is ejected into the aorta and travels through the systemic circulation with every heartbeat. (Chapter 21)

Cardiovascular disease (CVD) Damage to the heart and blood vessels or circulation, including circulation to the brain, kidney, and eyes. (Chapter 22)

Cascade impactor Device that uses multiple steps in determining aerosol particle sizes. (Chapter 3)

Catecholamines Group of similar compounds having sympathomimetic action; they mimic the actions of epinephrine. (Chapter 6, Chapter 21)

Central nervous system (CNS) System that includes the brain and spinal cord, controlling voluntary and involuntary acts. The brain and spinal cord make up the functional components of the CNS. The spinal cord provides nerve fibers that transport signals to and from the brain. The brain largely comprises three components: cortex, midbrain, and brainstem. (Chapter 5, Chapter 20)

Chemical name Name indicating the chemical structure of a drug. (Chapter 1)

Chlorofluorocarbons (CFCs) Liquefied gas (e.g., Freon) propellant used to administer medication from a metered dose inhaler (MDI). (Chapter 3)

Cholinergic (cholinomimetic) Parasympathomimetic agents causing stimulation of a receptor for acetylcholine. (Chapter 5, Chapter 7)

Cholinesterase inhibitors Drugs that block the activity of cholinesterase, an enzyme that inactivates the neurotransmitter acetylcholine. Acetylcholine is found at nerve terminals in both the central and the peripheral nervous systems. Cholinesterase inhibitors are used in the treatment of dementia to slow the progression of cognitive decline. (Chapter 20)

Chronic obstructive pulmonary disease (COPD) Disease process characterized by airflow limitation that is not fully reversible, is usually progressive, and is associated with an abnormal inflammatory response of the lung to noxious particles or gases. Diseases that cause airflow limitation include chronic bronchitis, emphysema, asthma, and bronchiectasis. (Chapter 1)

Chronotropic Agent affecting the rate of contraction of the heart. (Chapter 21, Chapter 22)

Circadian rhythms The approximately 24-hour cycle of biochemical, physiologic, and behavioral processes. *Circa* is Latin for "about," and *diem* is Latin for "day." (Chapter 22, Chapter 23)

Code name Name assigned by a manufacturer to an experimental chemical that shows potential as a drug. An example is aerosol SCH 1000, which was the code name for ipratropium bromide, a parasympatholytic bronchodilator. (Chapter 1)

Common cold Nonbacterial respiratory tract infection characterized by malaise and a runny nose. (Chapter 15)

Congestive heart failure (CHF) Failure of the heart to pump blood adequately, resulting in lung congestion and tissular edema. (Chapter 19)

Conscious sedation Method of sedation used during certain invasive procedures. The goals of conscious sedation are to decrease the level of consciousness and relieve anxiety and pain, while allowing the patient to follow verbal commands. Conscious sedation is achieved through the use of several classes of drugs, including benzodiazepines and narcotic analgesics. (Chapter 20)

Creatinine clearance Measurement of the renal clearance of endogenous creatinine per unit of time; considered to be an estimate of glomerular filtration rate (GFR) but overestimates GFR by 10% to 15%. It is used for drug-dosing guidelines. (Chapter 22)

Cyclic AMP (cAMP) Nucleotide produced by β_2-receptor stimulation; it affects many cells but causes relaxation of bronchial smooth muscle. (Chapter 6)

Cyclic GMP (cGMP) Nucleotide producing the opposite effect of cAMP; that is, it causes bronchoconstriction. (Chapter 6)

Cystic fibrosis (CF) Inherited disease of the exocrine glands, affecting the pancreas, respiratory system, and apocrine glands. Symptoms usually begin in infancy and are characterized by increased electrolytes in the sweat, chronic respiratory infection, and pancreatic insufficiency. (Chapter 1, Chapter 13)

d-(+)-Dimers Covalently cross-linked degradation fragments of the cross-linked fibrin polymer during plasmin-mediated fibrinolysis; the level increases after the onset of fibrinolysis and allows for identification of the presence of fibrinolysis. (Chapter 22)

Dead volume Amount of solution that remains in the reservoir of a small volume nebulizer once sputtering begins, causing a decrease in aerosolization. (Chapter 3)

Deposition Process by which particles deposit out of suspension to remain in the lung. (Chapter 3)

Diastolic blood pressure (DBP) Lowest pressure reached right before ventricular ejection. (Chapter 21)

Diuretic Drug that increases urine output. (Chapter 19)

Dose-ceiling effect Maximum dose of a drug beyond which it no longer exerts a therapeutic effect; however, toxic effects increase. (Chapter 22)

Downregulation Long-term desensitization of β receptors to β_2 agonists caused by a reduction in the number of β receptors. (Chapter 6)

Dromotropic An agent that influences the conduction of electrical impulses. A positive dromotropic agent enhances the conduction of electrical impulses to the heart. (Chapter 21)

Drug administration Method by which a drug is made available to the body. (Chapter 1, Chapter 2)

Dysrhythmia/arrhythmia Irregular (faster or slower) heartbeat; the term *arrhythmia* is used more frequently than *dysrhythmia*. (Chapter 21)

Edema Swelling resulting from abnormal accumulation of fluid in intercellular spaces of the body. (Chapter 19)

Efferent Signals that are transmitted from the brain and spinal cord. (Chapter 5)

Elasticity Rheologic property characteristic of solids; it is represented by the storage modulus G'. (Chapter 9)

Electroencephalography (EEG) Measurement and recording of the gross electrical activity of the brain. During EEG recordings, electrodes are typically placed across multiple scalp regions. The electrodes are connected to amplifiers and filters that detect, magnify, and record the electrical activity of the brain. (Chapter 23)

Emitted dose Dose released by an aerosol device. (Chapter 17)

Endogenous Refers to *inside*, produced by the body. (Chapter 11)

Enteral Use of the intestine. (Chapter 2)

Exogenous Refers to *outside*, manufactured to be placed inside the body (e.g., medication). (Chapter 11)

Expectorant Medication meant to increase the volume or hydration of airway secretions. (Chapter 9, Chapter 15)

Fasciculation Involuntary contraction or twitching of groups of muscle fibers. (Chapter 18)

Fibrin split or fibrinogen degradation products (FDPs) Small peptides that result after the action of plasmin on fibrinogen and fibrin in the fibrinolytic process. FDPs are anticoagulant substances that can cause bleeding if fibrinolysis becomes uncontrolled and excessive. (Chapter 22)

First-pass effect Initial metabolism in the liver of a drug taken orally, before the drug reaches the systemic circulation. (Chapter 2)

Flu Nonbacterial infection with rapid onset of symptoms, including fever, headache, and fatigue. (Chapter 15)

Gel Macromolecular description of pseudoplastic material having both viscosity and elasticity. (Chapter 9)

Generic name Name assigned to a chemical by the United States Adopted Name (USAN) Council when the chemical appears to have therapeutic use and the manufacturer wishes to market the drug. (Chapter 1)

Glomerular filtration Mechanism by which hydrostatic pressure forces fluid out of the glomerular capillaries and into the renal ducts. (Chapter 19)

Glomerular filtration rate (GFR) Volume of water filtered from the plasma by the kidney via the glomerular capillary walls into Bowman capsules per unit time; considered to be 90% of creatinine clearance and equivalent to inulin clearance. (Chapter 22)

Glycoprotein Protein with covalently attached oligosaccharide units. The principal constituent of mucus and a high-molecular-weight glycoprotein, it gives mucus its physical and chemical properties such as viscoelasticity. (Chapter 9)

Heterodisperse In reference to the size of particles in an aerosol, meaning the particles are of different sizes. (Chapter 3)

Hydrofluoroalkane (HFA) Nontoxic liquefied gas propellant used to administer medication from an MDI. (Chapter 3)

Hypersensitivity Allergic or immune-mediated reaction to a drug, which can be serious, requiring airway maintenance or ventilatory assistance. (Chapter 2)

Hypersomnia Presence of excessive sleepiness. Daytime sleepiness is so great that it leads to inappropriate daytime napping or sleep. Excessive sleepiness is not alleviated by prolonged sleep times or by napping. (Chapter 23)

Hypertensive emergency Blood pressures greater than 180/120 mm Hg, when the elevation of blood pressure is accompanied by acute, chronic, or progressing target organ injury. (Chapter 22)

Hypertensive urgency Blood pressures greater than 180/120 mm Hg without signs or symptoms of acute target organ complications. (Chapter 22)

Hypnotic Class of drugs used to induce sleep. (Chapter 23)

Hypovolemia Abnormally decreased volume of blood circulating in the body. (Chapter 19)

Idiosyncratic effect Abnormal or unexpected reaction to a drug, other than an allergic reaction, compared with the predicted effect. (Chapter 2)

Immunoglobulin E (IgE) Gamma globulin that is produced by cells in the respiratory tract. (Chapter 11, Chapter 12)

In vitro Mechanically simulating the clinical setting; testing in a laboratory. (Chapter 3)

In vivo Testing done on animals or humans; clinical testing. (Chapter 3)

Infant Child between the ages of 1 month and 1 year. (Chapter 17)

Inhalation Taking a substance, typically in the form of gases, fumes, vapors, mists, aerosols, or dusts, into the body by breathing in. (Chapter 2)

Inhaled or delivered dose Dose reaching the patient's mouth or artificial airway. (Chapter 17)

Inotrope Agents affecting the strength of muscular contraction. (Chapter 21, Chapter 22)

Intrinsic sympathomimetic activity (ISA) Having the ability to activate and block adrenergic receptors, producing a net stimulatory effect on the sympathetic nervous system. (Chapter 22)

LaPlace's law Physical principle describing and quantifying the relationship between the internal pressure of a drop or bubble, the amount of surface tension, and the radius of the drop or bubble. (Chapter 10)

Leukotrienes Chemical mediators that cause inflammation. (Chapter 12)

Local effect Limited to the area of treatment (e.g., inhaled drug to treat constricted airways). (Chapter 2)

Lung availability/total systemic availability ratio (L/T ratio) Amount of drug that is made available to the lung out of the total available to the body. (Chapter 2)

Lung dose Dose reaching the trachea and beyond. (Chapter 17)

Mast cells Connective tissue cells that contain heparin and histamine. (Chapter 12)

Mast cell stabilizers Also known as *cromolyn-like agents;* agents used prophylactically to treat the inflammatory response in asthma. (Chapter 12)

Mean arterial pressure (MAP) Pressure that drives blood into the tissues averaged over the entire cardiac cycle. (Chapter 21)

Methylxanthines Chemical group of drugs derived from xanthines. There are three methylated (CH_3) xanthines: caffeine, theophylline, and theobromine. (Chapter 8)

Monodisperse In reference to the size of particles in an aerosol, meaning all particles are the same size. (Chapter 3)

Mood stabilizer Drugs used primarily to treat bipolar disorders. (Chapter 20)

Mucin Principal constituent of mucus. Principal airway gel-forming mucins MUC2, MUC5AC, and MUC5B are proteins with attached oligosaccharide (sugar) side chains. (Chapter 9)

Mucoactive agent Term connoting any medication or drug that has an effect on mucus secretion. See *Mucokinetic agent, Mucolytic agent, Mucolytic expectorant, Mucoregulatory agent,* and *Mucospissic agent.* (Chapter 9)

Mucokinesis Therapeutic movement of excessive or abnormal secretions from the respiratory tract. (Chapter 15)

Mucokinetic agent Medication that increases ciliary clearance of respiratory mucus secretions. (Chapter 9)

Mucolytic agent Medication that degrades polymers in secretions. *Classic mucolytics* have free thiol groups to degrade mucin, and *peptide mucolytics* break pathologic filaments of neutrophil-derived DNA or actin in sputum. Classic mucolytics are ineffective for the therapy of airway disease and are not recommended, whereas dornase alfa seems to be effective for the therapy of cystic fibrosis and perhaps bronchiectasis. (Chapter 9)

Mucolytic expectorant Agent that facilitates removal of mucus by a lysing, or mucolytic, action. *Example:* dornase alfa. (Chapter 15)

Mucoregulatory agent Drug that reduces the volume of airway mucus secretion and seems to be especially effective in hypersecretory states, such as bronchorrhea, diffuse panbronchiolitis, cystic fibrosis, and some forms of asthma. (Chapter 9)

Mucospissic agent Medication that increases the viscosity of secretions and may be effective in the therapy of bronchorrhea. (Chapter 9)

Mucus Secretion, from surface goblet cells and submucosal glands, composed of water, proteins, and glycosylated mucins. The glycoprotein portion of the secretion is termed *mucin*. *Mucus* (noun) is the secretion; *mucous* (adjective) is the cell or gland type. (Chapter 9)

Muscarinic An agent that produces the effect of acetylcholine or an agent that mimics acetylcholine. Same as *cholinergic*. (Chapter 7)

Myasthenia gravis Autoimmune neuromuscular disorder characterized by chronic fatigue and exhaustion of muscles. (Chapter 18)

Nebulizer Device used for making a fine spray or mist, also known as an *aerosol generator*. (Chapter 3)

Neonatal Refers to period of time between birth and first month of life. (Chapter 17)

Nephrocalcinosis Renal lithiasis in which calcium deposits form in the renal parenchyma, resulting in reduced kidney function and the presence of blood in the urine. (Chapter 19)

Nephron Microscopic functional unit of the kidney, responsible for filtering and maintaining fluid balance. Each kidney has approximately 2 million nephrons. (Chapter 19)

Neuromuscular blocking agent (NMBA) Substance that interferes with the neural transmission between motor neurons and skeletal muscles. (Chapter 18)

Neuron (nerve cell) Basic functional unit of the nervous system that is specialized to transmit electrical nerve impulses and carry information from one part of the body to another. A neuron consists of a cell body, axons, and dendrites. (Chapter 18)

Neurotransmitter Chemical that is released from a nerve ending to transmit an impulse from a nerve cell to another nerve, muscle, organ, or other tissue, such as *acetylcholine* or *norepinephrine*. (Chapter 18, Chapter 20)

Nominal dose Dose in a delivery device. (Chapter 17)

Nonproprietary name Name of a drug other than its trademarked name. (Chapter 1)

Norepinephrine (NE) Naturally occurring catecholamine produced by the adrenal medulla that has properties similar to epinephrine. It is used as a neurotransmitter in most sympathetic terminal nerve sites. (Chapter 5)

Nosocomial pneumonia Pneumonia that is acquired in a health care setting. (Chapter 18)

Official name In the event that an experimental drug becomes fully approved for general use and is admitted to the *United States Pharmacopeia–National Formulary*, the generic name becomes the official name. (Chapter 1)

Off-label Use of drugs with no U.S. Food and Drug Administration (FDA)–approved labeling. (Chapter 17)

Oligosaccharide Sugar that is the individual carbohydrate unit of glycoproteins. (Chapter 9)

Orphan drug Drug or biologic product for the diagnosis or treatment of a rare disease (affecting fewer than 200,000 persons in the United States). (Chapter 1)

Ototoxicity Damage to the ear, specifically the cochlea or auditory nerve and sometimes the vestibulum, by a toxin. (Chapter 19)

Parasomnias Group of sleep disorders manifested by undesirable motor, sensory, or behavioral phenomena that occur during sleep. The *International Classification of Sleep Disorders, Revised (ICSD-R)* lists 24 parasomnias. More commonly encountered parasomnias include confusional arousals, sleep terrors, and sleepwalking. (Chapter 23)

Parasympatholytic Agent blocking or inhibiting the effects of the parasympathetic nervous system. (Chapter 5, Chapter 7)

Parasympathomimetic Agent causing stimulation of the parasympathetic nervous system. (Chapter 5, Chapter 7)

Parenteral Administration in any way other than by the intestine; most commonly used to describe injection (e.g., intravenous, intramuscular, or subcutaneous). (Chapter 2)

Pediatric Refers to period between 1 month and 18 years of age. (Chapter 17)

Penetration Refers to the depth within the lung reached by particles. (Chapter 3)

Percentage Part of the active ingredient that is in a solution containing 100 parts. (Chapter 4)

Peripheral nervous system (PNS) Portion of the nervous system outside the CNS, including sensory, sympathetic, and parasympathetic nerves. (Chapter 5)

Pharmacodynamics Mechanisms of drug action by which a drug molecule causes its effect in the body. (Chapter 1, Chapter 2)

Pharmacogenetics Study of the interrelationship of genetic differences and drug effects. (Chapter 1, Chapter 2)

Pharmacognosy Identification of sources of drugs from plants and animals. (Chapter 1)

Pharmacokinetics Time course and disposition of a drug in the body based on its absorption, distribution, metabolism, and elimination. (Chapter 1, Chapter 2)

Pharmacology Study of drugs (chemicals), including their origin, properties, and interactions with living organisms. (Chapter 1)

Pharmacotherapy Treatment of disease by drug therapy. (Chapter 22)

Pharmacy Preparation and dispensing of drugs. (Chapter 1)

Phlegm Purulent material in the airways. From the Greek word for inflammation. When expectorated, phlegm is called *sputum*. (Chapter 9)

Phosphodiesterase (PDE) Enzyme responsible for the breakdown of cyclic adenosine 3′,5′-monophosphate (cAMP). (Chapter 8, Chapter 21)

Pneumocystis jiroveci (formerly *carinii*) Organism causing *Pneumocystis* pneumonia in humans, seen in immunosuppressed individuals such as patients with human immunodeficiency virus infection. (Chapter 1)

Pneumocystis pneumonia (PCP) Interstitial plasma cell pneumonia caused by the organism *Pneumocystis carinii* (now known as *Pneumocystis jiroveci*). This pneumonia is common among patients with lowered immune system response. (Chapter 13)

Polydisperse In reference to the size of particles in an aerosol, meaning many different particle sizes. (Chapter 3)

Polysomnography Measurement and recording of EEG activity during sleep, typically coupled with measurement and recording of cardiorespiratory activity and eye movements. (Chapter 23)

Prescription Written order for a drug, along with any specific instructions for compounding, dispensing, and taking the drug. This order may be written by a physician, osteopath, dentist, veterinarian, and other health care providers but not by chiropractors or opticians. (Chapter 1)

Prodrug Drug that exhibits its pharmacologic activity when it is converted, inside the body, to its active form. (Chapter 6)

Prophylactic treatment Prevention of respiratory distress syndrome (RDS) in infants with very low birth weight and in infants with higher birth weight but with evidence of immature lungs who are at risk for developing RDS. (Chapter 10)

Prostaglandin One of several hormone-type substances circulating throughout the body. (Chapter 11)

Pseudomonas aeruginosa Gram-negative organism, primarily a nosocomial pathogen. It causes urinary tract infections, respiratory system infections, dermatitis, soft tissue infections, bacteremia, bone and joint infections, gastrointestinal infections, and various systemic infections, particularly in patients with severe burns and in patients who are immunosuppressed (e.g., patients with cancer or acquired immunodeficiency syndrome). (Chapter 1)

Reabsorption Return to the blood of most of the water, sodium, amino acids, and sugar that were removed during filtration; occurs mainly in the proximal tubule of the nephron. (Chapter 19)

Receptor Molecular structure inside or outside the cell component that combines with a drug to change or enhance the function of the cell. (Chapter 2, Chapter 18)

Renin Enzyme, also known as *angiotensinogenase*, released by the kidney in response to a lack of renal blood flow and responsible for converting angiotensinogen into angiotensin I. (Chapter 22)

Rescue treatment Retroactive, or "rescue," treatment of infants who have developed respiratory distress syndrome. (Chapter 10)

Reservoir device Global term describing or referring to extension, auxiliary, or add-on devices attached to MDIs for administration of medication. This term can include *spacer* and *valved holding chamber*. (Chapter 3)

Respiratory care pharmacology Application of pharmacology to the treatment of pulmonary disorders and more broadly, critical care. (Chapter 1)

Respiratory syncytial virus (RSV) Virus that causes the formation of syncytial masses in cells. This leads to inflammation of the bronchioles, which may cause respiratory distress in infants. (Chapter 1, Chapter 13)

Rheology Study of the deformation and flow (strain) of matter. (Chapter 9)

Schedule Amount of drug that is needed, based on a patient's weight. (Chapter 4)

Sedation Production of a restful state of mind, particularly by the use of drugs that have a calming effect, relieving anxiety and tension. (Chapter 18)

Sol Macromolecular description of the respiratory secretion in true solution, with the physical property of viscosity (usually referred to as the *periciliary layer*). (Chapter 9)

Solute Substance or active ingredient that is dissolved in a solution. (Chapter 4)

Solution Physically homogeneous mixture of two or more substances (liquid). *Buffer solution* refers to an aqueous solution able to resist changes of pH with addition of acid or base. *Isotonic solution* refers to a solution having equal concentrations inside and outside the cell. *Normal solution* refers to 1 gram-equivalent weight of solute per 1 L of solution. *Molal solution* refers to 1 mole of solute per 1000 g of solvent. *Molar solution* refers to 1 mole of solute per 1 L of solution. *Osmolal solution* refers to 1 osmole per kilogram of solvent. *Osmolar solution* refers to 1 osmole per liter of solution. (Chapter 4)

Solvent Substance, usually a liquid, used to make a solution. (Chapter 4)

Somatic motor neurons Part of the nervous system that controls muscles that are under voluntary control. (Chapter 18)

Spacer Simple tube or extension device with no one-way valves to contain the aerosol cloud; its purpose is simply to extend the MDI spray away from the mouth. (Chapter 3)

Sputum Expectorated secretions that contain respiratory tract, oropharyngeal, and nasopharyngeal secretions; bacteria; and products of inflammation, including polymeric DNA and actin. Purulent sputum contains very little mucin and is similar in composition to pus. (Chapter 9)

Stability Describing the tendency of aerosol particles to remain in suspension. (Chapter 3)

Status asthmaticus Exacerbation of asthma that does not respond to standard treatment. (Chapter 18)

Status epilepticus At least 30 minutes of continuous seizure activity without full recovery between seizures. (Chapter 18)

Steroid Also known as *glucocorticoid* or *corticosteroid*; an agent that produces an antiinflammatory response in the body. (Chapter 11)

Steroid diabetes Hyperglycemia (i.e., increased plasma glucose levels) resulting from glucocorticoid therapy; glucocorticoids break down proteins and fats to generate building blocks for gluconeogenesis. (Chapter 11)

Stimulant Drug that increases activity of the brain. Stimulants can be divided into two classes: amphetamines and respiratory stimulants. Amphetamines cause increased wakefulness, improved concentration, and appetite suppression. Respiratory stimulants include doxapram, xanthines, carbonic anhydrase inhibitors, salicylates, and progesterone. (Chapter 20)

Stimulant expectorant Agent that increases the production and presumably the clearance of mucus secretions in the respiratory tract. *Example:* guaifenesin. (Chapter 15)

Strength Amount of solute in a solution, usually expressed as a percentage. (Chapter 4)

Structure-activity relationship (SAR) Relationship between a drug's chemical structure and the outcome it has on the body. (Chapter 2)

Substitute neurotransmitter Neurotransmitter or hormone replacement that may be weaker or inert. (Chapter 22)

Sudden cardiac death (SCD) Episode of ventricular fibrillation, pulseless ventricular tachycardia, pulseless electrical activity, or asystole. (Chapter 21)

Surface tension Attraction of molecules in a liquid-air interface, such as the liquid lining in lung tissue and the air, pulling the surface molecules inward. (Chapter 10)

Surfactant Agent that reduces surface tension. (Chapter 10)

Sympatholytic Agent blocking or inhibiting the effect of the sympathetic nervous system. (Chapter 5)

Sympathomimetic Drugs that partially or completely mimic the effects of the sympathetic nervous system. *Note:* Tremor, tachycardia, and increased blood pressure can occur with their use, especially when taken orally. Rebound congestion can occur if used for longer than one day. (Chapter 5, Chapter 6, Chapter 15)

Synergism Drug interaction that occurs from combined drug effects that are greater than if the drugs were given alone. (Chapter 2)

Synergistic effect Effect of two chemicals on an organism is greater than the effect of either chemical individually. (Chapter 19)

Synergy Combined effect of two antimicrobials is greater than their added effect (i.e., $1 + 1 > 2$). (Chapter 14)

Systemic effect Pertains to the whole body, whereas the target for the drug is not local; possibly causing side effects (e.g., capsule of acetaminophen for a headache). (Chapter 2)

Systolic blood pressure (SBP) Peak pressure reached during ventricular ejection. (Chapter 21)

Tachycardia Overly rapid heartbeat, usually defined as greater than 100 beats/min in adults. (Chapter 21)

Tachyphylaxis Rapid decrease in response to a drug. (Chapter 2)

Therapeutic index (TI) Difference between the minimal therapeutic and toxic concentrations of a drug; the smaller the difference, the greater chance the drug would be toxic. (Chapter 2)

Therapeutics The art of treating disease with drugs. (Chapter 1)

Tolerance Decreasing intensity of response to a drug over time. (Chapter 2)

Topical In pharmacology, use of the skin or mucous membrane for drug administration (e.g., lotion). (Chapter 2)

Toxicology Study of toxic substances and their pharmacologic actions, including antidotes and poison control. (Chapter 1)

Trade name Brand name, or proprietary name, given by a particular manufacturer. (Chapter 1)

Transdermal Use of the skin for drug administration (e.g., patch). (Chapter 2)

Urine output Amount of urine produced in 24 hours. Normal urine output averages 30 to 60 mL/hr. (Chapter 19)

Valved holding chamber Spacer device with the addition of one-way valve to contain and hold the aerosol cloud until inspiration occurs. (Chapter 3)

Vasodilator Agent causing dilation of the blood vessels. (Chapter 21)

Vasopressor Agent causing contraction of the capillaries and arteries. (Chapter 21)

Ventricular fibrillation (VF) Cardiac condition in which normal ventricular contractions are replaced by coarse or fine, rapid movements of the ventricular muscle. (Chapter 21)

Virostatic Stopping a virus from replicating. (Chapter 13)

Virucidal Killing a virus. (Chapter 13)

Virus Obligate intracellular parasite containing either DNA or RNA that reproduces by synthesis of subunits within the host cell and causes disease as a consequence of this replication. (Chapter 13)

Viscosity Resistance of liquid to sheer forces; a rheologic property characteristic of liquids and represented by the loss modulus G''. (Chapter 9)

Xanthine Nitrogenous compound found in many organs and in the blood and urine. (Chapter 8)

Page numbers followed by "*f*" indicate figures, "*t*" indicate tables, and "*b*" indicate boxes.

Page numbers followed by "*f*" indicate figures, "*t*" indicate tables, and "*b*" indicate boxes.